HANDBOOK OF
GERONTOLOGICAL SERVICES

HANDBOOK OF GERONTOLOGICAL SERVICES

Edited by

Abraham Monk

Columbia University

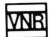 VAN NOSTRAND REINHOLD COMPANY
_____ New York

Copyright ©1985 by **Van Nostrand Reinhold Company Inc.**
Library of Congress Catalog Card Number: 84-20968
ISBN: 0-442-27806-3

Developed by Robert A. Rosenbaum.

Manufactured in the United States of America.

Published by Van Nostrand Reinhold Company Inc.
135 West 50th Street
New York, New York 10020

Van Nostrand Reinhold Company Limited
Molly Millars Lane
Wokingham, Berkshire RG11 2PY, England

Van Nostrand Reinhold
480 Latrobe Street
Melbourne, Victoria 3000, Australia

Macmillan of Canada
Division of Gage Publishing Limited
164 Commander Boulevard
Agincourt, Ontario MIS 3C7, Canada

15 14 13 12 11 10 9 8 7 6 5 4 3 2 1

Library of Congress Cataloging in Publication Data
Main entry under title:
Handbook of gerontological services.
   Includes index.
   1. Aged—Services for—United States—Handbooks, manuals,
etc.   I. Monk, Abraham.
HV1461.H34   1985   362.6'0973   84-20968
ISBN 0-442-27806-3

Contents

Part IV: Community-Based Services

Part V: Home-Based Services

Part VI: Long-Term Care and Institution-Based Services

Preface

The *Handbook of Gerontological Services* aims to meet the need for a comprehensive review of the types of social intervention methods and the range of services available to the elderly. Written from a practice perspective, the *Handbook's* primary concerns are the issues that service providers confront on a day-to-day basis, from the time a particular program is planned and developed until it comes into contact with its intended beneficiaries.

Handbooks usually have a pretension to universality, but no such claim will be made here. To delve into all existing services for the aged would have required extending the book beyond all reasonable limits. Selectivity thus became the inevitable imperative, but priority criteria were not easily agreed upon. It is safe to admit that services that are in high demand and are repeatedly used by increasing numbers of consumers do merit inclusion. Yet there are specialized services used by small minorities that constitute critical components in the continuum of care. These services cannot be overlooked because they fill a sensitive need and reinforce the effectiveness of the more general services. A third order of services may not be as widespread or of immediate strategical importance, but may be tapping needs not yet fully recognized. This book seeks to do justice to all three types, but only time will tell whether it strikes a good balance among these services.

The *Handbook* is intended for several audiences: professional service practitioners, informal caregivers, community action groups, policymakers and administrators, researchers, academicians, students in the field of aging, and, last but not least, the elderly who wish to learn about the myriad of service systems impinging upon their lives. For some readers, this book will offer practical information, the nuts and bolts of the "how-to" variety. Others may extrapolate basic leads for research and concepts for teaching. In all instances, the *Handbook* offers an inventory of the state of the art and of the creative ferment permeating the gerontological-services field. It is addressed to the wide audience of human service practitioners that staff the multidisciplinary teams in hospitals, long-term-care facilities, multipurpose senior centers, mental-health clinics, family-service agencies, unions, Area Agencies on Aging, personnel departments, and the world of industry and business at large. It should be borne in mind that services for the aging constitute a complex and challenging endeavor that requires the collaboration of many professions.

The *Handbook* is made up of seven parts.

Part 1. "Concepts and Issues" serves as a conceptual introduction to the issues of life span, human development, and old age. It also examines the attitudes toward old age among service workers and in society at large, the implications for practice of the family life, and the intergenerational contacts of older persons.

Part 2. "Client Evaluation" provides basic information on major instruments for psychological, medical, functional, and social assessment as well as on the most common disturbances in old age. It also underscores the relation between psychosocial and medical diagnostic procedures on one hand and the design of the treatment plan on the other.

Part 3. "Treatment and Intervention Modalities" begins with the facilitation of access to services and the case management procedures required to coordinate an individual treatment plan. Contributors then review individual casework methods, specialized casework and clinical approaches to individual services, group work and resocialization methods, and the macrosocietal strategies of community organization and social action.

Part 4. "Community-Based Services" begins the actual review of formally sponsored programs. The services in question are focused on the family domain, work and retirement, outpatient mental-health services, bereavement counseling, assistance to crime and abuse victims, legal advice, and, ultimately, the multifaceted content of senior centers.

Part 5. "Home-Based Services" considers the types of residential and living arrangements designed for the older person and the range of home-delivered services for the frail and homebound.

Part 6. "Long-Term Care and Institution-Based Services" includes the range of services for the chronically ill and the incapacitated. Attention is given to long-term-care facilities, services for the dying, respite and adult day-care programs, advocacy services for nursing-home residents, and protective legal and social services for those unable to fully assume responsibility over their lives.

Part 7. "Policy, Planning, and Operation of Services" wraps up the preceding exposition of services by venturing into a systematization of the services continuum. It also analyzes the intricacies of public funding, contracting, and monitoring the provision of services. The last chapter points to the growing relationship between information processing and program management. Although its premises are more generic than preceding chapters, their application to gerontological services may well serve as a paradigm of computer technology for other service fields.

The chapters included in Parts 4, 5, and 6 therefore present the services in a continuum from wellness to chronicity. While the authors treat their subjects according to their individual perspectives and the idiosyncrasy of the topic, for the most part they follow a certain structural uniformity. All chapters thus tend to address the following five topical areas:

Need—the epidemiological scope and characteristics of the problem addressed by the service in reference

Assessment—ways of diagnosing and measuring the problem and need under scrutiny, both at the community and individual level

Interventions—the range of services devised to cope with the problem of need and determination of how clients learn about the service and come in contact with it; the role performed by social workers in conjunction with other professionals and paraprofessionals; the skills required for the provision of services and the effectiveness of the most commonly practiced forms of intervention; the specific needs of ethnic and minority elderly and differential approaches of attending to their needs; finally, ways in which this service is coordinated with other services

Theory—an interpretation of the problem and needs addressed by each service in terms of social-science theory; extent to which practice and intervention skills reflect different conceptual interpretations

Policy—a critical examination of public policies mandating or regulating each service; funding mechanisms, appropriations, and participation of different levels of government in the planning and provision of each service

By utilizing this model, service-related factors such as assessment, policy, service provision, etc., are integrated in the presentation of each service. Policy issues, for instance, are examined in conjunction with, say, protective services or nursing-home care. A separate systematic presentation of all policies for the aged is therefore no longer needed.

The experts who contributed to the writing of this handbook bring to bear the vantage point of their day-to-day responsibilities. Some are front liners, the direct providers of the services they write about. Others are planners and administrators but still linked in a direct capacity with their assigned topics. Others are academic researchers with substantial familiarity with and deeply invested in their specialities. Some have written with almost exclusive reference to the settings where they carry out their practice. Others have adopted instead a comparative perspective that includes several settings.

In developing the content for this volume and in conducting the day-to-day relations with nearly thirty authors, I was fortunate in being assisted by Robert A. Rosenbaum. Although an outsider to the social-services field, he lent his expertise as a professional editor to expurgate the text of its imperfections and to put it into a language accessible to a wide audience. Ms. Susan Munger of Van Nostrand Reinhold Company deserves special thanks for her encouragement and patience. Finally, this book would not have been possible without the earnest commitment made by the authors. They undertook their assignments with a sense of mission and accepted our suggestions for repeated modifications and even extensive rewrites with collegial undertanding.

ABRAHAM MONK

Contributors

Sherry Berkman, D.S.W.
Assistant Research Social Worker
Neuropsychiatric Institute
University of California at Los Angeles
Los Angeles, Calif. 90024

Ann Burack-Weiss, M.S.S.W.
Training Consultant, Brookdale Institute on Aging and
    Human Development
Assistant Professor, Columbia University School of
    Social Work
New York, N.Y. 10025

Elias S. Cohen, J.D., M.P.A.
Vice President
Community Services Institute, Inc.
Narbeth, Pa. 19072

Raymond T. Coward, Ph.D.
Associate Professor
Department of Special Education, Social Work and
    Social Services
University of Vermont
Burlington, Vt. 05405-0160

Margaret E. Hartford, Ph.D.
Consultant on Retirement and Social Gerontology
Professor Emeritus of Gerontology and Social Work,
    University of Southern California
Los Angeles, Calif. 90089-0411

Nancy A. Hufnagel, M.S.W., J.D., LL.M.
Associate, Shanley & Fisher, P.C.
Morristown, N.J. 07960

Richard A. Kalish, Ph.D.
Visiting Professor of Health Science
Brooklyn College, City University of New York
Brooklyn, N.Y. 11210

Rosalie A. Kane, D.S.W.
Social Scientist
The Rand Corporation
Santa Monica, Calif. 90406

Lenard W. Kaye, D.S.W.
Associate Director
Brookdale Institute on Aging and Human Development
Columbia University School of Social Work
New York, N.Y. 10025

Jordan I. Kosberg, Ph.D.
Professor, Department of Gerontology
University of South Florida
Tampa, Fla. 33620

Howard Litwin, D.S.W.
Lecturer, Paul Baerwald School of Social Work
Hebrew University of Jerusalem
Mt. Scopus, Jerusalem 91905

Louis Lowy, Ph.D.
Associate Dean and Professor of Social Work and
    Gerontology
Boston University School of Social Work
Boston, Mass. 02215

Martin McCarthy, Ph.D.
Special Assistant for Information Systems Development
New Jersey Department of Higher Education
Trenton, N.J. 08625

Abraham Monk, Ph.D.
Brookdale Professor of Gerontology
Director, Brookdale Institute on Aging and Human
    Development
Columbia University School of Social Work
New York, N.Y. 10025

Gary M. Nelson, D.S.W.
Assistant Professor and Chairperson of the Aging
    Specialization
University of North Carolina School of Social Work
Chapel Hill, N.C. 27514

Eloise Rathbone-McCuan, Ph.D.
Associate Professor
Department of Special Education, Social Work and
    Social Services
University of Vermont
Burlington, Vt. 05405-0160

Edmund Sherman, Ph.D.
Associate Professor, School of Social Welfare
Faculty Research Associate, Ringel Institute of
    Gerontology
Nelson A. Rockefeller College of Public Affairs and Policy
State University of New York
Albany, N.Y. 12222

Susan E. Sherman, Ph.D.
Associate Professor, School of Social Welfare
Faculty Research Associate, Ringel Institute of
    Gerontology
Nelson A. Rockefeller College of Public Affairs and Policy
State University of New York
Albany, N.Y. 12222

Phyllis R. Silverman, Ph.D.
Associate Professor, Institute of Health Professions
Massachusetts General Hospital
Boston, Mass. 02114

Barbara Silverstone, D.S.W.
Executive Director
The New York Association for the Blind
New York, N.Y. 10022

Kenneth Solomon, M.D.
Adjunct Assistant Professor, Department of Psychiatry
University of Maryland School of Medicine
Staff Psychiatrist, Geropsychiatry Unit
Sheppard and Enoch Pratt Hospital
Baltimore (Towson), Md. 21204

Julia C. Spring, M.S.W., J.D.
Associate Clinical Professor
Columbia University School of Law
New York, N.Y. 10027

Raymond M. Steinberg, D.S.W.
Associate Director for Service System Design and
    Evaluation
Institute for Policy and Program Development
Andrus Gerontology Center
University of Southern California
Los Angeles, Calif. 90089-0191

Cynthia Stuen, A.M.
Director of Community Education
Brookdale Institute on Aging and Human Development
Columbia University School of Social Work
New York, N.Y. 10025

Miriam Teplitz, C.S.W.
Unit Administrator, Services to Older Adults
Peninsula Counseling Center
Woodmere, N.Y. 11598

Sheldon S. Tobin, Ph.D
Professor, School of Social Welfare
Director, Ringel Institute of Gerontology
Nelson A. Rockefeller College of Public Affairs and Policy
State University of New York
Albany, N.Y. 12222

Mario Tonti
Director of Community and Family Services
The Benjamin Rose Institute
Cleveland, Ohio 44115

Ron Toseland, Ph.D.
Assistant Professor, School of Social Welfare
Faculty Research Associate, Ringel Institute of
    Gerontology
Nelson A. Rockefeller College of Public Affairs and
    Policy
State University of New York
Albany, N.Y. 12222

Judith Treas, Ph.D.
Associate Professor of Sociology
University of Southern California
Los Angeles, Calif. 90089-0191

Judith Wineman, M.S.W., C.S.W.
Assistant Director, Retiree Service Department
International Ladies' Garment Workers' Union
New York, N.Y. 10001

PART I

CONCEPTS AND ISSUES

1

Gerontological Social Services: Theory and Practice

Abraham Monk, Ph.D.

Columbia University

Gerontological and geriatric specializations are emerging in practically all human-service professions, which is not surprising when we consider that American society is undergoing what Cowgill (1977) termed a "revolution of age," an unprecedented decline of mortality and fertility rates. The net effects are obvious: as fewer children are born and more adults survive into advanced senescence, the elderly are becoming a proportionally larger segment of society. Moreover, the average life expectancy is inching up relentlessly toward the ninth decade of life, and it is no longer uncommon to find two generations in retirement within the same family lineage. Retirement itself is a novel institution. It has created a life-style based upon economically nonproducing leisure roles that may eventually encompass a good third of a person's life span.

Initial professional responses to this demographic challenge were couched in a language of therapeutic pessimism and denials. Some practitioners felt that the aged were impervious to change, that their decline was irreversible, and that rehabilitative efforts on their behalf were altruistic but futile gestures. They similarly contended that there was no need for a separate geriatric specialization because the problems of the aged could be subsumed under more generic nosological entities or syndromes. One therefore dealt with arthritis, depression, or blindness in functional rather than in age-categorical terms.

No service discipline, however, could withstand for long the clamor of the elderly and their natural support networks seeking remediation for their multiple concerns. The public policies that ensued and the substantial apportionment of resources earmarked for those over age 65 became compelling inducements. Some professionals may have joined the new gerontological "bandwagon" for opportunistic reasons, while others have genuinely internalized an old-age consciousness, but their commitment to penetrate a barren and uncharted scientific domain was equally risky and praiseworthy.

The knowledge base at hand was initially too tenuous for guiding effective practice, and professions borrowed avidly from each other. No sooner did a breakthrough occur in one field than it was tested, metabolized, and incorporated into other disciplines. Because of this borrowing phenomenon, gerontologists soon developed a sense of kinship that on occasion transcended their primary occupational allegiances. Social workers working with the aged often sensed a greater affinity, and certainly interacted more frequently, with psychiatrists and nurses in the same field than with social workers specializing in a more remote area like criminal justice and probation. The resulting role blurring was not always harmonious. Nor it did preclude feuds about claims to territorial exclusivity. Professions are still far from a consensus on their respective domains, but they are more aware that the knowledge explosion in gerontology is not owned by any one discipline, that the state of the art is in constant flux, and that new information is relentlessly generated to replace what was upheld as valid only yesterday. Moreover, professions are realizing that they cannot singly contend with the multiple ramifications of old-age-related problems. Multidisciplinary collaboration is a pragmatic necessity, but practitioners in each service profession are simultaneously expected to be "multiskilled," competent in a wide range of diagnostic and treatment modalities as well as thoroughly informed about the service options offered by sister disciplines.

It should not be surprising, therefore, that this handbook incorporates skills shared by many human-service professions. It recognizes that all professionals wish to enable older persons to lead normal lives in their natural environments, and that they similarly want to assist in untangling situational problems as well as making irreversible chronic conditions more bearable. The successful provision of service, like the test of an effective therapist, ultimately depends on a keen understanding of the client for whom the service is intended. Because the elderly are so heterogeneous and because psychosocial theories underlying gerontological practice are so diverse, professional judgments must be, of necessity, eclectic and tentative. Gerontological practitioners find it a formidable enterprise to determine what all potential clients share in common, what may be specific to each group—racial, ethnic, religious, urban, rural, or socioeconomic—and ultimately what may be unique to each individual. This chapter aims to assist in this discerning function by exploring, *first*, how service providers initially approach their elderly clients; *second*, how theoretical frameworks guide the helping function; *third*, what critical issues and recurrent patterns are found in that function; and *fourth*, in what ways policy guides the provision of service.

PROFESSIONAL ATTITUDES TOWARD THE AGED

The first issue is an attitudinal one. First encounters in interpersonal relations are seldom neutral or devoid of emotional connotations. Providers of human services are no exception, and when entering the field of aging without proper training they will act as unconscious carriers of the negative images perpetuated by their culture. They may therefore begin by exhibiting a fear of aging itself, followed by a phobic reaction of disgust and rejection, and end with a rationalization that conceives all dysfunctions and pathologies as inevitable correlates of old age for which, obviously, nothing can be done. Adverse reactions toward aging may be systematized in four categories: disvaluation, marginalization, internalization, and normativity.

Disvaluation

Disvaluation is the result of derogatory biases that deny the social and personal significance of the older person. The old, according to Butler (1974), are perceived as unproductive, rigid, uninteresting, withdrawn, and senile. It is further implied that they are a parasitical population voraciously demanding more than they contributed to society. When combined, all these myths seem to lend respectability to "ageism," an active process of discrimination against older persons that Butler likens to the prejudices of race, gender, religion, and color. Ageism leads to a view of the elderly as less worthy, in cost-benefit terms, of receiving services. This line of reasoning may end with denying them their human dignity altogether. They are already robbed of their adult identities when referred to by service providers in seemingly affectionate terms as "children."

Marginalization

Older persons may be spared the traumatic effects of deliberate exclusion or discrimination, but they may still be ignored or forgotten. In a study of the images of old age in literature for adolescents, Peterson and Karnes (1976) found that, even when mentioned positively, the aged were not central characters. They were cast instead as peripheral shadows, unrelated to the mainstream of events. For the most part they were neither loved nor hated, simply unnoticed. Robertson (1976) examined the role of grandparents and similarly found that, although generally accepted by their grandchildren, they were not necessarily selected as role models.

There is more to marginalization, however, than sheer indifference or unawareness. The elderly who live alone are increasing in numbers. They are for the most part women. Some find it progressively more difficult to negotiate open spaces, stairs, distances, and public transportation. Others fear being assaulted and mugged. They become virtual recluses who sever their ties with the outside world unless assisted by the remnants of their natural support systems. They join, for the most part, the ranks of an invisible population seldom heard from again by social agencies and forgo services and benefits to which they may be rightfully entitled.

Internalization

One of the most devastating effects of prejudice occurs when victims end up accepting the prejudiced images of themselves and conforming their behavior to those images. Older persons may, for instance, introject the myths of rigidity and unproductivity and not trust themselves as capable of learning or doing new things. Their self-confidence is shattered, and the stereotypes become self-fulfilling prophecies. However, a study conducted by Louis Harris and Associates (1975) on behalf of the National Council on Aging did not find extensive evidence of internalization. The study established instead that the elderly are a substantially optimistic group harboring far more positive feelings about themselves than were attributed to them by younger respondents. They apparently resist the reinforcing properties of negative labels and retain a healthy self-esteem. Borges and Dutton (1976) discovered that optimistic outlooks toward life may even increase with age, and Ward (1977) found no relation between old-age identification and loss of self-esteem; among older males, achievement-related variables such as education and socioeconomic status affected feelings of self-regard far more than age. Negative views about one's old age, when manifested, seemed to be more an effect than a cause of deep-seated self-deprecation. In other words, people with low self-esteem will also feel bad about their old age, but not all those who age end up debasing themselves.

Service providers often find in their clinical experience certain behaviors that may suggest the internalization of dependence. The apparent helplessness exhibited by an elderly client may not be congruent, however, with his/her relatively good functional status. Brody et al. (1971) termed this behavior an expression of the "excess disability syndrome," often consisting of a manipulative strategy of feigning dependence in order to receive attention and ensure an uninterrupted flow of care.

Normativity

Logical derivatives from attitudes toward older persons are the culturally established norms that sanction what they should and should not do.

Norms prescribing age-appropriate behaviors are arbitrary and constantly changing, and they are made for all age groups. They tend, however, to be far more confining and restrictive for the older person. Neugarten, Moore, and Lowe (1965) suggest that this may be due to the fact that the elderly themselves ascribe greater importance to age norms. The young in turn tend to reject age as a valid yardstick by which to judge behavior.

Older persons may be ridiculed and dismissed as aberrant or senile for wearing youthful clothing, dating, or expressing sexual intimacy. Criticisms and sanctions leveled by their own peer group tend to be far more effective in inducing conformity to restrictive age norms than those imposed by professional outsiders. Negative attitudes are more visible in long-term-care facilities simply because of the numerically larger concentration of older persons in a single location and their intensive interaction with staff. Kayser-Jones (1981) systematized the most frequently reported complaints of staff abuse in four categories:

1. *Infantilization*—treating the patient as an irresponsible, undependable child
2. *Depersonalization*—providing services in an assembly-line fashion, disregarding the patients' individual needs
3. *Dehumanization*—not only ignoring elderly persons but stripping them of privacy and of their capacity to assume responsibility for their own lives
4. *Victimization*—attacking the older person's physical and moral integrity through verbal abuse, threats, intimidation, theft, blackmail, or corporal punishments

Gubrium (1980) found that even in the absence of such harsh forms of treatment, nursing-home residents may be affected by other subtle but equally demeaning exclusionary procedures. Staff, for example, will "plan ahead" without making the patient part of the decision-making process. They may also engage in "distancing," that is, treating the issues summarily and minimizing their importance in front of the client. "Subplotting" consists, in turn, of a series of codes and subterfuges aimed at limiting the range of issues to be shared with the patient. Most of these patterns or forms of staff-patient relations are typical, however, of all total or long-term-care institutions and are not limited to the elderly alone. They reflect for the most part administrative expediency by an overburdened and often ill-trained staff rather than a malicious intent to debase the patient. The institutionalized elderly, however, constitute an easy target: they are too feeble and decompensated to assert their rights or retaliate, and they are truly powerless after having lost their networks of friends and relatives outside the institution. The fact remains too that, in advanced cases of frailty or organic brain syndrome, staff must take over and make decisions for the patient. Adult children often find themselves in the same predicament, and Blenkner (1965) advised them to treat their ailing parents with "filial maturity," which consists of communicating to their elders that they can truly rely on the care of their offspring without having to feel dependent. There is no role reversal whereby the older person becomes the child of his/her own children. Filial maturity simply means offering support without exacting the price of submission.

Filial maturity ought not be confined exclusively to the family domain. It has a comparable place in the professional helping relationship as a form of "therapeutic maturity" that begins by precluding all condescension, pseudofamiliarity, and attacks on the older person's sense of privacy. Have professional helpers ever thought what it does to senior persons who were always addressed with deference by their last name to suddenly be called by their first names by a worker half their age or even the age of their grandchildren? Therapeutic maturity is therefore launched with the empathetic endeavor of reaching out to the clients' feelings of self-esteem and playing them out as one's own. It continues with the helpers reflecting on their own feelings and attitudes toward aging as a life process and toward the aged as people. The actual intervention that ensues requires an immersion in the knowledge base, the plethora of facts that constitute the discipline of gerontology and their underlying meanings. The latter is the function of theory because, unless guided by sound conceptual interpretations, practice is reduced to an aimless application of techniques.

THEORETICAL FOUNDATIONS OF PRACTICE

The last quarter of a century has been a period of relentless theoretical productivity as far as the field of aging is concerned. While a sign of serious investigative commitment, it could also be very disconcerting to new practitioners seeking to anchor their interventions in a less shifting interpretative ground. Unable to contend with so much change, some practitioners tend to set their minds and lock themselves in a chosen theory, holding its propositions as unshakable truths. This has been true for both academic schools and social agencies. Seasoned practitioners, for the most part, have extricated themselves from canonized dogmas and opted instead for a greater intellectual openness and pragmatic eclecticism.

Professional helpers were initially attracted to Cumming and Henry's (1961) theory of intrinsic disengagement because of its functionalist appeal. It gave the process of aging a "purpose" consisting of the realization and acceptance of the terminality of life in the way that is least disruptive to society. It defined the older person's withdrawal or separation as natural, irreversible, universal, and gradual, irrespective of individual or cultural idiosyncrasies. It added a libertarian connotation by asserting that disengagement freed the person from the yoke of day-to-day obligations. Disengagement, finally, was consistent with a clinical predilection for contracting in the therapeutic relation, because it entailed a tacit understanding between person and society to reduce their reciprocal expectations.

The "activity"-oriented theoreticians (Carp, 1968; Maddox, 1963; Rose,

1964) questioned whether disengagement is a natural process or whether it is culturally induced to make room for succeeding generations. The latter possibility, if true, is tantamount to systematic discrimination and therefore regarded as morally reprehensible. If disengagement leads to stripping the aged of the instrumental roles that enabled them to remain independent agents, clinical intervention should be primarily addressed to neutralizing any further victimization. It must also assist in generating compensatory new roles, as proposed by Rosow (1973), to replace those that have been lost.

Contracting also plays a central, implicit role in exchange theory (Blau, 1964; Dowd, 1975; Emerson, 1962). It hinges upon the older persons' capacity to perform their assumed obligations once power resources such as status, money, and skills have been substantially reduced or lost forever. Unable to offer such desirable attributes in return for social recognition, influence, or independence, the elderly become a powerless bunch. They have only one asset left to trade: submission and the recognition of dependence on those who master and control resources. This is the very last contract they can enter into to secure protection and guarantee survival. Social workers have found exchange theory a helpful tool for better understanding phenomena such as alienation, dependence, and depression among the aged. It also gives them a ready-made framework to legitimize self-help and coalitional program initiatives in community development.

The three theories under brief scrutiny—disengagement, activity, and exchange—implicitly state normative prescriptions of what life satisfaction or "good" aging is all about. From the disengagement perspective this consists of relinquishing social participation prior even to the onset of an inner sense of psychological detachment. For "activity" theory this involves harnessing new interactive skills, making oneself count, and shaping new roles. The exchange theory suggests in turn tapping one's hidden potentials and personal assets, joining forces with peers for mutual support, and entering into alliances with other disadvantaged groups. The three theories also give similar recognition, despite their conceptual disparities, to an omnipresent reality of loss. Rosenmayr (1982) criticized this concept of loss as a rather elementary form of reductionism and suggested paying attention instead to economic poverty as the underlying determinant of all forms of deprivation. Poverty in old age produces lack of stimulation, dependence on handouts and public assistance, illness, inadequate health care, and an overall shrinkage of opportunities. It also precipitates a "self-induced social deprivation," phenomenologically akin to disengagement, consisting of a passive and fatalistic resignation to one's fate, loss of all hope of ever being able to break the vicious circle of destitution and despondence.

The concept of life satisfaction has become for social workers and other service providers a powerful construct in its own right. It enables them to view a person's existence as striving for closure, in accordance with a script woven with values, expectations, and dreams—the ideals that confer meaning and purpose when a person approaching the end of life ponders whether it was all worth it. Even earlier, during middle age, crises often stem from a sense of discrepancy between a person's aspirations and what he or she has actually accomplished. The pursuit of unrealistic expectations that cannot come to fruition—like upward mobility or the highest rung of a career ladder—may lead to depression and alienation. Stock taking, in these circumstances, causes a sense of defeat, not satisfaction. The mission of clinical intervention in such an instance is, according to Parkes (1971), to facilitate change of the individual's values and expectations, what he terms the person's "assumptive world." Old expectations must be questioned and discarded and new ones formulated and tested. The perceived discrepancy between the "assumptive world" in question and life realities ought not to bring an irrevocable crisis but lead to new insights, an accommodation to new alternatives, and perhaps even the discovery of hidden potential.

While the preceding psychosocial theories gained popularity among gerontological practitioners, Erikson's (1959) model of the life cycle has for years dominated the teaching of human behavior and life-transition counseling. Similar interests in other stage-structured theories also increased. Group counseling at a time of life transitions is termed by Freud-Loewenstein (1978) a "strikingly effective" and a "preferred" method for dealing with people in crisis and populations at risk. Some developmental or stage theories conceive of life as a fixed and universal sequence of maturational processes, evolving in a hierarchy of more complex life tasks (Duvall, 1971; Loevinger, 1976; Piaget, 1976). For others, like Erikson (1959) and Levinson (1978), there is no such ascending hierarchy: each period of life has its distinct characteristics and a series of tasks or challenges that must be mastered for optimal growth, but each stage is not necessarily better than the preceding stage. Brennan and Weick (1981) identified five assumptions shared by most theories of adult human development.

1. Human development continues throughout life.
2. The life cycle consists of a series of discrete stages.
3. Transitions from stage to stage are often marked by crises.
4. Growth may occur as the possible outcome of such crises.
5. Adulthood must be understood in terms of a person's capacity to cope with new challenges and crises.

Although not explicitly admitting it, most psychological theories of human development have imitated biological epigenetic models. They assume that human beings unfold all their potentialities in early adulthood and begin thereafter an invariant process of decline. Lerner and Ryff (1978) found however that cognitive development may continue throughout life and does not necessarily slow down at any fixed point of the life cycle. The rigidity and resistance to new learning that is often associated with aging is not an intrinsic developmental process, according to Botwinick (1978), but a defensive posture, possibly a maladaptive form of coping behavior when having to contend with threatening circumstances. Furthermore, differences in learning capacity between young and old may be accounted for by initial training, not age, according to Labouvie-Vief (1982). The young can better handle new informational inputs because of their more updated levels of scientific, mathematical, and computer-related training. Even when acknowledging that basic intellectual capacities show decline, especially in very advanced age, Plemons, Willis, and Baltes (1978) point out that intellectual functions can be practiced and have a reserve capacity that can be "activated." Besides, slower mental processing among the aged does not mean that less information is being stored and retrieved. Erikson describes the last stage of life, "integrity," as the acceptance of one's life the way it has been, not the way one would like it to have been, and taking full responsibility for it without blaming others. Being satisfied with one's life confers upon a person his/her ultimate authenticity, the realization of having become one's true self. This is an aspiration, however, that not all will reach. Some will fall prey instead to Erikson's dialectic opposite of integrity, "despair," so often manifested in depression and negative life-review assessments.

Life-cycle theories in general, and Erickson's in particular, offer a naturalistic, nonpathological foundation for social intervention. Transitions from stage to stage, according to Levinson (1978), entail a rather complex set of tasks: accepting the losses that result from the ending of the preceding stage; reassessing the past; selecting those aspects one wants to continue; and formulating what course one wishes for the future.

Some of these tasks are unconscious, while others enter into the realm of awareness. They then produce emotional repercussions that oscillate from elation to panic or anxiety. In the latter case, as in all crises, the individual's coping skills may be strained beyond their limits. Rapoport (1967) advised in such instances to focus on the precipitating stresses. Her method of intervention consisted of fostering an adaptation to the new reality, reducing the anxiety by offering reassurance, relief from loneliness, a boost to the person's self-esteem, concrete information and advice as a sort of anticipatory guidance, and direct teaching of interpersonal skills. Yet the notion that the life cycle is organized in a sequence of stages and the hypothesis that both middle age and aging are characterized by pervasive crises and traumatic losses are far from receiving universal acceptance. Neugarten and Brown-Rezanka (1978-79) state that dominant themes and life concerns stay for life and reappear without a fixed order. The alleged predictability of life-cycle transitions is disregarded as unreliable and capricious. "Some of the old regularities in timing have disappeared and some of the social clocks that tell people whether they are on time or off time are no longer operating."

Pearlin (1982) argues in turn that, instead of a dominant theme, as proposed by Erikson, there may be multiple patterns of aging and that not all members of a cohort are exposed to the same conditions of life: "While moving an equal distance across the life span from the same temporal starting point may provide a basis for some common experiences, such commonalities are not sufficiently powerful to erase the profound differences that result from people having different origins and from the variations in their current social and economic experiences." Individual variability within a cohort may then be greater than the differences that separate cohort from cohort. Pearlin also disputes the view that the negative effects of life accumulate with age. For some, the gratifications and compensations found throughout the years, and especially in maturity, may well cancel out negative residues. In the balance sheet of life not all the aged come out losers. Some may even find themselves ahead of the game. Defining what constitutes a detrimental experience in contrast to a positive one depends on each person's psychological makeup and cumulative life history. The "empty nest" syndrome, for instance, that allegedly begins when the last child leaves the parental home is experienced by some as a source of desolation and grief, but others may exult and rejoice in their newly gained freedom. People of the same cohort may react differently to the same situations, and Pearlin adds that aging itself does not produce more distress than the challenges faced by the young, although he circumscribes this statement to the healthy elderly. A life-course approach, instead of a life-cycle one, views life transitions as a continuous, unin-terrupted process rather than as discrete segments of human experience. Even when conceptually isolating aging, youth, or middle age, each must be viewed in light of the entire life continuum, the pathways of a person's entire life, and how they were shaped in each instance by social and historical circumstances.

In sum, life-cycle theories succeed in better explaining intrapersonal life sequences. They may be less effective in explaining the interpersonal variability within the same cohort and even less in explaining differences across historical periods and cultural circumstances. Those who challenge the assumption that the life cycle is organized in fixed stages, as if these stages were ontological absolutes, do not mean to imply that defined life transitions do not exist. They contend instead that such transitions may be experienced differently by different people in different times and circumstances. The bottom line consists in relating to elderly clients, as with clients of any age, in terms of their personal uniqueness, without forcing them into preconceived conceptual schema. Theories and derived classifications will always remain tentative and partial explanations of reality. While offering a convenient framework for making a puzzling and confusing world more intelligible, they should not be received as immovable belief systems.

THE HELPING FUNCTION

The philosophical affirmation that all human beings have a right to complete their expected life cycle and that no stage of life is more valuable or more deserving of service inputs than others are the central premises of gerontological practice. This belief proceeds with the clinical recognition of each person's unique personality and coping patterns. Consequently, older persons should not be "homogenized" as if they were all alike.

Even when committed to the principle of individualization, however, service providers find it necessary to anchor their practice in some regularities or constancies characteristic of large populations. Practice-related taxonomies center, for the most part, on the functional capacities of older persons. While such taxonomies are too numerous to be reviewed here, the one outlined by the Gerontological Society (1978) for the Health Care Finance Administration can be cited as an example. It identified four target groups: the "unimpaired," the "minimally impaired," the "moderately impaired," and the "severely impaired" elderly. These classifications constitute a linear continuum from minimal to maximal impairment, taking into account some chronological parameters as well as the auspice of preventive, supportive, and protective services.

The category of "severely impaired" comprises people usually in their late 70s and older who exhibit advanced and multiple conditions such as osteo-arthritis, cancer, Parkinson's disease, paralysis, and cerebral vascular disease. A high incidence of confusion, disorientation, depression, and behavioral disorders is also present. The severely impaired have, for the most part, lost the capacity for self-care, and family supports, even when available, are not adequate to the need. Continuous and comprehensive long-term care is therefore required in either nursing homes or chronic-care hospitals, but homecare is not excluded if round the clock and properly monitored.

The "moderately impaired" are typically in their mid 70s or older. They are no longer self-sufficient; although not bedridden, they may be afflicted by the same conditions as the preceding group. Some may also have suffered mild strokes, heart failure, and amputations as well as visual and hearing impairments. They also exhibit memory loss and confusion, especially when subject to stress. While most individuals in this group can take care of some of their needs, they must be placed under medical, nursing, and social-work supervision at home or in a protected environment. It is in this group that social workers find the greatest resistance to any interposed support that may suggest surrendering one's independence.

The "minimally impaired" tend to be in their late 60s and early 70s. Their illnesses may be acute and may cause temporary activity restrictions. Chronic impairments are, however, mild and do not impede continuity of life-style. There are signs of progressively advancing disability due to heart and circulatory disorders, arthritis, and visual defects. Occasional forgetfulness, while not serious in itself, may provoke anxiety and self-consciousness. Although these individuals can take care of themselves, they can also profit from community-based preventive services.

The "unimpaired elderly" are found in the youngest group, ranging from early to late 60s. They have minimal sporadic functional limitations and are fully capable of meeting all their needs. Major problems relate to the retirement transition and possible reduction in standard of living. Services are needed to assure continuity of interests, prevention of postponement of the onset of disabilities, and life enrichment.

Classifications based on functional ability and health status are commonly used because they offer a rationale for either institutional placement or community-based care decisions. Other classifications take into account the personality style in adjustment to retirement. Reichard, Livson, and Peterson (1962) found three well-adjusted and two poorly adjusted types among men. The positive types were:

1. *Mature.* They enter into old age without neurotic conflicts, exhibiting genuine satisfaction with whatever comes and without regretting the past.
2. *Rocking chair.* These individuals are the good disengagers, opting for a nonobligatory life and welcoming the freedom from responsibility. They find pleasure in "doing nothing."
3. *Armored.* Anxiously concerned about their waning resources, they ward off anxiety with compulsive activity. They make good adjustments as long as they can sustain intense activity levels.

The negative types were:

1. *Angry.* They despair over their failure to achieve life goals and blame others for it.
2. *Self-hating.* They experience a similar sense of failure but blame themselves for how their life turned out. Both these types exhibit high rates of depression, low self-regard, alienation, and feelings of worthlessness.

Reichard, Livson, and Peterson's typology is only one example of a number of psychosocial classifications evolved through analysis of empirical data. It has served to alert practitioners against simple dichotomic notions that all "disengagement-prone" behavior is bad and that an infusion of multifaceted program activities is a suitable prescription for all.

Classifications are auxiliary tools and should be used only as part of an overall evaluation procedure. Too literal an adherence to a typology based on functional ability, for instance, may lead, according to Illich (1975), to "structural iatrogenesis," namely, the possibility that health professionals, by appending a sick or disabled label on people, may destroy their resources for handling their deficits in an autonomous way. Determinations of who is capable and who is impaired are not easy to make. As Larson (1964) pointed out:

One can seldom say, for example, that on this day or in this week, an adult who had previously been able to meet and resolve the problems of every day living with reasonable prudence became incapable of doing so. Moreover loss of capability may be uneven . . . an older person may be "childish" in his conversation but regular in meeting his financial obligations.

A comprehensive evaluation therefore goes beyond the fixed parameters of established classifications and taps for strengths and decrements into areas such as: self-care, physical and mental health, functional capacity, coping skills, present and past roles, occupational status, work and life satisfaction, family status, interpersonal relations, primary support systems, housing and environmental context, and economic conditions, including benefits that may accrue to a person for reasons of vesting, maturity of insurance plans, age, and proven need.

When an individual service plan is needed, social workers should keep in mind that, contrary to commonly held assumptions, many older persons can be helped with insight therapy. Prolonged forms of treatment may not be practical or feasible in all circumstances, and Oberleder (1966) suggests that interventions with the elderly should not be directed to changing their personality makeup but to alleviating their anxiety and maintaining adequate functioning. Verwoerdt (1981) similarly views psychotherapy as being supportive because regression and transference are not dealt with or interpreted. The basic goal then is to strengthen existing coping skills. A client's defenses should be understood as mechanisms to ward off an adverse reality and the anxiety it produces. Because older persons experience multiple and almost simultaneous stresses, defense mechanisms are not necessarily maladaptive in all instances. Some may be positive because they enable the person to contend with those blows. Ford (1965) observed, for instance, that denial gives the person a chance to reorganize, delay, or postpone dealing with a crisis until he or she can marshal inner or external resources more effectively. The same may be said about "withdrawal," when the person avoids taking risks and abandons the field. It may not be too high a price to pay in order to retain one's selfhood. Manipulation and aggression may also be interpreted on occasion as signs of vitality. They are proactive behaviors revealing a capacity to assess the environment and to increase personal gains. The plan of treatment capitalizes on the older person's remaining strengths and coping resources, but it may also offer sincere reassurance, particularly when progressive disabilities have set in. It is much easier to accept one's dependencies when realizing that one is not alone and that others care. In any event, treatment objectives should be scaled down to a realistic expectation level, commensurate with the person's remaining strengths. Any improvement, regardless of how imperceptible, is an auspicious indicator of therapeutic effectiveness. It may produce the added benefits of enhancing the person's sense of control over his/her life and improving his/her battered self-esteem.

Rowlings (1981) observed that treatments for the elderly consist, for the most part, of the management of their dependence and the management of risk. The former is commonly handled through case-management systems. The latter requires sheltered environments, community-based services, and preventive therapies. In addition, a "quality of life" orientation should be geared to enriching the overall circumstances of a person's life and adding more opportunities and alternatives. This is primarily attained through policy analysis, policy development, social planning, and community organization. It begins at the individual level with helping people obtain better and more suitable resources, a subject to be reviewed in the next section.

APPLYING SOCIAL POLICY

Social Security constitutes the leading source of income for older persons. Medicare covers nearly half of their acute health-care costs, and Medicaid foots almost 60 percent of the nursing-home bill. No other age group is so dependent on public entitlements, yet older persons are intimidated by complex eligibility requirements and the voluminous paperwork required to apply for a given benefit. There is the agony of waiting for decisions and not knowing how to seek redress when an application is disallowed on obscure statutory grounds. Overcome by sheer physical exhaustion, discouraged by transportation costs, long lines, and the hurried expedience of clerical personnel, many seniors simply give up and do not press for their rights. Social workers stepping in to facilitate access to services and to restore the provision of entitlements are similarly bewildered by the sheer number of programs addressed to the aged. The House Select Committee on Aging found between 50 and 200 federal programs with major assistance commitments to older persons (U.S. Congress, 1977). Must an effective social worker become proficient in all of them? Kutza (1981) notes, to everybody's relief, that there are only eight programs that constitute the core of the aging-focused policies: Social Security (Old Age and Survivors Insurance), tax allowances and benefits, Medicare, Older Americans Act services, Medicaid, Supplemental Security Income, food stamps, and housing subsidies. Ultimately, a geriatric practitioner ought to have a good working knowledge of only four: Social Security (OASI), Supplemental Security Income (SSI), Medicare (Title XVIII), and Medicaid (Title XIX). Only one piece of legislation is exclusively aimed at the elderly: the Older Americans Act, which focuses for the most part on the coordination of existing resources and the planning of new ones. Social workers approach the myriad of programs for the aged wondering whether their clients qualify for services and how those who are entitled can obtain those benefits. A generic prescription for policy application therefore includes the following considerations:

1. *Eligibility.* To whom is the program addressed? Who is entitled to apply for benefits and who does not qualify? Are there any retroactive eligibility provisions that compenstate for services rendered prior to the application?
2. *Proof of eligibility.* What evidence must clients submit in order to establish whether they qualify for the benefits?
3. *Adequacy.* Are the benefits obtained commensurate with the client's needs? Assuming they meet those needs only partially, are there any

other programs that can be used as backup or supplement? What is the best possible "package" of benefits that can be set up on behalf of a client?

4. *Costs.* Are there any known or hidden costs, deductibles, premiums, or "spend down" requirements the client must bear before becoming eligible for a specific benefit?

5. *Application.* What steps must the client follow in order to apply for a specific benefit? What is the waiting time, how quickly are applications acted upon, and how long does it take to obtain benefits?

6. *Confidentiality.* Are the client's rights to privacy assured during the application and service-delivery process? Do clients have access to their files?

7. *Quality assurance.* Are the program personnel properly trained and equipped to deliver the benefits? Have quality standards and evaluative procedures been instituted to monitor the service-delivery process?

8. *Plan of service.* Are clients involved in determining an eventual plan of service? What are the possible limitations or changes in duration, type, and level of service that may be subsequently introduced? Who has the authority to effect such changes?

9. *Due process.* How can the client request a review of a denial or termination of benefits? What are the mechanisms of appeal and grievance hearing? What information must the client submit when initiating an appeal?

10. *Advocacy.* If the program does not properly address a problem or does not reach its intended target population, how can clients and social workers bring this fact to the attention of policymakers? What are the best strategies for creating awareness and bringing about community pressure to effect change?

11. *Policy formulation.* What are the best possible alternatives to a deficient or obsolete policy? What are their estimated benefits and what is their economic, political, and administrative feasibility?

Concerning the last two items—advocacy and policy formulation—it is to the social worker's advantage to know how existing policies evolved, whether they share a common pattern, and what future awaits them.

Policies for the aged, as for any other problem area, resulted from breakdowns in the provision of critical services by the voluntary or private sectors, thus forcing a reluctant government to intervene. As more needs were identified, additional remedial actions had to be sanctioned and instituted. This is the proverbial incrementalism of all policymaking in America, a step-by-step course guided by the pressures of interest groups and the circumstantial convenience of political agendas. There is no underlying commitment to a comprehensive and long-range strategy, and Estes (1979) suggests that many of the resulting policies are deliberately ambiguous precisely to avoid making definite value decisions.

Incrementalism, however, has its advantages too: it permits trial-and-error adjustments, and it does not freeze providers in an ideological corner.

Value preferences, of course, enter into consideration when policymakers must contend with basic dilemmas: Are social policies for the aged meant to provide a floor of protection only, or should they seek to upgrade the quality of older persons' lives? Should they emphasize an income or a service strategy? Should services be universally responsive to all older persons or residually limited to those in greater need?

Should programs be based on a social-insurance model, thus providing benefits in direct relation to a person's previous contributions, or should they seek to reduce income disparities by redistributing both money and resources? Is there a reason for separate programs for the elderly, or should they be integrated in a comprehensive service strategy for all needy members of society? Each of these questions merits an extensive discussion that would exceed the intent of this chapter. The issues, however, are more than academic since they touch upon the future scope and even the survival of the programs for the aged. The question whether there should be special separate services for the aged, for instance, received widespread attention at the time of the 1981 White House Conference on Aging, when those in favor of dismantling the network of gerontological services argued that services should exist to handle problems in general, regardless of the ages of those affected. Attacking problems separately for each age group results in a debilitated and fragmented strategy. Insisting on separate policies may lead to negative labeling, stigmatization, or token symbolic measures that fall short of the mark.

Advocates of an age-categorical approach claim, in turn, that doing away with the present system will not produce the alleged age "integration." It will lead instead to a functional specialization along disease or organ criteria. As in the traditional medical model, it will treat symptoms of dysfunctions but seldom the whole person, and may overlook the fact that illnesses in younger age groups are for the most part acute and episodic while chronicity is the dominant expression of pathology in old age. The very goals of treatment for the latter can no longer be restoration of health, as for the young, but compensation for loss of function. Moreover, older persons are often afflicted by a cluster of chronic conditions that might include arthritis, diabetes, deafness, recent widowhood, loss of income, absence of immediate relatives, and so on. These multiple conditions interact and combine in unpredictable ways, and they cannot be attacked piecemeal as separate functional entities.

The discussion may become superfluous when we take into account that the elderly tend to lose out when mixed with other age groups but are strengthened by peer interaction. Landmark initiatives concerning services for the aged in the United States were invariably spearheaded through age-categorical, not universalistic, programs. The four major public programs relevant to the aged—

Social Security, Medicare, Supplemental Security Income, and nutrition (Older Americans Act) — began as "age specific" programs. Whenever generic programs were launched without making special provisions for older persons, the latter ended up discouraged at having to compete with the young for access to these services. In other instances they could not obtain the universal service because of deliberately discriminatory service practices. A study by the U.S. Commission on Civil Rights (1977) found that many community mental-health centers adopted an administrative policy of limiting older persons to no more than 5 percent of their caseloads, despite the fact that older persons constitute nearly 12 percent of the population and possibly 20 percent of the population at risk.

There are recommendations to resolve the impasse by keeping services age-integrated until age 75 and then offering age-categorical services to the older cohort. The reasoning behind such an arrangement is expedient but not very rational. Some services, like preretirement counseling or occupational retraining, do not make sense at age 75. They are not needed at age 25, either, but may be useful only for those in the age 50 to 60 cohort.

Ideally, services should be organized in a two-tiered system: both universalistic and particularistic. A hospital may provide general outpatient services, but certain ailments may require the input of a pediatrician and other ailments the input of a geriatric specialist. A school system offers high-school education for all, but a middle-aged adult who wishes to complete the requirements for a high-school diploma may need a didactic approach different from that targeted for adolescents. Besides, it is unlikely that an older person would feel comfortable in a class with teenagers. Age-categorical services have the advantage of being more individualizing. They employ differential assessment methods and a more profound understanding of the issues, crises, and developmental potentialities of each stage of the life cycle. Social policies will have to make special allowance for these specialized services, whether free standing or as parts of universal programs, even when advocating greater closeness of generations and more effective utilization of primary support networks.

In essence, the application of social policy to practice goes beyond the knowledge and negotiations of entitlements. It requires as well an understanding of (1) the underlying philosophy of such policies, (2) the political climates that foster the adoption of new ideas or force the retraction of a too progressive advance, (3) the emerging issues that require societal intervention, and (4) the process that leads to the adoption of new policies, from grass-roots organization to lobbying, legislative drafting, and mobilization of political support.

Social workers are not passive implementers of programs even when seeking to maximize their potential benefits on behalf of elderly clients. They also assist in formulating the policies that authorize those programs. They take the lead in protecting good ongoing programs, when jeopardized, and in recommending changes when other programs are no longer adequate.

A MANPOWER AGENDA

Working with the aged, as it has unfolded in this chapter, is no light matter. It starts with an attitudinal self-appraisal and emotional preparation followed by the systematic learning of a vast knowledge base that encompasses theory, normal and pathological human development, and social-policy issues. It finally requires the acquisition of a complex battery of practice skills, some of which give greater emphasis to institutional and sheltered care while others are addressed to the well or minimally impaired aged. Where does such preparation take place? Gerontological services are not in the forefront of the educational agenda of schools of health and social services, and most specialists have to improvise on their jobs. In a manpower report submitted by Elias Cohen to the Senate Special Committee on Aging on behalf of the Gerontological Society, attention was drawn precisely to the fact that only 10 percent and perhaps a maximum of 20 percent of the professionals of all disciplines primarily or exclusively serving the elderly have any formal training in gerontology or geriatrics (U.S. Congress, 1973). While the report does not disaggregate by occupational groups, there is no reason to believe that training levels of social workers have been markedly better. Even when gerontological training was on an ascending course during the late 1960s and 1970s, thanks to an abundance of the Title IV-A training funds of the Older Americans Act, relatively few graduate schools of social work rushed to generate full-fledged teaching concentrations on the subject. Those funds were practically gone, for all practical purposes, in the early 1980s, and whatever is left can support only short, in-service and nondegree-oriented workshops, usually under the aegis of Area Agencies on Aging. Only a handful of schools of social work offer systematic training in aging that goes beyond a couple of elective courses. Some do so on their own, while others succeed in engaging the support of private foundations. The gap left by the withdrawal of federal funding has not been filled.

This is rather paradoxical when we consider the mind-boggling level of demand for gerontological social workers forecast for the next fifteen or twenty years. The U.S. Labor Department's 1982 list of the top twelve high-demand occupations, as reported by *Newsweek,* placed "geriatric social work" in second place, with an estimated employment of 700,000 by 1990, behind only industrial-robot engineering. Future estimates take into account not only the growing number of older persons, from about 24 million in 1980 to 35 million in 2000, but also the internal changes in the composition of the 65-plus cohort. Demographic projections estimate that the 75-and-older group, which represented 38 percent of the total aged in 1980 or about 9 million people, will rise to 44 percent or 15.4 million people by the turn of the century. Estimates of the proportion of the frailest and most dependent among the age group 75 and older range from 9 to 20 percent, depending on the definition of functional impairment (U.S. Bureau of the Census, 1977). In any case, frail older persons, those who find it difficult to cope with the vicissitudes of life for easons of health, economics, housing, and family supports, are the fastest growing segment of the elderly population. Services connected with the provision of long-term care for that group, whether community- or institution-based, will obviously follow suit.

There will also be an emerging demand at the other end of the age spectrum. During the late 1960s and early 1970s retirement before age 65 became a desirable option for nearly half of all prospective retirees. In recent years a reverse trend emerged, aimed at abolishing mandatory retirement altogether or at least at gradually postponing it, as a means of restoring fiscal viability of the Social Security system. Early retirement had already lost some of its appeal due to the inflation of the late 1970s, which substantially eroded the purchasing power of fixed-pension benefits. However, with inflation rates dropping while endemically high unemployment rates persist, early retirement may regain its position as a favored alternative for older workers. Gerontological practitioners may then be confronted with vast numbers of leisured, younger retirees whose value primacy is no longer work but active exploration and search for self-renewal. Social workers will then have to come to terms with a new culture of leisure, centered around a sense of self-directedness, lifelong learning pursuits, and quality-of-life concerns.

Working with the aged holds many promises, but it will take time until these latent career opportunities will be fully realized. In the meantime practitioners must attend to their clients' service needs without always having available a ready-made and comprehensive service system. It is often up to them to design or even improvise new services. It is also their ultimate challenge to propose new legislation and advocate service reforms. Idealistic practitioners may find this a highly creative and pioneering task, but it is also a very demanding one in which the signs of "combat fatigue" show at an early stage. Excitement and frustration go with building a new field of service.

REFERENCES

Blau, P. M., (1964). *Exchange and power in social life*. New York: Wiley.

Blenkner, M. (1965). Social work and family relationships in old age. In E. Shanas and G. F. Streib (Eds.), *Social structure and the family: Generational relations*. Englewood Cliffs, N.J.: Prentice-Hall.

Borges, M. A., and Dutton, L. J. (1976). Attitudes toward aging: Increasing optimism found with age. *Gerontologist*, **16**(3), 220-224.

Botwinick, J. (1978). *Aging and behavior* (2nd ed.). New York: Springer.

Brennan, E. M., and Weick, A. (1981). Theories of adult development: Creating a context for practice. *Social Casework*, **62**(1), 13-19.

Brody, E. M., Kleban, M. H., Lawton, M. P., and Silverman, H. A. (1971). Excess disabilities of mentally impaired aged: Impact of individualized treatment. *Gerontologist*, **11**(2), 124-133.

Butler, R. N., (1974). Successful aging and the role of the life review. *Journal of the American Geriatrics Society*, **22**(12), 529-535.

Carp, F. M. (1968). Some components of disengagement. *Journal of Gerontology*, **23**(3), 382-386.

Cowgill, D. O. (1977). The revolution of age. *Humanist*, **37**(5), 10-13.

Cumming, E., and Henry, W. E. (1961). *Growing old: The process of disengagement*. New York: Basic Books.

Dowd, J. J. (1975). Aging as exchange: A preface to theory. *Journal of Gerontology*, **30**(5), 584-594.

Duvall, E. M. (1977). *Marriage and family development* (5th ed.). New York: Harper & Row.

Emerson, R. M. (1962). Power-dependence relations. *American Sociological Review*, **27**(1), 31-41.

Erikson, E. H. (1959). Identity and the life cycle. *Psychological Issues*, **1**(1), 18-171.

Estes, C. L. (1979). *The aging enterprise: A critical examination of social policies and services for the aged*. San Francisco: Jossey-Bass.

Ford, C. S. (1965). Ego-adaptive mechanisms of older persons. *Social Casework*, **46**(1), 16-21.

Freud-Loewenstein, S. (1978). Preparing social work students for life-transition counseling within the human behavior sequence. *Journal of Education for Social Work*, **14**(2), 66-73.

Gerontological Society. (1978). *Working with older people: A guide to practice*. Rockville, Md.: U.S. Department of Health, Education and Welfare.

Gubrium, J. F. (1980). Patient exclusion in geriatric settings. *Sociological Quarterly*, **21**(3), 335-347.

Illich, I. (1975). *Medical nemesis: The expropriation of health*. London: Calder & Boyars.

Kayser-Jones, J. S. (1981). *Old, alone, and neglected: Care of the aged in Scotland and in the United States*. Berkeley: University of California Press.

Kutza, E. A. (1981). *The benefits of old age: Social welfare policy for the elderly*. Chicago: University of Chicago Press.

Labouvie-Vief, G. (1982). Individual time, social time and intellectual aging. In T. K. Hareven and K. J. Adams (Eds.), *Aging and life course transitions: An interdisciplinary perspective*. New York: Guilford Press.

Larson, N. (1964). Protective services for older adults. *Public Welfare*, **22**(4), 247-251, 276.

Lerner, R. M., and Ryff, C. D. (1978). Implementing the life-span view: Attachment. *Life-Span Development and Behavior*, **1**, 1-44.

Levinson, D. J., et al. (1978). *The seasons of a man's life*. New York: Knopf.

Loevinger, J. (1976). *Ego development: Conceptions and theories*. San Francisco: Jossey-Bass.

Louis Harris and Associates. (1975). *The myth and reality of aging in America*. Washington: National Council on the Aging.

Maddox, G. L. (1963). Activity and morale: A longitudinal study of selected elderly subjects. *Social Forces*, **42**(2), 195-204.

Neugarten, B. L., and Brown-Rezanka, L. (1978-79). *Midlife women in the 1980s*. Paper submitted to the House Select Committee on Aging. Quoted in U.S. Congress. House. Select Committee on Aging. *Women in midlife — Security and fulfillment* (2 vols.). Washington: Government Printing Office.

Neugarten, B. L., Moore, J. W., and Lowe, J. C., (1965). Age norms, age constraints, and adult socialization. *American Journal of Sociology*, **70**(6), 710-717.

Oberleder, M. (1966). Psychotherapy with the aging: An art of the possible? *Psychotherapy: Theory, Research and Practice*, **3**(3), 139-142.

Parkes, C. M. (1971). Psycho-social transitions: A field for study. *Journal of Social Science and Medicine*, **5**(5), 101-115.

Pearlin, L. I. (1982). Discontinuities in the study of aging. In T. K. Hareven and K. J. Adams (Eds.), *Aging and life course transitions: An interdisciplinary perspective*. New York: Guilford Press.

Peterson, D. A., and Karnes, E. L. (1976). Older people in adolescent literature. *Gerontologist*, **16**(3), 225-231.

Piaget, J. *The child and reality: Problems of genetic psychology*. New York: Penguin, 1976.

Plemons, J. K., Willis, S. L., and Baltes, P. B. (1978). Modifiability of fluid intelligence in aging: A short-term longitudinal training approach. *Journal of Gerontology*, **33**(2), 224-231.

Rapoport, L. (1967). Crisis-oriented short-term casework. *Social Service Review*, **41**(1), 31-43.

Reichard, S., Livson, F., and Peterson, P. G. (1962). *Aging and personality*. New York: Wiley.

Robertson, J. F. (1976). Significance of grandparents: Perceptions of young adult grandchildren. *Gerontologist,* **16**(2), 137-140.

Rose, A. M. (1964). A current theoretical issue in social gerontology. *Gerontologist,* **4**(1), 46-50.

Rosenmayr, L. (1982). Biography and identity. In T. K. Hareven and K. J. Adams (Eds.), *Aging and life course transitions: An interdisciplinary perspective.* New York: Guilford Press.

Rosow, I. (1973). The social context of the aging self. *Gerontologist,* **13**(1), 82-87.

Rowlings, C. (1981). *Social work with elderly people.* London: Allen & Unwin.

U.S. Bureau of the Census. (1977). Projections of the population of the United States: 1977 to 2050. *Current Population Reports,* Series P-25, No. 704. Washington: Government Printing Office.

U.S. Commission on Civil Rights. (1977). *The age discrimination study.* Washington: The Commission.

U.S. Congress. House. (1977). Select Committee on Aging. *Fragmentation of services for the elderly.* Washington: Government Printing Office.

U.S. Congress. Senate. (1973). Special Committee on Aging. *Training in gerontology.* Washington: Government Printing Office.

Verwoerdt, A. (1981). *Clinical geropsychiatry* (2nd ed.). Baltimore: Williams & Wilkins.

Ward, R. A. (1977). The impact of subjective age and stigma on older persons. *Journal of Gerontology,* **32**(2), 227-232.

2

Life Span, Human Development, and Old Age*

Judith Treas, Ph. D.

University of Southern California

Sherry Berkman, D.S.W.

University of California at Los Angeles

The transition from middle years to old age has many markers. With the sixty-fifth birthday, one joins the age group we somewhat arbitrarily associate with old, but many 65-year-olds do not think of themselves as aged. Indeed, many Americans continue to refer to themselves as middle-aged well into the seventh and eighth decades of life. For most of us, the subjective sense of our own aging arises not from chronological age but rather from more concrete changes in our lives. From a physical standpoint, one may be aware of a decline in stamina, a twinge of arthritis, or the diagnosis of a chronic disease. From a social perspective, one's activities, commitments, and relations to others may change. For example, one may become a great grandparent, a retiree, or a resident of a nursing home. Alternatively, the signs of one's own aging may be manifest in the changes in the world in which we live. Lifetime friends may grow old and die. The old neighborhood may deteriorate or become unexpectedly chic. Contemporary tastes in clothes, music, and morals may seem increasingly bizarre.

The later years of life call upon us to negotiate a myriad of changes—some gradual, some abrupt, some anticipated, and others unforeseen. In the context of coping with these changes, we are challenged to come to terms with our own

*Preparation of this chapter was supported by the Andrew W. Norman Institute for the Advanced Study of Gerontology and Geriatrics.

aging. To these new demands, we bring a life-span legacy of experience, resources, and response patterns. In this way, the latter years of lafe present both a vehicle for continuity and a forum for change.

SOCIALIZATION

The social psychology of aging has long emphasized adult socialization as the mechanism by which older persons adapt to the changes thrust upon them. In other words, the rights, responsibilities, rewards, and rules of late-life social roles are learned. Some roles are mastered by trial and error. Other roles (e.g., widowhood) benefit from anticipatory socialization—studying how people in the role act and undertaking role rehearsals—beginning long before the role is actually assumed. As Rosow (1974) noted, however, socialization to old age is problematic, because behaviorial expectations are only vaguely defined, because there is little motivation to learn a role that is not valued, and because few formal vehicles for socialization exist.

Take a case in point. Popular media, a potential mechanism for late-life socialization, offer two dominant portrayals of the elderly. The down-and-out stereotype pictures the impoverished elder, bereft of kin and beset by major health problems and severe functional limitations. This stereotype does not fit the objective circumstances of most older lives, and few would feel any incentive to adopt abject behavior. On the other hand, the media constantly confront us with the case of the elder who makes no concessions to old age. The 80-year-old mountain climber, the ageless silent-film star, and the octogenarian industrialist are posed as models of aging worthy of imitation. Unfortunately, this stereotype also affords few useful guidelines to the conduct of later life; it fails to confront the fact that for most of us old age is both a continuation of a prosaic existence and an encounter with new circumstances (e.g., health problems) to which we must accommodate.

If there are deficiencies in societal provisions for socialization to the transitions of old age, it is in part because late-life change is novel in its scope and predictability. As Treas and Bengtson (1982) point out, improvements in mortality rates have led to a "democratization" of middle age, old age, and even advanced old age. In 1900, for example, only one-half of Americans could expect to survive from age 20 to age 65. By 1976, fully 84 percent of women and 70 percent of men were reaching old age. Survival into old age—once a chancy proposition—has become commonplace. Lengthening lifetimes have given rise to a long empty-nest phase in the family life cycle as well as a postmarital stage of independent living apart from kin. Changing work patterns have meant that today's elderly experience the leisure life-style of retirement unknown to earlier generations.

The changes of late life have come to be inevitable for broad segments of the

American population, and this situation is historically unique. We will live years and even decades with retirement, widowhood, or chronic illness. The lessons of our youth and the examples of our own parents' aging are scarcely relevant to the era of extended lifetimes that we can look forward to. At the same time, our social institutions exhibit a cultural lag in their failure to provide opportunities for socialization to the transitions of the later years. The dearth of mental-health and rehabilitative services targeting older Americans points to a societal shortsightedness; we fail to appreciate the many years over which older persons can expect to recoup the costs of intervention programs.

That so many older persons successfully negotiate the transitions of old age in the absence of cultural models has led gerontologists to question the idea that individuals are passive learners of societally scripted roles (Gubrium and Buckholdt, 1977; Marshall, 1980b; Neugarten and Hagestad, 1976). Newer conceptions of adjustment to old age emphasize the elderly as interacting with a social environment to fashion their own roles. Keith (1982), for example, describes how the residents of a French retirement home reacted to the young director's attempt to cover up the death of an aged resident. Out of this incident, they created new norms by requesting through the Residents Committee that deaths be announced in the dining hall and that transportation be provided to the funeral.

To sum up, growing old poses significant life changes, and the aging of the American population has made these changes of ever greater concern. The broader society may be faulted for failing to identify appropriate models of aging as well as for failing to provide formal social institutions for socialization and resocialization in the later years. Despite a lack of guideposts to the later years of the life cycle, the elderly do adapt and even grow with the changes and challenges posed by old age. Collectively and individually, they negotiate new roles in keeping with the new circumstances in which they find themselves. They also draw upon the coping strategies, support networks, and experiences that have served them well in earlier years.

COPING

If sociological thinking has moved away from the idea of the individual as the passive learner of static roles, so have psychological paradigms come to emphasize the individual as activist. Lazarus (1980) notes the shift in psychology away from viewing behavior as a passive response to external stimuli or internal drives. Instead, an interest in perception has led to the recognition that cognition mediates human adaptation to environmental demands. What is more, a dialectical perspective on change has stressed that individuals continually alter their environments in a way to require further adaptation (Riegel, 1977).

Coupled with greater attention to individual differences, these perspectives have informed psychological thinking on how we cope with stresses like those encountered in the transitions of old age.

As Lazarus (1980) argues, stressful situations may be those *judged* by the individual to involve harm or loss—either as a potential threat or as an accomplished fact. Old age certainly calls upon individuals to confront losses—the death of one's spouse, a drop in income, a decline in mobility, the loss of a socially esteemed job—although not all losses will be evaluated as uniformly harmful and stressful by the person to whom they occur. One may welcome retirement from a job, and the death of one's spouse following a lengthy illness may call forth feelings of relief as well as regret. Still other stressful situations may be defined as challenges presenting opportunities for new growth, achievement, and enhanced self-esteem. For example, Myerhoff (1978) documents the pride that aged Jews in Venice, California take in getting along on fixed incomes and in a changing neighborhood. Unfortunately, the emphasis in the gerontological literature on the losses of old age has diverted attention away from the positive impetus to change that is afforded by many of the transitions of later life.

Coping is behavior directed toward dealing with feelings and problem-solving. The capacity for coping depends on personal resources and personal style. George (1980) identifies financial assets, health, social supports, and education as resources that may cushion the impact of stress or facilitate adaptation to new circumstances. Certain stable personality traits are also thought to contribute to coping. Chronic anxiety, poor impulse control, and denial may inhibit the realistic appraisal of situations, as well as the formulation and implementation of adaptive responses. Openness to new experiences suggests a flexibility that contributes to coping.

Studies of personality in later life have developed typologies that suggest the variation that exists in personal coping styles (Lowenthal, Thurnher, and Chiripoga, 1975; Neugarten, Havighurst, and Tobin, 1968). For example, Neugarten and associates (1968) distinguish "integrated" copers from the "passive-dependent," who just take things as they come; the "armored defended" with defensively denying coping styles; and the least successful "unintegrated" types. There is convincing evidence that personality traits do not change with age, at least for adult white males (McCrae, Costa, and Arenberg, 1980). This stress on stable personality structures suggests that the threats and challenges of old age are met with adaptive behavioral repertoires developed over a lifetime.

In contrast with the traditional notion of stable dispositions are processual paradigms in which personality serves continually to sort out experiences and guide behavior. Haan (1977) has pointed out that very different adaptational responses derive from just a limited number of generic ego processes. Coping is just one mode of expression for such processes, with denial and fragmentation representing alternative modes. According to Haan (p. 34):

Coping involves purpose, choice, and flexible shift, adheres to intersubjective reality and logic, and allows and enhances proportionate affective expression; defensiveness is compelled, negated, rigid, distorting of intersubjective reality and logic, allows covert impulse expression, and embodies the expectancy that anxiety can be relieved without directly addressing the problem; fragmentation is automated, ritualistic, privatistically formulated, affectively directed, and irrationally expressed in the sense that intersubjective reality is clearly violated.

For example, a generic process like selective awareness would take the form of concentration when coping is involved, denial when defensive modes of expression are at play, and fixation when dysfunctional fragmentation is manifested. Different modes of expression may come into play at different times, and any mode's success as an adaptational mechanism may depend on the particular situation. Denial may provide a refreshing "time out" from problem solving. Fixation may be rewarded as an admirable single-minded commitment.

This processual notion of freewheeling personality organization would seem to conflict with the finding that adult personality structure exhibits stability even in the face of aging. However, as McCrae and associates (1980, p. 882) emphasize, a "succession of phenotypically different behaviors may be needed at different ages to express the same enduring disposition."

Other research by McCrae (1982) lends further credence to the situational nature of coping. McCrae's research challenges the notion that aging brings a greater reliance on denial and distortion (Guttman, 1970) as well as the idea that the coping styles of the aged are necessarily more effective and more firmly grounded in reality (Vaillant, 1977). Cross-sectional age comparisons did not suggest that older persons resorted to different coping mechanisms than did the young. To the extent that older persons employed different mechanisms, such differences could be largely accounted for by age differences in the kinds of stresses encountered. Older people deal with health-related losses while their juniors face challenges associated with work and family. Controlling for type of stress, age differences were found for only two "theoretically immature" coping mechanisms. The middle-aged and the aged were less likely to draw on hostile reactions or escapist fantasies. In short, older persons seem to rely on the same strategies as younger folks for solving problems and dealing with emotions.

How *successfully* one deals with perceived stress — be it a loss, a threat, or a challenge — depends on the dynamic properties of the individual *and* his/her environment. Lawton and Nahemow (1973) pose an instructive "environmental press" model of aging and adaptation in which outcomes of individual-environmental transactions depend on the demands (or press) of the environment and the capacities (or competence) of the individual. Mediating such transactions are personality style and environmental cognition. Tremendous environmental demands, of course, may overwhelm even the most competent older person. Because they provide little stimulation, environments that place few demands on the individual may also lead to poor outcomes in terms of maladaptive behavior and negative feelings. As the environmental-press model suggests, coping is the product of the fit between the person and his/her environment, and an appropriate level of stress may actually contribute to well-being. There is some indication that this appropriate level of stress may be lower for older persons than for the young, however. In later stages of life, multiple life events or role transitions seem to be more problematic than at earlier life-cycle stages (Lowenthal, Thurnher, and Chiriboga, 1975).

CRITICAL EVENTS

Old age is characterized by changes that may warrant the label of "critical events." That is to say that these changes are demanding ones, implying stress and requiring personal and social reorganization on the part of the individual. Some critical events are idiosyncratic. They may be of tremendous significance to the individual, but they are not commonplace among the older population. A mugging or the deeply felt death of a pet are examples that come to mind. Other critical events touch many more lives. To a greater or lesser extent, events such as retirement or widowhood define old age in our minds. Let us briefly consider a few of these critical transitions.

Retirement

It is tempting to think of retirement as an event, perhaps symbolized by the awarding of a gold watch. Atchley (1975), however, has emphasized that retirement is a process epitomized by a seven-stage sequence beginning long before the last work day and likely continuing until death. As one moves closer to retirement, the prospect becomes less remote and perhaps even frightening. The worker may begin to plan for this eventuality and to try on leisure roles. After retirement, the euphoria of a newfound sense of freedom may give way to a letdown. Eventually, long-term adjustments are undertaken that serve the retiree until death, incapacitating illness, or a new job intervenes.

Retirement demands that we restructure our time, build social relationships outside a work setting, accommodate a drop in income, and forge an identity that is not linked to our occupation. As problematic as this seems, research on adjustment to retirement suggests high levels of satisfaction at least for those who retire in relatively good health and with adequate income. This may reflect several factors: that many jobs are themselves unsatisfying, that compulsory retirement carries no stigma of incompetence, and that a leisure-oriented retirement role for the healthy, middle-class aged is fairly well defined and socially approved. Friedmann and Orbach (1974) review the research literature to debunk the notion that retirement leads to declines in physical and mental health or to disruptions in family or social relationships. This is not to deny that retirement may be a wrenching experience to some, especially to those who are heavily invested in their work, who lack outside interests, or who have had difficulty making other life transitions. If retirement is a critical event, however, it is one that leads to successful resolution for most individuals.

Widowhood

In contrast to retirement, widowhood constitutes a critical event fraught with adjustment problems in the short term and over the long haul. Bereavement, for example, is commonly characterized by symptoms that might be taken as indicators of serious psychopathology under any other circumstances (e.g., crying, angry outbursts, insomnia, weight loss). The experience of mourning, however, is typically seen as an essential aspect of adjustment to the loss of a spouse. The outcome of this life transition is by no means assured, and the widowed are more vulnerable to mortality, morbidity, suicide, and mental illness than are their still-married counterparts.

Some of the negative consequences of widowhood derive from the loss of a significant other and the accompanying social roles. With widowhood, the surviving spouse ceases to be confidant, helpmate, sex partner, and companion. Although prescriptions for adjustment to widowhood typically call for the substitution of other meaningful roles, prospects for remarriage are typically poor, especially among the aged (Treas and VanHilst, 1976). Contacts with in-laws drop off, and the social-support system of elderly widows is limited largely to grown offspring (Lopata, 1979). Other negative consequences of widowhood may have to do with the fact that it is associated with declining incomes. One study found that the morale of widowed women was much like that of their married counterparts once their lower incomes, poorer health, or older age were taken into account (Morgan, 1976).

Some evidence suggests that adjustment to widowhood may be easier for those who anticipate their loss (Marshall, 1980a). Older women seem to adjust more readily than younger ones. Since men are not as likely to survive a spouse, they evidence greater adjustment difficulties. Thus mental preparation and anticipatory socialization may facilitate bereavement and the building of a new life.

Residential Relocation

Although the aged are not as likely to move as are younger persons, late-life circumstances may occasion a change of residence. Urban renewal, condominium conversion, and rising rents displace some older people while others voluntarily seek out the leisure life-style of a retirement community. Changes in health, income, or social supports may necessitate the move to a nursing home or to an offspring's household. Some moves may lead to a stimulating change of scene and a better life, but positive outcomes are by no means assured. How well older people cope with the potential stresses of a move depends on a number of factors, not the least of which are their own capacities and vulnerabilities.

Studies of involuntary transfers of the institutionalized elderly have raised the issue of "relocation trauma" — that is, increased mortality, especially among the most impaired. Several studies now indicate no significant differences in mortality rates for relocated and nonrelocated seniors (Borup, Gallego, and Heffernan, 1979), although relocation, whether voluntary or involuntary, is associated with a decline in health status (Ferraro, 1983). The nature of the move itself may well influence adaptation as well. A national sample of "normal" older persons demonstrated that morale declined when the elderly moved from a better to a worse residential environment (Schooler, 1975). Lieberman and Tobin considered four longitudinal studies in which moves ranged from voluntary admissions to nursing homes to mass transfers between institutions (Lieberman, 1975). They concluded that the amount of environmental change was the best predictor of adaptive outcome, regardless of individual differences in coping styles, personal resources, and perceptions of stress.

LIFE STAGES

As the discussion of "critical events" suggests, aging brings certain predictable changes that typically engender stress and require adaptational response. Among students of the life span, an ongoing debate centers on whether the second half of life affords so many common experiences and shared preoccupations as to warrant generalizing from chronological age to life-cycle stage. Recent developmental models embracing the notion of stages have pointed to "transitions," "passages," "seasons," and "turning points." As these terms imply, stage theories often assume a more or less predictable ordering of personal concerns over the life cycle. They stress a certain age-related inevitability to critical developmental challenges. Perhaps most importantly, many theories suggest a social-psychological differentiation of the life cycle in which personal growth is to be found in breaks with previous ways and in resolutions of new concerns.

There are abundant examples of adult development models in which stages figure prominently (Erikson, 1963; Havighurst, 1972; Levinson, 1978; Gould, 1978; Sheehy, 1976; Buhler, 1968). For instance, drawing on psychoanalytic theory, Erikson (1963) identified concerns dominating the second half of life. In middle years, the challenge to ego is the establishment of generativity, that is, a stake in future generations. In old age, the task is to cultivate ego integrity, permitting one a sense of satisfaction and resolution in looking back over life. Informed by Erikson's ideas, Havighurst (1972) pointed to specific developmental tasks forced upon individuals at particular ages by physical maturation and the expectations of Western culture. Among the tasks confronting the old are adjusting to retirement, declining health, and widowhood. Achieving a task "on time" contributes to personal happiness, to societal approval, and to achievement of subsequent tasks.

Levinson's (1978) model deals with inevitable changes in the underlying pattern and meaning of an individual's life—his "life structure." In this formulation, periods of stability are punctuated by periods of transition. For example, Levinson and his associates direct particular attention to the transition of middle age in which youthful aspirations must usually be reconciled with more modest accomplishments. The upshot of this transition is an era in which men report taking pride in the accomplishments of their juniors and focusing less on work and more on family domains. In other words, life's circumstances undermine the existing life structure, leading to the construction of a new one.

Although stage models of adult development are undeniably fascinating and insightful, this approach has been criticized on a number of grounds. One criticism stems from the fact that stage theories tend to imply a broad applicability. Such theories, however, have typically been inspired by small, even clinical, populations. There is little evidence, for example, that Levinson's model may be generalized to women or that Havighurst's developmental tasks hold outside the middle class (Huyck and Hoyer, 1982).

Neugarten (1979) has provided one of the most extensive criticisms of stage theories of adulthood. She hypothesizes, first, a movement toward an age-irrelevant society in which age provides fewer inviolable norms for behavior. In a world in which grandmothers attend college while their middle-aged sons drop out of the labor force, it makes less sense to talk about an invariant succession of stages. Second, she argues that psychological preoccupations are not tidily resolved and permanently abandoned for new themes. Some concerns and challenges are salient at many different points in one's life. "Identity is made and remade; issues of intimacy and freedom and commitment to significant others, the pressures of time, the reformulation of life goals, stocktaking and reconciliation and acceptance of one's successes and failures—all these preoccupy the young as well as the old" (p. 891). Third, personality changes are unlikely to occur swiftly in response to an age-related life event. Instead, changes transpire gradually, in part because the mind is never concerned with only the present, but also brings the past to bear on any situation.

From a social-phenomenological perspective, Gubrium and Buckholdt (1977) certainly agree that interpretations of the present are colored by considerations of the past and future. They question, nonetheless, the usefulness of life stages as well as other paradigms that have dominated the study of aging (pp. 8-9):

For us, changes, stages, and development have no existence save what people make of them in word and deed. The important questions are not how people *respond to* life or *proceed through* stages, but how they negotiate and generate the reality and meaning of change, stages, and development; how the come to have a sense of them as things separate from themselves . . . ; and how they subsequently respond to them as real things.

This perspective is concerned with more than how people come to identify stresses, initiate responses, or define themselves as old. From this point of view, the professional expert looms large in creating our commonplace understandings of growing older. Of interest is how stage theorists themselves construct the theories that laypersons use to make sense of their lives. Also of concern is how such theories are applied by social workers and other professionals whose evaluations of clients may themselves influence the course of lives.

SOCIAL SUPPORTS IN OLD AGE

Although aging brings many changes that demand personal adaptations, a lifetime of social relationships typically affords us ongoing support in confronting the challenges of the later years. Family, friends, and neighbors provide us with social continuity, guideposts for behavior, inputs to self-esteem, and direct assistance. In the words of Kahn and Antonucci (1981), they serve as convoys through the life cycle.

Family life may assume particular significance in old age, because death and disability take their toll on age peers, because blood is thicker than water in times of adversity, and because imminent death increases the importance of inter-generational claims on immortality. The family arena is one that furnishes meaningful social roles to the elderly at a time when other areas of life (e.g., work) are characterized by role loss. For example, Rosenthal, Marshall, and Synge (1980) have discussed succession to the role of family head. In addition, the mutual socialization of family members assures a comfortable compatibility between the generations in terms of values, attitudes, and behavior (Bengston, 1975). The aged's "developmental stake" in younger relations may even serve to color their perceptions, minimizing whatever differences may exist (Bengston and Kuypers, 1971).

The exchange of goods and services between generations has been amply documented (Bengston and Treas, 1980). Although older family members are apt to give as well as receive, services provided the frail and dependent elderly by their relations are of considerable consequence—sometimes making the difference between community living and institutionalization. Caring for the impaired elderly can impose considerable costs upon caretaking kin, however. For this reason, gerontological attention has shifted from preoccupation with the needs of the elderly to a concern with the problems of a "sandwich generation" of middle-aged caretakers torn between competing demands of a job, aging parents, and other family members (Brody, 1981).

Considerable attention has focused on the question of what, if anything, distinguishes the roles of family members from those of the elderly's friends. Blau (1973) argues that friendship, being based on common needs and voluntary relations of equals, is more important to older people's self-esteem than are intergenerational bonds. Litwak and Szelany (1969) pose the notion of functional differentiation, with kin suited to long-term commitments like custodial care, neighbors dealing with emergencies close at hand, friends offering counsel on contemporary matters, and professionals furnishing technical advice. Cantor (1980), however, posits a "hierarchical compensatory model." Regardless of the task, she maintains, family members are preferred for support. If kin are not available, friends and neighbors are called upon with public and private agencies serving as last resorts. While assigning varying degrees of importance to nonrelatives, the literature suggests that relationships outside the family can also help individuals deal with the changes associated with growing older.

Despite these generalities, research tends to indicate the existence of ethnic differences in family relationships and in social networks of the elderly. Valle (1976), for example, calls attention to cultural differences such as family structure, role expectations, place of the elderly in society, use of nonkin/institutional assistance, and the meaning of aging, illness, and death. Black and Hispanic elderly tend to provide greater help to their children than do whites (Cantor, 1979) and probably rely more upon support from informal social networks (Manson, Murray, and Cain, 1980). However, the ties between elderly Hispanic women and their children and grandchildren have been found to be significantly stronger than those of either elderly whites or blacks (Andrus Gerontology Center, 1977).

Cultural differences are also evident in the use of resources such as mutual-aid associations and helping agents (e.g., *curanderos*, healers, medicine people). Valle and Mendoza (1978), for example, describe the natural helping systems of the elderly Latino population they studied, and the unique use of key natural helpers, *servidor communicativos* (communitywide service brokers), who act both as translators and liaisons, linking the person in need with the general community and complex governmental systems. For those elderly isolated by language, physical limitations, or cultural barriers, the assistance of such brokers, who are aware of resources and able to successfully negotiate bureaucracies, may be critical.

SOME IMPLICATIONS FOR SOCIAL-WORK PRACTICE

What can social workers learn from recent research on adult development? Perhaps foremost is a reiteration of the fallacy of defining old age in purely chronological terms. There is no magical age barrier that separates seniors from nonseniors, nor is there any validity in viewing all postretirement individuals as having identical needs and problems. For example, despite conventional stereotypes, only 5 percent of the nation's seniors (persons 65 and older) are institutionalized. Even that group can hardly be considered homogeneous in terms of needs: estimates indicate that half of the patients exhibit some type of mental illness (many in fact have lived in mental hospitals for most of their adult lives), between one-third and one-half have disorders of the circulatory system (heart disease, stroke, and disorders associated with stroke), about one-fourth are somewhat physically handicapped by permanent stiffness, and approximately 15 percent have digestive disorders (Gottesman and Hutchinson, 1979).

Consistent as this evidence of heterogeneity may be with the traditional social-work value of client individualization, it is all too frequently ignored by agencies that establish rigid age-eligibility requirements and promote programs tailored to the needs of "the elderly" as if they comprised a uniform group. Perhaps it makes more sense to view the aged not as a separate and distinct entity but as individuals occupying a particular position on a developmental continuum. Thus behaviors exhibited in old age can be viewed in the context of lifelong patterns of accommodation and adaptation. This period of life can be characterized as evolutionary rather than as terminal, requiring the resolution of certain key tasks (e.g., adjustment to loss and one's own impending illness and death) and the exercise of different behaviors and coping mechanisms (Butler and Lewis, 1982; Neugarten, 1968, 1976).

Similarly, old age can be characterized not only as a period marked by frequent loss and change but as a unique time of life offering the potential for growth and development (Ryff, 1982). For too long, social workers and other mental-health professionals have discriminated against the elderly, viewing them as emotionally rigid and intellectually stagnant, likely to profit little from interventions and offering few prospects for change (Butler and Lewis, 1982; Monk, 1981). Current research indicates that rigidity, fixation, and denial are neither the exclusive province of the elderly nor are they necessarily the hallmark of aging. Seniors are able to develop insight into their motivations and alter their behavior, using coping mechanisms that do not differ appreciably from those of younger individuals faced with similar stresses.

While such stresses may arise from a variety of sources, they are frequently precipitated by the occurrence of certain critical events that require personal reorganization and the development of different coping mechanisms and behaviors. Frequently mentioned precipitators are retirement, widowhood, and residential relocation, but even the loss of a pet or a change in rooms can require alternative forms of adaptation or adjustment. The impact of these critical events can be lessened through certain anticipatory activities that allow the individual to resolve some of his/her feelings prior to the actual occurrence of the event. Thus an elderly man's move to a nursing home can be resolved more successfully if he is actively involved in the decision-making process, if he is provided with several alternatives, and if he receives counseling and orientation prior to his relocation. Furthermore, the incorporation of familiar objects from his previous home (e.g., family photos, plants, a comfortable chair) within his new living arrangements will make the transition smoother (Brody, 1979).

Another means of helping the elderly deal with such stressful situations is through the use of informal support systems. Current research indicates that the family is still the major provider of social and emotional support to its aging members, even when they require long-term care (e.g., Brody, 1981; Shanas, 1979, 1980). Thus, even when seniors reside in long-term-care settings, kin should be encouraged to become involved in assessment, goal setting, and service-delivery activities (Brubaker and Brubaker, 1982). This coordinating or sharing of services provided by societal organizations *and* the family conserve or supplement formal resources while reducing the burden placed upon the family (Streib, 1972).

Filial support is not always readily available or possible. Long-standing intergenerational conflict, unresolved feelings toward parental aging and dependency, and competing personal demands can affect a child's willingness to help his/her parent (Lowy, 1979; Johnson, 1978; Brubaker and Brubaker, 1982). Variables such as a child's proximity to a parent and the impact of caretaking upon the caretaker's own life also influence the extent of filial behavior (Houser and Berkman, 1981). While caring for an elderly parent can negatively affect an offspring's life-style, straining the emotional, financial, and physical resources of kin, positive benefits may be realized as well, primarily in the form of improved parent-child relationships (Houser, 1982).

In order to minimize the adverse aspects of helping, certain services (e.g., transportation, housekeeping) can be provided institutionally, while families are encouraged to continue to provide emotional and social support. Although this strategy is intended to encourage kin involvement without overburdening individual family members, its execution requires a high investment in time and energy on the part of a worker willing to adopt a case-management approach.

A worker may also be called upon to help clarify behavioral expectations. A middle-aged daughter's idea of appropriate behavior for a 70-year-old widow may not correspond at all with the behavior exhibited by her mother. Far from being a placid, dependent elder, this widow may be campaigning for the Gray Panthers, protesting rent increases, or maintaining her own home in the face of serious physical limitations. In these situations, it is the worker's responsibility to help members of both generations clarify, articulate, and communicate their feelings and expectations to arrive at a greater understanding of the perceptions and motivations of the other. This task is made easier by an appreciation of the different developmental agendas faced by persons at different stages of the life cycle.

Old age can be "the last of life for which the first is made" (Browning).

Whether it is a rewarding period can be due in part to the ability of the individual, the family, and society to deal with the unique challenges offered. By providing education, clarification, and direction, the gerontological social worker has a crucial role in helping the elderly and their families derive their "maximum growth potential" (Monk, 1981).

REFERENCES

Andrus Gerontological Center. (1977). *Social and cultural aspects of aging: Community survey report.* Los Angeles: The Center.

Atchley, C. (1975). *The sociology of retirement.* Cambridge, Mass.: Schenkman.

Bengtson, V. L. (1975). Generation and family effects in value socialization. *American Sociological Review,* **40**, 358-371.

Bengston, V. L., and Kuypers, J. A. (1971). Generational differences and the developmental stake. *Aging and Human Development,* **2**(1), 249-260.

Bengston, V. L., and Treas, J. (1980). The changing family context of mental health and aging. In J. E. Birren and K. W. Schaie (Eds.), *Handbook of mental health and aging.* Englewood Cliffs, N.J.: Prentice-Hall.

Blau, Z. S. (1973). *Old age in a changing society.* New York: New Viewpoints.

Borup, J. H., Gallego, D. T., and Heffernan, P. (1979). Relocation and its effects on mortality. *Gerontologist,* **19**(2), 135-140.

Brody, E. M. (1979). Social work and long-term care facilities. In E. M. Brody (Ed.), *A social work guide for long-term care facilities.* Washington, D.C.: U.S. Department of Health, Education, and Welfare.

Brody, E. M. (1981). "Women in the middle" and family help to older people. *Gerontologist,* **21**, 471-480.

Brubaker, T. H., and Brubaker, E. (1982). *Family support of older persons in the long-term-care setting: Recommendations for practice.* Paper presented at the Annual Meeting of the National Council on Family Relations, Washington, D.C.

Buhler, C. (1968). The developmental structure of goal setting in group and individual studies. In C. Buhler and F. Massarik (Eds.), *The course of human life.* New York: Springer.

Butler, R. N., and Lewis, M. I. (1982). *Aging and mental health.* St. Louis: C. V. Mosby.

Cantor, M. H. (1979). The informal support system of New York inner city elderly: Is ethnicity a factor? In D. E. Gelfand and A. J. Kutzik (Eds.), *Ethnicity and aging.* New York: Springer.

Cantor, M. (1980). *Caring for the frail elderly: Impact on family, friends and neighbors.* Paper presented at the Annual Meeting of the Gerontological Society of America, San Diego.

Erikson, E. (1963). *Childhood and society.* New York: Norton.

Ferraro, K. F. (1983). The health consequences of relocation among the aged in the community. *Journal of Gerontology,* **38**(1), 90-96.

Friedmann, E. A., and Orbach, H. L. (1974). Adjustment to retirement. In S. Arieti (Ed.), *American handbook of psychiatry* (2nd ed.), vol. 1. New York: Basic Books.

George, K. (1980). *Role transitions in later life.* Monterey, Calif.: Brooks/Cole.

Gottesman, L. E., and Hutchinson, E. (1979). Characteristics of institutionalized elderly. In E. M. Brody (Ed.), *A social work guide for long-term care facilities.* Washington, D.C.: U.S. Department of Health, Education, and Welfare.

Gould, R. (1978). *Transformations: Growth and change in adult life.* New York: Simon & Schuster.

Gubrium, F., and Buckholdt, R. (1977). *Toward maturity.* San Francisco: Jossey-Bass.

Guttman, D. L. (1970). Female ego styles and generational conflict. In J. M. Bardwick, E. Douvan,

M. S. Horner, and D. L. Guttman (Eds.), *Feminine personality and conflict*. Belmont, Calif.: Brooks/Cole.

Haan, N. (1977). *Coping and defending: Processes of self-environment organization*. New York: Academic Press.

Havighurst, R. (1972). *Developmental tasks and education* (3rd ed.). New York: David McKay.

Houser, B. B. (1982). *Filial crisis among the adult children of older women*. Paper presented at the Annual Meeting of the National Council on Family Relations, Washington, D.C.

Houser, B. B., and Berkman, S. L. (1981). *Filial expectations, outcomes and crises*. Paper presented at the 61st Annual Meeting of the Western Psychological Association, Los Angeles, Calif.

Huyck, M. H., and Hoyer, W. J. (1982). *Adult development and aging*. Belmont, Calif.: Wadsworth.

Johnson, E. S. (1978). "Good" relationships between older mothers and their daughters: A causal model. *Gerontologist*, **18**(3), 301-306.

Kahn, R. L., and Antonucci, T. C. (1981). Convoys of social support: A life-course approach. In S. B. Kielser, J. N. Morgan, and V. K. Oppenheimer (Eds.), *Aging: Social change*. New York: Academic Press.

Keith, J. (1982). *Old people as people: Social and cultural influences on aging and old age*. Boston: Little, Brown.

Lawton, M. P., and Nahemow, L. (1973). Ecology and the aging process. In C. Eisdorfer and M. P. Lawton (Eds.), *Psychology of adult development and aging*. Washington, D. C.: American Psychological Association.

Lazarus, R. S. (1980). *The stress and coping paradigm*. In L. A. Bond and J. E. Rosen (Eds.), *Competence and coping during adulthood*. Boston: University Press of New England.

Levinson, D., with Darrow, C., Klein, E., Levinson, M., and McKee, B. (1978). *The seasons of a man's life*. New York: Knopf.

Lieberman, M. A. (1975). Adaptive processes in later life. In N. Datan and L. H. Ginsberg (Eds.), *Life span developmental psychology: Normative life crises*. New York: Academic Press.

Litwak, E., and Szeleny, I. (1969). Primary group structures and their function: Kin, neighbors, and friends. *American Sociological Review*, **34**, 465-481.

Lopata, H. Z. (1979). *Women as widows: Support systems*. New York: Elsevier North Holland.

Lowenthal, M. F., Thurnher, F., and Chirboga, D. (1975). *Four stages of life*. San Francisco: Jossey-Bass.

Lowy, L. (1979). *Social work with the aging: The challenge and promise of the later years*. New York: Harper & Row.

McCrae, R. R. (1982). Age differences in the use of coping mechanisms. *Journal of Gerontology*, **37**(4), 454-460.

McCrae, R. R., Costa, P. T. Jr., and Arenberg, D. (1980). Constancy of adult personality structure in males: Longitudinal, cross-sectional and times of measurement analyses. *Journal of Gerontology*, **35**(6), 877-883.

Manson, S. M., Murray, C. B., and Cain, L. D. (1980). *Ethnicity, aging and support networks: An evolving methodological strategy*. Paper presented at the 33rd Annual Meeting of the American Gerontological Society.

Marshall, V. W. (1980a). *Last chapters: A sociology of aging and dying*. Monterey, Calif.: Brooks/Cole.

Marshall, V. W. (1980b). *State of the art lecture: The sociology of aging*. Presented at the 9th Annual Scientific and Educational Meeting, Canadian Association of Gerontology, Saskatoon, Saskatchewan.

Monk, A. (1981). Social work with the aged: Principles of practice. *Social Work*, **26**(1), 61-67.

Morgan, L. A. (1976). A re-examination of widowhood and morale. *Journal of Gerontology*, **37**(4), 454-460.

Myerhoff, B. (1978). *Number our days*. New York: Dutton.

Neugarten, B. L. (Ed.). (1968). *Middle age and aging*. Chicago: University of Chicago Press.

Neugarten, B. L. (1976). Middle age and aging. In B. B. Hess (Ed.), *Growing old in America*. New Brunswick, N.J.: Transaction.

Neugarten, B. (1979). Time, age, and the life cycle. *American Journal of Psychiatry,* **136**(7), 887-894.

Neugarten, B., and Hagestad, G. (1976). Age and the life course. In R. H. Binstock and E. Shanas (Eds.), *Handbook of aging and the social sciences.* New York: Van Nostrand Reinhold.

Neugarten, B. L., Havighurst, R. J., and Tobin, S. S. (1968). Personality patterns of aging. In B. L. Neugarten (Ed.), *Middle age and aging.* Chicago: University of Chicago Press.

Riegel, K. F. (1977). History of psychological gerontology. In J. E. Birren and K. W. Schaie (Eds.), *Handbook of the psychology of aging.* New York: Van Nostrand Reinhold.

Rosenthal, C. J., Marshall, V. W., and Synge, J. (1980). The succession of lineage roles as families age. *Essence,* **40**(3), 179-193.

Rosow, I. (1974). *Socialization to old age.* Berkeley: University of California Press.

Ryff, C. D. (1982). Successful aging: A developmental approach. *Gerontologist,* **22**(2), 209-214.

Schooler, K. K. (1975). Response of the elderly to environment: A stress-theoretic perspective. In P. G. Windley and G. Ernst (Eds.), *Theory development in environment and aging.* Washington, D.C.: Gerontological Society.

Shanas, E. (1979). The family as a social support system in old age. *Gerontologist,* **19**(2), 169-174.

Shanas, E. (1980). Older people and their families: The new pioneers. *Journal of Marriage and the Family,* **42**(1), 9-15.

Sheehy, G. (1976). *Passages: Predictable crises of adult life.* New York: Dutton.

Streib, G. F. (1972). Older families and their troubles: Familial and social responses. *Family Coordinator,* **21**(1), 5-19.

Treas, J. and Bengtson, V. L. (1982). The demography of mid- and late-life transitions. *Annals of the American Academy of Political and Social Sciences,* **464**, 11-21.

Treas, J., and VanHilst, A. (1976). Marriage and remarriage rates among older Americans. *Gerontologist,* **16**, 132-136.

Vaillant, G. E. (1977). *Adaptation to life.* Boston: Little, Brown.

Valle, R. (1976). *Natural helping networks.* San Diego: Campanile Press.

Valle, R., and Mendoza, L. (1978). *The elder Latino.* San Diego: Campanile Press.

PART II

CLIENT
EVALUATION

3

Assessing the Elderly Client

Rosalie A. Kane, D.S.W.

The Rand Corporation, Santa Monica, Calif.

Multidimensional assessment is a crucial component of service to the elderly. Regardless of where they work, human-service professionals must develop strategies to collect, weigh, and interpret relevant information about the client. Properly used, assessment becomes a decision-making tool. The major clinical purpose of assessment is to facilitate decisions about the type and amount of services that should be offered to a particular client. Periodic reassessments then determine whether the services or treatments should be continued, discontinued, or changed.

Human-service professionals, and social workers in particular, are no strangers to the concept of assessment. Social workers have been taught to assess the client thoroughly, sensitively, and almost continuously. They are conditioned to consider both social history and current functioning. They are urged to take a family-centered approach. And, above all, a social worker's assessment deals with both the *person* and the *environment* in which the person functions. All these familiar principles pertain to geriatric assessment. What then is so special about assessment of the aged?

First, the assessment of an older client is likely to be complex. The history-taking is complicated because seniors have accumulated more life experiences to take into account. Assessment of current functioning is complicated because such functioning is usually a product of interacting physical, mental, and social factors, making interpretation of observed or reported behavior difficult. The process of assessment can also be complicated by compromised communication abilities of older clients or even by the generation gap that sometimes yawns between the assessor and the assessed. Despite these complexities, assessment takes on a powerful imperative with elderly clientele. As the general population becomes proportionately older and the numbers of persons in their late 70s and 80s increases, the pressure on social programs will also increase. Service providers must allocate types of resources and services according to an equitable and justifiable formula, and assessment is the key to that allocation.

A second characteristic of assessment of the elderly is its emphasis on measurement. The reliance on uniform instruments is perhaps the most troublesome feature to social workers, who may be more comfortable drawing conclusions from unfettered clinical judgment. The aging field has spawned hundreds of assessment instruments, including many that yield one or more summary scores (Kane and Kane, 1981). Some instruments measure a single attribute (e.g., social involvement, ability for self-care), whereas other multidimensional assessment tools cover several aspects of physical, mental, and social functioning. Some instruments are essentially questionnaires that elicit the client's self-report, whereas others use ratings and observations made by professionals. Some screening tools can be completed in a matter of minutes, but some assessments take several hours and involve the participation of a multidisciplinary team. The professional is challenged to choose an instrument wisely and to use it well, which may require consideration of issues of reliability and validity that were formerly the exclusive province of the researcher or program evaluator.

This chapter presents some specific purposes of assessment, discusses appropriate content for assessment of an older person, offers criteria for selecting an assessment tool, reviews some commonly used instruments, and concludes with practical issues relevant to making assessments of older persons and their families.

PURPOSE OF FORMAL ASSESSMENTS

Formal assessments take a toll in time and energy for both workers and clients. If performed, analyzed, and used consistently, they represent a distinct budget item. Nevertheless, uniform, systematic assessment approaches are critical to serving the elderly. They are used for screening and casefinding, for care planning, and for monitoring and quality assurance. Furthermore, clinically derived assessment often forms the basis for program evaluation and research. At each clinical step, the assessment organizes the worker, provides a checklist for items that might be forgotten, and offers a comparison point against which to observe improvement or deterioration.

Screening and Casefinding

Screening is a brief assessment procedure that triggers a fuller assessment in specified circumstances. It is often appropriate to screen large populations of older persons to identify those needing a particular service. For example, an Area Agency on Aging might want to know who in its catchment area would benefit by an activities program or by respite services for caregivers of the frail elderly. Or, to take another common example, a hospital social-work department that realistically could offer counseling to only some of the many older hospital patients might wish to choose those clients systematically rather than let caseloads fill up haphazardly. In each instance, a screening tool is needed. Obviously such a screening process should be brief, inexpensive, and yet capable of pinpointing the target group of interest.

Screening requires consideration of two epidemiological terms: sensitivity and specificity. A sensitive screen tends to pick up most persons with the targeted condition but may at the same time pick up "false positives," who are dropped after later assessment. In contrast, a specific screen will tend to eliminate persons without the targeted condition, thus minimizing false positives; however, the specific test may have a high rate of false negatives, meaning that persons with the condition of interest will *not* be identified in the screening. The desirable sensitivity or specificity of the test will depend on the frequency, severity, and remediability of the condition sought. For instance, when screening for elder abuse, a life-threatening condition with relatively low frequency and with the possibility of effective action, one prefers a sensitive tool. It is important to pick up all true cases, and sorting out the false positives is unlikely to become onerous. But when screening for depression among the bereaved, a common phenomenon, a specific test will be more useful since the second-stage assessment and the elimination of false positives could be prohibitively expensive. Those individuals planning screening tests must take these issues into account in setting the thresholds for action.

Determining eligibility for a service or benefit requires a special type of screening. Especially in the case of long-term-care services for the frail elderly, clients often need to meet a measurable threshold of income, disability, or both before receiving service. For example, to be eligible for nursing-home care under Medicare, the beneficiary must be deemed to require "skilled" care as defined by the legislation. Equity demands a uniform approach to eligibility testing. But the service provider must distinguish *eligibility* for a service from *need* for that service. For example, an elderly man may be eligible for Title XX homemaking services on the basis of his income and his restricted ability to ambulate and care for the household. But he may not need that service because his spouse provides it, just as she has done for the past forty years. Eligibility categories are usually defined rather broadly, but the subsequent full assessment of those eligible for services should determine what mix of services (if any) is appropriate for the particular case. Rarely will the situation be as clearcut as in the example. More often, the program must struggle to forge decision rules for determining the desirability of offering a particular service once formal eligibility is established.

Care Planning and Service Delivery

A comprehensive assessment forms the basis for decisions about intervention. From such an assessment, the professional decides whether a problem exists, whether needs are unmet, and what type and quantity of assistance should be recommended. The advantages of collecting information according to a routine format are compelling:

1. In the case of a team of providers (multidisciplinary or otherwise), everyone can gain the same view of the client and communication is enhanced.
2. In the case of complex problems, a consistent assessment format can enhance the likelihood that the assessor will review most relevant information.
3. Those serving older people need to identify *change* on dimensions of interest. For the elderly, a change in functioning (e.g., a drop in the amount of social contact) may be more important than the actual description of functioning (e.g., the absolute amount of social contact). Even if no services are deemed necessary, the initial assessment offers a baseline against which subsequent change can be observed.
4. If resources are scarce, caregivers will be able to compare the functional abilities, social needs, and social resources of clients and offer services where they would seem to have most benefit.
5. A comprehensive assessment touching on a variety of important dimensions allows the worker or the team to make a judgment about the reasons for a problem and therefore to decide how to intervene. For example, on self-care dimensions, two clients may show identical failure to cook and eat their meals, but further assessment on cognitive and affective dimensions might show memory loss in one and depression in the other. The treatment plan would differ markedly for those two individuals.

A common complaint is that the sophistication of assessment outstrips the variety in service prescriptions. Sometimes this results from the entrenched habits or lack of imagination in the human-service professionals and agencies. Sometimes the problem is a genuine paucity of service in the community. To guard against the former, professional personnel should spend time consciously developing decision rules (sometimes called algorithms) that outline the type of services to be used, given specific assessment results. Time should be set aside for creative "brainstorming" about the kinds of innovative service packages that could be pieced together in specific circumstances.

Monitoring and Quality Assurance

Another purpose of assessment is ongoing monitoring of the service. Such monitoring can be done by the individual provider to establish whether a particular intervention (e.g., day care or group therapy) is having its desired effect. Often monitoring is also done by an umbrella organization that has responsibility to authorize payment for a particular service. The latter agency needs to keep sufficient track of the client to know whether the need for the service continues and whether changes on significant dimensions would suggest a different service package.

Too often, assessment (like diagnosis) is reserved for the front end of an association with a client. Thus social service or rehabilitation records may show extensive multidisciplinary workups and team interpretation of the data, but the subsequent record is often comparatively important because changes can be precipitous and unpredictable.

In some circumstances, client assessments are used as a form of quality assurance. This is particularly true in residential settings where the condition of the older person is construed as a positive outcome of care. Monitoring for quality assurance requires careful consideration of the outcomes that the program should reasonably be expected to influence. Quality assurance may also require that functioning be assessed in terms of actual performance (i.e., what the client does) rather than capacity to perform (i.e., what the client is capable of doing). For example, if a client is capable of ambulating and bathing by herself but is permitted neither to go outside the nursing home nor to take a bath without supervision, one could hardly applaud the nursing home for fostering a higher quality of life as reflected by increased independence. Assessors need to be clear about whether they should measure capacity, actual performance, or both.

Assessment as an End in Itself

Later chapters in this book discuss one-stop intake programs and case-management services. In such programs, skilled assessment and subsequent case planning is the major part of the service offered. Legislation is periodically introduced at the federal or state level to allow Medicaid funding for comprehensive assessments before nursing-home placements are permitted. Inherent in such policy is the idea that the review entailed in the comprehensive assessment is a worthwhile benefit to the client, resulting in plans that are more humane and less costly than placement in a nursing home.

It is, of course, possible to oversell assessment; nobody is cured by diagnosis, nor are anyone's problems solved by assessment. However, caregivers conducting an assessment and clients participating in an assessment can generate more imaginative solutions to problems. For example, a client typically reviews his/her resources and considers sources of assistance as part of the assessment; this process serves as a review and an organizer for the client as well as for the worker.

CONTENT OF ASSESSMENT

Function versus Diagnosis

In assessing the elderly, an accurate medical and/or psychiatric diagnosis is essential. Medical diagnosis for elderly patients is often inadequate. Treatable medical conditions can be easily missed, and many physicians currently in practice have not been trained to distinguish aspects of normal aging from pathological processes, which could lead to both undertreatment and over-treatment (Kane, Ouslander, and Abrass, 1984). Geriatric assessment units, where a specially trained team thoroughly assesses physical functioning, identify an average of 3.5 treatable conditions, undiagnosed in previous medical care (Rubenstein, Abrass, and Kane, 1981). Senile dementia is an overused diagnosis (Garcia, Redding and Blass, 1981) and is sometimes bestowed without a careful examination of physical (e.g., infections, high drug dosages), emotional (e.g., depression), or environmental causes of confusion. For all these reasons, a social worker or other multipurpose assessor should establish whether a creditable geriatric workup has been done and arrange for one if necessary (particularly in the context of "old-old" clients—those over 75—seeking long-term care). Perhaps in time, geriatrically sensitive medical workups will become the norm, but for the next decade at least, adequate medical diagnosis cannot be taken for granted.

Similarly, psychiatric diagnosis should not be short-circuited. Although DSM-III describes many of its diagnostic entities as having a typical onset in adolescence or early adulthood (e.g., schizophrenia, most affective disorders, substance abuse), the document acknowledges that new cases can develop in later years (American Psychiatric Association, 1980). Reactive disorders (including both posttraumatic stress and adjustment disorder) can appear at any age and can harken back to much earlier stimuli. Personality disorders, although appearing early, are lifelong phenomena and may become more troublesome to others with the dependencies of old age. In addition, DSM-III gives considerable direct attention to organic mental disorders and the differential diagnosis between delirium and chronic dementias further explicated by Sloane (1980).

Unfortunately, older persons tend not to receive mental health services, especially diagnostic and treatment services, on an outpatient basis (Task Panel on Elderly, 1978). True age-specific prevalence figures for psychiatric disorders are therefore hard to determine. Recently Dohrenwend and his colleagues (1980) estimated that 18 to 25 percent of persons over 65 suffer from functional (i.e., nonorganic) mental disease, particularly affective disorders. The assessor will be less likely to omit a psychiatric diagnosis if the older person has a history of mental illness; however, the possibility of new incidence or existence of a previously unrecognized psychiatric condition must be considered. Many of these conditions are eminently treatable.

The complexity of psychiatric diagnoses among older people is highlighted by a series of chapters in the research book *Handbook of Mental Health and Aging* (Birren and Sloane, 1980). Miller (1980) describes the differential diagnosis between dementia and functional disorders and discusses "terminal drop" and the phenomenon of declining cognitive ability in the months before death. Lawton, Whelihan, and Belsky (1980) review the problems of personality tests for older people and raise many cautions about validity. (Dye's discussion of the same topic in another volume (1982a) abstracts and critiques the most common personality tests used with the elderly, including tests of personality rigidity, and is a good resource for further information on available tests). Post (1980) offers a lucid discussion of paranoid, schizophrenic, and schizophreniclike states in the elderly, describing little-studied phenomena such as the "senile recluse" as well as the range of paranoid-type disorders, with and without hallucinations, with and without affective components. Post's discussion is recommended for a cogent account of clinical pictures.

Although careful medical and, if appropriate, psychiatric diagnosis is a crucial part of the assessment of older clients, diagnosis is insufficient for care planning. Older persons tend to accumulate chronic diseases, and a simple list of active diagnoses does not explain the *functional* abilities of the individual. Nor does it accurately predict the need for services. Two people with diabetes, osteoarthritis, or even schizophrenia may manifest very different functional abilities.

Functioning is a product of an individual's abilities, motivation, and environment (with environment construed broadly to include the physical environment, the task expectations, and the availability of social support). Any individual can experience large increases or decreases in functional performance with environmental changes. For example, a previously competent person might be rendered incompetent in a foreign country where an unfamiliar language is spoken. Conversely, a somewhat inept person may be rendered competent by a secretary or household staff. Those assessing the elderly must examine both actual abilities and environmental issues. In moving from assessment data to a plan, the assessor must consider ways to increase capacity and motivation (e.g., educational approaches; physical therapy, occupational therapy, or psychotherapy; medical treatments; prosthetic devices) and ways to render the environment less complicated or demanding. Because the older person is vulnerable to environmental insult and sudden, far-reaching changes in social support, the environmental component of the functional assessment should not be neglected.

Multidimensional Assessment

Figure 3-1 summarizes components of a thorough, multidimensional assessment of the functioning of an older person. Each box represents a domain worthy of separate assessment, but the various domains are related. A change in one domain is likely to be accompanied by a change in others, and thus the etiology of functional impairment is often difficult to determine. Considerable agreement can be obtained on the domains for inclusion, though different authorities subdivide or title them differently. Figure 3-1 suggests nine content areas for assessment: physical, emotional, cognitive, self-care capacity (ADL and IADL), social, environmental, service use, value preferences, and finally, burden on the support system.

Physical Factors

Even those without medical training can gather useful information about a client's health. Determining the diagnoses the client has accumulated, the drugs the client uses, and his hospital- and physician-utilization patterns will present a composite picture of health status. Pain and discomfort is also important to gauge, although instruments to do so are rudimentary. Kane et al. (1983a, b) have developed an approach to measuring pain and discomfort among nursing-home residents, using headache, joint pain, itching, dizziness, and chest pain as indicators. Physical conditions highly relevant to functional ability and not usually the province of an internist or general practitioner include vision, hearing, dentition, and podiatric status. The assessor might determine whether impairment exists in any of these areas, whether full evaluation and treatment has been sought, and when applicable, whether the client has appropriate prostheses and devices. Finally, self-report of physical health has been shown to be a good predictor of mortality (Mossey and Shapiro, 1982). Assessors should be warned, however, that although the measures discussed in this section will afford a capsule view of cumulative morbidity, they will not account for etiology of problems and do not substitute for a geriatric workup. In fact, if the assessors determine that the individual is taking ten or more prescription or nonprescription drugs and has accumulated numerous diagnoses, referral to a geriatric assess-

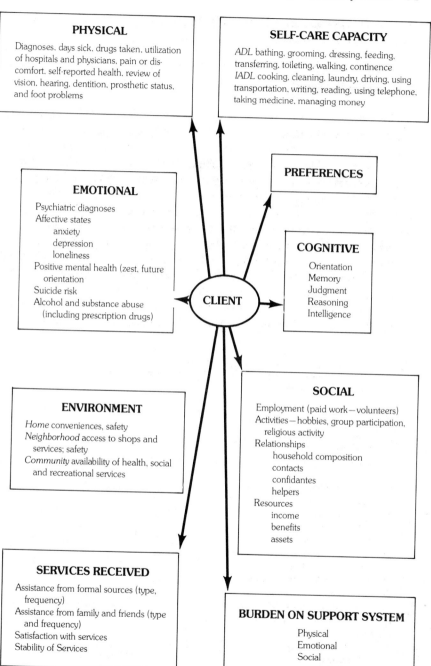

Figure 3-1. Components of a multidimensional assessment.

ment unit might be indicated. (This is especially true if the evaluation of self-care capacity shows substantial impairment as well.)

Emotional Factors

The emotional category includes a review for functional psychopathology, particularly affective disorders. Several short batteries of questions have been developed to screen for depression. Most often used with the elderly are the Zung Self-Rated Depression Scale (Zung, 1965) and the Beck Inventory of Depression (Beck et al., 1961). (Both are shown in Table 3-1.) Common indicators of depression such as appetite loss, fatigue, insomnia, palpitations, and sexual disinterest may be masked by physical and social circumstances of the elderly. Some recommend that the assessment emphasize indicators of dysphoric mood rather than psychophysiological signs of depression (Gallagher, Thompson, and Levy, 1980). Positive well-being is sometimes measured through scales such as Life Satisfaction Index (LSI) (Havighurst, Neugarten, and Tobin, 1961) or the Philadelphia Geriatric Morale Scale (Lawton, 1972), although there is some overlap between the common measures of depression and the common measures of morale. (See Table 3-2 for these two morale scales.)

Table 3-1. Examples of Scales to Measure Affective Status

Zung Self-Rated Depression Scale

1. I feel downhearted and blue.[a]
2. Morning is when I feel the best.
3. I have crying spells or feel like it.
4. I have trouble sleeping at night.
5. I can eat as much as I used to.
6. I still enjoy sex.
7. I notice that I am losing weight.
8. I have trouble with constipation.
9. My heart beats faster than usual.
10. I get tired for no reason.
11. My mind is as clear as it used to be.
12. I find it easy to do the things I used to.
13. I am restless and can't keep still.
14. I feel hopeful about the future.
15. I am more irritable than usual.
16. I find it easy to make decisions.
17. I feel that I am useful and needed.
18. My life is pretty full.
19. I feel that others would be better off if I were dead.
20. I still enjoy the things I used to do.

[a]For each item, the respondent rates the statement as "a little of the time," "some of the time," "good part of the time," or "most of the time."

Modified Beck Depression Inventory[b]

1. I do not feel sad.
   I feel sad.
   I am sad all the time and can't snap out of it.
   I am so sad or unhappy that I can't stand it.
2. I am not particularly discouraged about the future.
3. I do feel like a failure.
4. I get as much satisfaction out of things as I used to.
5. I don't feel particularly guilty.
6. I don't feel I am being punished.
7. I don't feel disappointed in myself.
8. I don't feel I am any worse than anyone else.
9. I don't have thoughts of killing myself.
10. I don't cry any more than usual.
11. I am no more irritated now than I ever am.
12. I have not lost interest in other people.
13. I make decisions about as well as I ever could.
14. I don't worry that I look worse than I used to.
15. I can work about as well as I used to.
16. I can sleep as well as usual.
17. I don't get any more tired than usual.
18. My appetite is no worse than usual.
19. I haven't lost much weight, if any, lately.
20. I am no more worried about my health than usual.
21. I have not noticed any recent change in my interest in sex.

[b]Each item has 4-5 responses, representing a range of mood; the respondent picks the one most appropriate. We included all four responses only for item no. 1.
Sources: Zung scale adapted from W. W. K. Zung. (1965). A self-rating depression scale. *Archives of General Psychiatry,* **12**, 73-70. Beck inventory from A. T. Beck et al. (1961). An inventory for measuring depression. *Archives of General Psychiatry,* **4**, 53-63.

Table 3-2. Examples of Scales Measuring Subjective Well-Being in the Elderly

Philadelphia Geriatric Center Morale Scale

1. Things keep getting worse as I get older. (No)[a]
2. I have as much pep as I did last year. (Yes)
3. How much do you feel lonely? (Not much)
4. Little things bother me more this year. (No)
5. I see enough of my friends and relatives. (Yes)
6. As you get older, you are less useful. (No)
7. If you could live where you wanted, where would you live? (Here)
8. I sometimes worry so much that I can't sleep. (No)
9. As I get older, things are (better, worse, the same) than/as I thought they'd be. (Better)
10. I sometimes feel that life isn't worth living. (No)
11. I am happy now as I was when I was younger. (Yes)
12. Most days I have plenty to do. (No)
13. I have a lot to be sad about. (No)

[a]The correct answer, shown in parentheses, is scored one point.

(*continued*)

Table 3–2. (*Continued*)

14. People had it better in the old days. (No)
15. I am afraid of a lot of things. (No)
16. My health is (good, not so good). (Good)
17. I get mad more than I used to. (No)
18. Life is hard for me most of the time. (No)
19. How satisfied are you with your life today? (Satisfied)
20. I take things hard. (No)
21. A person has to live for today and not worry about tomorrow. (Yes)
22. I get upset easily. (No).

Life Satisfaction Index (LSI-A)

Here are some statements about life in general that people feel differently about. Would you read each statement in the list and, if you agree with it, put a check mark in the space "agree." If you do not agree, put a check mark in the space under "disagree." If you are not sure one way or the other, put a check mark in the space "?."

1. As I grow older, things seem better than I thought they would be. (Agree)
2. I have gotten more of the breaks in life than most of the people I know. (Agree)
3. This is the dreariest time of my life. (Disagree)
4. I am just as happy as when I was younger. (Agree)
5. My life could be happier than it is now. (Disagree)
6. These are the best years of my life. (Agree)
7. Most of the things I do are boring or monotonous. (Disagree)
8. I expect some interesting and pleasant things to happen to me in the future. (Agree) *
9. The things I do are as interesting to me as they ever were. (Agree)
10. I feel old and tired. (Disagree)
11. I feel my age, but it doesn't bother me. (Agree)
12. As I look back on my life, I am fairly well satisfied. (Agree)
13. I would not change my past life, even if I could. (Agree)
14. Compared to other people my age, I've made a lot of foolish decisions in my life. (Disagree)
15. Compared to other people my age, I make a good appearance. (Agree)
16. I have made plans for things I'll be doing a month or a year from now. (Agree)
17. When I think back over my life, I didn't get most of the important things I wanted. (Disagree)
18. Compared to other people, I get down in the dumps too often. (Disagree)
19. I've gotten pretty much what I expected out of life. (Agree)
20. In spite of what people say, the lot of the average man is getting worse, not better. (Disagree)

Sources; Moral scale adapted from M. P. Lawton. (1972). The dimensions of morale. In D. Kent, R. Kastenbaum, and S. Sherwood (Eds.), *Research planning, and action for the elderly.* New York: Behavioral Publications. Life satisfaction index adapted from R. J. Havinghurst, B. L. Neugarten, and S. S. Tobin. (1961). The measurement of life satisfaction. *Journal of Gerontology,* **16**, 134-143.

Suicidal ideation should be assessed directly whenever evidence of depression or despair is found. (The incidence of completed suicides in persons over age 65, particularly among men, is high and probably underreported.) Although assessors may be uncomfortable asking, older persons will respond willingly and reliably to the question "How often have you thought of killing yourself?" with response categories such as "never," "occasionally," "often," and "almost all the time" (Kane et al., 1983*b*).

Cognitive Factors

A cognitive appraisal is important whenever the assessor suspects that memory and intellectual functioning are impaired. Several tests have been developed to assess memory and cognitive function. The best-known brief tests ascertain orientation for place, time, and person; recent and remote memory; and calculation. Table 3-3 presents the Short Portable Mental Status Questionnaire, which is part of a larger instrument developed at Duke University (1978). Other instruments tap higher levels of functioning by presenting simple problems and checking abstract thinking through proverb interpretation; the Folstein Mini-Mental Status Questionnaire (Folstein and McHugh, 1975) is an example. Dye (1982b) abstracts and critiques seventeen measures of intellectual functioning that have been applied to the elderly, including elaborate batteries. On the other end of the spectrum, simpler tests of cognitive ability have been developed for nursing homes, using indicators like knowledge of the season of the year, the next meal, and the location of one's room (Lawton, 1972). These have the advantage of not relying on information about the date and current events that may seem somewhat irrelevant to nursing-home residents.

Two cautions about brief mental-status assessments. First, such assessments are sometimes used to determine whether a client is capable of answering the rest of the questions on an assessment instrument. Decision rules often state that if a client gets a specified number of questions incorrect, a significant other

Table 3-3. Short Portable Mental Status Questionnaire (SPMSQ)

Short Portable Mental Status Questionnaire (SPMSQ)

1. What is the date today (month/day/year)?
2. What day of the week is it?
3. What is the name of this place?
4. What is your telephone number? (If no telephone, what is your street address?)
5. How old are you?
6. When were you born (month/day/year)?
7. Who is the current president of the United States?
8. Who was the president just before him?
9. What was your mother's maiden name?
10. Subtract 3 from 20 and keep subtracting from each new number you get, all the way down.

0-2 errors = intact
3-4 errors = mild intellectual impairment
5-7 errors = moderate intellectual impairment
8-10 errors = severe intellectual impairment

Allow one more error if subject had only grade school education.
Allow one fewer error if subject has had education beyond high school.
Allow one more error for blacks, regardless of education criteria.

Source: Duke University. (1978). Center for the Study of Aging and Human Development. Multidimensional functional assessment: The OARS methodology. Durham, N.C.: Duke University.

will provide the remaining information. However, cognitive abilities are spotty, and persons making errors on the Short Portable Mental Status Questionnaire are capable of reliably answering other questions, particularly those pertaining to their activities, relationships, moods, and preferences. And certainly nobody else is likely to give an accurate answer to this type of question! It is dangerous to eliminate the client as a source of further information on the basis of a marginal cognitive score.

The second caution is that the assessor should supplement information from short tests with other kinds of information. The historical onset of the cognitive impairment is important, as is the presence or absence of personality change or antisocial behavior. The differential diagnosis between pseudodementia (i.e., depression presenting with dementia symptoms) and true cognitive loss is assisted by information about suddenness of onset and accompanying behavior (see Salzman and Shader, 1979, for tabular comparisons of pseudodementia and true dementia). Furthermore, the planning for and with the client with memory loss is influenced by other factors such as social intactness and appropriateness. It is also useful to look for strengths in the behavior of the person with cognitive impairment. If that individual takes care of someone else, for example, he is exhibiting positive signs of cognition that should counterbalance any test score (Gurland et al., 1982).

Social Factors

As Figure 3-1 shows, the social assessment should take into account social activities, social relationships, and social resources. Activities include interests and hobbies that can be pursued in solitude and those that involve participation in social or membership groups. Relationships include the frequency of human contact and interaction, the availability of necessary assistance from others, and access to a trusted confidante. Although a minimum threshold of social activity and contact is probably intrinsically good (e.g., associated with feelings of well-being, good sleeping patterns, lessened depression), the major goal is for the individual to have *meaningful* activities and social contacts. Simple counts do not tell the story—the person with four friends is not twice as well off as the person with two friends. The person with balanced activities is not better off than the tennis or bridge fanatic. Certainly the person who participates in a range of activities that he perceives as tedious and unfulfilling has not achieved social well-being. Therefore, social well-being has a subjective as well as an objective component; the assessor should determine whether the activities and contacts are satisfying to the individual. The importance of a pet in promoting social well-being should not be discounted nor should the seriousness of the loss of a pet be underestimated.

Work should not be forgotten, even if the person is retired. Because our identities are so enmeshed with our work, the assessor should know what kind of work the individual did and where his/her skills lie. This is particularly true for men in the elderly cohorts, and women increasingly identify with their work. A knowledge of work history and general abilities may suggest volunteer involvements compatible with the individual's physical capabilities and interests. Certainly the assessment of a person bound for or already in a nursing home should not neglect the occupational component. Demonstration projects in nursing homes (see, for example, Jorgensen and Kane, 1976) have shown that individuals with utilizable skills, such as a concert pianist or an expert gardener, often have no opportunity to use them in the nursing-home environment because no one is aware of the person at that human level. On a positive note, Laufer and Laufer (1982) describe how nursing-home residents with foreign-language skills became adjunct instructors to local college students and formed mutually important relationships through that exchange. This type of model program shows the payoff from assessments that try to encapsulate the abilities, interests, and skills older people have developed in a lifetime of work and community involvement.

In a social assessment, baseline values become especially important. Typically, for example, social isolation is measured by the absolute amount of face-to-face, telephone, and even mail contact between the older person and others in a particular (or typical) week. But some people are more gregarious than others. Social contact amounting to a daily telephone call and two or three outings or visits during a week might be a comfortable pattern for some people and represent an alarming narrowing of social contact for others. With repeated assessment, it might be important to inquire whether the information given represents a change.

Environmental Factors

The environmental assessment has not been well developed or standardized. There is increasing awareness of the importance of assessing the adequacy of the immediate environment, both home and neighborhood, in terms of safety factors, convenience, and manageability for a person with other impairments. Often household equipment or renovation can make a person more functional in a particular setting. In the neighborhood, the proximity to shops, buses, beauty parlors, libraries, parks, and pharmacies may be important. Delivery policies of nearby businesses may also be important. So far, instrumentation on environment tends to concentrate on the perceived adequacy of residential or institutional environments (Windley, 1982). Research by Carp and Carp (1982) on perceptions of the elderly about ideal features of a residential neighborhood might ultimately lead to yearly checklists for that neighborhood.

Self-Care Capacity

Self-care capacity is based on functional performance, which, as already indicated, is a product of a person's physical and mental capabilities, his psychological motivation, and the environmental pressures. Therefore, the entire physical, emotional, cognitive, and environmental assessment will yield information about the ability of the individual to sustain an independent life-style. But a more direct way of tapping into this content is to assess self-care performance directly. Two acronyms come into prominence in this functional assessment: ADL (activities of daily living) and IADL (instrumental activities of daily living).

ADL activities refer to basic self-care skills such as bathing, feeding, dressing, transferring into and out of bed or onto and off the toilet, walking or using a wheelchair, and grooming oneself. Continence is often included in an inventory of ADL activities, although it is a physiological function. One of the most parsimonious and frequently used ADL measures is the Katz ADL scale (Katz et al., 1963), a six-item scale that divides each function only two ways (independent and dependent; see Table 3-4). In contrast, other approaches gather more information. For instance, ability to eat can be broken down further to distinguish complete independence from need for some assistance with cutting meat, from need for special equipment, and from complete dependence. Similarly the function itself can be broken down into component parts: for example, drinking from a cup, eating from a plate. The level of detail required will depend on the type of organization sponsoring the assessment and its purpose. Usually it is useful to distinguish between independence with the help of equipment and independence with the help of another person. If one can move with a walker, one has gained a degree of independence over the person who requires another individual to help with the walking. Value judgments are involved in assessing ADL capacity—for example, if the speed and competence with which dressing is performed does not meet the abstract standards of a particular assessor, the person might be deemed dependent. An ADL assessment also varies as to whether the information comes from the report of the client, the report of a relative, the rating of a caregiver, or actual observation of the client. Some assessment tools use simulated equipment, allowing the client to demonstrate the capacity to perform certain skills (e.g., butter bread, use the telephone) (Kuriansky et al., 1976).

IADL functions are more complex activities that support independence. Typically cooking, cleaning, doing laundry, using transportation or driving, telephone use, self-medicating abilities, and money management are included. Some assessors also examine the capacity for heavy work such as major cleaning or gardening. IADL performance is rendered more or less difficult by the kind of equipment that the client has at his disposal (compare a washtub to an automatic washing machine to a coin laundry down three flights of stairs).

Table 3-4. Katz Index of ADL

Index of Independence in Activities of Daily Living

The Index of Independence in Activities of Daily Living is based on an evaluation of the functional independence or dependence of patients in bathing, dressing, going to the toilet, transferring, continence, and feeding. Specific definitions of functional independence and dependence appear below the index.

A   Independent in feeding, continence, transferring, going to toilet, dressing, and bathing.
B   Independent in all but one of these functions.
C   Independent in all but bathing and one additional function.
D   Independent in all but bathing, dressing, and one additional function.
E   Independent in all but bathing, dressing, going to toilet, and one additional function.
F   Independent in all but bathing, dressing, going to toilet, transferring, and one additional function.
G   Dependent in all six functions.
Other   Dependent in at least two functions, but not classifiable as C, D, E, or F.

Independence means without supervision, direction, or active personal assistance, except as specifically noted below. This is based on actual status and not on ability. A patient who refuses to perform a function is considered as not performing the function, even though he is deemed able.

Bathing (sponge, shower or tub)
Independent: assistance only in bathing a single part (as back or disabled extremity) or bathes self completely
Dependent: assistance in bathing more than one part of body; assistance in getting in or out of tub or does not bathe self

Dressing
Independent: gets clothes from closets and drawers; puts on clothes, outer garments, braces; manages fasteners; act of tying shoes is excluded
Dependent: does not dress self or remains partly undressed

Going to toilet
Independent: gets to toilet; gets on and off toilet; arranges clothes, cleans organs of excretion (may manage own bedpan used at night only and may or may not be using mechanical supports)
Dependent: uses bedpan or commode or receives assistance in getting to and using toilet

Transfer
Independent: moves in and out of bed independently and moves in and out of chair independently (may or may not be using mechanical supports)
Dependent: assistance in moving in or out of bed and/or chair; does not perform one or more transfers

Continence
Independent: urination and defecation entirely self-controlled
Dependent: partial or total incontinence in urination or defecation; partial or total control by enemas, catheters, or regulated use of urinals and/or bedpans

Feeding
Independent: gets food from plate or its equivalent into mouth (precutting of meat and preparation of food, as buttering bread, are excluded from evaluation)
Dependent: assistance in act of feeding (see above); does not eat at all or parenteral feeding

Source: S. Katz, A. B. Ford, R. W. Moskowitz, B. A. Jackson, and M. W. Jaffee, 1963, "Studies of Illness in the Aged. The Index of ADL: A Standardized Measure of Biological and Psychosocial Function," *Journal of the American Medical Association* **185**, 94 ff.

IADL performance also depends somewhat on learned abilities — homemaking skills for men and money-management skills for women may be lacking in the cohorts now elderly. Such skills can be developed, however, as part of a plan. A plan can also be directed at simplifying the activities so that they can be performed within an individual's reduced capacities (e.g., presorted medication doses, telephone modifications, step-reducing devices).

Services Received

The assessor must contrast the client's needs uncovered by the assessment with the services the client is presently receiving. Knowledge of the extent to which the client needs and receives assistance not only gives guidance for care planning but permits estimation of the cost of service. This part of the assessment should separate several aspects of assistance:

1. It should distinguish assistance from agencies or paid personnel and assistance dependent on volunteer labor of family and friends.
2. It should distinguish between services purchased by the individual and services reimbursed under a benefit or insurance program.
3. It should identify both the *actual services* needed and the *source* of that assistance. In our pluralistic form of social organization, similar services can be received from a variety of agencies and programs (both residential and community-based). A true picture of the service pattern requires "disaggregating" discrete services (e.g., homemaking assistance, financial-planning assistance, shelter, recreation) from the source of that assistance. As part of Duke University's OARS methodology (Duke University, 1978), services were disaggregated into twenty-four discrete functions. (See Table 3-5 for the service list and the applicable unit of measurement.) The Cleveland GAO study (U.S. Comptroller General, 1977) used this method to study the relationship between functional impairment and use of services.
4. It should distinguish services purchased on a discretionary basis from services needed to maintain functioning.

If the client receives considerable long-term-care service from family and friends, the assessment should examine components of that "informal support." It is useful to know how much time is actually being given by family and neighborhood helpers and how much of that time is needed to maintain functioning. "Personal time dependency" is a phrase coined by Gurland and his colleagues (1978) to express the essence of the long-term-care dilemma. One goal of the care plan is to decrease "personal time dependency," which, in the long run, is likely to create a burden on the support system.

Table 3-5. Disaggregated Long-Term-Care Services

Category of Service	Unit of Measurement
Basic maintenance	
Transportation	Passenger round trips
Food, groceries	Dollars
Living quarters (housing)	Dollars
Supportive	
Personal care	Contact hours
Continuous supervision	
Checking services	
Meal preparation	Meals
Homemaker-household	Hours
Administrative, legal and protective	Hours
Remedial	
Social/recreational	Sessions
Employment	Number of times provided
Sheltered employment	Hours of employment
Education — employment related	Training session hours
Remedial training	Number of sessions
Mental health	Sessions
Psychotropic drugs	
Nursing care	Contact hours
Medical	Number of visits/dollars
Supportive devices and prostheses	Dollars
Physical therapy	Sessions
Relocation and placement	Moves
Systematic multidimensional evaluation	Hours
Financial assistance	Dollars or dollar equivalent
Coordination, information and referral services	Hours

Source: Adapted from Duke University. (1978). Center for the Study of Aging and Human Development. *Multidimensional functional assessment: The OARS methodology.* Durham, N.C.: Duke University.

The assessor should also examine the stability of the assistance that the individual is receiving. Some persons may be at the end of their financial benefits. Others may enjoy excellent help from the family, but the family support may rest on one individual alone. The services received by such people lack depth. For example, someone may be depending on one son alone, and if he were transferred to another community no backup assistance would be available (Kulys and Tobin, 1980). The assessor should know which proportion of the caseload has support systems that are one deep.

Burden on Support System

Closely related to the previous category is the assessment of burden on the support system. Presently there are no widely used instruments to tap this dimension, although some investigators are doing work that should isolate features of burden. Often the caregiver is also over 65 (a postretirement "child," a sibling, or, most frequently, a spouse). In such instances, each older person in the constellation is assessed individually. It may be that the amount of care needed by a husband is beyond the physical and emotional capability of the wife. The service plan may be directed then to providing some respite or assistance for the primary caregiver.

Families in the so-called "middle generation" who struggle with responsibilities related to minor children as well as to aging parents may be experiencing enormous cumulative pressures. Intuitively one would expect that pressure to be a function of the extent of multiple physical and financial demands and the duration of those demands. However, no good instrumentation has emerged to measure this phenomenon and to identify middle-generation families who are more burdened than others. Research does report certain phenomena related to an elderly relative in the household that strain the family's endurance: incontinence and night wandering are most notable and should be flagged as signs that the family needs help even before such help is demanded. Another elusive factor is the relationship of spouses as affected by care given to one or another spouse's parents, and such reactions are probably conditioned by the affectional ties between parents and their adult children, the formative experience of middle-generation husband and wife with grandparents in their own original households, and personal concepts of duty and religious responsibility.

Preferences

Assessment of the preferences of the older person is of paramount importance and may be the most neglected aspect of a multidimensional assessment. Long-term-care arrangements (be they in institutions or in the community) involve compromise with the ideal. Even if funds were not constrained, a program that sets out to achieve a maximum goal in one area (say, ADL and IADL capacities) may need to compromise on pain relief and even social well-being. If such trade-offs must be made, surely the opinion of the older person should be sought about what should be maximized and what aspects of well-being should be traded off (Kane and Kane, 1982). Some older persons may wish to emphasize physical safety and freedom from risk of accidents more than goals of independence, but others may prefer to accept the risks of falling or the knowledge that services will be incomplete at home rather than to accept the dependence and "quality of life" loss inherent in nursing-home placement. Unfortunately, these issues are seldom put squarely to the persons most concerned. The value preferences and risk-aversion of professionals and family members often dictate the ultimate plan.

Of course, the professional cannot be irresponsible and allow the older person to take risks that are dangerous to the entire community. Even here, however, it is important that a double standard not develop. For example, if a teenager of a middle-aged adult leaves on a faucet or forgets his keys, there is no particular cause for alarm. Few housewives have *never* burned the bottom out of a kettle. However, if such an event occurs once or twice for a person over age 75, the question about ability for self-care is often raised.

CRITERIA FOR AN ASSESSMENT TOOL

The nine areas of multidimensional assessment pose an enormous challenge. Somehow the assessment, with the help of standardized tools, needs to be streamlined and organized so that it generates accurate, useful information with relative speed. Several criteria should be considered in choosing and using an assessment tool.

Reliability

Reliability simply means that, in the absence of real change, repeated assessments will yield the same results. Factors that may make assessment of the elderly unreliable include changes in the way an assessment is done from one assessor to the next (interrater reliability) or from one time to the next (intrarater or intertemporal reliability). In programs serving the elderly, the whole staff must speak the same language, and it is imperative that they use uniform definitions and approaches for their assessment. Merely using a standard instrument does not assure reliability, especially if each worker rates abstract factors like depression, social support, or self-concept according to personally developed criteria. Few assessment tools for the elderly have undergone rigorous tests of reliability (Kane and Kane, 1981; Mangen and Peterson, 1982).

Validity

Validity is the ability of the instrument to measure what it sets out to measure. Reliability is necessary but not sufficient for validity. A false bathroom scale, for example, can yield 100 percent reliability but 100 percent inaccurate results. Similarly, all nurses aides might in good faith agree that a client was incapable of self-care, but their rating could be invalid. Some factors that affect the validity of a measure are the opportunity for raters to make observations, the anxiety of the person being assessed, or the familiarity of the testing environment. A client may be incapable of self-care in a hospital, but that test may not validly reflect his abilities when at home with familiar surroundings and equipment. Because physical, mental, and social factors are so intertwined in the elderly, an effort to measure one component may be rendered invalid by one of the others. For example, a tool to measure cognitive impairment may produce a poor score, but actually the individual's physical status (e.g., deafness) may have produced the result. Finally, many scales are used to measure abstract aspects of well-being in the elderly, and those scales may not be valid reflections of the dimension being measured. The social worker should always go back to the actual questions used to measure an abstraction (say, social isolation, loneliness, or family burden) and see if, at least on the face of it, the measure seems to tap all aspects of the phenomenon.

Suited to Population

Assessment procedures must be appropriate for measuring change in the particular population being assessed. Some tools will fail to pick up changes that have great meaning for better or worse for clients already substantially impaired because the instrument is not calibrated finely enough. For example, a community planner might find it sufficient to divide people into those who are not bedbound, but the person who is bedbound experiences great differences in quality of life, depending on his ability to sit up and move in bed. Similarly, on social dimensions, instruments used in nursing homes should be able to pick up finer nuances of difference at the lower end of the functional spectrum than those used, for example, in a multipurpose senior center.

Because the elderly population is so diverse, many agencies will need the capacity to assess persons with wide-ranging functional abilities. (This is particularly true of one-stop assessment centers.) "Branching techniques" should be developed so that, on the basis of a particular response or observation, the assessor eliminates some procedures and turns to others. It is frustrating and embarrassing for people if they are asked to perform procedures that are obviously too difficult or too simple. It is also time-consuming to go through elaborate processes to prove the obvious.

Practical

Assessment procedures should be comfortable for the assessor to use and the client to undergo. Questions should be ordered to fit clinical criteria about interview flow. As much as possible, expensive equipment should be eliminated and instruments developed that can be used by persons without extensive professional training.

In developing practical approaches, the assessor should not underestimate the ability of the older person himself to make systematic observations. For screening and for monitoring, the older person is an important aide. Generally speaking, no one has better opportunity or more motivation to make the observation. (The latter point is tempered somewhat by the human tendency to prevaricate to protect a status or benefit or to prevent a feared outcome such as being sent to a nursing home.) The ability of paraprofessional aides (e.g., homemaker/home-health aides or nursing-home attendants) to make important observations should also not be discounted. Such personnel need to know what to look for, when, how often, and why. They also need to be provided with convenient formats for recording that recognize the minimal literacy in the English language of many such personnel.

EXAMPLES OF MULTIDIMENSIONAL TOOLS

Most states have developed multidimensional assessment tools to gauge the need for nursing-home care. Some of these measures are merely descriptive, but others, such as New York's DSM-III, yield a score upon which action is taken. For the most part, the measures used to determine nursing-home placement are easily manipulated to generate the desired result. Various monitoring groups such as state nursing-home inspection agencies and professional standards review organizations (PSROs) have developed patient-specific assessment tools designed to provide baseline information about the nursing-home residents and form the foundation for a nursing-care plan (Kane et al., 1979). Many are modeled after efforts of the Department of Health and Human Services to develop a minimum standard for recordkeeping in nursing homes (U.S. DHEW, 1978; Jones, McNitt, and McKnight, 1974). Typically they contain sections to be completed by each member of the multidisciplinary team. Such tools are useful formats for uniform recording but do not produce any scores through which clients can be compared.

Some multidimensional assessment tools do produce a single score that takes into account physical, mental, and social dimensions of functioning. The Sickness Impact Profile (SIP) is such a device (Bergner et al., 1976). The tool was designed from a health perspective and was not particularly designed for the elderly. In all probability, the information is too condensed to be useful for care planning.

Gerontologists have produced multidimensional instruments that yield several scores in different domains. The CARE battery (Burland et al., 1977-78) is one such example. The best known multidimensional assessment technique in gerontology is the OARS methodology, developed by the Older Americans Resource and Service Center at Duke University (1978). OARS collects information in five areas (physical health, ADL capacity, mental health, social well-being, and economic well-being); information is gathered through an interview with the client or (if the client fails a brief cognitive test) a significant other.

The instrument takes an average of ninety minutes to administer and, with training, interviewers achieve reliability of judgment when presented with the same interview stimulus.

The scores in the OARS instrument are derived from clinical judgment as refined by reviewing responses to the questions on the instrument. After the administration, the assessor rates each of the five areas on a six-point scale ranging from excellent functioning to totally impaired. The assessor is reminded which responses to read over for each rating and is given anchoring statements. The scores can then be added up for an overall score (i.e., two score of six would be the most independent, and thirty the most dependent) or the person can be rated according to the number of domains impaired. The domain scores can also be examined separately.

The OARS instrument represents one of the best-studied and most widely accepted approaches to gerontological assessment. Nonetheless, it still presents some unresolved problems: (1) it is inadequate to assess functioning at the lower end of the spectrum; (2) the score still relies on judgment rather than on a numerical treatment of the individual questions in each domain; and (3) in summary treatments, all domains are considered equal and independent.

INTERVIEWING CONSIDERATIONS

Finally, some practical considerations are important for eliciting reliable and valid information from older persons, particularly those with physical impairments. Some are common sense, but others may be overlooked because they are embedded in the instrument and its language or procedures.

Older persons may have visual, hearing, or communication difficulties. The pace should be geared to the client's abilities. If visual prompts are used, they should be oversize. The room should be quiet and the interviewer should sit so that his lips can be observed and he should speak slowly (though not necessarily loudly). Privacy should be arranged; many older persons do not speak as comfortably about matters of bodily function as does the current generation. If the assessment is long, it may need to be broken into component parts so as not to tire the client. Many of these guidelines pertain to clinical encounters with the elderly as well as with the initial assessment. Besdine (1982) provides an excellent review of the physical conditions that promote a good diagnostic encounter with an older person.

Sometimes the very language of the instrument is inappropriate to the age group or the cultural cohort. Psychological jargon has crept into the general language, but is not as familiar to older persons. Even concepts like "service" may be unfamiliar to a large number of elderly middle-class respondents, whereas they could readily describe help that they needed or received. Some words also are unsuited to many older ears. In our own work in nursing-home assessments, we needed to change the word "anxious" to "tense" because the former was heard as "ancient." Similarly, we had to reword a question about satisfaction with the word "residence" because it sounded as though we were inquiring about satisfaction with the other "residents."

CONCLUSION

The assessment of an older client must be suited to the purpose. Screenings may touch on several dimensions of functioning, but should not be long and cumbersome. Comprehensive assessment must touch on multiple dimensions of functioning; at the end, the assessor should be left with a composite picture of what the client does and can do and a sense of the etiology of any impaired functioning. A service plan should flow naturally from a good assessment, and that plan should consider ways of improving capacity, changing motivation, or changing the environment. Possible burden on the caregiving constellation must be part of the assessment, and the preferences of the individual client should not be forgotten in the zeal for neat, measurable packages.

Whenever possible, it is recommended that agencies employ uniform assessment techniques. The eventual goal for the gerontological fields is a common language with shared empirical referents that can be used across settings. In areas where no good instrumentation currently exists (e.g., assessment of environment, family burden, or client preference), it is important that these aspects of functioning be assessed routinely and with common general questions. Only through the systematic accumulation of clinical information will it be possible to develop measurement tools in these presently underdeveloped areas. Even in areas where we now have useful tools (e.g., measurement of ADL, cognitive abilities, and depression), it is important to subject those measures to tests of continued clinical relevance. The assessment tools must always serve their users rather than take on an independent existence.

REFERENCES

American Psychiatric Associations. (1980). *Diagnostic and statistical manual of mental disorders* (3rd ed.). Washington: APA.

Beck, A. T., Ward, C. H., Mendelson, M., Mock, J., and Erbaugh, J. (1961). An inventory for measuring depression. *Archives of General Psychiatry,* **4**, 53-63.

Bergner, M., Bobbitt, R. A., Kressel, S., Pollard, W. E., Gilson, B. S., and Morris, J. R. (1976). The Sickness Impact Profile: Conceptual formulation and methodology for the development of a health status measure. *International Journal of Health Services,* **6**, 393-415.

Besdine, R. (1982). The data base of geriatric medicine. In J. W. Rowe and R. Besdine (Eds.), *Health and disease in old age.* Boston: Little, Brown.

Birren, J. E., and Sloane, R. B. (Eds.). (1980). *Handbook of mental health and aging.* Englewood Cliffs. N.J.: Prentice-Hall.

68 R. A. Kane

Carp, F. M., and Carp, A. (1982). The ideal residential area. *Research on Aging*, **4**, 411-439.

Dohrenwend, B. P., Dohrenwend, B. S., Gould, M. S., Link, B., Neugehauer, R., and Wunsch-Hitzig, R. (1980). *Mental illness in the United States: Epidemiological estimates.* New York: Praeger.

Duke University. (1978). Center for the Study of Aging and Human Development. *Multidimensional functional assessment: The OARS methodology.* Durham, N.C.: Duke University.

Dye, C. J. Personality. (1982 a). In D. J. Mangen and W. A. Peterson (Eds.), *Research instruments in social gerontology,* vol. 1: *Clinical and social psychology.* Minneapolis: University of Minnesota Press.

Dye, C. J. (1982 b). Intellectual functioning. In D. J. Mangen and W. A. Peterson (Eds.), *Research instruments in social gerontology,* vol. 1: *Clinical and social psychology.* Minneapolis: University of Minnesota Press.

Folstein, M. F., and McHugh, P. R. (1975). Mini-mental state: A practical method for grading the cognitive state of patients for the clinician. *Journal of Psychiatric Research,* **12**, 189-198.

Gallagher, D., Thompson, L. W., and Levy, S. M. (1980). Clinical psychological assessment of older adults. In L. Poor (Ed.), *Aging in the 1980's: Selected contemporary issues in the psychology of aging.* Washington: American Psychological Association.

Garcia, C. A., Redding, M. J., and Blass, F. P. (1981). Overdiagnosis of dementia. *Journal of the American Geriatric Society,* **29**, 407-410.

Gurland, B. J., Dean, L. L., Copeland, J., Gurland, R., and Golden, R. (1982). Criteria for the diagnosis of dementia in the community elderly. *Gerontologist,* **22**, 180-186.

Gurland, B., Dean, L., Gurland, R., and Cook, D. (1978). Personal time dependency in the elderly of New York City: Findings from the US-UK cross-national geriatric community study. In Community Council of Greater New York, *Dependency in the elderly of New York City: Policy and service implications of the US-UK cross-national geriatric community study.* New York: Community Council of Greater New York.

Gurland, B., Kuriansky, J., Sharpe, L., Simon R., Stiller, P., and Birkett, P. (1977-78). The Comprehensive Assessment and Referral Evaluation (CARE): Rationale, development, and reliability. *International Journal of Aging and Human Development,* **8**, 9-42.

Havighurst, R. J., Neugarten, B. L., and Tobin, S. S. (1961). The measurement of life satisfaction. *Journal of Gerontology,* **16**, 134-143.

Jones, E., McNitt, B., and McKnight, E. (1974). *Patient classification for long-term care: User's manual.* (HRA 75-3107) Washington: Government Printing Office.

Jorgensen, L. A., and Kane, R. L. (1976). Social work in the nursing home: A need and an opportunity. *Social Work in Health Care,* **1**, 471-482.

Kane, R. A., and Kane, R. L. (1981). *Assessing the elderly: A practical guide to measurement.* Lexington, Mass.: D. C. Heath.

Kane, R. A., Kane, R. L., Kleffel, D., Brook, R. H., Eby, C., Goldberg, G. A., Rubenstein, L. Z., and VanRyzin, J. (1979). *The PSRO and the nursing home,* vol. 1: *An assessment of PSRO long-term care review.* Santa Monica, Calif.: Rand Corporation.

Kane, R. L., and Kane, R. A. (1982). *Values and long-term care.* Lexington, Mass.: D. C. Heath.

Kane, R. L., Bell, R., Riegler, S. Z., Wilson, A., and Kane, R. A. (1983a). Assessing the outcomes of nursing-home patients. *Journal of Gerontology,* **38**, 385-393.

Kane, R. L., Bell, R., Riegler, S. Z., Wilson, A., and Keeler, E. (1983b). Predicting the outcomes of nursing-home patients. *Gerontologist* **23**, 200-206.

Kane, R. L., Ouslander, J. G., and Abrass, I. (1984). *A manual of geriatric medicine.* New York: McGraw-Hill.

Katz, S., Ford, A., Moskowitz, R., Jackson, B., Jaffe, M., and Cleveland, M. A. (1963). The index of ADL: A standardized measure of biological and psychosocial function. *Journal of the American Medical Association* **185**, 914-919.

Kulys, R., and Tobin, S. S. (1980). Older people and their "responsible others." *Social Work,* **25**, 138-145.

Kuriansky, J. B., Gurland, B. J., Fleiss, J. L., and Cowan, D. W. (1976). The assessment of self-care capacity in geriatric psychiatric patients. *Journal of Clinical Psychology,* **32,** 95-102.

Laufer, E. A., and Laufer, W. S. (1982). From geriatric resident to language professor: A new program using the talents of the elderly in a skilled nursing facility. *Gerontologist,* **22,** 551-554.

Lawton, M. P. (1972). The dimensions of morale. In D. Kent, R. Kastenbaum, and S. Sherwood (Eds.), *Research, planning and action for the elderly.* New York: Behavioral Publications.

Lawton, M. P., Whelihan, W. M., and Belsky, J. K. (1980). Personality tests and their uses with older adults. In J. E. Birren and R. B. Sloane (Eds.), *Handbook of mental health and aging.* Englewood Cliffs, N.J.: Prentice-Hall.

Mangen, D. J., and Peterson, W. A. (Eds.) (1982). *Research instruments in social gerontology,* vol. 1: *Clinical and social psychology.* Minneapolis: University of Minnesota Press.

Miller, E. (1980). Cognitive assessment of the older adult. In J. E. Birren and R. B. Sloane (Eds.), *Handbook of mental health and aging.* Englewood Cliffs, N.J.: Prentice-Hall.

Mossey, J. M., and Shapiro, E. (1982). Self-rated health: a predictor of mortality among the elderly. *American Journal of Public Health,* **72**(8), 800-808.

Post, F. (1980). Paranoid, schizophrenia-like and schizophrenic states in the aged. In J. E. Birren and R. B. Sloane (Eds.), *Handbook of mental health and aging.* Englewood Cliffs, N.J.: Prentice-Hall.

Rubenstein, L. Z., Abrass, I. B., and Kane, R. L. (1981). Improved patient care on a new geriatric evaluation unit. *Journal of the American Geriatric Society,* **29,** 531-536.

Salzman, C., and Shader, R. I. (1979). Clinical evaluation of depression in the elderly. In A. Raskin and L. F. Jarvik (Eds.), *Psychiatric symptoms and cognitive loss in the elderly: Evaluation and assessment techniques.* Washington: Hemisphere Publishing Corporation.

Sloane, R. B. (1980). Organic brain syndrome. In J. E. Birren and R. B. Sloane (Eds.), *Handbook of mental health and aging.* Englewood Cliffs, N.J.: Prentice-Hall.

Task panel reports submitted to the President's Commission on Mental Health. (1978). Washington: Government Printing Office.

U.S. Comptroller General. (1977). *The well-being of older people in Cleveland, Ohio.* Washington: Government Printing Office.

U.S. Department of Health, Education, and Welfare. (1978). *Working document on patient care management: Theory to practice.* Washington: Government Printing Office.

Windley, P. G. (1982). Environments. In D. J. Mangen and W. A. Peterson (Eds.), *Research instruments in social gerontology,* vol. 1: *Clinical and social psychology.* Minneapolis: University of Minnesota Press.

Zung, W. W. K. (1965). A self-rating depression scale. *Archives of General Psychiatry,* **12,** 63-70.

4

Mental Health and the Elderly

Kenneth Solomon, M.D.

Sheppard and Enoch Pratt Hospital
Baltimore, Md., and University of Maryland
School of Medicine

Older individuals are more likely to demonstrate evidence of acute or chronic psychopathology than are individuals in any other stage of life. Indeed, Post (1968) suggests that 20 to 30 percent of the elderly have psychiatric disorders. Older people make up a large percentage of new admissions and the majority of long-term-stay clients in state hospitals and other institutions. Approximately 5 percent of the elderly are institutionalized because of psychopathologic or behavioral difficulties (Redick, Kramer, and Taube, 1973).

Psychiatric dysfunction in the elderly is not caused by the biologic changes that occur with aging, although some changes in the biochemistry and physiology of the brain may increase the vulnerability of the elderly to certain psychologic dysfunctions and organic neurologic disease. Rather, the development of psychopathologic dysfunction in the elderly arises from the interaction of the triggers of current psychosocial stressors and the older person's lifelong learned ability to cope adaptively with stress.

STRESS AND COPING IN THE ELDERLY

New psychiatric symptoms in the elderly are always triggered by current stress. The elderly have a characteristic set of psychodynamic responses to stress, regardless of its biologic, psychologic, or social nature (Goldfarb, 1968, 1974; K.

Solomon, 1981a, 1981b, 1982a, 1982c, 1983a, b, c). As this stress is experienced by older people, it leads to a sense of diminished mastery over their environment and therefore to increased feelings of helplessness and ambivalence about dependency needs. These feelings may produce two affects. One is fear, as the older person worries about what is to become of him/her as he/she works to resolve the stress. The other affect is anger at self or others, anger over what has happened to the older person as well as anger at experienced powerlessness and loss of mastery. These affects, also conceptualized as flight or fight, are mediated biologically by the general adaptation syndrome, which triggers the organism to either cope or to become biologically exhausted (with subsequent illness or death) (Selye, 1950). Whether the person feels fear or anger or a mixture of the two depends on how that person has responded to stress throughout his/her life. The basic stress response does not change with increasing age.

Acute and Unexpected Stress

The stress experienced by the older person may be acute and unexpected or chronic. The events that cause acute, unexpected stress may be grouped into three major categories, all characterized by loss.

The first set of losses is in the social support system. They include loss of spouse, siblings, friends, parents, children, other relatives, and neighbors. The most psychologically devastating of these is the loss of a spouse (Guttmann, Grunes, and Griffin, 1979; Homes and Rahe, 1967; Wolff, 1977).

A second set of losses concerns social role and involves a shift from institutional to tenuous and informal roles and a shift as well in gender roles. By their very nature, tenuous and informal roles, which exist at the whim of the primary group or society, are sources of stress for the elderly (Rosow, 1976). Particularly stressful for men is the loss of opportunities for the expression of gender-role expectations (K. Solomon, 1982b, 1982c; Solomon and Hurwitz, 1982).

The third major set of losses falls into a miscellaneous group that includes loss of health, independence, adequate income, mobility, adequate housing, and leisure activities. These losses are the result of societally determined changes, such as retirement (Friedmann and Orbach, 1974; Sheppard, 1976), and chronic diseases that inhibit the functioning of the older person (Wilson, 1970).

Chronic Stress

Besides these actue episodic stressors, chronic stressors arise from the "victimization" of the elderly (K. Solomon, 1983a, b). This victimization has four dimensions: economic, attitudinal, role, and physical. Like all chronic situations in which the individual is "one down," the individual feels oppressed, angry, despondent, and helpless and may turn the anger onto himself/herself or explosively outward towards others or society at large (Brody, 1974).

Economic victimization includes not only illegal "ripoffs" and fraudulent schemes but also legal and sanctioned policy, such as inadequate pensions, the effects of inflation, and business practices that bilk the elderly consumer of needed funds.

Physical victimization includes abuse of the older person by his/her children or spouse as well as the effects of crime against person and property. It also includes much of the poor treatment that the elderly frequently receive from health-care givers in the form of inadequate diagnostic evaluations, inappropriate medication or surgery, and inadequate care in custodial institutions.

Attitudinal victimization is the result of the stereotyping of the elderly (Ryan, 1976; Tuckman and Lorge, 1953a). As Butler (1975) and Solomon and Vickers (1979) note, stereotyping leads to misdiagnosis and the provision of inadequate and irrelevant services. Individual needs of the elderly are not identified, and their individuality is lost. This contributes to the learned helplessness of many older individuals, especially in the health-care setting (Maier and Seligman, 1976; Seligman, 1975; K. Solomon, 1979c, 1982e).

Role victimization comes with the shift from institutional to tenuous and informal social roles. The elderly may then lapse into a state of rolelessness with subsequent alienation, anomie, apathy, and psychopathologic symptomatology if they are unable to adopt even tenuous or informal roles (Akisal and McKinney, 1975; Bibring, 1961; K. Solomon, 1981a).

THE PSYCHOGERIATRIC EVALUATION

Before an intervention can be planned for the older individual with significant psychologic dysfunctions, a complete psychogeriatric evaluation is necessary. The goal is to get as much information as possible for a comprehensive understanding of the person's psychosocial state. The evaluation requires examination of the person's current stresses, his/her psychodynamic response to these stresses, the responses of various social subsystems that interact with the individual, and the strengths and weaknesses of the individual's personality. The evaluation also includes the elimination of any treatable medical causes of symptoms that may be present.

The psychogeriatric evaluation has eleven components. While it is presented in its entirety in this chapter, it is not expected nor required that any individual member of the geriatric team be responsible for the entire evaluation. Many authors have examined the roles of various mental-health professionals and have divided them into two major categories: generalist and specialist. Generalist roles are those clinical roles that are not limited by disciplinary boundaries or training. Rather, these roles are used by all professionals in the fulfillment of various professional tasks. They are discussed in more depth elsewhere (Cohen, 1973; Smith, 1972; K. Solomon, 1979b, 1982d). Specialist roles allow for differentiation of professionals on the team and utilization of specific skills, knowledge, and personality traits of these professionals in the total care of the individual (Harris and Solomon, 1977; Howard, 1979; Pons, 1979; Romaniuk, 1979). Most work accomplished in the psychosocial aspects of caring for the elderly person in a mental-health/human-service setting utilizes generalist skills of all members of the team. The psychogeriatric evaluation is one task that can be largely completed using only generalist skills.

The components of the psychogeriatric evaluation are:

1. History of the Present Episode

One needs to know exactly what the client is feeling and experiencing, how long the problem has been going on, what seemed to trigger it, what makes it better (even temporarily), what seems to make it worse, and what interventions the client, family, and mental-health personnel have tried to improve this particular problem. It is in the history of the present episode that one asks specific questions regarding the various symptoms needed to make a diagnosis as well as to assess blocks to need satisfaction, including presence or absence of vegetative, depressive, psychotic, phobic, and obsessive-compulsive symptoms.

2. Past Psychiatric History

One not only needs to ask if the client has had inpatient or outpatient psychiatric treatment in the past, but whether he/she has received intervention for emotional problems from other personnel such as psychologists, social workers, psychiatric nurses, and clergy. In addition, a history of receiving "nerve pills" or other psychotropic drugs from a family physician is important. This information will help clarify the client's ability to cope and his/her coping mechanisms. The presence of a history of a severe psychiatric disability would be an indication either for a prescription of specific interventions (especially psychopharmacologic) that have been successful in the past (Ayd, 1975) and the avoidance of interventions that have been unsuccessful.

3. Past and Present Medical Status

The client's medical history is necessary to assess his/her overall functional capabilities and to know what problems to expect in the future. The presence or absence of certain medications may impair or enhance the overall treatment process. This history may also hint at certain somatic disorders or medications that may be causing the psychopathology noted in the client (e.g., depression secondary to hypothyroidism or toxic psychosis secondary to antidepressants).

4. Drug History

The client's use of drugs must be ascertained, which not only includes prescription medications, but also over-the-counter drugs and street drugs. Many older people have problems with alcohol or drugs, which may interfere with their overall functioning as well as with the treatment program or which may otherwise cause specific psychiatric disorders. Besides alcohol, the most commonly abused drugs in the elderly are over-the-counter "nerve pills," benzodiazepines, marijuana, barbiturates, amphetamines, and legal narcotic analgesics; the use of these drugs must be specifically ascertained.

5. Psychosocial Evaluation

The purpose of the psychosocial evaluation is to gather information about the client's past coping skills, factors that may enhance or inhibit psychiatric and physical rehabilitation, and to assess other stresses and resources in the patient's environment.

The psychosocial evaluation begins with a family history, which includes information about the client's parents, siblings, and children. The evaluation includes the medical and psychiatric histories of these individuals, and what kind of relationships these people had and have with each other and with the client. The family history also includes occupational and social-class background of the client's parents, their immigration status, and the relationship between the parents.

In the developmental history, the client's meeting of developmental landmarks is assessed. The examiner also gathers information about the client's life as a child.

In the educational history, one asks questions about the client's level of education and use of this education. Why the client stopped or continued educational pursuits at different times in his/her life is ascertained. The client's interest in lifelong learning, vocational rehabilitation, and attitudes toward education are also assessed.

In the client's occupational history, the examiner looks at the jobs the client has held, his/her ability to hold a job, and the kind of work he/she is interested in. One also examines for exposure to occupational hazards that might have diagnostic or therapeutic implications.

In the marital and sexual history, one examines these relationships as a major resource and stress. These factors need to be examined regardless of marital status, sexual orientation, or sexual exclusivity or nonexculsivity. If the client has never married or cohabited, the reasons need to be assessed. The entire spectrum of the individual's interpersonal relationships is examined in this way. One also ascertains the client's interest in and level of sexual activity with its obvious implications for treatment.

One then looks at the client's current financial situation, which not only includes examination of his/her sources of income but which also includes other social services that substitute for income. These sources include food stamps, health insurance coverage, and Title III nutrition programs.

The examiner then investigates the client's current housing, which is examined for the presence or absence of barriers and to see how the house can be made barrier-free. Thus housing becomes both a stress and a resource to the individual.

How the client uses leisure time is also assessed. This factor is important not only to provide relaxation for the client but also to gather information about the client's ability to relax, experience positive affects, and develop meaningful rather than just time-consuming activities.

In planning intervention, knowledge of the client's premorbid personality is crucial. This information will tell the therapist what kind of defenses and coping mechanisms the person uses. The examiner will also learn how the person has satisfied various needs in the past and whether or not the person has been capable of adapting to stress in the past. It will clarify other psychologic stresses and resources the individual brings into the rehabilitation situation and helps to assess the risk of the individual developing major psychopathology in the future. For example, those with labile personality disorders are at risk for developing depression and those with stable personality disorders are at risk for developing either depression or paraphrenia when stressed in old age (Solomon, 1981b; Weiss, 1973). Those without personality disorders are more likely to cope successfully with stress. At the same time that one assesses the premorbid personality of the client, one examines the entire environment to assess other stresses and resources that are present.

6. Review of Systems

While a review of systems has traditionally been part of the medical examination, it can be done by any professional. During the review of systems, the examiner asks about various symptoms of disease, including pain, visual problems, bowel habits, diet and appetite, sleep, and sexual functioning. Formal guides to a review of systems have been published elsewhere (Adams, 1958; Delp, 1968; Friedland, 1967; Judge and Zuidema, 1963).

7. Physical Examination

The physical examination should be complete, including a rectal and pelvic examination. Although this must be done by a physician, nurse practitioner, or physician's assistant, the mental-health/human-service worker must be apprised of this information in order to understand the problems of the older person and plan appropriate interventions.

8. Neurologic Examination

As many older individuals in the rehabilitation setting have or are suspected to have neurologic disease, a thorough neurologic examination must be done. This examination does not have to be done by a neurologic consultant since all physicians and other health professionals who do physical examinations are trained to do neurologic examinations. This information must be transmitted to the members of the team.

9. Mental-Status Examination

The mental-status examination has fifteen parts in addition to observation of the client during the conduct of the psychogeriatric examination. Delineation of psychopathologic symptoms is necessary for an accurate assessment of the psychosocial status of the older client. Accurate, value-free descriptions of behavior, without labels, are the backbone of the mental-status examination. In reviewing the mental-status examination, one can easily see many forms of behavior that vary from the expected normative behavior of the client. These variations are not necessarily psychopathologic. For example, a sad affect would be very appropriate to someone who has recently had a cerebrovascular accident but would not be appropriate for someone who has just won a lottery.

There are several descriptions of the conduct of the mental-status examination (MacKinnon, 1980; Menninger, 1962; Stevenson and Sheppe, 1974). The parameters of the mental-status examination will be discussed in turn.

First one notes the client's appearance. How is the person dressed? Is the person in a bed or wheelchair or ambulatory? What is his/her posture? Are there any other signs that might indicate the possibility of physical disease? Appearance is either appropriate or inappropriate for the client's medical condition and social setting. For example, it would not be generally considered appropriate for a client to wear pajamas to an outpatient appointment but it would be appropriate to wear them in a hospital. The social context of a client's appearance must be taken into account. The same holds true for posture, which may be relaxed, tense, indicative of physical pathology, or bizarre and unusual as in some psychotic individuals.

One then notes the client's level of consciousness and alertness. The level of consciousness may be normal or the client may be hyperalert with wide eyes and furtive scanning of the environment or drowsy, sleeping, obtunded, semicomatose, or comatose.

The third part of the examination is evaluation of the client's attention span. The client may have marked difficulty paying attention because of distractability or hearing deficit. On the other hand, a client may be demonstrating denial or selective inattention, and may, for unconscious reasons, not attend to the examiner. Selective inattention is usually under some conscious control, but denial is not. Distractability is usually noted in severe psychotic or cognitive disorders.

Mood is ascertained by asking the client how he/she feels and what is his/her underlying mood. For example, is he/she happy, sad, angry? Mood may be euthymic; it may be happy or sad within the realm of human experience. Or the client may experience extremes of mood including elation or euphoria on the one hand or severe depression on the other. The client may be angry or hostile or be experiencing anxiety or fear.

Associated with mood is the fifth parameter of the mental-status exam, affect. This is the behavioral manifestation of the underlying mood, and is usually ascertained through examination of the client's facial expression. Is the facial expression angry, sad, happy, dull, or blunted? Also, the examiner wants to know if the affect corresponds to the expressed thought content. The client's affect may be appropriate or inappropriate. Inappropriate affect is affect that does not fit the underlying mood or the content of the person's thoughts. If inappropriate, it may also be blunted or flattened, which is when the person does not facially express underlying feelings.

Sixth, one examines the level of activity. Is it normally active, hyperactive, or hypoactive? Are there tremors or other abnormal movements? The client may demonstrate psychomotor retardation, in which all physical functions are slowed up, or psychomotor agitation, in which he/she is restless or agitated. Mild agitation may be manifested by mild finger tapping and hand wringing. Severe agitation is manifested by difficulty staying still for more than a few moments, which must be differentiated from akathisia, which is a common Parkinsonian symptom.

One then examines the quality of the client's speech. One considers the quantity, volume, tone, inflection, speed, and understandability (coherence). Speech may be incoherent or indistinct because of aphasia or dysarthria. It may be rapid or slow, monotonous or inflected, too low or too loud. It may or may not be appropriate to the situation, content, or affect.

The examiner then considers the client's thought process. Is it rational, logical, and oriented toward a goal? Does the client attempt to answer questions in a reasonably concise manner? Is the client able to express himself/herself or is there evidence of receptive or expressive aphasia? Deficiencies of thought include paucity of thought, which is a relative lack of expressed thought. Perseveration occurs when the same thought is repeated over and over again, regardless of its relevance to the question asked. Other disorders of thought process include a loss of the normal logical pathways. When mild, this is called tangentiality, in which the client seems to constantly digress from topic, or circumstantiality, in which the client "beats around the bush" but eventually answers the question. More severe loss of logical aspects of thought is called loose associations or derailment. When severe, the client's speech may be almost impossible to understand. This situation is called a word salad. In addition, the client may use neologisms, newly invented words that may have idiosyncratic meanings known only to the client.

Next, one examines the content of the client's thought. What is it that the person is specifically thinking and is it relevant to the business at hand? Disturbances of thought content include vagueness, compulsive repetition, or obsessive intrusion of a thought alien to the client's ego. The client may demonstrate idées fixes, which are unshakeable, encapsulated ideas that may or may not be delusional. The client may also be preoccupied with phobic ideas or fantasies. He/she may demonstrate delusions, which may be reasonable logical beliefs but which are not based in reality. Delusions are frequently paranoid in the elderly. They may be encapsulated or limited to only a samll part of the client's life and not affect the client's functioning in other ways, or they may be unencapsulated, global, and severely disruptive. They may be organized into a delusional system or they may be disorganized. The client may also demonstrate confabulation or the creation of "factual" information to cover up memory deficits, which must be differentiated from willful lying. Depressive thought content, including self-deprecation, statements of irrational guilt, and feelings of helplessness, hopelessness, worthlessness, and uselessness may also be demonstrated. Finally, certain specific Schneiderian first-rank symptoms of schizophrenia are included as disturbances of thought. These symptoms include thought insertion (the belief that an outside force or person is putting thoughts in the client's head), thought control (the belief that an outside force is controlling the client's thoughts), behavioral control (a similar belief associated with behavior), thought withdrawal (the belief that an outside force is taking thoughts out of the clients head), and thought broadcasting (the belief that people are able to hear the client's thoughts). Schneiderian first-rank symptoms are believed to be pathognominic of schizophrenia in younger people (Kendell, Brockington and Leff, 1979), but have no specific pathognomonic consequence in the elderly.

In examining perception, one examines the client's ability to understand the spoken and written word as well as looking for unusual perceptual experiences. Many major disorders of perception are pathophysiologic in nature and include receptive aphasias and the results of major sensory deficits.

Another common disorder of perception is the illusion, in which things are perceived in ways that do not match the reality. The optical illusion is an example with which everyone is familiar. Misperceptions are another form of perceptual disorder, in which something is misidentified as something it is not. The most severe perceptual disorders are hallucinations, in which the client creates sensory inputs not based in the external environment. These hallucinations may be auditory, visual, olfactory, gustatory, tactile, or kinesthetic. Specific Schneiderian perceptual symptoms include the experience of hallucinating two voices communicating with each other or a single voice keeping up a running commentary on the client's behavior.

Memory is examined, in part, during the process of obtaining a history, a process that allows the examiner to ascertain the accuracy of the client's recent and remote memory. Questions about the client's activities over the few days prior to the examination test for recent memory. To test for immediate recall, one gives the client three items to remember and checks back with him/her several minutes later to see if they are recalled. Memory disturbances includes specific amnesias and hypomnesias as well as more global disturbances of immediate recall, recent memory, and remote memory, and the part processes of registration, retention, recognition, and recall.

One then tests for orientation. Does the client know the day of the week, date, month, year, and season? Does the person know the name of the place he/she is in, the address, the floor, the room number? Can the client give a reasonable account of himself/herself? Is the client aware of the present situation? In other words, does the client understand the environmental parameters surrounding him/her? Difficulty with orientation is called disorientation and is marked by the client's inability to identify the time, the place, or basic information about himself/herself.

One assesses the client's level of intelligence by examining his/her ability to perform higher cortical functions. Can the client serially subtract seven from a hundred? Can the client follow simple instructions? Can the client read and write a simple sentence? How well does the client interpret proverbs? Are these proverbs interpreted abstractly or concretely? The proverbs I usually use are: "You can lead a horse to water but you can't make it drink" and "People in glass houses shouldn't throw stones." Can the client identify similarities and differences between items such as an apple and an orange? Disorders of intelligence may include life long intellectual deficits, as in mentally retarded individuals, or acquired intellectual deficits. The latter may be specific, like dyslexia, or global, as in dementia, and include difficulties following simple instructions, reading, calculating, and writing sentences. These disorders may also include loss of the ability to abstract proverbs, which is partially dependent upon the educational level and cultural background of the client.

One tests judgment by assessing what the client would do in hypothetical situations. The situations I use are: What would the client do if he/she found a letter lying on the ground in front of a mailbox, and what would the client do if he/she smelled smoke while at the movies. These questions give the examiner information about client's ability to integrate environmental cues and choose between several alternative behaviors. Difficulties of judgment include impulsivity, the failure to take the consequences of one's behavior into account prior to action.

The final part of the mental-status examination is the assessment of the client's level of insight, which is accomplished by asking the client why he/she feels he/she has developed the specific emotional, behavioral, or cognitive difficulty. Levels of insight range from a complete denial of all symptoms to the ability to identify symptoms but not their consequences or etiology, to the ability to identify symptoms and consequences but not their etiology, to insight as to the nature and cause of the psychosocial difficulties. The level of insight will often determine the type of intervention planned with the client.

10. Laboratory Examination

The specific laboratory examination is dependent upon the nature of the psychologic difficulty considered. For geriatric clients who develop psychopathology, the laboratory examination should include a complete blood count; renal, liver, and thyroid function studies; electrolytes; fasting blood sugar; electrocardiogram; chest x-ray; serology for syphilis; and serum concentrations of drugs that the client is taking. In addition, if a diagnosis of brain failure is being considered, the client should also have vitamin B_{12} and folate blood levels assessed, with an electroencephalogram and computerized axial tomography of the head. Other specific laboratory evaluations may also be necessary.

11. Social Examination

This examination is the final part of the psychogeriatric evaluation. It includes information gathered from review of the client's chart and from discussions with social-service staff, nursing staff, family members, neighbors, and other important individuals in the client's life. It will corroborate the history the client gives the examiner and will also give the examiner insight into other symptoms that the client may be unwilling or unable to discuss. It will also help assess and enlist the interpersonal resources available to the client. If feasible, the social examination should include a tour of the client's home to assess resources, stresses, and barriers in the environment.

THE MAJOR PSYCHIATRIC DYSFUNCTIONS

Depression

Depression is the most common psychiatric disturbance in the elderly. Estimates of the incidence of depressive episodes that significantly interfere with life functioning in persons 65 and over range from 15 percent to 68 percent, with most researchers noting an incidence of 30 to 40 percent (Ban, 1978). This finding compares with a 10 percent incidence of depression in the general population (Sartorius, 1975), making depression three to six times more frequent in the elderly than in the young. The prevalence of depression in the elderly in the community has been estimated by Blazer and Williams to be approximately 15 percent (Blazer and Williams, 1980). The frequency of depression in the elderly is associated with the many stresses that they face. The elderly may also be biologically predisposed to the development of depression.

Description

Depression is manifested by sad mood (or its equivalent) and various vegetative disturbances (American Psychiatric Association, 1980). There is a change in appetite (usually loss but occasionally increase) and change in the sleep cycle (usually difficulty falling asleep, difficulty remaining asleep, and early morning awakening, but occasionally hypersomnia). The client demonstrates either psychomotor agitation or retardation and may complain of anxiety, weakness, or feeling slowed up, but not sadness. The client feels fatigued, even after adequate sleep, and feels that he/she does not have the energy or the motivation for rehabilitation and other tasks. The client feels guilty and blames himself/herself for these problems. The client has difficulty concentrating and demonstrates a cognitive disturbance manifested by a disturbance of recent memory and immediate recall, concrete thinking, pervasive doubt, and what the author has described as "viewing the world through gray-colored glasses." In addition, the depressed individual manipulates himself/herself and others into situations that will guarantee failure (Bonime, 1966; Kovacs and Beck, 1978) and then internalizes the guilt and anger at others who do not respond to these manipulations. The severely depressed person may verbalize suicidal feelings, ideation, or plans. As suicide is one of the leading causes of death in the elderly (Weiss, 1974), the examiner must always ask the client about suicidal ideation. Some severely depressed individuals will also demonstrate a variety of psychotic symptoms, including delusions and hallucinations.

The phenomenology of depressive disorders in the elderly varies with the premorbid history of the older person. Many elderly present the classic semiology of depression, including sad mood, psychomotor agitation, guilt, self-deprecation, hopelessness, worthlessness, helplessness, appetite and weight disturbance, sleep disturbance, and suicidal ideation. However, many elderly exhibit psycho-motor retardation without guilt, anger, and self-deprecation. Those elderly with a premorbid history of an affective disorder of difficulty in handling conflicts about hostility and dependency are more likely to develop a depressive picture that fits the classic description. The elderly with good premorbid histories who suffer a multitude of losses are likely to experience predominantly affective loss, leading to a clinical picture more consistant with a retarded depression. Loss and grieving are not as intimately associated with anger as they are in younger individuals; this lack of association contributes to the clinical picture just noted.

Depression is the major psychiatric disturbance that may be fatal; the major reason is suicide. One-fourth of all suicides in the United States occur in individuals over 65. The rate of suicide in white men over 65 is three times that of white men aged 25. White men over 75 have the highest incidence of successful suicide, followed by white men 65 to 74 and white women over 65 (Weiss, 1974). The elderly are the only age group in which successful suicides outnumber suicide attempts; when the elderly are suicidal, they are likely to be successful.

Death of the depressed elderly person may also result from major physiologic consequences of the depression, even in the absence of suicidal intent. The appetite disturbance that accompanies depression may lead the older person to withdraw from food and drink. Severe fluid and electrolyte disturbances may rapidly develop, which may be fatal because of secondary pneumonia or seizures. The immobility caused by depression may lead to the development of decubitus ulcers, which may become secondarily infected, leading to sepsis. Thus depression in an older person is potentially more dangerous and the need for treatment more urgent than in a younger person.

Etiologic Factors

The etiology of depression is unclear at this time. Certain factors make depression more likely to occur in the elderly. Biologically, increased turnover of neurotransmitters may lead to a relative unavailability of these chemicals in the parts of the brain associated with modulation of mood. This biologic vulnerability may be the substrate for psychosocial factors discussed above to become triggers for the development of depression.

Diagnosis

The diagnosis of depression involves the differentiation of depression from physical diseases, particularly dementia. Depression is probably the most common cause of pseudodementia in the elderly (Libow, 1973); since depression is treatable and many of the dementias are not, an accurate diagnosis is absolutely essential. One difficulty in differential diagnosis is that depressive symptoms may be noted in the demented individual early in the course of the brain disease. The severely depressed individual, especially one with a retarded depression, may be so anergic as to make it impossible to differentiate between depression and dementia. Kahn (1978) has noted that many cognitive changes, primarily deficits of immediate recall and recent memory, occur in the depressed individual. In addition to the cognitive changes, there are severe difficulties of attention that may seem to be a memory deficit. The anergic, depressed individual may be so retarded that he/she may become incontinent and unable to care for basic bodily needs. Because of anergia, the depressed individual may think more concretely than in the premorbid state, which may also give the impression of a loss of cognitive functioning. Agitation and an inability to respond to the examiner may lead to a false impression of cognitive disturbance. Secondary physiologic changes may lead to delirium, with subsequent missed diagnosis of the underlying depression.

Endocrine disorders may present as an affective disturbance indistinguishable from a major depressive disorder (Whybrow and Hurwitz, 1976). Depression is commonly seen in clients with chronic renal disease, anemia, and brain tumors, and as a result of head trauma. Mood changes, lethargy, fatigability, weight loss, and sleep disturbances are seen in a myriad of systemic diseases and as side effects of many medications, especially hormones, psychotropic drugs, and antihypertensive medications.

The diagnosis of depression is made by a combination of inclusion and exclusion criteria (American Psychiatric Association, 1980). These criteria include at least four of the following eight:

1. Appetite/weight disturbance
2. Sleep disturbance
3. Disturbance in activity level
4. Cognitive disturbance
5. Disturbance in energy level
6. Disturbance in usual interests
7. Disturbance of attention
8. Suicidal ideation/plans/behavior

Other features that should be noted include mood disturbance of at least two weeks duration. Exclusion criteria—that is, that the depression is not part of a physical disorder or other major psychiatric disorder or that it is not a normal grief reaction—should be noted. It is absolutely essential to differentiate between depression (a major disturbance) and sadness (a universal experience).

Once the diagnosis of depression is made, treatment should be rapidly and aggressively instituted because of the potentially fatal outcome of this disturbance. A combination of pharmacotherapy with antidepressant medication (or, if the client has delusions or hallucinations, with antipsychotic medication), psychotherapy (especially of the cognitive-behavioral orientation), and environmental manipulation is indicated.

Alcoholism and Chemical Dependency

Combined, these two sets of disorders probably affect 10 to 25 percent of the elderly population. In spite of the relatively frequent use (as anecdotally reported; good epidemiologic data do not exist) of alcohol, marijuana, barbituates, stimulants, tranquilizers, and narcotics by the elderly, virtually nothing is known about these disorders in the elderly.

There seem to be two groups of elderly alcoholics. One group consists of those alcoholics who have managed to live to age 65 without dying of hepatic disease, esophageal varices, or other sequelae of ethanol addiction. This group is psychodynamically and behaviorally no different from younger chronic alcoholics.

The second group of alcoholics are the reactive alcoholics, those who may or may not have been premorbid social drinkers but who, after experiencing a series of stresses in old age, begin to drink heavily for the first time. Some differences have been noted between male and female alcoholics who begin to drink for the first time in later life. Men tend to drink alone rather than with friends, and the major reason they give for their drinking is self-medication to cope with severe losses. Many of these men have been extremely dependent on someone whom they have lost, and they have become severely depressed. They are unable to cope with many of the stresses of daily life without the use of alcohol. Their alcohol use rapidly accelerates to an addiction, frequently in a matter of months.

Women tend to drink in the company of others. Many of these women have been somewhat compulsive and dependent individuals who have characterologically been unable to express anger. In the presence of stress, usually the loss of a significant other, they use alcohol to release the hostile feelings that they have repressed and suppressed for a lifetime.

One difficulty with treating elderly reactive alcoholics is that many of the facilities available to alcoholics do not seem to be appropriate for these individuals. Treatment of the underlying depression, which is quite common, is an absolute necessity for successful treatment of the alcoholism. Many elderly reactive alcoholics do not find Alcoholics Anonymous to be relevant, as they have never hit "rock bottom" and their life histories have been quite different from those of typical AA members. The use of disulfiram may not be a safe adjunctive treatment because of the presence of hepatic, cardiac, or renal disease. The use of individual and group phsychotherapy and treatment of the underlying depression with antidepressants are probably the most useful therapeutic modalities for these patients.

Brain Failure

The third most common psychiatric disorder in the elderly is brain failure, which denotes a functional neurologic loss. Brain failure has four mutually nonexclusive dimensions, and the clinical presentation of any individual may be conceptualized as a mixture of factors on these axes. These axes are continua, and an individual may shift on any or all of them at any time during the course of the disease.

One axis is the symptomatologic. One terminus is delirium, which is a disorder of attention and which is associated with an altered state of consciousness. The other terminus is dementia, which is a disorder of memory and which is associated with a normal state of consciousness. Some people with dementia may also have symptoms of delirium and vice versa. The second axis is the time of onset of symptoms and ranges from acute and sudden, as seen in drug toxicity or a cerebrovascular accident, to very slow, chronic, and insidious, as seen in Alzheimer's or Creutzfeldt-Jakob disease. The third axis is that of etiology, from completely extrinsic, as in head trauma, to completely intrinsic, as in multi-infarct dementia. Finally, there is the prognostic axis, ranging from completely reversible to completely irreversible.

It has been estimated that approximately 6.2 percent of individuals over age 65 will develop brain failure. At age 65, the incidence is 2 to 3 percent, which gradually increases to approximately 20 percent at age 80 (Kay, 1977). It then levels off and remains at 20 percent for the rest of the life cycle. Although only 5 percent of the elderly are institutionalized, the diagnosis of dementia is present in 50 percent of institutionalized elderly (Redick, Kramer, and Taube, 1973). However, approximately one of every four individuals who present with evidence of brain failure has a completely treatable cause of the disorder.

Clinical Features

The primary signs and symptoms of brain failure are those symptoms that are completely attributable to the neurological deficit *per se* and include memory loss, aphasias, agnosias, apraxias, and disorientation. There are also secondary symptoms. These symptoms are part of the individual's attempts to adapt to or cope with the loss of functioning, personality traits that become accentuated into symptoms when previously acquired coping mechanisms are lost, and the consequences in and response of the environment and support network to the individual with brain failure.

In early dementias, depression is frequently seen and may cloud the diagnostic picture (K. Solomon, 1982f). The depressive symptoms develop from the individual's grief over loss of functioning and memory as a body part. This loss, like the loss of any other body part, is experienced as a narcissistic injury and requires that the individual work it through and find new modes of functioning (Kolb, 1975).

Anxiety is also frequently seen, with a constant worry of what will happen to the self or family or with fears that children will inherit the disease. This anxiety has a strong existential component and is frequently relieved by honest sharing of prognostic information with the elderly client.

Psychotic symptoms may develop as the dementing individual attempts to reestablish psychologic homeostasis. The individual with brain failure has difficulty remembering and integrating parts of the environment, which may be further accentuated by the presence of a visual or hearing deficit. The person may then develop delusions to explain what is happening to him/her and to the world around him/her. The presence of a sensory deficit may further lead these individuals to create their own sensory input in the form of hallucinations, a form of sensory deprivation psychosis (P. Solomon, 1961).

Confabulation may also be noted. As the individual attempts to reestablish psychic homeostasis, he/she "invents" a reality that is plausible and that allows for denial of the unpleasant blanks in memory.

As the individual loses cognitive capabilities, he/she may act in ways that cause the family, neighborhood, and community alarm (Mace and Rabins, 1982). He/she becomes more dependent on others in the community to successfully manage activities of daily living, which may lead to anger, recriminations, guilt, overdependency, helplessness, inappropriate attempts at maintaining autonomy, or denial by the family, community, or the demented client. The secondary family problems not only cause anxiety and depression in themselves, which further complicate the clinical picture, but may lead to major family psychopathology, including the development of psychiatric symptoms in other members of the family. Behavioral difficulties, although derived from sources in the individual's premorbid personality, become a constant source of difficulty for the client and the caregivers.

Diagnosis and Treatment

Twenty-five percent of individuals with brain failure have a treatable cause of the symptomatology. If the symptoms are not treated within a reasonable time, permanent brain disease may occur secondarily. Therefore, it is incumbent upon the evaluating physician to do a thorough evaluation of all individuals with brain failure. This includes a complete history, especially looking for hints of drug toxicity (including alcohol and over-the-counter drugs) and a nutritional history. It includes complete physical and neurologic examinations. Laboratory work recommended includes a urinalysis; blood tests to rule out hematologic, hepatic, renal, and thyroid diseases; a chest x-ray; and an electrocardiogram. Other laboratory studies to rule out other treatable causes of dementia (pseudo-dementia) include vitamin B_{12} and folate blood levels, serology for syphilis, an electroencephalogram, and computerized tomography (CT scan) of the head. If a full evaluation is otherwise negative, and if there is cortical and central atrophy on cranial tomography, one can make a presumptive diagnosis of Alzheimer's disease (which cannot be proved except at autopsy). The history, examination, and results of laboratory tests will lead to a specific diagnosis for almost all causes of reversible and irreversible brain failure. If the history and examinations reveal hints of another condition that may lead to pseudodementia, other tests (e.g., blood levels of various drugs, angiography, lumbar puncture) must also be performed.

Whenever possible, treatment is aimed at the specific cause of the brain failure. However, if that is not possible, treatment must be symptomatic with an emphasis on maintaining environmental homogeneity and helping the person continue to function at maximum levels. The use of cognitive-acting drugs, such as cerebral vasodilators or dihydrogenated ergot alkaloids, is not recommended, as the clinical efficacy of these drugs has never been demonstrated.

Paraphrenia

Paraphrenia is a diagnosis rarely made in the United States, although there is no paucity of paranoid elderly encountered in clinical practice. This diagnosis is frequently subsumed under other labels. Paraphrenia is a paranoid psychosis that develops in an older person without a premorbid history of major psychiatric problems and in the absence of organic brain disease. Premorbidly, most individuals with paraphrenia have been schizoid, aloof, or suspicious (Isaacs, 1973); however, they have never evidenced frank psychotic symptomatology. In some individuals, the paranoid ideation is limited to only certain sharply delineated areas of thought. In other individuals, it is a more global and systematized delusional process. Schneiderian symptoms may be present, which has frequently led to a misdiagnosis of late-onset schizophrenia. However, schizophrenia rarely begins after age 35 and has a poor prognosis. Paraphrenia rarely begins prior to age 55, and its prognosis is excellent. The paranoid delusions frequently have more than a kernel of truth in them and indeed may be so plausible that a thorough evaluation of the person's social history may be necessary for the examiner to be thoroughly convinced that the individual is dealing with delusion rather than reality. In about two-thirds of cases of paraphrenia, the paranoid symptomatology develops as a defense against a potentially overwhelming depression. In these cases, treatment of the psychotic symptomatology frequently leads to the elucidation of depressive symptomatology that had been masked by the paranoid ideation. Treatment of the subsequent depression is then necessary. Kay, Cooper, and Garside (1976) have noted that sensory deficits occur in approximately 70 percent of elderly individuals with paranoid ideation; investigation and correction of this problem are an important part of the diagnosis and intervention of clients with paraphrenia. Paraphrenia is treated with a combination of reality-testing, supportive psychotherapy, and antipsychotic medication.

Mania

Mania is much less common than depression in the elderly. In some ways, it is the extreme opposite of depression, as the manic individual's mood is elated or euphoric. He/she demonstrates extreme impulsivity, diminished need for sleep, increased energy, psychomotor agitation, and rapid speech. Many manic individuals are quite hostile and may be overtly paranoid. Some also demonstrate hallucinations or delusions. Older manic individuals are less likely to demonstrate the physical hyperactivity and rapid speech than younger people, so that the mood disturbance becomes the paramount sign of the disorder. The treatment of mania is also psychopharmacologic, psychotherapeutic, and sociotherapeutic.

Personality Disorders

Personality disorders affect approximately 5 percent of the elderly (K. Solomon, 1981b) and are lifelong maladaptive interpersonal behavior patterns that may become evident for the first time or intensified in old age. Individuals with personality disorders may seek or be referred for therapy for the first time in old age because their social network has either broken down or is no longer willing or able to put up with the maladaptive behavior or because they have become uncomfortable with their behaviors. There is some "maturing out" of the more impulsive labile disorders, such as narcissistic and borderline disorders, as they become less affectively and behaviorally intense. These individuals, especially if dependent, are prone to the development of depression when under stress in late life. Individuals with a stable disorder, such as the obsessive-compulsive, paranoid, or schizoid disorders, tend to remain stable or become worse throughout life. These individuals are prone not only to the development of depression but also to paraphrenia and other psychotic syndromes of late life because they are no longer able to control their environment and have a cognitive style of doubt, guardedness, and suspiciousness.

Neuroses

Neuroses, phobias, and anxiety disorders are syndromes that are rare in the elderly. When they do occur, they are frequently indicative of an underlying depression or organic problem. However, an occasional individual may develop neurotic symptoms for the first time when his/her adaptational mechanisms break down because of psychosocial problems. Therapy for both personality disorders and neuroses is long-term individual or group psychotherapy or psychoanalysis.

Other Psychiatric Disturbances

All psychiatric disturbances that occur at a younger age may also occur in the elderly. Elderly schizophrenics with chronic symptoms have been noted to have a somewhat diminished affective intensity to their psychotic symptomatology (Verwoerdt, 1976). They frequently have developed and maintained some kind of social stability that allows for fairly consistent daily functioning, even in the presence of psychotic symptomatology (Zusman, 1966). The same is also true of those who are mentally retarded, although psychotic symptomatology is absent and their functioning frequently depends on an institutional environment. Sexual dysfunctions may also occur for the first time in old age. Besides demythologizing and education, treatment follows the techniques developed by Masters and Johnson (1970).

PSYCHOPATHOLOGIC SYMPTOMS OF MEDICAL DISEASES AND MEDICAL SYMPTOMS OF PSYCHOPATHOLOGY

Psychopathologic Symptoms

Memory Loss

As just stated, causes of memory deficit are legion; indeed, almost any disease listed in standard medical textbooks can cause reversible or irreversible memory loss and loss of intellectual functioning in the elderly (Libow, 1973). The major reversible causes are depression; drug intoxication (alcohol, marijuana, and over-the-counter drugs); side effects of medication, malnutrition, and hypovitaminoses; reversible neurologic diseases (especially the sequlae of head trauma); hypothyroidism or hyperthyroidism; other endocrine disorders; cardiovascular disease; severe and acute systemic infections; and any severe acute medical disease. As the usual symptoms of these various diseases often are not present in the elderly (Exton-Smith and Overstall, 1979) — for example, an older person may not experience pain with a heart attack or symptoms of diminished metabolism with hypothyroidism — referral to a physician in all cases of memory loss is absolutely necessary for a complete evaluation.

Depression

While depression may seem to be a reasonable response to real life situations in the elderly, it may be a result of side effects of medication, neurologic disease, endocrine disorders (especially thyroid disease), infections (even minor ones), and chronic illness. Indeed, the majority of clients with Alzheimer's disease also experience concurrent depression, and the differentiation of these two disorders may be difficult if not impossible (K. Solomon, 1982f).

Psychotic Symptoms

Hallucinations are common side effects of a variety of medications, head trauma, other neurologic disorders, endocrine disorders, and any severe acute illness. Paranoid symptoms may be seen in a variety of acute and chronic neurologic diseases, as a manifestation of drug toxicity, and in a variety of endocrine diseases, infections, and post traumatic states, as well as masking depression.

Medical Symptoms

Fatigue

Fatigue is a common symptom of any chronic illness, anemia, malignancies, infectious processes, and as a side effect of medications. It is also a common symptom of depression, Alzheimer's disease, and a variety of labile personality disorders and neuroses.

Constipation

Constipation is seen in a variety of gastrointestinal diseases, as side effects of medications, and as a common complaint of older people who are unaware that the older gastrointestinal tract normally slows down its functioning. Constipation is also frequently seen as a vegetative symptom of depression, obsessive-compulsive personality, and neurotic disorders.

Difficult or Rapid Breathing

Difficulty in breathing or shortness of breath is commonly seen in a variety of pulmonary and cardiovascular diseases. It is also frequent symptom of anxiety (along with hyperventilation) and labile personality disorders.

Weakness

Weakness is part of a variety of chronic musculoskeletal and many neurologic diseases of an acute or chronic nature. It is also a common complaint in Alzheimer's disease, in depression, and in labile personality disorders.

Pain

Pain may be indicative of localized disease or may be referred from disease elsewhere in the body. When accompanied by other physical concommitants of pain (e.g., sweating, facial grimacing, pallor) and if acute in onset, it is almost always due to bodily disease. Chronic pain has both psychologic and physiologic components, and the etiology may be difficult to ascertain. Aside from a legion of chronic physical conditions causing pain, chronic pain is a common symptom of depression, personality disorders, and schizophrenia.

Sleep Difficulties

Although the most common cause of sleep difficulties is depression, this symptom is commonly seen as a result of any chronic illness, the use of hypnotics, the presence of pain or respiratory difficulties, as a response to any acute biologic or psychosocial stress, and the presenting symptom of the primary sleep disorders, especially sleep apnea. It is a frequent end-result of boredom, as the individual takes naps during the day, then goes to bed early, and having had a good night's sleep during the day, still expects to sleep until the usual waking hour. Dreams and nightmares may be side effects of a variety of medications, especially psychotropic drugs.

PRINCIPLES OF INTERVENTION

The goal of intervention is to change symptoms into adequate coping, adaptation, and growth by reversing the psychodynamic schema just cited. Most of this can be accomplished by members of the team, utilizing generalist skills. As Rogers (1959) has pointed out, the major qualities of a good psychotherapist are not technical skills but rather empathy (the ability to psychologically put oneself in the other person's place), unconditional positive regard (the ability to accept the client as he/she is; this is not the same as liking the client), and genuineness (accepting oneself as one is).

Based on the sequence of psychodynamic events outlined earlier in this chapter, intervention should follow a predictable sequence of events. There is some overlap in the sequence to allow for maximal therapeutic flexibility when working with the elderly person with a psychologic disturbance. These principles of intervention hold whether or not the disturbance is primarily organic or functional in nature.

Intervention is divided into two phases. The first is the phase of crisis intervention and may be easily accomplished by mental-health-care workers. This is the reversal of the psychodynamic sequence of events noted in the early part of the chapter. The second phase of therapy is relevant only for those individuals who have a lifelong history of inadequate coping skills or those who wish to pursue further personal growth; it consists of long-term psychotherapy and should be done by a psychotherapist.

Crisis Intervention

The first step in therapy is a direct attack on the symptoms. If the person has psychotic symptoms (mania, delusions, hallucinations), catastrophic reactions, or organically based agitation that has been uncontrolled by nonpharmacologic measures, antipsychotic medication (Table 4-1) is indicated. Antipsychotic medications should not be used as the treatment of symptoms of anxiety, as there is no evidence that these medications are efficacious for these problems (K. Solomon, 1976; K. Solomon and Hart, 1978). Nor should they be used in the treatment of organically based symptoms until the underlying causes of the symptoms are elucidated. If the client meets the criteria for a diagnosis of major depressive disorder, antidepressant medication (Table 4-2) is indicated. Antide-

Table 4-1. Antipsychotic Drugs

I. Phenothiazines

  A. *Aliphatic*
    1. Chlorpromazine (Thorazine)
    2. Promazine (Sparine)
    3. Triflupromazine (Vesprin)

  B. *Piperidine*
    1. Thioridazine (Mellaril)
    2. Mesoridazine (Serentil)
    3. Piperacetazine (Quide)

  C. *Piperazine*
    1. Prochlorperazine (Compazine)
    2. Trifluoperazine (Stelazine)
    3. Butaperazine (Repoise)
    4. Perphenazine (Trilafon)
    5. Fluphenazine (Prolixin, Permitil)
    6. Acetophenazine (Tindal)

II. Thioxanthenes
    1. Chlorprothixene (Taractan)
    2. Thiothixene (Navane)

III. Butyrophenones
    1. Haloperidol (Haldol)

IV. Dihydroindolones
    1. Molindone (Moban, Lidone)

V. Dibenzoxazepines
    1. Loxapine (Loxitane, Daxolin)

Table 4-2. Antidepressant Drugs

I. Tricyclics

  A. *Iminobenzyls*
    1. Imipramine (Tofranil, Presamine, Imavate, Janimine, W. D. D., SK-Pramine)
    2. Trimipramine (Surmontil)
    3. Desipramine (Norpramin, Pertofrane)

  B. *Dibenzoheptadienes*
    1. Amitriptyline (Elavil, Endep)
    2. Nortriptyline (Aventyl, Pamelor)
    3. Protriptyline (Vivactil)

  C. *Dibenzoxepins*
    1. Doxepin (Sinequan, Adapin)

  D. *Dibenzoxazepines*
    1. Amoxapine (Asendin)

(continued)

Table 4-2. (*Continued*)

II. Tetracyclics
    1. Maprotiline (Ludiomil)
    2. Trazodone (Desyrel)

III. Monoamine Oxidase Inhibitors
    1. Isocarboxazid (Marplan)
    2. Tranylcypromine (Parnate)
    3. Phenelzine (Nardil)

pressants should not be used in the treatment of anxiety nor for adjustment disorders, sadness, or grief reactions. If the client is manic, lithium is the treatment of choice.

One must be careful with psychopharmocologic agents in the elderly. The reasons for this can be elucidated by pharmacokinetics of drugs in the elderly (Friedel, 1977). Both therapeutic effects and side effects increase as the concentration of free drug in the blood increases. It takes less medication to provide higher blood levels in the elderly because of changes in the factors responsible for the maintainance of the concentration of drugs in the blood. The absorbed dose may be somewhat erratic, as gastrointestinal motility is diminshed, leading to an increased opportunity for the drug to be absorbed. However, arterial blood flow and transport enzyme activity are diminished, leading to decreased absorption. Because of changes in liver enzyme activity and renal function, the time it takes to metabolize and eliminate the drug is extended, resulting in an increased concentration of the drug in the blood. Since there is proportionally more fat tissue than water in the older body, and psychopharmacologic agents (lithium excepted) are all fat-soluble, this too leads to increased concentration of the drug in the blood. Furthermore, the amount of free drug in the blood also increases as the concentration of albumin diminishes with age (Greenblatt, 1979), reducing plasma binding of the drug. In addition, the central nervous system is more sensitive to the effects of these drugs, and the barrier protecting the brain from drugs is weakened with age, increasing the effects of these drugs in the older person.

Psychotropic drugs have many side effects. Commonly occurring side effects include oversedation, constipation, dry mouth, dizziness, a "drunken" gait, falls, increased anxiety, cognitive disturbances, psychotic symptoms, depression, a metallic taste in the mouth, heartburn, and indigestion. Less common are disturbances of liver function, changes in heart rhythm, allergic reactions (especially skin rashes), increased sensitivity to sunlight, difficulty controlling body temperature in hot environments, increased vulnerability to seizures, anemia, difficulty urinating, high fever, disturbances of endocrine function, increased risk of infections, and sudden death. Specifically, antipsychotic drugs also commonly produce a variety of neurologic side effects resembling Parkinson's disease (tremor, increased muscle tone, difficulty with coordination, gait disturbances, a mask-like face) and a chronic neurologic disorder called tardive dyskinesia, manifested by involuntary wiggling of the facial and tongue muscles, fingers, arms, toes, and torso, and facial grimacing. Thus psychotropic drugs cannot be prescribed with impunity, since they are far from benign. On the other hand, they should always be prescribed when indicated, for therapy will not be of benefit unless the client is capable of responding to it, something precluded by the presence of severe psychopathology.

A variety of nonpharmacologic techniques may be used in the treatment of anxiety. For episodic anxiety, the breathing exercises used in Lamaze childbirth (Bing, 1962) are of help. For more continuous anxiety or tension, relaxation exercises such as described by Jacobson (1938) and Wolpe (1969) may be of help. For some clients, cognitive behavior therapy (Kovacs and Beck, 1978), regular strenuous physical exercise (e.g., jogging or swimming), transcendental meditation, tantric or other forms of yoga, massage or other body work, sex (including masturbation), or biofeedback may also be of benefit in mastering anxiety. Acupressure to the junction of the mastoid process and base of the skull may be helpful in the treatment of tension headache. Because of the unproven efficacy of benzodiazepines (K. Solomon, 1976; K. Solomon and Hart, 1978) and other antianxiety agents such as hydroxyzine or meprobamate (Greenblatt and Shader, 1971), these drugs probably have little place in the treatment of the elderly. However, the sedation caused by benzodiazepines may be helpful as an adjunct treatment for chronic anxiety if nonpharmacologic interventions have not been successful (Table 4-3).

If the older person demonstrated phobic, compulsive, or obsessive symptoms, the use of traditional behavior-modification techniques is indicated (Schaefer and Martin, 1969; Wolpe, 1969). Sexual dysfunctions may be treated by sexual therapies developed by Masters and Johnson (1970). Hypnosis may also be used for specific neurotic symptoms. Acting up, whether it be aggressive, dependent, or helpless, is managed with behavioral paradigms that emphasize environmental manipulation and limit-setting of the inappropriate behavior.

Following the direct attack on symptoms, the therapist next helps the client ventilate the underlying affect. This involves giving the client permission to feel

Table 4-3. Benzodiazepines

1. Chlordiazepoxide (Librium, Libritabs, SK-Lygen)
2. Diazepam (Valium)
3. Oxazepam (Serax)
4. Clorazepate (Tranxene, Azene)
5. Prazepam (Vestran, Centrax)
6. Lorazepam (Ativan)
7. Halazepam (Paxipam)
8. Alprazolam (Xanax)

fear, anger, or loss and to verbalize these feelings. Permission must be especially given to individuals who are afraid of antagonizing the therapist if they get angry at the therapist. It should be made clear that it is "OK" to be angry at members of the team and to direct this anger at them rather than toward oneself. Clients who are particularly labile in expressing affect must learn how to channel affect into verbal communication conducive to therapy. Those who do not express affect must be pushed to do so. Ventilation is sometimes enhanced through the use of movement, poetry, art, or music therapies.

The next step is the minimization of helplessness and dependency. The major modalities used in this part of therapy are environmental manipulation and behavioral techniques. The client is given graduated behavioral tasks that the therapist knows he/she can definitely manage. At first these tasks should be graded according to the individual's current level of functioning. For example, severely depressed individuals may be required just to get out of bed by a certain time. A better-functioning individual may be required to attend a senior center or take care of certain tasks in his/her environment. It is frequently necessary to enlist the aid of family members or other resources in the community to aid in the accomplishment of these tasks. This is especially true if the individual suffers from brain failure. Remotivation and rehabilitative therapies are also quite useful at this juncture in therapy. The patient must internalize feelings that counter helplessness and dependency.

Regaining mastery requires that the client have control over his/her life. That requires choice and options. The client must be told that he/she is responsible for his/her behavior. This responsibility is more than just an existential statement, for without responsibility there can be no need to master and manipulate one's environment. Mastery requires that the older person have choice. The client should be allowed to make all decisions for himself/herself. In an institution, this includes decisions regarding clothing, menu, visitors, activities, and therapeutic goals. The client should not be cut off from his/her network, but must use this network to help maintain autonomy and mastery. The older person must be encouraged to take risks and to try out new options that may not be comfortable for the therapist yet may be comfortable for the older person. For the individual without brain failure, however, these choices require that the therapists give and even create options appropriate for the individual's problems, so that he/she may be able to choose from a wide range of options to resolve the problems that led to the development of the symptomatology.

The last step in this phase of therapy is to attempt to reverse the stress. Losses in the social-support system are frequently managed by helping the individual create a new support system. For example, the older person may attend a senior center, reestablish contact with other family members and friends, or find a new job. Loss of role requires that the individual seek out new meaningful roles, give positive valence to old roles, realign himself/herself with old interests, or attempt to create new roles. The memory deficits of brain failure may be partially reversed with reality orientation and other modalities (Ernst et al., 1978; Stephens, 1969). Specific stresses that can be reversed through appropriate use of the human-service delivery system should be tackled early, as these stresses usually affect basic activities of daily living. A major goal, however, is not to use this system to *do for* the older person (and thus create further dependency and helplessness) but to teach the older person how to advocate for himself/herself and control the human-service delivery system (and thus further mastery, choice, and self-responsibility). For the older person who has previously functioned well, this is frequently all the therapy that is necessary.

Psychotherapy

For those older persons who wish to continue their self-examination and grow or for those individuals with a lifelong history of inadequate coping skills, one then enters the second stage of intervention, the stage of psychotherapy. Older individuals are quite motivated for help, and resistances are fewer. As such, they are quite amenable to various psychotherapeutic modalities.

Therapeutic Modalities

If the problems are primarily intrapsychic, a form of individual psychotherapy is the treatment of choice. For those who are psychologically minded, an insight-oriented psychotherapy (psychoanalysis, psychoanalytically oriented psychotherapy, Gestalt therapy, transactional analysis, client-centered psychotherapy, or existential therapy) is the treatment of choice, occasionally augmented with a movement therapy, such as Feldenkrais or dance therapy, massage therapy, neurolinguistic programming, or art therapy. If the problems are primarily interpersonal, group psychotherapy, family therapy, or marital therapy is indicated. For those individuals who are not good candidates for an insight-oriented psychotherapy, such as those with an overlay of somatization, those who are not psychologically minded, or those who cannot tolerate a transference relationship, long-term supportive psychotherapy may also aid in coping with future stress.

Some technical modifications of psychotherapy may become necessary in working with this age group. Because some clients may fatigue easily, it may be wise to limit sessions to thirty minutes rather than the traditional fifty minutes for these clients. Sessions should be scheduled at such times as to maximize the older person's alertness and diurnal and other biologic rhythms, as well as special travel needs. Many elderly rely on public transportation, limit their driving to daylight hours because of limitations in night vision, or avoid nocturnal excursions into or out of high-crime areas. Taking the history requires a much longer time because there are more years of experience. History-taking should emphasize an assessment of the person's lifelong strengths and how he/she coped with stress (Butler, 1974) so that these techniques may be utilized and reinforced during psychotherapy. As older persons have frequently had many years of self-examination, it may be possible to start psychotherapy at a level of insight that is deeper than with younger clients. In addition, older persons are aware of their limited life span and are more motivated for psychotherapy than are younger persons (LeShan and LeShan, 1961). Because of this, resistances are diminished, which allows for a more rapid identification and working through of major dynamic issues, followed by willingness on the part of the older person to put these insights and affective changes into their behavioral repertoire. Interpretations thus may be given earlier in therapy and concentration on resistances may be minimized.

Techniques of Gestalt therapy and transactional analysis may be particularly helpful in working with an older person with a personality disorder. If there is a degree of somatization, identification of the emotional concomitants of the somatization may be translated into verbal affective statements. For example, somatic pain may first be concretized so that the older person is asked what his/her stomach is feeling. The person is then asked, using a Gestalt technique (Perls, 1969), to translate that into a statement about what he/she is feeling and own the statement and feeling. That statement is then used as a bridge to the identification of the underlying affective state. Once that underlying affective state is identified, the person's maladaptive responses to it can be further identified in a way consistent with supportive or insight-oriented therapy. Because many older people with unresolved dependency issues behave in a childlike way, various transactional analytic techniques, as well as responses to the individual as an adult and pointing out the childlike ways in which he/she behaves, may be a particularly helpful form of interpersonal insight (Maxwell and Falzett, 1974). It is particularly important for the therapist at this stage not to behave in a parental way.

Group psychotherapy with older persons can be quite successful in promoting therapeutic changes (Goldfarb, 1971). It tends to work better when the groups are homogeneous and consist only of older people because many older persons have a reluctance to share in a mixed-age group in which they may be the only older person and in which younger clients dominate. However, in a geriatric therapy group, this is generally not so. In addition, because older psychiatric clients are more likely to be women, there are frequently not enough men in the group to dominate it, thus allowing for greater intimacy and sharing. The group may be utilized to be supportive, to confront, and to suggest specific behavioral modifications, as well as to give insight and feedback on the interpersonal aspects of the individual's personality disorder. Group psychotherapy is partic-ularly helpful in individuals with dependent personality disorders or passive-aggressive personality disorders because the group is frequently unwilling to tolerate the pathologic behavior, thus forcing change in the maladaptive responses to stress with the support and advice of the group. In addition, as there is an element of social isolation in many elderly clients, the group brings to the client a consistent social network that can be expected to be helpful in times of crisis (K. Solomon and Zinke, 1981).

Family or couple psychotherapy may consist of a behaviorally oriented approach in which the family is used as behavioral engineers to modify—with classical reinforcement, extinction, or punishment paradigms—the behaviors of the identified client. Or a communications, functional, or structural model may be utilized to help clarify the person's needs and to help the family members or spouse behave in a way that maximizes appropriate response-outcome. With the relatively nonverbal individual with interpersonal difficulties living at home, utilization of a family member or a substitute for a family member, such as a home-health aide, as an intervenor may be an important element in family or behavioral therapy.

For clients with severe dependency needs or for those who are schizoid, day hospitalization or attendance at special social groups for the elderly may be helpful. These social groups may involve nonthreatening activities and may allow for the gradual desensitization of the older withdrawn individual to a social network that may be supportive. Day hospitalization may allow clients to structure their lives. In the context of nonthreatening recreational activities, plus therapeutically oriented groups and individual sessions, moderate success can result with a severely disturbed older person with a dependent, schizoid, or schizotypal personality disorder. In addition, ancillary social and rehabilitative services may be necessary and helpful within the context of any of the therapeutic modalities. There may be a need to teach budgeting, shopping, or advocacy skills, especially for the chronically dependent or schizoid individual. Assurance that the older person is receiving appropriate and complete social services such as food stamps, Medicare, etc. may become an important part of developing the therapeutic alliance as well as a way of minimizing some of the social and day-to-day stresses on the client that would interfere with ongoing therapy.

Transference Issues

Major transference issues develop during the course of any psychotherapy. A particularly important one in working with the elderly is the development of dependency upon the therapist. The therapist is frequently perceived as a consistently caring and nurturing individual (a perfect mother), who is always helping out and who frequently does so in concrete ways. The older person, especially one with conflicts around dependency needs, may transfer dependency from family or social network to the therapist and may expect the therapist to make all major and minor life decisions for the client. Some therapists, such as Goldfarb (1968, 1974), encourage the dependency in the hope that the client will identify with the therapist and incorporate the therapist's superego as his/her own, thus leading to changes in maladaptive interpersonal paradigms. Thus, even after termination of therapy, the dependency is encouraged so that therapeutic headway may continue. Others therapists, myself included, emphasize growth and autonomy on the part of the older client and tend to de-emphasize dependency. In therapy with older clients, I prefer to emphasize choice, responsibility, and risk-taking behaviors to try out new interpersonal skills that are necessary to maximize autonomy and independent functioning on the part of the older client.

Parentification of the therapist is an important form of transference in psychotherapy for the elderly with personality disorders. In many ways this parentification is no different from the parentification seen in the context of any transference relationship, in which the therapist is seen as if he/she were various significant others in the client's life. However, because the parents of older clients are frequently either deceased, ill, or dealing with many of the same stresses as the older client, parentification brings out many unresolved psychodynamic issues related to loss, separation, and parent/child relations that have been repressed for several generations. Thus parentification becomes an important part of the therapeutic involvement as it rapidly brings up important dynamic issues that are dealt with by the usual psychotherapeutic modalities of explanation, clarification, questioning, and interpretation (Bibring, 1954; Olinick, 1954). Goldfarb (1968, 1974) emphasized parentification without interpretation, so that the elderly client will identify with the therapist to facilitate the incorporation of the therapist's superego. I prefer to interpret it, so as to foster resolution of the conflicts noted immediately preceding.

On the other hand, however, the client is usually older and frequently quite significantly older than the therapist. The individual may infantilize the therapist and may relate to the therapist either as a child or a grandchild. This brings up important therapeutic issues, especially intergenerational issues and issues of control and dependency, for the therapist is seen as if he/she were the patient's own child or grandchild.

Countertransference Issues

Countertransference issues are many in psychotherapy with older individuals. As just mentioned, adherence to stereotypes may lead to an inappropriate denial of the therapeutic growth potential of the older client as well as the inappropriate reinforcement of dependency and helplessness of the older client. In addition, working with the older client may bring up many anxieties and stresses about the therapist's own aging, which leads both to status inconsistency and to a state of cognitive dissonance (Festinger, 1957). A frequent response to these states in dealing with the elderly is to reinforce the stereotypes of older people (K. Solomon, 1979a), which then becomes a therapeutic blind spot in working with older clients. Stereotyping and the subsequent development of learned helplessness can be combatted through a variety of educational and experiential techniques that emphasize issues of the therapist's own aging, demythologizing, correction of cognitive dissonance, and the development of nonstereotyped attitudes towward the elderly. (K. Solomon, 1983a, K. Solomon and Vickers, 1980, 1981).

Because of the age differential between therapist and client, the therapist may parentify the client, which may have important consequences as the therapist may fear bringing up certain dynamic issues because they are unresolved between him/her and his/her parents. The therapist may not allow himself/herself to experience anger at the client and therefore may allow the client to act out or to continue various forms of maladaptive behavior rather than confronting the effects of the behaviors. The therapist may be overly gentle or may avoid dealing with issues related to sexuality in the older client because of countertransference problems.

On the other hand, the therapist may infantilize the older client. The infantilization may take the form of being overly helpful and reinforcing dependency on the part of the client. This may lead to a crisis in therapy as the therapist has to deal with his/her own relationship with his/her children. Infantilization also diminishes the growth potential or therapy as well as leading to a gentleness in therapy that may be inappropriate.

Other issues that the therapist must deal with when doing psychotherapy with older people are the issues of illness and death. Older persons miss sessions when they become acutely ill or suffer exacerbations of chronic medical illness that may or may not require hospitalization. The vulnerability of the client, the therapist, and the therapy then become important issues with which the therapist, too, must work and leads to many existential questions, such as limits, attitudes, *weltanschauungen,* and the meaning of life, which the therapist may not have worked thorough with himself/herself. Illness interrupts the flow of therapeutic sessions and, if accompanied by brain changes such as delirium, may actually lead to a major therapeutic reversal; it may take months of therapy to regain premorbid levels of psychologic functioning. Medical illness also leads to the prescription of drugs that may adversely interact with either the person's psyche or with psychotropic medications that may be prescribed.

Dying may be an acute or a chronic, protracted process. In any case, it may lead to the therapist being unable or unwilling to work with the client during his/her final hours, when the therapist may be most needed. The therapist may be angry at the client for leaving and may take out his/her anger by missing or canceling sessions, being late for sessions, or prematurely terminating therapy. The therapist has to experience and work with his/her own grief over the loss of the client. The loss is not only that of the individual client, but also loss and grief as a generic life issue. Because death is a frequent occurrence in the life of the therapist working with the elderly, the therapist must confront his/her own finitude and limits of his/her own life.

WHEN TO CALL THE PHYSICIAN

All clients with major psychopathology who have not had a thorough medical evaluation should be evaluated by a physician, who can complete the physical examination, neurologic examination, and laboratory examination portions of the psychogeriatric examination. If there is any question about the possibility of drug interactions, drug side effects, or medical diseases that may cause psychopathology, or if information about the client's medical condition and prognosis are germane to the therapeutic process, referral to a physician is also necessary. Referral is necessary whenever the client develops new medical symptoms, even if the therapist suspects that these symptoms are psychogenic in origin. A geropsychiatrist should see the client if the client has symptoms of major psychopathology for which psychopharmacologic intervention is necessary or if the mental-health worker simply feels the need for counsultation and another opinion, even if things are going well therapeutically. In choosing medical/psychiatric consultants, it is important to choose a physician with skills working with the elderly and with positive attitudes toward this age group.

REFERENCES

Adams, F. D. (1958). *Physical diagnosis.* Baltimore: Williams and Wilkins.

Akisal, H. S., and McKinney, W. T. Jr. (1975). Overview of recent research in depression: Integration of ten conceptual models into a comprehensive clinical frame. *Archives of General Psychiatry,* **32**, 285-305.

American Psychiatric Association (1980). *Diagnostic and statistical manual of mental disorders* (3rd ed.). Washington: American Psychiatric Association.

Ayd, F. J. Jr. (1975). Treatment-resistant patients: A moral, legal and therapeutic challenge. In F. J. Ayd, Jr. (Ed.), *Rational psychopharmacotherapy and the right to treatment.* Baltimore: Ayd Medical Communications.

Ban, T. (1978). The treatment of depressed geriatric patients. *American Journal of Psychotherapy,* **32**, 93-104.

Bibring, E. (1954). Psychoanalysis and the dynamic psychotherapies. *Journal of the American Psychoanalytic Association,* **2**, 745-770.

Bibring, E. (1961). The mechanism of depression. In P. Greenacre (Ed.), *Affective disorders.* New York: International Universities Press.

Bing, E. (1962). *Six practical lessons for an easier childbirth.* New York: Bantam.

Blazer, D., and Williams, C. D. (1980). Epidemiology of dysphoria and depression in an elderly population. *American Journal of Psychiatry,* **137**, 439-444.

Bonime, W. (1966). The psychodynamics of neurotic depression. In S. Arieti (Ed.), *American handbook of psychiatry* (1st ed.), vol. 3, New York: Basic Books.

Brody, E. B. (1974). Psychosocial aspects of prejudice. In S. Arieti et al. (Eds.), *American handbook of psychiatry* (2nd ed.), vol. 2. New York: Basic Books.

Butler, R. N. (1974). Successful aging and the role of life review. *Journal of the American Geriatrics Society,* **12**, 529-532.

Butler, R. N. (1975). *Why survive? Being old in America.* New York: Harper & Row.

Cohen, R. E. (1973). The collaborative co-professional: Developing a new mental helath role. *Hospital and Community Psychiatry,* **24**, 242-246.

Delp, M. H. (1968). Study of the patient. In M. H. Delp and R. T. Manning (Eds.), *Major's physical diagnosis.* Philadelphia: Saunders.

Ernst, P., Beran, B., Safford, F., and Kleinhauz, M. (1978). Isolation and the symptoms of chronic brain syndrome.*Gerontologist,* **18**, 468-474.

Exton-Smith, A. N., and Overstall, P. W. (1979). *Geriatrics.* Baltimore: University Park Press.

Festinger, L. (1957). *A theory of cognitive dissonance.* Stanford: Stanford University Press.

Friedel, R. O. (1977). Pharmacokinetics of psychotherapeutic agents in aged patients. In C. Eisdorfer and R. O. Friedel (Eds.), *Cognitive and emotional disturbance in the elderly.* Chicago: Year Book Medical Publishers.

Friedland, E. (1967). Clinical clerk case study outline. Buffalo: State University of New York at Buffalo.

Friedmann, E. A., and Orbach, H. L. (1974). Adjustment to retirement. In S. Arieti et al. (Eds.), *American handbook of psychiatry* (2nd ed.), vol. 1. New York: Basic Books.

Goldfarb, A. I. (1968). Clinical perspectives. In A. Simon and L. J. Epstein (Eds.), *Aging in modern society.* Washington: American Psychiatric Association.

Goldfarb, A. I. (1971). Group therapy with the old and aged. In H. I. Kaplan and B. J. Sadock (Eds.), *Comprehensive group therapy.* Baltimore: Williams & Wilkins.

Goldfarb, A. I. (1974). Minor maladjustments of the aged. In S. Arieti et al. (Eds.), *American handbook of psychiatry* (2nd ed.), vol. 3. New York: Basic Books.

Greenblatt, D. J. (1979). Reduced serum albumin concentration in the elderly: A report from the Boston Collaborative Drug Surveillance Program. *Journal of the American Geriatrics Society* **27**, 20-22.

Greenblatt, D. J., and Shader, R. I. (1971). Meprobamate: A study of irrational drug use. *American Journal of Psychiatry* **127**, 1297-1303.

Gutmann, D., Grunes, J., and Griffin, B. (1979). *The clinical psychology of later life: Developmental paradigms.* Paper presented at the 32nd Annual Meeting of the Gerontological Society, Nov. 29, Washington, D.C.

Harris, M., and Solomon, K. (1979). Roles of the community mental health nurse. *Journal of Psychiatric Nursing and Mental Health Services* **15**, 35-39.

Holmes, T. H., and Rahe, R. H. (1967). The social readjustment rating scale. *Journal of Psychosomatic Research* **11**, 213-218.

Howard, M. (1979). *The community mental health nurse and geropsychiatry.* (1979). Paper presented at the 32nd Annual Meeting of the Gerontological Society, Nov. 26, Washington, D. C.

Isaacs, A. D. (1973). Geriatric psychiatry. *Practitioner* **210**, 86-95.

Jacobson, E. (1938). *Progressive relaxation.* Chicago: University of Chicago Press.

Judge, R. D., and Zuidema, G. D. (1963). *Physical diagnosis: A physiologic approach.* Boston: Little, Brown.

Kahn, R. L. (1978). *Learned helplessness and cognitive impairment in the elderly.* Paper presented at the 31st Annual Meeting of the Gerontological Society, Nov. 19, San Francisco.

Kay, D. W. K. (1977). The epidemiology and identification of brain deficit in the elderly. In C. Eisdorfer and R. O. Friedel (Eds.), *Cognitive and emotional disturbances in the elderly.* Chicago: Year Book Medical Publishers.

Kay, D. W. K., Cooper, A. F., and Garside, R. R. (1976). The differentiation of paranoid from affective psychoses by patients' premorbid characteristics. *British Journal of Psychiatry,* **129**, 207-215.

Kendell, R. E., Brockington, I. F., and Leff, J. P. (1979). Prognostic implications of six alternative definitions of schizophrenia. *Archives of General Psychiatry,* **36**, 25-31.

104   K. Solomon

Kolb, L. C. (1975). Disturbances of the body-image. In S. Arieti et al. (Eds.), *American handbook of psychiatry* (2nd ed.), vol. 4. New York: Basic Books.

Kovacs, M., and Beck, A. T. (1978). Maladaptive cognitive structures in depression. *American Journal of Psychiatry*, **135**, 525-533.

LeShan, L., and LeShan, E. (1961). Psychiatry and the patient with a limited life span. *Psychiatry* **24**, 318-322.

Libow, L. S. (1973). Pseudo-senility: Acute and reversible organic brain syndromes. *Journal of the American Geriatrics Society*, **21**, 112-121.

Mace, N. L., and Rabins, P. V. (1982). *The 36-hour day: A family guide to caring for persons with Alzheimer's disease, related dementing illnesses, and memory loss in later life*. Baltimore: John Hopkins University Press.

MacKinnon, R. A. (1980). Psychiatric history and mental status examination. In H. I. Kaplan, A. M. Freedman, and B. J. Sadock (Eds.), *Comprehensive textbook of psychiatry* (3rd ed.), vol. 1. Baltimore: Williams & Wilkins.

Maier, S. F., and Seligman, M. E. P. (1976). Learned helplessness: Theory and evidence. *Journal of Experimental Psychology: General* **105**, 3-46.

Masters, W. H., and Johnson, V. E. (1966). *Human sexual response*. Boston: Little, Brown.

Masters, W. H., and Johnson, V. E. (1970). *Human sexual inadequacy*. Boston: Little, Brown.

Maxwell, J., and Falzett, B. (1974). *OK childing and parenting*. El Paso: Transactional Institute of El Paso.

Menninger, K. A. (1962). *A manual for psychiatric case study* (2nd ed.). New York: Grune & Stratton.

Olinick, S. L. (1954). Some considerations of the use of questioning as a psychoanalytic technique. *Journal of the American Psychoanalytic Association*, **2**, 57-66.

Perls, F. (1969). *Gestalt therapy verbatim*. Lafayette: Real People Press.

Pons, S. L. (1979). *Roles of the community geropsychiatric social worker.* Paper presented at the 32nd Annual Meeting of the Gerontological Society, Nov. 26, Washington, D.C.

Post, F. (1968). Psychological aspects of geriatrics. *Postgraduate Medical Journal*, **44**, 307-318.

Redick, R. W., Kramer, M., and Taube, C. A. (1973). Epidemiology of mental illness and utilization of psychiatric facilities among older persons. In E. W. Busse and E. Pfeiffer (Eds.), *Mental illness in later life*. Washington: American Psychiatric Association.

Rogers, C. R. (1959). A theory of therapy, personality and interpersonal relationships as developed in client-centered framework. In S. Koch (Ed.), *Psychology: A study of a science*. New York: McGraw-Hill.

Romaniuk, M. (1979). *A look at the psychologist's role on a community geropsychiatry team.* Paper presented at the 32nd Annual Meeting of the Gerontological Society, Nov. 26, Washington, D.C.

Rosow, I. (1976). Status and role change through the life span. In R. H. Binstock and E. Shanas (Eds.), *Handbook of aging and the social sciences*. New York: Van Nostrand Reinhold.

Ryan, W. (1976). *Blaming the victim*. New York: Vintage.

Sartorius, N. (1975). Epidemiology of depression. *WHO Chronicles*, **29**, 423.

Schaefer, H. H., and Martin, P. L. (1969). *Behavioral therapy*. New York: McGraw-Hill.

Seligman, M. E. P. (1975). *Helplessness*. San Francisco: W. H. Freeman.

Selye, H. (1950). *The physiology and pathology of exposure to stress*. Montreal: Acta.

Sheppard, H. L. (1976). Work and retirement. In R. M. Binstock and E. Shanas (Eds.), *Handbook of aging and the social sciences*. New York: Van Nostrand Reinhold.

Smith, F. S. (1972). *Definition of a generalist* (mimeo.). Albany: Capital District Psychiatric Center.

Solomon, K. (1976). Benzodiazepines and neurotic anxiety: Critique. *New York State Journal of Medicine*, **76**, 2156-2164.

Solomon, K. (1979a). The development of stereotypes of the elderly: Toward a unified hypothesis. In E. P. Lewis, L. D. Nelson, D. H. Scully, and J. S. Williams (Eds.), *Sociological research symposium proceedings (IX)*. Richmond: Virginia Commonwealth University.

Solomon, K. (1979b). *The geropsychiatrist and the delivery of mental services in the community.* Paper presented at the 32nd Annual Meeting of the Gerontological Society, Washington, D.C.

Solomon, K. (1979c). Social antecedents of learned helplessness of the elderly in the health care setting. In E. P. Lewis, L. D. Nelson, D. H. Scully, and J. S. Williams (Eds.), *Sociological research symposium proceedings (IX)*. Richmond: Virginia Commonwealth University.

Solomon, K. (1981a). The depressed patient: Social antecedents of psychopathologic changes in the elderly. *Journal of the American Geriatrics Society.* **29**, 14-18.

Solomon, K. (1981b). Personality disorders in the elderly. In J. R. Lion (Ed.), *Personality disorders: Diagnosis and management* (2nd ed.). Baltimore: Williams & Wilkins.

Solomon, K. (1982a). The elderly patient. In J. A. Spittell, Jr. (Ed.), *Clinical medicine*, vol. 12, *Psychiatry.* Hagerstown: Harper & Row.

Solomon, K. (1982b). The masculine gender role: Description. In K. Solomon and N. B. Levy (Eds.), *Men in transition: Theory and therapy.* New York: Plenum.

Solomon, K. (1982c). The older man. In K. Solomon and N. B. Levy (Eds.), *Men in transition: Theory and therapy.* New York: Plenum.

Solomon, K. The roles of the psychiatric resident on a community psychiatric team. (1982d). *Psychiatric Quarterly,* **54**, 67-76.

Solomon, K. (1982e). Social antecedents of learned helplessness in the health care setting. *Gerontologist,* **22**, 282-287.

Solomon, K. (1982f). The subjective experience of the Alzheimer's patient. *Geriatric Consultant,* **1**, 22-24.

Solomon, K. (1983a). Intervention for the victimized elderly and sensitization of health professionals: Therapeutic and educational efforts. In J. I. Kosberg (Ed.), *The abuse and maltreatment of the elderly.* Boston: Wright-PSG.

Solomon, K. (1983b). Victimization by health professionals and the psychologic response of the elderly. In J. I. Kosberg (Ed.), *The abuse and maltreatment of the elderly.* Boston: Wright-PSG.

Solomon, K. (1983c). Assessment of psychosocial status in the aged. In O. L. Jackson (Ed.), *Clinics in physical therapy,* vol. 6, *Geriatrics.* New York: Churchill Livingstone.

Solomon, K. (1984). The geriatric patient with cognitive dysfunction. In L. Robinson (Ed.), *Psychological aspects of care of hospitalized patients.* Philadelphia: F. A. Davis.

Solomon, K., and Hart, R. (1978). Pitfalls and prospects in clinical research on antianxiety drugs: Benzodiazepines and placebo—A research review. *Journal of Clinical Psychiatry,* **39**, 823-831.

Solomon, K., and Hurwitz, R. (1982). *Stress, coping, and the older gay man.* Paper presented at the 59th Annual Meeting of the American Orthopsychiatric Association, Apr. 2, San Francisco.

Solomon, K., and Vickers, R. (1979). Attitudes of health workers toward old people. *Journal of the American Geriatrics Society,* **27**, 186-191.

Solomon, K., and Vickers, R. (1980). *Stereotyping the elderly: Changing the attitudes of clinicians.* Paper presented at the 33rd Annual Meeting of the Gerontological Society of America, Nov. 25, San Diego.

Solomon, K., and Vickers, R. (1981). *Stereotyping the elderly: Further research on changing the attitudes of clinicians.* Paper presented at the 34th Annual Meeting of the Gerontological Society of America and the 10th Annual Meeting of the Canadian Association on Gerontology, Nov. 10, Toronto.

Solomon, K., and Zinke, M. R. (1981). *Group psychotherapy with the depressed elderly.* Paper presented at the 58th Annual Meeting of the American Orthopsychiatric Association, Mar. 31, New York.

Solomon, P. (1961). *Sensory deprivation.* Cambridge: Harvard University Press.

Stephens, L. (1969). *Reality orientation: A technique to rehabilitate elderly and brain damaged patients with a moderate to severe degree of disorientation.* Washington: American Psychiatric Association.

Stevenson, I., and Sheppe, W. M. Jr. (1974). The psychiatric examination. In S. Arieti et al. (Eds.), *American handbook of psychiatry* (2nd ed.), vol. 1. New York: Basic Books.

Tuckman, J., and Lorge, I. (1953). Attitudes toward old people. *Journal of Social Psychology* **37**, 249-260.

Verwoerdt, A. (1976). *Clinical geropsychiatry.* Baltimore: Williams & Wilkins.

Weiss, J. A. M. (1973). The natural history of antisocial attitudes: What happens to psychopaths? *Journal of Geriatric Psychiatry,* **6**, 236-242.

Weiss, J. A. M. (1974). Suicide. In S. Arieti et al. (Eds.), *American handbook of psychiatry* (2nd ed.), vol. 3. New York: Basic Books.

Whybrow, P. C., and Hurwitz, T. (1976). Psychological disturbances associated with endocrine disease and hormone therapy. In E. J. Sachar (Ed.), *Hormones, behavior, and psychopathology.* New York: Raven Press.

Wilson, R. N. (1970). *The sociology of health: An introduction.* New York: Random House.

Wolff, C. T. (1977). Loss, grief, and mourning in adults. In R. C. Simons and H. Pardes (Eds.), *Understanding human behavior in health and illness.* Baltimore: Williams & Wilkins.

Wolpe, J. (1969). *The practice of behavior therapy.* New York: Pergamon Press.

Zusman, J. (1966). Some explanations of the changing appearance of psychotic patients: Antecedents of the social breakdown syndrome concept. *Milbank Memorial Fund Quarterly,* **44** (Suppl.), 366-396.

PART III

TREATMENT AND INTERVENTION MODALITIES

5

Access Assistance and Case Management

Raymond M. Steinberg, D.S.W.

Andrus Gerontology Center
University of Southern California

How do older people and their families find their way to the vast array of
programs and services such as those described in this handbook? How does the
complex and often overloaded service system reach out and facilitate the
elderly's search for help in trouble, in the maintenance of independence, and in
the enrichment of the quality of life? This chapter addresses a number of
interventions aimed at making connections between those who most need an
available service and the service (or combination of services) that is most
appropriate to their needs and entitlements. Some of these intervention programs
(such as case advocacy and case management) not only connect those who
seek service with responsible agencies but also serve such supplementary
functions as broadening public awareness about problems and remedies,
monitoring effective service delivery, assisting agencies in reaching or working
with hard-to-serve clientele, and documenting needs for improving the community's service-delivery system.

Access assistance and case management will be discussed from a variety of
professional perspectives: the front-line practitioner dealing directly with clients,
the program planner or agency administrator, and the interagency-system
coordinator. Since this is a program domain in which there is very little
standardization of jargon or uniformity in standards of program or practice,
alternative names for services will be listed, alerting the reader to variations
across the country.

NEED

The need to facilitate access to appropriate services in behalf of elderly clients must be viewed from three perspectives, that of the overall system of services, that of the individual program that must supplement its own resources through coordination with other programs, and that of the client. In spite of a very large number of programs in each locality that purport to link clients to services and to coordinate service delivery to individuals and families, the needs for access assistance and case management with the older adult population remain largely unmet (Bertsche and Horejsi, 1980; U.S. General Accounting Office, 1978, 1979a). Many older persons are not connecting at all with services they need, others are finding partial or incoherent combinations of services, and others are receiving services that are, at best, failing to address their most important problems or, at worst, having harmful effects on their well-being. While some deficiencies are the result of gaps in available services, ineffective services, and clients whose resistive behavior works against their own best interests, a great many of the problems can be traced to mismatches between persons and services.

The Service System Level

In the United States there is no centralized authority with absolute control over what services are set in place and whom they are required to serve. It may be said that we tend to have a nonsystem. In this chapter the word *services* is given its broadest possible connotation, referring not only to psychosocial and medical services, but also to housing, home helps, nutrition, transportation, income assistance, education, etc. No one agency can rationalize the planning, interlinking, and distribution of this vast and intricate maze. Access assistance and comprehensive case management are necessary, and must be custom-designed for each locality for a variety of reasons (Aiken et al., 1975; American Health Planning Assn., 1982; Callahan, 1980; Coward, 1979; Holmes et al., 1979; Horejsi, 1978; John, 1977; Kahn, 1970, 1976; Steinberg, 1978; Taietz, 1970; Tobin et al., 1976).

Each Locality's Service System Is Complex

Human-service programs are offered not only by governmental agencies but also by nonprofit voluntary agencies (such as those subsidized by United Way). In addition, many similar programs are provided by proprietary agencies (for profit) to clients who can afford to pay or who are covered by insurance for that kind of service. Usually "function follows funding"—that is, different funding sources subsidize particular kinds of services to selected groups in the population. These categorical funding patterns from a multiplicity of sources result in fragmentation, duplication, and gaps in the array of services available in a locality. At the same time, growth in consumerism (which increases demands for excellence in service) as well as professionalism (which sometimes promotes differentiated turfs) have tended to increase agency specialization.

Services Are Not Standardized

Each locality in the United States has its unique history in the development of its human-service system. Variations occur based on local values, economic circumstances, population size, and pure accident. Therefore, which services were set in place by which sponsor over history will influence today's distribution of functions and the constraints placed on service delivery. In the 1960s and 1970s the federal government played a strong role in promoting needed services around the country to reduce discrepancies between localities in quality and quantity of services. One example was the Older Americans Act, which promoted the development of state units on aging and Area Agencies on Aging (AAAs) and through these planning and coordinating entities established nationwide networks of such programs as nutrition (congregate and home-delivered meals), information and referral, legal services, and nursing-home ombudsmen. While these federal initiatives did much to reduce the inequities among communities (especially the 1973 Comprehensive Services Amendments to the Older Americans Act of 1965 and Title XX of the Social Security Act), the act was also a mandate to decentralize the planning and monitoring of new programs. This decentralization (or "federalism") approach, which continues into the 1980s, permits local adaptation in the organization and policies of service programs that receive federal subsidy. Consequently, what is known as "home chore" in one locality may be referred to as "attendant care" or "homemaker" in another. Numerous national trade associations attempt to act as standard-setting bodies through education and persuasion, but they usually do not have power to impose minimum-quality controls on their member agencies. State governments have authority to enforce standards in some kinds of services, such as nursing homes. However, enforcement personnel are usually in short supply and standards are not uniform from state to state.

Programs Are Constantly Changing

Much of the rapid change in services to the aging in recent years can be traced to the decentralized "seed money" programs of the Older Americans Act. In addition, exposés of discrimination against the elderly in service delivery (U.S.

Commission on Civil Rights, 1977) and the growing political impact of "gray power" resulted in mandates to serve the elderly in other federally initiated programs such as mental health and public-service employment. The rising national and local consciousness of the elderly resulted in numerous privately sponsored and supported programs through service clubs, religious groups, and employment-related associations. State governments also instituted state-level older American acts and passed legislation to reform long-term care with goals of cost containment and deinstitutionalization. At the same time, tax-payer revolts have directly and indirectly caused cutbacks in agency budgets while increasing the conditions that contribute to individual needs (such as delayed care and reduced income). All these influences have resulted in constantly shifting policies, procedures, and levels of service at the local level. These changes make it difficult for laymen and most professionals to keep up to date about what services are available.

Resources to Meet Human Needs Are in Short Supply and Cannot Be Wasted

The United States is clearly not yet committed to universal coverage for social services as has been the case in public education. Therefore social-service planners have had to "make do" with scarcities of resources (Kahn, 1969, 1970; Kane and Kane, 1980; Kutza, 1980). Faced with hard choices in setting priorities, professional planners and their boards of directors, advisory bodies, and task forces have had to address such questions as the following: Of all the kinds of services that people need, which ones will be maintained? Of all the kinds of people who need services, which people will be eligible for service first? If we cannot serve people for as long as they need the services, what should be the limits of duration of a service to a given individual? To what extent should service recipients (or their families) be required to pay at least a part of the cost (Monk, 1979)? Since high-quality service usually costs more, what should be the minimum standard of acceptability? The decisions that local communities make about these priorities will affect their array of services. Since the resulting variations cannot be anticipated in any text for national distribution, laymen and professionals must reorient their knowledge of programs in terms of their locality and in terms of variations between subareas of their community.

The Program Level

Programs Need to Reach Their Appropriate Target Populations

Usually an agency has far more people apply for service than it can serve. If the agency fails to screen applicants, it may fail to meet the goals for which it was established. Numerous evaluations have shown, for example, that alternatives to institutionalization, such as adult day-care and protective services, did not reach their intended target population—those at risk of institutionalization (Holmes and Hudson, 1975; Horowitz and Estes, 1971; John, 1977; Steinberg and Jurkiewicz, 1980; Weissert, Wan, and Livieratos, 1980). Other programs, such as new community-care organizations, developed long waiting lists that included people with more urgent needs than those who had entered the program during its initial months (Quinn, 1975). At the same time, many service providers fail to include an equitable number of elderly or minority elderly if they do not make special efforts to do so (Group for the Advancement of Psychiatry, 1971; Holmes et al., 1979). Therefore, it is important for each agency that other agencies and community leaders who refer clients are well aware of what the agency offers and who can and cannot be served. The same agency, in turn, has a responsibility to refer those it cannot serve to a more suitable program.

Programs Must Be Concerned with the "Whole Person" and Obtain Supplementary Services That Their Clients Need

There is increasing recognition of the fact that when one area of functioning becomes impaired in old age there is likely to be a domino effect on other areas of independent functioning. The interrelationships of problems and the interdependencies of solutions result in the need for agencies that serve the elderly to connect their clients with other agencies, to work in multidisciplinary teams, and to maintain other coordinative linkages with a network of agencies (Duke University, 1973; Rao, 1977; White, 1980). For example, a home-delivered meals program may be serving an elder who is physically mobile but too depressed to prepare her own meals or go out to a congregate meals site. Arthritis pains contribute to the depression. Consequently, a viable long-range solution may involve a physician, a physical therapist, a mental-health clinic, and a transportation or escort service as well as family counseling with relatives.

The Client Level

Many Older Persons Are Not Socialized to Trust or Utilize Human-Service Agencies

It must be kept in mind that many of today's elders were not born in the hospital and that in their youth there were few human-service programs. Obtaining help from outside the family was considered shameful. Many of today's elders were immigrants from countries where government officials were deeply mistrusted or where a personal introduction by an influencial friend was necessary to get a response. For some of these immigrants, language problems constitute a barrier to appropriate service. Therefore, in addition to the confusing maze of service programs and entitlements, there is a built-in attitudinal resistance to seeking help from public programs (Cuellar and Weeks, 1980; Guttman, 1980; Nuttbrock and Kosberg, 1980; O'Brien and Wagner, 1980). It is not true that people resist service more as they grow older. It is rather a matter of which era they were raised in. Thus some who are now the "young old," who participated in the labor and civil-rights movements, who were helped to survive in the New Deal or Great Society programs of the 1930s and 1960s, or who spent many work years anticipating Social Security benefits, are less prone to reject services now or in the future when needs may arise. The relatively broad participation of elders in such activities as AAA advisory councils, silver-haired legislatures, senior advocacy organizations, and special housing projects, combined with higher educational levels, will increase senior demands for service as each successive age cohort encounters personal needs for help.

Older Persons, and Their Significant Others, Do Not Know What Service Options Are Available to Them

Not only the elders but their middle-aged children as well tend to hold on to old stereotypes that older people inevitably go to nursing homes or homes for the aged, or that an older person who fails to be 100 percent capable in independent living will be whisked off to a mental institution by officials (Louis Harris and Associates, 1975). Slowly the public media and word of mouth are getting the message out that community-based and home-based services can be provided and that the older person has a right of choice to be in the least restrictive environment. Many private practitioners to whom elders and their families turn for advice—physicians, lawyers, and clergy—are not well informed about these alternatives, and some do not have the time to seek out information. As a result, many elders remain unserved or served in an inappropriate way.

Older Persons Need to Be Steered Away from Services That Can Be Harmful in Their Particular Cases

In most cases, access to services improves the conditions of older people if an appropriate match is made (Perlman, 1975; U.S. General Accounting Office, 1977a, 1979b, 1982). The right match depends on accurate assessment of clients. There is striking evidence of the potential benefits of services. The General Accounting Office (GAO), which is the research arm of Congress, applied the Duke University OARS assessment tool for a vast longitudinal study of the well-being of older people in Cleveland (U.S. General Accounting Office, 1977b, 1979a). Persons who had not received needed help in 1975 *and* who were receiving all help needed in 1976 were compared, by GAO, with others who did not receive such help in either year. In terms of percentages, more than eight times as many recipients (73.5 percent) improved in health status as compared with nonrecipients (8.9 percent), while about five times as many non-recipients (18.9 percent) worsened compared with service recipients (3.8 percent). The GAO found that "older people who receive assessment and referral are more likely to receive other appropriate services."

However, if there is a mismatch of people and services the results can be deadly. Numerous studies have shown that from 10 to 30 percent of people in nursing homes could have been cared for at home or at a lesser cost group-care setting. Other research has shown little or no difference in health, physical functioning, or social supports between those who enter institutions and those who do not (Branch and Jette, 1982). Some of the difference can be explained in terms of differences in people's value preferences (Brody, 1969; Steinberg and Carter, 1983). Other differences have been documented in the way people are assessed and placed, often with misinformation about the options and the limitations of agency and family time to make alternative arrangements. Experimental demonstration-program evaluations such as those of the Georgia Alternative Health Services Project (Skellie and Coan, 1980; U.S. General Accounting Office, 1982) have shown that, given particular levels of impairment, elders who avoid long nursing-home stays through the use of home services may live as much as two years longer or feel more satisfaction with their lives (Hodgson and Quinn, 1980; Stassen and Holohan, 1980).

Another kind of mismatch was identified by Sherwood and Morris (1981) in their evaluation of an emergency alarm and response system for the aged (Lifeline; see next section on interventions). In this Boston experiment, Lifeline users, on the average, needed only one nursing-home day for every thirteen days used by persons without the Lifeline service. But when the evaluators looked more closely at which users benefited most, they found that those who benefited from the program were those who were functionally impaired and *not* socially isolated, while the functionally impaired *and* socially isolated (who were assumed to need it most) were *harmed by the use of the service.* Sherwood and Morris state:

. . . too often, based on "needs assessment," professionals dispense services to those they *think* need them, without having hard evidence on which clients, in fact, would be most benefitted, and which would be harmed by the use of the service.

Frankfather, Smith, and Caro (1981), in evaluating New York's Family Support Program, drew attention to the problems of a lack of fit between the value preferences of the elderly clients, family members, and service providers. They reported that usually the providers' preference prevailed, and concluded:

The professionals' method of negotiating [care plans] indicates a need for more-stringent user protection. It is important to retain some program discretion, especially for the severely disabled without agents. It is also *important to protect users from distortion or abuse of preference* [emphasis added].

Among many examples provided by that evaluation were cases in which clients complained of bugs in their residence. Workers reportedly preferred to arrange for traumatic and costly relocation of housing rather than simply calling for an exterminator service, which was what the client really wanted!

In this section we have reviewed needs for access assistance and case management from the levels of the service system, programs, and clients. At all three levels there must be an optimum fit between services and the particular older persons who may need or want them. Given the great array of different services and different individual seekers of service, and given the great variation between United States communities, there can be no one linking mechanism that solves all problems of access and case coordination. In the next section we will examine the many different approaches to assessment and intervention. A given community will usually develop a unique mixture of linking services for various purposes and with various degrees of depth and length of involvement with older clients.

INTERVENTIONS

There is a wide spectrum of ways by which agencies attempt to connect the people who need services with appropriate programs. No one of these ways is the best way. Rather, there are a variety of options that accomplish different purposes for different need populations.

The range of program types or interorganizational linkages for access assistance includes the following:

Public information campaigns and special events
Outreach, friendly visitors, and senior companions
Routine referrals and referral agreements
Information and referral programs
Facilitative services such as transportation and escort
Colocation and outstationing
Emergency-assistance programs
Specialized case advocacy
Comprehensive assessment centers
Case management
Protective services and guardianship
Automated interagency client-tracking system
"Total care" ranging from life-care communities to "social and health maintenance organizations" (SHMOs) (i.e., few, if any, referrals are needed because all services are offered "in house")

The above is a continuum of increasing responsibility and increasing involvement in the many dimensions of a client's life. Each level of responsibility may be short term or long term; some must be responsive to changing needs over time. Three kinds of programs in the just-cited inventory (protective services, legal services, and total-care organizations) are discussed in other chapters and therefore will not be discussed here.

The relative depths of transactions between worker and client in the eleven kinds of programs just listed range from simple provision of a specific piece of information (such as a telephone number) that has been explicitly requested to a long-term supportive relationship dealing with intimate and threatening aspects of the client's life and involving numerous significant others who are part of the client's social network and professional treatment team.

In the following overview of the way these kinds of programs facilitate access to services and/or coordinate service delivery, only brief mention will be made of the corresponding assessment required—that is, what the worker needs to know about the client in order to assist in making a match between the service and the requirements of the client. Following this overview of interventions, we will discuss some of the generic issues in assessment for access assistance.

Information Campaigns and Special Events

There are a number of strategies used by agencies to build broad public awareness of their existence and functions. Human-interest stories in newspapers and TV interviews or documentaries usually produce a temporary wave of new requests for information or service, and also are thought to be remembered by a larger audience that does not react until a need arises. Another common technique is for a central coordinating agency (Area Agency on Aging, United Way, or city department) to produce a *directory of services* for the elderly in an abbreviated form suitable for wide distribution. Sometimes the distribution is aimed at the seniors themselves through program sites, branch banks, supermarkets, or door-to-door delivery. While such distributions have a general public-relations and educational value, they are not a cost-effective way to reach those with the greatest needs in a way that is timely and that motivates older people to take the first step toward needed help. In some communities, effective distributions of services directories have been made to selected "gatekeepers" whose daily jobs often call for connecting people in trouble to services— clergymen, sheriffs, mortitians, druggists, bartenders, mail carriers, firefighters—as well as to health and social-service workers. In a few communities, aging advocates have been able to arrange for such listings to be included in the telephone directory as a special section.

Another approach is to stage a special event that attracts older persons who do not necessarily have prior contacts with services and that provides opportunities for *person-to-person interaction*. These special events are often in the form of a "health fair" at a shopping center, a presentation and display at neighborhood or ethnic-association meetings, or a mobile information unit whose stops at given places are widely advertised in advance. While these events may have only moderate and long-range value in identifying new clients, they sometimes reach out and establish relationships with clients who would be overlooked and at the same time give agency personnel a humbling reminder of how difficult it is to explain professional service programs to lay publics and potential consumers (and, of course, how hard it is for consumers to sort out services and service jargon).

Outreach, Friendly Visitors, and Senior Companions

While there are a number of different uses for the term *outreach* in the aging network, we will limit the discussion here to the use of persons who go out into the community to gatherings of seniors and to homes in order to introduce potential new clients to the services of their agency. Outreach workers are sometimes asked about services that they do not provide, and at these times they are informally drawn into information and referral (I&R), which is discussed below. Most times, however, their function is to promote participation in the program or programs that they represent. Their role is to say "You need what we've got" rather than "What do you need and I'll help you find it." An important additional role of outreach workers is to follow up with participants who have dropped out of the program. This special interest in the client not only helps many clients to resume participation (or find another more appropriate service) but also keeps the agency informed about why clients drop out. In outreach work with the elderly it is especially important that return contacts be made (Brickner et al., 1976; Foley, 1976; Steinberg, 1979). Some older persons will reject offers of service the first time due to lack of trust and to be sure that their right to refuse will be respected. They sometimes respond more positively the second time around if the service is suitable.

Occasionally the term outreach is used by agencies to indicate any ongoing or follow-up contact with clients that is made in the clients' homes or other locations outside the program site or agency offices. Examples of this kind of outreach are friendly visitors and senior companions who provide a personal, socialization experience to homebound individuals. They are "dynamic listeners" and although they may be an adjunct of another program (family service, case management, community mental-health service, or senior center) their mission is not to sell any program. Yet they do facilitate access to services when they encounter a crisis and report it, or when their friendly conversation helps the client to think through a course of action about which he/she has had ambivalent feelings. Such workers, whether they are volunteers or paid paraprofessional service employees, are usually trained to recognize situations that call for professional assistance.

A variation of friendly visiting is telephone reassurance through which communications are maintained with vulnerable older persons by volunteers (Match, 1972; Van Coevering, 1973). Daily or semiweekly telephone calls are initiated by the volunteer to clients who have consented to this service. While the primary value of this service is informal social interaction, when crises arise the telephone-reassurance worker refers to information on file as to which agency or relative should be called to the scene.

Routine Referrals and Referral Agreements

Access to service for the client is frequently the result of referral from one agency (which does not offer the needed service) to another (which is presumed to offer the appropriate service). It is extremely important that the agency worker refer clients to the appropriate place—otherwise there is "ping-ponging" of help-seekers, which discourages them and which consumes the time of workers in other agencies who must again refer the client on to a more suitable agency (Frankfather, 1977; U.S. General Accounting Office, 1978). A good referral is one in which the practitioner not only gives accurate identifying information about the other agency but also explains to the client what the other agency provides and what steps the client may expect to take to obtain the service.

Since in most communities it is difficult for a single worker to keep up to date about all other agencies, several methods are used. Most of all, the workers in an agency must be familiar with the community's information and referral (I&R) agency and use it as needed for consultation about resources. In addition, nonprofessional personnel, such as receptionists who respond to callers, must be oriented to the importance of their response to the feelings and actions of callers and must know when to pass the call or visitor to a professional worker. Some larger agencies establish a position of "resource developer" or "coordinator" who is knowledgeable about community services and whose job includes creative responses to unusual requests or gaps in services. This community-services coordinator provides new information to agency workers through bulletins, personal presentations at staff meetings, and in-service training sessions.

When a given agency is frequently involved in referrals to or from another specific agency, it is desirable to formulate a written referral agreement that specifies for workers in both agencies what each offers and what the referral and intake procedures are for eligible applicants. These formal agreements, if well disseminated can simplify the process for both workers and clients. In any case, formal understandings are made more effective when there is also informal interpersonal interaction among workers across agencies. Such relationships can be cultivated through professional associations, interagency meetings, and agency "open house" special events to which other agencies' workers are invited.

Information and Referral Programs (I&R)

Information and referral agencies specialize in maintaining up-to-date inventories of all human services available in their service areas. In many cases, these inventories are periodically published as service directories. An increasing number of I&Rs have converted their resources inventories to automated data bases that can be searched quickly in accord with callers' need categories, geographic locations, and preferences. At the same time, I&R programs train their own staff members to be especially skillful at short-term interactions with help-seekers. Help-seekers may be the person who needs help, a significant other, or an agency worker who is obtaining the information in behalf of the person who needs help. Many times, sorting out the problems presented, and listening carefully for evidence of underlying or related problems that the caller finds difficult to recognize or express, requires sensitive handling of communications (Abbott, 1979; Burkhardt, 1979; Morrow, 1966; Ogg, 1969). At other times, only a simple answer to a simple question is needed. The following are the most common interventions for I&R workers:

Simple informational response is a transaction to provide the name, location, or telephone number of an agency explicitly identified by requestor.

Explanation response answers requestor's question about the "why" or "how to" searching for appropriate resources, without referring to a specific agency.

Unassisted referral involves brief assessment of the requestor's problem, data verification, if necessary, and direction to one or more appropriate resources.

Assisted referral involves assessment of the client's problem and active participation of the worker to link the client to appropriate resources through facilitation or advocacy (e.g., conferencing calls, negotiating access or eligibility, contacting significant others, or accompanying client to service).

Crisis handling, which usually involves a client in a panic or life-threatening situation, calls for the worker to aggressively maintain contact with the client, take immediate action in behalf of a client who cannot cope, and/or obtain prompt acceptance of responsibility of the case by a specialized agency or practitioner.

I&R programs may be age-generic (all ages) or may specialize in senior services. They may be centralized, serving from one office an entire county or state, or may be decentralized to towns and neighborhoods. I&R workers sometimes have professional education and experience, while others are paraprofessionals or indigenous volunteers serving neighbors or peer participants in another senior program.

Each variation is associated with corresponding strengths and weaknesses. For example, age-specific programs have been shown to gain better acceptance and use by elders (Applied Management Sciences, 1975), but sometimes senior-to-senior outreach extends only to the elderly who are already affiliated with organizations, bypassing the homebound and isolated (Dennen and Sykes, 1979; Opinion Research Corp., 1975). In addition, many new I&Rs for seniors, developed under the Older Americans Act, have been underfunded, inadequately staffed, and unmonitored for performance or effectiveness. Long-established professional programs operated from a central office have been evaluated as providing more accurate referrals but failing to be used adequately by minority elderly, while neighborhood-based paraprofessionals reached underserved population groups but failed to clarify problems and make appropriate referrals (Newcomer, 1976). On the other hand, volunteers and paraprofessionals can be trained and supported with professional consultation (in addition to being provided with directories) so that they better handle the *process* of I&R as well as the content (Mouton, 1972).

Facilitative Services Such as Transportation or Escort

In many cases involving a frail or isolated older person, knowing about the agency and being accepted into a program or service are not enough to make that resource accessible to the older person. In such cases, transportation or escort must get the client to the agency. In many communities the Area Agency on Aging (AAA) has established a dial-a-ride service or has teamed with other coordination agencies to provide transportation for all segments of the service area and for numerous kinds of programs. Other programs recruit volunteers to accompany elders to medical appointments or to a service location that is unfamiliar or otherwise hard to reach. In addition, some programs develop transportation and escort capacities for service to their own clients who regularly need assistance to attend congregate-meals sites, senior centers, or clinics.

An alternative way to make services more accessible for older persons who have difficulties of mobility is to provide home visits. Such a bridge of service delivery is common with visiting-nurse, meals-on-wheels, home-chore, and case-management services.

Colocation and Outstationing

When two or more agencies share an office or program facility and advertise the joint effort as a multiservice or multipurpose center, accessibility for clients may be enhanced (National Institute of Senior Centers, 1978). Colocated service centers are a convenience for ambulatory clients who may need more than one service. Clients often save travel time. Familiarity with the location of one service facilitates the older person's acceptance of an additional service. The multipurpose center is more visible to new clients and to community leaders who refer elders for service. When workers of various agencies are in proximity to each other, they become familiar with other programs through interagency meetings and informal contacts, thereby improving referrals and case coordination. For some programs the shared location not only offers economies of common reception areas, restrooms, telephone systems, and equipment but also permits workers to be located close to their client populations.

Such centers, however, do not enhance accessibility if, in order to find a big enough property for many agencies, a compromise location is selected that is distant from target populations and inconvenient with respect to public transportation and parking. Centers that have a dominant constituency of well, active older persons will have to make special efforts to ensure that the frail elderly are also welcomed and served (Jacobs, 1976). Conversely, locations that are associated with the sick and frail will have to overcome resistances of the relatively unimpaired elders toward participation in programs aimed at them. In rural areas it may be more desirable to have various agencies scattered throughout the service area rather than geographically concentrated, so that all residents have easy access to at least one agency, which in turn can help clients access the rest of the delivery system (Steinberg, 1978).

Outstationing involves the locating of a worker from one agency at the facility of another agency. Outstationing can be scheduled by appointment or on a routine part-time or full-time basis. Outstationed personnel provide the services of their own agency rather than a joint program with other agencies. It may also be that outstationed workers serve a different population than the host agency.

While outstationing most often occurs in service agencies, government buildings, or nonprofit community centers, there may also be arrangements in shopping centers, branch banks, or transportation terminals in order to reach concentrations of older persons. Another variation of outstationing is the use of a mobile unit that travels either to clients' homes or to visible neighborhood focal points. Mobile units have a certain pizzazz (i.e., innovative image) and attract attention for a while, but generally they have not proven cost-effective as a service-delivery base for older persons (except for library books and possibly for food shopping).

Emergency Assistance Programs

Emergency-assistance programs provide immediate crisis intervention in the form of short-term material assistance, protection, or counseling. Brief counseling is usually limited to reducing panic, clarifying issues, and helping clients to choose an effective course of action to solve the immediate problem. Once the crisis has been faced, or as part of remedying the crisis, the emergency-assistance worker must either convince the client to follow up with another agency or, with client consent, directly make arrangements for another agency to assume longer-range responsibility to help. These programs may be broadly defined as "hot lines," or may be organized around a special focus such as rape or abuse, crime victims' assistance, suicide prevention, or medical emergencies.

An extension of this kind of service is the Lifeline emergency alarm and response system. Lifeline is a twenty-four-hour service that allows disabled home-bound persons to call for help instantly. Some of the rented electronic devices will also call for help automatically if there is an absence of activity for a predetermined period of time. When the alarm is sounded, the sponsor agency, usually a hospital, contacts a nearby friend or relative to verify the situation. When necessary, the appropriate agency is rushed to the home. This kind of service is also known as EARS, which stands for Emergency Alarm and Response System.

At this point it is important to note that many emergencies of elders are detected and responded to by persons who are not part of the formal social-service network. Formal service agencies can build public awareness of what the "good Samaritan" can do when detecting an emergency and cultivate relationships with those who may frequently detect social and medical crises (Collins and Pancoast, 1976; Oglesby, 1968). Such community persons include the clergy; law-enforcement officers; milk, mail and newspaper delivery persons; pharmacists; mortitians; lawyers; and bartenders. Some I&Rs, as well as special emergency programs, place small signs in public telephone booths. In a few cities that have city-sponsored emergency phone numbers (such as 911), prior arrangements are made to have calls dealing with a social-service need channeled to the I&R or emergency-assistance agency.

A final example of a short-term crisis intervention is that of the hospital discharge department or medical social-service unit. While discharge from the hospital or emergency ward can be considered the recovery from a crisis, for some older persons recuperating from an illness or accident the pending return to one's own home is fraught with new needs. Meeting these needs becomes a crisis, especially when the physician fails to give sufficient advance notice so that home services can be arranged before discharge. These home services may be a combination of help from relatives and friends as well as from homecare providers to shop and prepare meals; provide personal care, if needed; arrange for nursing visits; and adapt the home environment in consideration of new impairments of the client. Failures to make these arrangements, either due to lack of time or gaps in available services, often result in inappropriate institutionalization.

Specialized Case Advocacy

Some programs have been established to serve populations with special needs by assisting their clients to obtain fair shares of available resources and by instructing other service agencies on how to respond to the special needs of their constituency. These programs also tend to handle grievances about quality of care and to contest denials of service. Among those who assist elderly clients are agencies that focus on the deaf, the blind, non-English-speaking groups, isolated rural enclaves, ex-offenders, the developmentally disabled, and the mentally ill. Many professional associations and labor unions provide individual case advocacy for their retired members. Other case advocates operate under the auspices of a religious congregation, community corporation, or housing authority (Bokser, 1982; Felton, Wallach, and Gallo, 1974).

Ombudsmen to troubleshoot grievances of older persons who are residents of nursing homes and other forms of domiciliary care are now established in every state (U.S. Administration on Aging, 1982). Legal-service programs not only take cases to court but also assist individuals in appeals before administrative bodies (Holmes and Holmes, 1979). In these examples, and unlike case management, the role of the worker is primarily to help the client get what he/she wants and not to assess the other kinds of needs of the client or to investigate alternative solutions. It is certainly within the role of the ombudsman and public-service lawyer to act as mediator, especially when the client's demands are unreasonable or when a misunderstanding has occurred. An important dimension of these two services, as well as of the other previously mentioned special-interest and I&R programs, is that the experience gained (in working with many individuals with similar problems or who have encountered similar barriers in accessing community services) will lead from case advocacy to class action. This class action takes many forms. It may indeed lead to court action, but may also take the form of testimony to the legislature, reports to planning and allocation bodies, or public exposés through the media. In these ways, the program aids a large population (in addition to its own clients) that may be encountering similar barriers in access to services.

Comprehensive Assessment Centers

A relatively new modality in the continuum of care is comprehensive geriatric assessment centers. Their purpose, like those of other modalities described in this chapter, is not to deliver treatment or monitor care but rather to clarify what level of care and what combination of interventions are needed by clients. Many of these centers arose from the growing recognition that many older patients are misdiagnosed (U.S. Commission on Civil Rights, 1977) or are unnecessarily institutionalized (U.S. Federal Council on Aging, 1978; U.S. General Accounting Office, 1977a, 1979b). Comprehensive psychosocial and medical assessment is well developed in many rehabilitation programs, adult day health-care centers, and Veterans Administration facilities, but in such settings assessment focuses for the most part on the conditions that the agency itself is capable of treating or influencing. Free-standing assessment centers (i.e., with no functions to follow up with the client after the assessment and referral phase) are viewed as having no vested interest in the diagnosis, hence are trusted to bring extra diagnostic skills and objectivity to the process as compared with service providers, who are viewed as defining people's problems by what their agency has to offer.

Some assessment centers assume responsibility for linking clients to a case-management program or a specific service provider in follow up to the assessment (Hageboeck, 1981). Others carry a principal function of diverting clients from an intended institutionalization or, at least, making the client or his caretakers aware of less restrictive environments in which suitable care can be provided. Increasingly, state Medicaid agencies are requiring "mandatory prescreening" by an assessment program before authorizing expenditures to place an older person in a nursing home. Similarly, many states require a complete, independent assessment before allowing persons to be committed to a mental hospital. In the context of this chapter it may be said that assessment programs prevent the wrong kind of service from being too accessible to persons who don't really need them and to whom they may do harm.

Case Management

Case management is a valuable and versatile approach to meeting the service needs of the homebound elderly and other persons with complex situations that place them at risk of institutionalization. It may be provided on a short-term or long-term basis. In different settings it may be known as "service management," "case coordination," "resource coordination," "casework," or "public-health nursing." It is most often performed by social workers or community-health nurses, with a great variety of staffing patterns involving gerontologists, psychologists, allied health professionals, paraprofessional case aides, and volunteers.

In view of the rapidly increasing use of this approach, buttressed by legislative efforts for cost containment and deinstitutionalization of the frail elderly (see "Need" and "Policy" sections), we will describe case management in some depth. (See also Austin, 1983; Beatrice, 1981; Carter et al., 1980; Duke University, 1973; Gottesman, Ishizaki, and MacBride, 1979; Steinberg and Carter,

1983). In many communities case management is located in a free-standing "channeling agency" or "community-care organization." In other communities it is found within service-providing agencies such as home-health agencies, senior multipurpose centers, family-service agencies, hospitals, and I&Rs, but separated organizationally from other service-delivery units of those sponsors.

The functions within case-management programs are in no way unique to this type of program. It is rather the breadth of facilitative functions and the depth of involvement in effective referral that characterize case management as a distinct service. While little uniformity exists in the way case management is structured or in the types of personnel who are involved at each stage of the helping process, eleven functions are commonly performed:

1. Casefinding, to identify and reach the particular target population that is most appropriate for the objectives and capacities of the program
2. Prescreening, in order to enroll those who can benefit most from the case-management program without excessive waiting time (while others are referred to other appropriate direct services)
3. Intake, in order to assure that the nature of the service is understood by clients, to demonstrate that the personnel are competent and interested in the client, and to engage the client to participate in the problem-solving process in his own behalf
4. Comprehensive assessment, to understand the client as a whole person and to be aware of strengths and needs in his situation and social network
5. Goal setting, to clarify expectations about what is to be achieved
6. Care planning, to arrange an individualized package of services and supportive activities suitable to the client's needs and values and within the constraints of available resources
7. Capacity building, to maximize the potential of the client and significant others to function independently and, when necessary, to obtain, coordinate, and monitor services on their own (this may range from simple modeling of telephone inquiries to arranging family-network meetings and providing supportive counseling)
8. Care monitoring, to make certain that high-quality services are found and delivered in a timely and coordinated way, and that the client suitably utilizes the offered services
9. Reassessment, to keep current regarding the status of the client and the appropriateness of the care plan
10. Termination, to phase out the case-management service when it is no longer necessary for the well-being of the client
11. Maintaining intermittent contact directly with the client or through continuing providers, to remain accessible to former clients in the event that case management is needed at a later time

Three attributes of case management and the elderly merit further description. First, the *assessment* covers physical as well as psychosocial conditions. It also considers environmental and economic circumstances. It takes stock of the problem that first brought the client to the agency's attention (i.e., the presenting problem) but also examines the interrelationships of problems and the informal social supports that are actual or potential sources of help. In order to maintain comprehensiveness and objectivity, many programs require workers to use a structured questionnaire or "assessment tool" (Kane and Kane, 1981). Whether the worker uses such a tool or a clinically oriented case record, there is usually no requirement to record the client's value preferences and life-style. Yet all good clinicians learn to take the client's values and life experiences into account when proposing a care plan.

Second, the *care plan*, or service plan, is also comprehensive. What is the desired outcome? What is to be done by the client (such as signing documents, informing relatives, requesting services directly, self-care, etc.)? What is to be done by family members, friends, or neighbors? What is to be done by the case manager? What is to be obtained from other agencies (in what sequence, for what duration, how paid for, whether additional specialized assessment is needed, what services would be desirable but are not available)? And what events will trigger a new step in the plan—reassessment, a new plan, or termination? The care plan is not only a record for the case manager but also serves as a frame of reference for the client, significant others, and participating service providers.

Third, following assessment and care planning, the facilitating and monitoring of service delivery (i.e., *implementation of the care plan*) becomes the most important and time-consuming part of the job. In working with clients and their significant others, case managers often do the following:

Give information about services to come
Model behaviors in how to secure services
Provide consultation on understanding problems, seeking solutions, carrying out plans for change, and evaluating changes
Confronting client if he or she is exacerbating his or her own problem
Teaching self-help and family monitoring of home serivces
Arranging for intermittent respite for informal caregivers
Preparing for reductions or termination of services
Less often, helping out with a specific task—doing it for them

In working with service providers in behalf of the client, the case manager has a multiplicity of tasks. These include:

Keeping up to date about programs and their intake requirements
Informing involved agencies about the case manager's work with the client

Providing information from the assessment and care plan
Negotiating for appropriate levels of service (which may include contracts
  for purchase of service if the program or client can afford to pay)
Giving encouragement to providers who accept "tough" or unusual cases
Monitoring the quality of care, including taking corrective action when necessary
Mediating conflicts between two or more providers or with the client
Creating a new service for the client or a class of clients, if not available in
  the community
Identifying and reporting systematic barriers to service accessibility (Eggert,
  Bowlyow, Nichols, 1980)
Troubleshooting arrangements with landlords, utility companies, zoning or
  sanitation officials
Obtaining outside consultation regarding specialized needs of the client

The tasks of a case manager are diverse and complex. The needs of clients, especially those in community-based long-term-care programs, are broad and constantly changing. Therefore, most case-management programs cannot offer to serve all on a first-come, first-served basis. They are generally restricted to a defined target population. However, the service has proved to be sufficiently valuable and therefore is being developed in many settings, for many levels of need, and for all income levels through the proprietary sector (for profit) as well as through the governmental and voluntary (nonprofit) sectors.

Automated Interagency Client Tracking System

In most programs using a client-tracking system, the purpose is to record, monitor, and report about the clients being served by one or several programs. To the extent that such systems permit the identification of unmet service needs, on an individual or aggregate basis, they may be viewed as a means for enhancing clients' access to services. For example, when fully operational, an automated system can alert each worker about all the clients who are scheduled for reassessments, or all clients whose service plans called for a particular service but who did not receive it. It can alert the administrator or planner to systematic gaps in available services, agencies with excessive delays in responding to referred clients, or cases in which costs of care are extremely high (Block and Richardson, 1979; Bowers and Bowers, 1977; Quinn, 1976; Steinberg and Carter, 1983).

All such systems maintain in coded form information about the client (usually obtained in an assessment or enrollment in a program) including the services needed by that client and the services being obtained. Some systems may also maintain information about the activities of workers with respect to specific clients and other work not specific to individual clients such as supervisory conferences, public-relations activities, and preparation of resource inventories.

In a few localities, where an Area Agency of Aging serves a relatively small and rural population, the AAA has attempted to include in its automated information system a complete inventory of all elders in its area, extending beyond current users of service. This inventory augments the lists of persons who receive service with additional names obtained from voting registrations, newspaper articles, and outreach contacts. With the help of such an inventory of elders, nonusers as well as users of service are sent periodic newsletters or announcements of special events.

These automated systems for client tracking more often fail than succeed. Their failures do not have to do with technological issues but rather with human factors and interorganizational difficulties such as finding commonly acceptable definitions of terms, resolving doubts concerning client confidentiality, allowing sufficient time for staff participation in the planning, and promptly demonstrating to information providers that the system is being used to facilitate their work and enhance service to clients. In those programs where the human factors and interorganizational issues have been carefully anticipated during the developmental phases of an automated system, both front-line workers and administrators find that client-tracking systems do facilitate the organization and evaluation of their work. From the client perspective, advantages of connecting with new services or enhancing the services they receive may be outweighed by potential threats to their rights of privacy, especially in an interagency system in which access to client information is not strictly controlled.

In this section we have briefly reviewed a wide range of programs for improving access to needed services. The methods vary with respect to their degree of involvement in the lives of their clients and therefore they require different degrees of knowledge about the needs and resources of their clients. In the next section we will review some common characteristics of assessment of client needs, wants, and resources.

ASSESSMENT

Specific methods of assessment are as varied as the methods of intervention outlined in the previous section. The distinguishing characteristics are (1) the depth and breadth of information about the client required for the intervention, (2) the relative formality and uniformity of the assessment process, and (3) the uses that are to be made of the assessment information.

First, the breadth and depth of information about the client should be limited to areas of concern that the program can help. There are two exceptions to this general rule. The agency may also need to know or account for aggregated data about which elders are and are not reaching the program. Therefore identifying information, such as place of residence, ethnicity, sex, and source of referral, may not be essential to an adequate response but may be requested of the client on order to evaluate equity of service and referral pathways. The second exception is when an inquiry or application for service has been addressed to one agency but must be referred to another more appropriate agency. In these cases, the worker may need to "assess" the client in areas beyond the agency's usual scope in order to determine what other agency would be most suited to the client's concern.

In general, assessments deal with the following:

What does the client want? (i.e., the presenting problem)
What does the client need?
What problem(s) is the client ready to work on first?
What strengths does the client have, personally and in a natural support system?
Which subsidized services does the client have entitlement to?
Which helps can the client afford to obtain in the marketplace?
What are the client's value preferences, reasonable goals, and abilities to use information alone?
What have been the client's previous experiences with services that may affect current motivations and expectations?

The expansion upon this short generic list by programs that engage in comprehensive and long-term involvements with clients usually occurs in the categories of client needs and strengths (such a psychosocial, medical, environmental, and economic).

The second variation is the relative formalization or standardization of the assessment process. Most programs use an open-ended, clinically oriented interview. There is a growing trend toward seeking uniformity in intake or assessment to assure that all necessary information is obtained from every client. This uniformity is obtained through use of a structured questionnarie, sometimes known as an "assessment tool" (Kane and Kane, 1981; Pfeiffer, 1973). Such tools not only attempt to ensure that all workers, regardless of education or experience, obtain relevant information, but also make possible objective ratings of levels of need among clients for purposes of tracking client progress over time and for purposes of program evaluation and workload distribution. Those programs that maintain long-term contact with clients may permit workers to engage in a cumulative process of assessment based on numerous successive interviews with the client (as trust and attention span improve). On the other hand, short-term interventions and demonstration research experiments tend to require the full, standardized assessment to be completed before care planning or service delivery begins.

The third consideration in assessment scope and method is how the information is to be used. There is the naive myth that eventually the field of gerontology will develop a single assessment tool that will meet the needs of all agencies so that information about the elderly and program evaluations can be compared. Similarly, the social-welfare community has often tried to develop a universal intake form that would make it unnecessary for different agencies to bother clients with the same questions—an effort that does not last long and that has proved to be unworkable in most communities (Calvert and McCaslin, 1972; Macro Systems, 1977; Mountain Plains Federal Regional Council, 1976).

Assessment for different purposes calls for varying approaches. Among the reasons for variation are the following:

Some are for research purposes, others are for clinical purposes (Kane and Kane, 1981).

Some are for a broad view of different needs, others are for diagnosis of specific impairments in order to develop a treatment plan in that specific area (Downing, 1979).

Some are for none of the above purposes, but rather to track clients' continuity of service through the system, to coordinate care, and identify gaps in service availability (U.S. General Accounting Office, 1979a).

Some are used for prescreening to determine whether or not a given older person meets the criteria (such as income, level of risk, and motivation) to be accepted into the program.

In addition to reflecting these different purposes, assessments must not be so unnecessarily lengthy as to place an excessive burden on the energies of the client, nor be intrusive of the client's privacy by extending into content areas that are beyond the program's capacity to provide assistance.

It is important that assessment for clinical purposes begin as much as possible with interviewing and observing the older client. This practice demonstrates to family members and other caregivers, as well as to clients, that although old, the client is assumed to be in charge of his or her problem-solving. It is also important that interviewers dealing with the elderly develop special skills in coping with possible sensory deficits, fatigue, desire to reminisce, and inability to recall on the part of the client, and possible ageist biases of the interviewer (Libow and Sherman, 1980).

THEORY

The spectrum of levels of intervention described in this chapter, the diversity of personnel who perform the functions, and the lack of uniformity in the organizational contexts in which they are conducted, all suggest a lack of common theoretical bases. There are, however, commonly accepted principles of practice that apply to the many different kinds of programs discussed in this chapter. Among these principles are:

The client's right of self-determination
Partializing problems in complex cases
Beginning where the client is
Involving all persons who will be affected by any proposed change

There is a body of theory that supports the coexistence in a given community of multiple approaches to access assistance, variability in the structure of programs from community to community, and a variety of responses for different sets of help-seekers.

Much of contingency theory has been developed in the analysis of organizations and systems of organizations. Weiner (1978, 53) summarized contingency theory as based on two assumptions: there is no one best way to organize and anyway of organizing is not equally effective (for all purposes or all environments). He further noted much research on administrator or worker style and concluded that "there is no one best way or style far surpassing others in effectiveness." March and Simon (1958, 39), in discussing research primarily focused on business organizations, stated that "Rigidity of [organizational] behavior increases the amount of difficulty with clients . . . and complicates the achievement of client satisfaction—a near-universal organizational goal."

Theories comparable to organizational contingency theory may be found in social-service and clinically oriented literature (Aiken et al., 1975; Cartwright and Zander, 1960; Kahn, 1969, 1976). For example, differentiation of worker roles (and program roles within the system) was outlined by Demone (1978) in terms of the change agent, the lobbyist, the ombudsman, the coordinator, and the advocate. Similarly, Demone differentiated approaches to change as consensus, process, collaboration, and Westley enabling, brokering, conferences, co-optation, and campaign. Lippett, Watson, (1958) developed a set of generic guidelines based upon numerous helping disciplines at various levels of practice (individual, group, and community). The authors described the phases that lead to "choosing an appropriate helping role" as (1) a diagnostic clarification of the problem, (2) assessment of the client motivation and capacity to change, (3) assessment of the change agent's motivations and resources, and (4) selecting appropriate change objectives. The particular community problems for which a program was established, as well as the particular needs and preferences of individual clients, will influence program design and clinical approaches.

Rothman (1974) summarized the findings from social-science research into "generalizations" and formulated "action guidelines" for practitioners. These generalizations have relevance for the programs in this chapter at all three levels of perspective: the client level, the program level, and the service-system level. The following examples relate to statements made earlier in this chapter.

The nature of an organization's goals may have a direct impact on its structure and leadership patterns (p. 138).

Organizations employing indigenous workers are successful in reaching clients who were not previously receiving services (p. 186).

Different client populations prefer different styles of participation. These preferences may change over time. (p. 382).

The rate of adoption of an innovation is directly related to the extent to which it is diffused in a manner compatible with the target system's norms, values, and customs. Innovations with a compatible diffusion process will have a higher adoption rate than innovations with an incompatible diffusion process (p. 446).

Different modes of communication are used by different adopters. Relatively early adopters of innovations tend to use mass media information sources whereas later adopters tend to use face-to-face information sources. The rate of adoption of an innovation is related to the degree to which information is passed through the appropriate communication mode (p. 448).

In the above quotations, the term "adopters of innovation" may be compared with this chapter's concerns about assisting older persons to utilize services with which they are unfamiliar. There must not only be a good match between the problem and the solution but also flexibility and sensitivity to adjust to the norms, values, and customs of each client. The above generalizations may also be viewed in the context of introducing a new kind of program (such as a community-care organization) into a community. Not only must the new program take into account preexisting programs, it must also be initiated with the appropriate communication mode (local advocates vs. outside consultants or research reports, etc.) and awareness of the norms and customs that prevail in the community.

POLICY

Several kinds of trends in the United States are reinforcing the need for and growth of access-assistance and case-management programs. First, there are broad trends in human-service policy. These broad trends are then reflected in specific pieces of governmental legislation and in comparable changes in approaches of the private sector. A third category of trends has to do with societal changes, including developments within and between the professions.

The four principal broad influences are (1) deinstitutionalization, (2) decentralization, (3) cost containment, and (4) the continuation of categorical approaches to social-services funding and delivery. The trend that favors deinstitutionalization, while sometimes motivated by cost containment, also obtains its impetus from public scandals regarding poor conditions within many institutions, recognition that community-based alternatives are essential to rehabilitation, and growing attention to patients' rights. This trend has been reinforced by court decisions that communities and agencies must provide to handicapped or ill clients the "least restrictive environment" (Cohen and Staroscik, 1982; Pfeiffer, 1973). Consequently, greater demands are placed on I&R and case-management programs to be aware of alternative services and to avoid premature referrals to institutions that may be avoidable.

The trend of federal policy toward decentralization of social-program choice and administration is previously discussed in the "Need" section of this chapter. Decentralization policies are sometimes known as *new federalism* (in the Nixon and Reagan administrations) but also developed momentum during the New Frontier and Great Society years of the 1960s (Kennedy and Johnson administrations). By encouraging local decision-making in allocations and plans for services, these federal policies recognized the unique variations from community to community, thus making the need for locally based information and referral as important as ever. At the same time, many of the legislative bills and grants-in-aid regulations mandated that some funds be set aside for I&R programs without regard for eligibility on the basis of income. Among the laws that encouraged the growth of I&R (and sometimes a proliferation of duplicative I&Rs) were the Older Americans Act (especially the 1973 comprehensive services amendments) and the Social Security Act Amendments of 1975 (which established Title XX). On the other hand, as the trend to decentralization takes the form of block grants in which minimum-required services are not specified, there are no mandates to continue I&R and other types of access-assistance programs.

The taxpayers' revolt of the late 1970s heightened the public demand for cost containment in both health and social services. The subsequent cutbacks and new approaches in social services placed new burdens on I&Rs to keep up to date on services available and to troubleshoot a new large volume of clients who had been dropped by diminishing programs or who had become the unemployed "new poor." Cost-containment advocates also looked to case management as a way to prevent overutilization of costly medical and long-term-care resources whenever it might be feasible to substitute less costly care at home or in the community. Cost containment is not only a concern of government but has also commanded the attention of private health-insurance companies, employer coalitions, and employee groups that must pay for the insurance. This part of the private sector is watching, and sometimes experimenting with, case-management approaches that may reduce the length of hospital stays and the overuse of skilled-nursing facilities by substituting homecare.

In spite of numerous strategies to decategorize human services, with consequent fragmentation of target populations and programs, the dominant trend continues to be categorical assistance such as for the poor, for the handicapped, for persons with particular kinds of illnesses, and for persons at specific levels of chronological age. Thus the patchwork of programs, each with its limiting boundaries, requires the existence, in each community, of experts for identifying and accessing appropriate services. While these functions are primarily carried by nonprofit agencies supported with public and United Way funds, there is a trend toward proprietary, private-practice agencies in which assessment and service-brokerage assistance is provided for a fee.

Cutting across the above general trends is the rapid ascendency of policies and legislation that directly and indirectly promote the use of case management in behalf of the frail elderly. Among the important benchmarks of this trend were the following:

The U.S. Federal Council on Aging (1978) developed its Public Policy and the Frail Elderly, which called for entitlement to assessment and case management for all persons over age 75.

The Secretary's Committee on Mental Health and Illness of the Elderly (U.S. Department of Health, Education, and Welfare, 1977) recommended a network of geriatric "assessment" centers to overcome problems of misdiagnosis and failures of the mental-health system to provide appropriate services and placements for the elderly.

Building on the experiences of such programs as Massachusetts's home-care corporations and Pennsylvania's service management, as well as demonstration research projects such as Triage (Connecticut) and Access (Rochester, N.Y.), the Administration on Aging funded numerous research projects and pilot programs in case management and established a national network of long-term-care gerontology centers to provide training and technical assistance in the development of local and state programs.

The U.S. General Accounting Office (1977a, 1978, 1979b, 1982) issued a series of reports to the Congress that generally promoted the use of improved I&R and case management.

The U.S. Congress, in 1978, mandated a joint demonstration involving AoA and the Health Care Financing Administration (HCFA) entitled Channeling Agencies, which not only established case-management programs in ten cities but also funded numerous additional states for long-term-care system development.

Numerous state legislatures established programs aimed at "alternatives to premature institutionalization" and at cost containment focused on case management, including New York (Nursing Homes without Walls), Utah, California, Arkansas, Washington, Maine, etc.

A variety of long-term-care reform bills were considered by Congress, raising public consciousness and resulting first in the establishment of Medicaid waivers (Omnibus Budget Reconciliation Act of 1981) that promoted case-managed alternative services programs. Each year thereafter new bills have been considered for expanding home-health care or amending Medicare so that case management and alternative services can become reimbursable and more widely available.

Finally, other trends, not necessarily reflected in public policy, deserve mention because they either adversely or favorably affect the development of access assistance and case-management programs. Perhaps as a consequence of the rapid growth and great variability of these programs, there has been a general inability to arrive at minimum program standards or practitioner qualifications. Therefore the control of the quality of these services has been very uneven, if not nonexistent. An influence toward improving quality of programs and practice is the previously mentioned growing consumerism among the elderly and tendencies to litigation on the part of all service consumers who encounter malpractice. Another force toward maintaining higher standards is the increasing entry of the proprietary sector into human services and competition between providers. This is not to imply that proprietary (for fee) services are of higher quality than the nonprofits but rather that consumers will exercise their choices. The increased opportunities for choice, especially for consumers who can afford to pay the full cost of service, mean that I&Rs and case managers must keep aware of all these choices and deal with dilemmas of maximizing quality while remaining cost-conscious.

Also noted previously is the probability that new cohort groups entering the ranks of "the elderly" will be more socialized to the existence of services and more demanding of their rights of access. And as stated many times in other chapters of this book, the numbers of elderly in the population are increasing at a great rate. More people will be needing and wanting services, which are not expected to increase at a commensurate rate. Well-informed I&R workers and case managers will be needed to ration resources and to link help-seekers with the finite supply of services.

In the specific instance of case management, there has been a preeminence of social workers as practitioners and administrators. Two kinds of trends may change the configuration of staffs and relative career opportunities among the professions. First is the emergence of nurses and others in comprehensive assessment and care planning with the elderly. The role of case coordinator, of course, is part of the tradition of the public-health nurse (Jamme, 1905), whose training and experience bridge the social, environmental, and medical components of assessment and care. A new wave of professionals with degrees in gerontology is moving into case management, bringing particular knowledge and skills for working with the elderly. In addition, paraprofessional aides have demonstrated their competence to establish rapport and to deal with instrumental and environmental needs of elders. A parallel trend in schools of social work to view case management as a less-than-professional area of practice (because it minimized therapeutic counseling and emphasizes functional needs) may further reduce the proportion of social-work leadership in these programs.

Meanwhile, the experience of community-care organizations and channeling agencies demonstrates that social-work skills are highly desirable in order to bring a high level of clinical expertise to the problem-solving processes of client-oriented, participative care planning (Kirschner, 1979; Wasser, 1966). Increasing work with the multiply impaired elderly and their families has highlighted the importance of dealing with mental-health needs and sensitive value preferences. Social work also has a history of moving from private troubles to social issues (Morris, 1977), just as case management calls for dealing with service-system development as well as case-by-case practice. All access-assistance programs, including case management, call for providing technical assistance to and maintaining interorganizational linkages with a wide range of human-service agencies in behalf of individual clients and groups of clients. Thus competence in community organization and group work, as well as casework, are required. In summary, and in spite of trends to the contrary, quality-access assistance and case management demand professional generalists.

This section has presented a broad overview of policy and practice trends that affect current and future programs in access assistance and case management. It is likely that the names and locations of these programs may change over time, but on balance the trends point to continuity and much growth in this area, which has been a key component of the American human-service delivery system for over a century (Button, 1918; Carter, 1978; Falconer, 1926; Reynolds, 1919; Seidl et al., 1983; Steinberg, 1982).

REFERENCES

Abbott, K. (1979). Information and referral. In M. B. Holmes and D. Holmes (Eds.), *Handbook of human services for older persons.* New York: Human Sciences Press.

Aiken, M., et al. (1975). *Coordinating human services.* San Francisco: Jossey-Bass.

American Health Planning Association. (1982). *A guide for planning long term care health services for the elderly.* Washington: The Association.

Applied Management Sciences. (1975). *The study of the perspective of relative benefits of age-segregated versus age-integrated I&R services presently operating: Aggregate report.* Silver Springs, Md.: AMS.

Austin, C. D. (1983). Case management in long-term care: Options and opportunities. *Health and Social Work,* **8**(1), 16-30.

Beatrice, D. F. (1981). Case management: A policy option for long-term care. In J. J. Callahan, Jr., and S. S. Wallack (Eds.), *Reforming the long-term-care system.* Lexington, Mass.: Lexington Books.

Bertsche, A. V., and Horejsi, C. R. (1980). Coordination of client services. *Social Work,* **25**(2), 94-98.

Block, A. H., and Richardson, D., Jr. (1979). *Developing a client based feedback system for improving human service programs.* Rockville, Md.: Project Share.

Bokser, K. (1982). *Senior resident advisor program: A first step in a continuum of care.* New York: New York City Housing Authority, Office for the Aging.

Bowers, G. E., and Bowers, M. R. (1977). *Cultivating client information systems.* Washington: Project Share.

Branch, L. G., and Jette, A. M. (1982). A prospective study of long-term care institutionalization among the aged. *American Journal of Public Health,* **72**(12), 1373-1379.

Brickner, P. W., et al. (1976). Outreach to welfare hotels, the homebound, and the frail. *American Journal of Nursing,* **76**, 762-764.

Brody, E. (1969). Follow-up study of applicants and non-applicants to a voluntary home. *Gerontologist,* **9**(3), 187-196.

Burkhardt, J. E. (1979). Evaluating information and referral services. *Gerontologist,* **19**(1), 28-33.

Button, G. L. (1918). Value of registration to organizations which do not keep adequate records. *Proceedings of the National Conference of Social Work,* **45**, 324-329.

Callahan, J. J., Jr. (1980). Delivery of services to persons with long-term-care needs. In J. Meltzer et al. (Eds.), *Policy options in long-term care.* Chicago: University of Chicago Press.

Calvert, W. R., and McCaslin, R. (1972). *Central intake: Coordination or confusion.* Houston: Texas Research Institute of Mental Sciences.

Carter, G. W. (1978). Service coordination: A recycling of tested concepts. In R. M. Steinberg (Ed.), *Case coordination and service integration projects: Client impact, program survival and research priorities.* Los Angeles: Andrus Gerontology Center, University of Southern California.

Carter, G. W., et al. (1980). *Case coordination with the elderly: The experiences of front-line practitioners.* Los Angeles: Andrus Gerontology Center, University of Southern California.

Cartwright, D., and Zander, A. (Eds.). (1960). *Group dynamics: Research and theory* (2nd ed.). Evanston, Ill.: Row, Peterson.

Cohen, E., and Staroscik, L. S. (1982). *Community services and long term care: Issues of negligence and liability.* Philadelphia: Temple University Long Term Care Gerontology Center.

Collins, A. H., and Pancoast, D. L. (1976). *Natural helping networks: A strategy for prevention.* Washington: National Association of Social Workers.

Coward, R. T. (1979). Planning community services for the rural elderly: Implications from research. *Gerontologist,* **19**(3), 275-282.

Cuellar, J., and Weeks, J. (1980). *Minority elderly Americans: A prototype for area agencies on aging: Executive summary.* San Diego: Allied Home Health Association.

Demone, H. W. Jr. (1978). *Stimulating human services reform.* Washington: Project Share.

Dennen, T., and Sykes, T. M. (1979). *An analysis and evaluation of information and assistance programs for the elderly in the state of Washington.* Olympia: Washington Department of Social and Health Services.

Downing, R. (1979). Assessment and case coordination workers roles. In R. Downing, *Three working papers.* Los Angeles: Andrus Gerontology Center, University of Southern California.

Duke University Center for the Study of Aging and Human Development. (1973). *Guidelines for an information and counseling service for older persons.* Durham, N. C.: The Center.

Eggert, G. M., Bowlyow, J. E., and Nichols, C. W. (1980). Gaining control of the long term care system: First returns from the ACCESS experiment. *Gerontologist,* **20**(3), 356-363.

Falconer, D. P. (1926). The social service exchange: A tool for county cooperation. *Proceedings of the National Conference of Social Work,* **53**, 477-479.

Felton, G. S., Wallach, H. F., and Gallo, C. L. (1974). New roles for new-professional mental health workers: Training the patient advocate, the integrator, and the therapist. *Community Mental Health Journal,* **10**(1), 52-65.

Foley, L. M. (Ed.). (1976). *Stand close to the door.* Sacramento: School of Social Work, California State University.

Frankfather, D. (1977). *The aged in the community: Managing senility and deviance.* New York: Praeger.

Frankfather, D. L., Smith, M. J., and Caro, F. G. (1981). *Family care of the elderly: Public initiatives and private obligations.* Lexington, Mass.: Lexington Books.

Gottesman, L. E., Ishizaki, B., and MacBride, S. M. (1979). Service management—plan and concept in Pennsylvania. *Gerontologist,* **19**(4), 379-385.

Group for the Advancement of Psychiatry. Committee on Aging. (1971). *The aged and community mental health: A guide to program development.* New York: The Group.

Guttman, D. (1980). *Perspective on equitable share in public benefits by minority elderly: Executive summary.* Washington: School of Service, Catholic University of America.

Hageboeck, H. (1981). *Training the trainers manual: Iowa gerontology model project.* Iowa City: University of Iowa.

Hodgson, J. H. Jr., and Quinn, J. L. (1980). The impact of the Triage health care delivery system on client morale, independent living and the cost of care. *Gerontologist,* **20**(3), 364-371.

Holmes, D., and Hudson, E. (1975). *Evaluation report of the Mosholu-Montefiore day care center for the elderly in the northwest Bronx.* New York: Community Research Applications.

Holmes, D., et al. (1979). The use of community-based services in long-term care by older minority persons. *Gerontologist,* **19**(4), 389-397.

Holmes, M. B., and Holmes, D. (Eds.). (1979). *Handbook of human services for older persons*. New York: Human Sciences Press.

Horejsi, C. R. (1978). Client services coordination: Training and retraining for social workers in rural areas. *Human Services in the Rural Environment*, **3**(3), 6-19.

Horowitz, G., and Estes, C. (1971). *Protective services for the aged*. Washington: U.S. Administration on Aging.

Jacobs, B. (Ed.). (1976). *Working with the impaired elderly*. Washington: National Council on the Aging.

Jamme, M. R. (1905). The district nurse in co-operative work. *Proceedings of the National Conference of Charities and Corrections*, **32**, 280-284.

John, D. (1977). *Managing the human service "system": What have we learned from services integration?* Denver: Center for Social Research and Development, University of Denver.

Kahn, A. J. (1969). *Theory and practice of social planning*. New York: Russell Sage Foundation.

Kahn, A. J. (1970). Perspectives on access to social services. *Social Work*, **15**(2), 95-101.

Kahn, A. J. (1976). Service delivery at the neighborhood level: Experience, theory, and fads. *Social Service Review*, **50**(1), 23-56.

Kane, R. A., and Kane, R. L. (1980). The extent and nature of public responsibility for long-term care. In J. Meltzer et al. (Eds.), *Policy options in long-term care*. Chicago: University of Chicago Press.

Kane, R. A., and Kane, R. L. (1981). *Assessing the elderly: A practical guide to measurement*. Lexington, Mass.: Lexington Books.

Kirschner, C. (1979). The aging family in crisis: A problem in living. *Social Casework*, **60**(4), 209-216.

Kutza, E. (1980). Allocating long-term-care services: The policy puzzle of who should be served. In J. Meltzer et al. (Eds.), *Policy options in long-term care*. Chicago: University of Chicago Press.

Libow, L. S., and Sherman, F. (1980). *The core of geriatric medicine: A guide for students and practitioners*. St. Louis: Mosby.

Lippett, R., Watson, J., and Westley, B. (1958). *The dynamics of planned change*. New York: Harcourt, Brace & World.

Louis Harris and Associates. (1975). *The myth and reality of aging in America*. Washington: National Council on the Aging.

Macro Systems. (1977). *Analysis of the constraints to implementation of a single eligibility application for income security programs*. Macro Systems.

March, J. G., and Simon, H. A. (1958). *Organizations*. New York: Wiley.

Match, S. K. (1972). *Establishing telephone reassurance services*. Washington: National Council on the Aging.

Monk, A. (1979). Family supports in old age. *Social Work*, **24**(6), 533-538.

Morris, R. (1977). Caring for vs. caring about people. *Social Work*, **22**(5), 353-359.

Morrow, K. R. (1966). A basic program for referral services. *Rehabilitation Literature*, **27**(7), 197-202.

Mountain Plains Federal Regional Council. (1976). *Assessment of SPAARS (single purpose application and automatic referral system)*. Colorado: The Council.

Mouton, L. (1972). *Project referral network: Information and referral at the grass roots*. Los Angeles: Los Angeles County I&R Service.

National Institute of Senior Centers. (1978). *Senior center standards: Guidelines for practice*. Washington: National Council on the Aging.

Newcomer, R. J. (1976). *Evaluating information and referral services for the homebound elderly: A comparison of telephone and peer contact systems: Final report*. Springfield, Va.: U.S. National Technical Information Service.

Nuttbrock, L., and Kosberg, J. I. (1980). Images of the physician and help-seeking behavior of the elderly: A multivariate assessment. *Journal of Gerontology*, **35**(2), 241-248.

O'Brien, J. E., and Wagner, D. L. (1980). Help seeking by the frail elderly: Problems in network analysis. *Gerontologist*, **20**(1), 78-83.

Ogg, E. (1969). *Tell me where to turn: The growth of information and referral services*. New York: Public Affairs Committee.

Oglesby, W. B. Jr. (1968). *Referral in pastoral counseling*. Englewood Cliffs, N.J.: Prentice-Hall.

Opinion Research Corporation. (1975). *An evaluation of outreach of the nutrition program for the elderly.* Washington: U.S. Administration on Aging.

Perlman, R. (1975). *Consumers and social services.* New York: Wiley.

Pfeiffer, E. (Ed.). (1973). *Alternatives to institutional care for older Americans: Practice and planning.* Durham, N.C.: Duke University Center for the Study of Aging and Human Development.

Quinn, J. (1975). Triage: coordinated home care for the elderly. *Nursing Outlook,* **23**, 570-573.

Quinn, R. E. (1976). The impacts of a computerized information system on the integration and coordination of human services. *Public Administration Review,* **36**(2), 166-174.

Rao, D. B. (1977). The team approach to integrated care of the elderly. *Geriatrics,* **32**(2), 88-96.

Reynolds, W. S. (1919). Case conference, need and plan. *Proceedings of the National Conference of Social Work,* **46**, 336-339.

Rothman, J. (1974). *Planning and organizing for social change: Action principles from social science research.* New York: Columbia University Press.

Seidl, F. W., et al. (1983). *Delivering in-home services to the aged and disabled.* Lexington, Mass.: Lexington Books.

Sherwood, S., and Morris, J. (1981). *A study of the effects of an emergency alarm and response system for the aged.* Boston: Department of Social Gerontological Research, Hebrew Rehabilitation Center for the Aged.

Skellie, F. A., and Coan, R. E. (1980). Community-based long-term care and mortality: Preliminary findings of Georgia's alternative health services project. *Gerontologist,* **20**(3), 372-379.

Stassen, M., and Holohan, J. (1980). *Long term care demonstration projects: A review of recent evaluations.* Washington: Urban Institute.

Steinberg, R. M. (1978). Functional components and organizational issues in rural service systems for the aged. In D. A. Watkins and C. O. Crawford (Eds.), *Rural gerontology research in the northeast.* Ithaca, N.Y.: Northeast Regional Center for Rural Development, Cornell University.

Steinberg, R. M. (1979). Impact of minority aging research on services for minority elderly. In E. P. Stanford (Ed.), *Minority aging research.* San Diego: Campanile Press.

Steinberg, R. M. (1982). Case service coordination: Senior center issues. In B. Jacobs and R. P. Flaum (Eds.), *Senior centers: Helping communities serve older persons.* Washington: National Council on the Aging.

Steinberg, R. M., and Carter, G. W. (1983). *Case management and the elderly.* Lexington, Mass.: Lexington Books.

Steinberg, R. M., and Jurkiewicz, V. (1980). *A national directory of case coordination programs for the elderly 1979-1980 with findings from the national survey.* Los Angeles: Andrus Gerontology Center, University of Southern California.

Taietz, P. (1970). *Community structure and aging.* Ithaca, N.Y.: Department of Rural Sociology, Cornell University.

Tobin, S. S., Davidson, S. M., and Sack, A. (1976). *Effective social services for older Americans.* Ann Arbor: Institute of Gerontology, University of Michigan—Wayne State University.

U.S. Administration on Aging. (1982). *The long term care ombudsman program: National summary of state ombudsman reports for FY 1981: Executive summary.* Washington: U.S. Administration on Aging.

U.S. Commission on Civil Rights. (1977). *The age discrimination study.* Washington: The Commission.

U.S. Department of Health, Education and Welfare. (1977). *Report of the secretary's committee on mental health and illness of the elderly.* Washington: The Department.

U.S. Federal Council on Aging. (1978). *Public policy and the frail elderly.* Washington: The Council.

U.S. General Accounting Office. (1977a). *Home health—the need for a national policy to better provide for the elderly.* Washington: General Accounting Office.

U.S. General Accounting Office. (1977b). *The well-being of older people in Cleveland, Ohio.* Washington: General Accounting Office.

U.S. General Accounting Office. (1978). *Information and referral for people needing human services: A complex system that should be improved.* Washington: Comptroller General of the United States.

U.S. General Accounting Office. (1979a). *Conditions of older people: National information system needed.* Washington: General Accounting Office.

U.S. General Accounting Office. (1979b). *Entering a nursing home: Costly implications for Medicaid and the elderly.* Washington: General Accounting Office.

U.S. General Accounting Office. (1982). *The elderly should benefit from expanded home health care but increasingly these services will not insure cost reductions.* Washington: General Accounting Office.

Van Coevering, V. R. (1973). *Guidelines for a telephone reassurance service.* Ann Arbor: Institute of Gerontology, University of Michigan.

Wasser, E. (1966). *Creative approaches in casework with the aging.* New York: Family Service Association of America.

Weiner, M. E. (1978). *Application of organization and systems theory to human services reform.* Washington: Project Share.

Weissert, W. G., Wan, T. T. H., and Livieratos, B. B. (1980). *Effects and costs of day care and homemaker services for the chronically ill: A randomized experiment.* Hyattsville, Md.: U.S. Department of Health, Education and Welfare.

White, M. (1980). *Toward a conceptual framework for case coordination program design: Lessons from the past, guidelines for the future.* Unpublished doctoral dissertation, School of Social Work, University of Southern California.

SOURCES OF INFORMATION

National Clearinghouse on Aging, Administration on Aging, U.S. Department of Health and Human Services, 300 Independence Avenue, S.W., Washington, D.C. 20201. Examples of materials that have been distributed (subject to supply) and that are available through Clearinghouse repositories of the microfiche collection located in all parts of the country are the following titles: *I&R Services: Follow UP; I&R Services: Information-Giving and Referral; I&R Services: Interviewing and Information Giving; I&R Services: Reaching Out; I&R Services: Referral Procedures; I&R Services: The Role of Advocacy; I&R Services: A Training Syllabus; I&R Services: Volunteer Escort Service; Planning for the Elderly in Natural Disaster; Older Americans Health Fair Training & Orientation Guide; I&R Program Configuration; A Guide for Statewide Planning.*

Project Share: A National Clearinghouse for Improving the Management of Human Services. For reference searches or other questions, address Ms. Eileen Wolff, Project Officer, Project Share, P.O. Box 2309, Rockville, Md. 20852 (tel. 301-251-5170). Examples of Project Share's subject index that are relevant to this chapter are: case coordination methods; case management; client access to service system; client advocacy; communication and public information services; consumer access to services; consumer complaints processing and investigation and advocacy services; outreach techniques; service accessibility to clients; staff outstationing; transportation for disabled or older adults; use of case coordinators; victim advocacy programs/services.

National Technical Information Service (NTIS), 5285 Port Royal Road, Springfield, Va. 22161. This is a useful central source for obtaining copies of those references in this chapter that were prepared or funded by a federal agency.

6

Casework Services

Edmund Sherman, Ph.D.

State University of New York at Albany

Today's casework service is characterized by a number of different theoretical orientations. This chapter is not intended to describe these orientations or models as much as it is to show how they have been adapted to work with the elderly. Hopefully, this approach will serve the purpose of making the content more prescriptive than descriptive for the practitioner-reader.

OVERVIEW

There are several ways of defining, and in so doing distinguishing, casework from other interventions within the broad arena of service provisions that comprise gerontological practice. Fischer's (1978) identification of casework as the branch of social work "whose defining characteristic is the provision of individualized services" has the virtue of brevity. It also identifies casework as a social-work method, which serves to differentiate it from individualized services provided by other professional disciplines. However, in order to serve the purposes of this chapter, there is need of a definition or characterization that delineates certain crucial elements in casework practice. Helen Harris Perlman's (1957) characterization of casework seems to do this very well. Essentially, she sees casework as a process of helping people deal with their problems through

(1) the provision of resources, (2) the problem-solving work, and (3) the therapeutic relationship.

It is largely in terms of elements (2) and (3) that one is apt to see differences among the several casework-treatment models to be outlined in this chapter. There is general agreement in the casework literature on the need for the provision of "hard" and "soft" services. The importance of the linkage, brokerage, and advocacy roles of caseworkers cannot be overestimated when it comes to the reality of practice with older persons, a population with particularly great social, economic, and medical needs. Also, it must be distinguished from case management, which may include casework but which also encompasses the ongoing provision of concrete assistance to the elderly and often, as well, to family caregivers.

Although there have been changes in the relative emphasis on the provision of resources over the years, the major development in casework with the aged has been in the areas of problem-solving work and the therapeutic relationship, which represent, in short, the counseling aspects of casework service. These changes or developments are to a large degree related to changing social-work conceptions of aging and work with the aged, as well as to a growing diversification of direct-practice orientation and methods in social work generally. Whatever the reasons, these changes have been rather dramatic over the past fifteen years.

It should be added quickly that these changes have been largely in terms of approach rather than in volume of casework service. Lowy (1979), who described casework mostly in terms of its counseling function in settings such as family-service agencies, public-welfare departments, and mental-health clinics, noted that only in a minority of cases are such services available to the community aged living in their own homes. The situation is certainly no better in residential settings and institutions such as nursing homes and other long-term-care facilities as far as employment of professionally trained caseworkers is concerned (Garner and Mercer, 1980). Much of this, of course, is due to attitudes on the part of many social workers about working with the elderly in such settings, a fact that was dramatically highlighted by Kosberg (1973) ten years ago and that still holds true to a large extent.

Nevertheless, some important events and changes have taken place with respect to casework with the elderly that need to be placed into some kind of historical perspective. They have to do with new theoretical and research perspectives on aging, the call for accountability and evaluation of the effectiveness of services, and above all a changing attitude among social workers. Evidence for this was found by Cormican (1980), who reviewed three traditional social-work journals (Social Casework, Social Service Review, and Social Work) for five years from the beginning of 1970 through 1974. He found a marked change even within that brief period. The findings indicated that social workers began that period with an essentially negative view of aging. They tended to view aging as a process of losses and to emphasize protective services. In the middle of this period a more positive view of aging emerged, with an emphasis on counseling services. By the end of the period there was a recognition of the diversity of the aging process and of the need for differential treatment and services. This change in general social-work thinking was also reflected in casework in particular.

Casework, especially casework within the context of protective services, had to undergo a wrenching reappraisal in that period as a result of the findings reported by Blenkner, Bloom, and Nielsen (1971) from the research and demonstration project of protective services under the auspices of the Benjamin Rose Institute of Cleveland. The predominant service provided within the project (treatment) group was more intensive casework counseling (provided in 82 percent of those cases), and yet the treatment group demonstrated a higher mortality rate and a higher rate of institutionalization than did the control group. This was one of the eleven controlled studies reviewed by Fischer (1973), who came to the conclusion that casework was no more effective than no intervention at all. In fact, the higher mortality and institutionalization in the Cleveland study suggested to him that casework might even be more harmful than no intervention.

Later, using more sophisticated statistical techniques, Berger and Piliavin (1976) reanalyzed the data from the Cleveland study and found that the experimentals were significantly more debilitated and at risk than the controls on the basis of combined age, mental status, and physical functioning *before* treatment. Thus the difference in survival or mortality rates could not be attributed to the experimental (casework) condition. Although the reanalysis did not account for the higher rate of institutionalization, there was some retrospective reasoning among the professionals involved in the project that institutionalization had been viewed as a legitimate and often appropriate protective service among trained practitioners who preferred not to take the great risks involved in leaving alone many elderly people who wished to continue in their marginal and dangerous way of life (Wasser, 1971). In addition, a similar study that was somewhat more advanced in terms of research methodology was conducted in England, and it showed markedly different findings (Goldberg, 1970). The special project groups, which also had casework as the core of service delivery, showed significantly more positive measures of morale, activity level, and social need with no higher rates of mortality or institutionalization.

Nevertheless, the findings of the Cleveland study brought about a great deal of soul searching and reappraisal through the 1970s concerning the role of casework in protective services, the status and use of institutional care within the spectrum of service, and the need for more accountability and demonstration of the effectiveness of casework services.

These developments combined with the changing views of aging and the emergence of different theoretical orientations toward casework practice have made for a much more diversified range of services and approaches in the casework repertoire of the early 1980s.

The casework treatment models to be presented here represent the dominant ones in social work with the elderly at the present time. Some models are much more indigenous to social work than others, some are more recent than others, and some are more prevalent and appropriate in particular kinds of practice settings and with particular problems of aging. One major factor in differential use is the community/institution dimension. Casework approaches, even within the same theoretical orientations, can vary in important respects in work with aged clients in institutional settings as opposed to work with clients in their own homes.

As noted earlier the major differences in the models to be presented are with respect to the problem-solving work and the therapeutic relationship, particularly with respect to the nature and the objectives of these two elements of casework. In a sense, then, each model can be viewed as prescriptive for the application of particular treatment procedures and techniques within its own frame of reference so practitioner-readers with a strong single theoretical preference can use it that way. At the same time it should be apparent to the reader that a great deal of commonality exists among the models in terms of actual skills, techniques, and methods used in practice with respect to certain kinds of problems. In fact, there appears to be much convergence occurring in actual practice. Where these convergences and commonalities occur will be noted in the course of presenting each model.

However, it is also evident that the different treatment models can represent *alternative* ways of approaching the same problem and that certain of these alternatives have been found to be more appropriate and effective in dealing with the problem. Furthermore, it is also evident that approaches and techniques from different models can *complement* one another and can be used very effectively in conjunction with one another. The implications of these points will be considered later under "Future Directions."

TREATMENT MODELS

The Psychodynamic Model

The psychodynamic model has been perhaps the most influential model for the longest period of time with respect to casework with the aging. It is largely Freudian and psychoanalytic in its theoretical origins, and it is represented to a large extent in the psychosocial casework theory of Florence Hollis (1972) and more recently Francis Turner (1978). The first and most complete explication of this model for work with older persons was done by Edna Wasser in *Creative Approaches to Casework with the Aging* (1966).

Essentially, this model incorporates concepts from ego psychology with respect to adaptation (Hartmann, 1958), as well as Erikson's (1963) developmental tasks and psychosocial crises. When applied to the elderly, this ego-psychological framework provides a particular perspective that has been concisely summed up as follows:

The aged person is constantly making an adaptation to his environment in minor as well as major ways. Indeed, it is in the later years that losses and changes are most likely to occur, when the individual has less psychic and physical energy to deal with crises and maintain equilibrium. A breakdown may be manifested in regressive behavior; there may be a breakdown of instinctual drives and disturbances in the executive functions of the ego (Wasser, 1966, p. 17).

This brief quote incorporates a number of key ideas that greatly influence both assessment and intervention. Foremost is the concept of loss, and the specific ego problem is one of coping with progressive losses: physical, financial, and social status, and above all loss of significant object relations, which leads to loss of cathexis and its resultant impoverishment of ego. This has been referred to as "depletion," which can have profound emotional effects, from lowered self-esteem and guilt to depression and despair. Therefore attempts at "restitution" are made, which might include rather regressive adaptations on the part of the ego. Stanley Cath's (1963) psychological construct of depletion-restitution balance is central to this model. Essentially, the construct holds that efforts to strike a balance between external and internal depleting and restorative forces go on throughout life, especially in old age. Efforts at restitution that appear to be regressive have to be seen as defenses against depletion anxiety, which probably has its roots in dread of abandonment.

What is particularly important about this is that in practice the caseworker might have to shore up defenses that would be considered maladaptive for younger persons. In fact, mechanisms such as regression and denial can be adaptive rather than pathological in old age, as can dependency. This means dependency based on a realistic appraisal of limitations. Thus an elderly woman with heart trouble who lives alone will accept outside help with heavy housekeeping tasks, despite her prior sense of accomplishment and independence in carrying out such tasks.

Consequently, the caseworker will eschew some of the uncovering, insight-oriented techniques such as confrontation and deeper interpretation. The emphasis is definitely not on getting behind the defenses but rather on supporting many of them. Wasser (1966, pp. 25-26) put it rather succinctly: "Treatment of the older persons gives priority to supportive techniques. In helping the client build on his remaining strengths, supporting his useful defenses, and relieving his inner and outer stress, the caseworker encourages his capacity for self-mobilization."

Warmth (including physical expressions), encouragement, promoting realistic feelings of hope, positive reinforcement of coping efforts, and acceptance of regressive and dependent behavior are all to be heavily drawn upon in casework with the elderly. Furthermore, these techniques are apt to be appropriate throughout the course of long-term treatment with many elderly, unlike work with younger persons in which supportive techniques are more heavily used in the early stages of treatment. With the elderly these supportive procedures are frequently intended to help the client to feel better, more comfortable, stronger, and better able to cope over the long haul as well as immediately.

Nelsen (1980) proposed four types of supportive procedures that she sees as necessary conditions for change: protection, acceptance, validation, and education. Each has particular relevance for casework with the older client.

Protection involves the worker literally *taking over* for the client in some area of functioning. For example, in the case of confused elderly persons living alone whose utilities have been shut off for nonpayment due to mental confusion, the worker would have to step in and take over the contacts and payments necessary to obtain the utilities. Other such actions would probably have to be undertaken by the worker *for* rather than *with* the client in this protective-service situation. It might even be necessary, depending on the physical and mental status of the client, for the worker to take over completely by arranging for institutional placement. This was reflected in the Cleveland study in which this particular model was used in the treatment condition. However, it should be emphasized that the primary emphasis in this model was and is still very much on maintaining the older person in his or her home situation of choice. Thus the model calls for use of the entire range of concrete services that can maintain the older person at home: financial, medical, homemaker, transportation, and so on. Not only do these meet material, social, and health needs, but "they can help make restitution for the losses [the client] has suffered and they can sustain him until he can mobilize his own forces" (Wasser, 1971, p. 45).

Acceptance, in Nelsen's scheme, means providing confirmation that the client is worthy and valued despite occasional wrong behavior. In an elderly client this is apt to mean such confirmation in the face of regressive or possible aberrant behavior.

The supportive technique of validation is feedback to clients indicating *in what ways* they are good, strong, or likely to be effective. Because of depletion and lowered self-esteem, older people need to know positive attributes and aptitudes, past and present.

Education is a supportive procedure that involves teaching clients how to cope by providing information about and modeling different ways to behave, communicate, control emotions, and so on. An example might be the situation of an older person whose increased dependency and anger is being expressed inappropriately and is alienating family members who are needed for support and nurturance. The worker might teach the client how to express dependency needs appropriately, assertively, rather than aggressively by angry demands. Further, the worker might indicate how the client can suppress angry feelings in the context of the family but ventilate them in sessions with the worker. The family, too, can be taught how to understand and cope with these restitutional behaviors. It should be noted at this point that the family is seen as the primary restitutional resource for the older person, just as it is apt to be a source of some depletion through insensitivity, nonresponsiveness, and dysfunctional interactions.

The therapeutic relationship, Perlman's third element of casework, is markedly different in this model than in the others to be presented. Issues of transference and countertransference are immediately taken into account, and transference is seen as an inevitable factor in the relationship. Whether to encourage or discourage it and to what extent are key questions for treatment planning. It has already been noted that a certain amount of dependency is seen as appropriate and functional for older persons, and such dependency needs will be met by the worker directly or indirectly and frequently in conjunction with the client's family. In general, there will be an evolution in the treatment process from the development of trust in an initially dependent sort of relationship to the degree of independence of which the client is capable in terms of ego functioning. This frequently involves a certain amount of identification by the client with the worker as a model for problem-solving, which should then develop into a self-identification based upon new or recovered ways of coping effectively (Wasserman, 1974).

The goals and course of relationship with the institutionalized elderly are apt to be different. Goldfarb (1981) has indicated that independence cannot be a realistic goal in such cases; instead the aim should be simply to make the person less dependent. Therefore, the worker should accept the role of surrogate parent and allow the person to grow more independent in a secure relationship.

The therapeutic use of reminiscence has become an integral part of psychodynamic work with the elderly ever since Butler's (1963) explication of the role of reminiscence in the life-review process. Much of the social-work treatment literature on reminiscence has been on its use with individuals and groups in institutional settings (Ingersol and Goodman, 1980; Ingersol and Silverman, 1978; Lewis and Butler, 1974; Liton and Olstein, 1969), but it can just as appropriately be used in casework with aged individuals living in the community (Kaminsky, 1978; Lowy, 1979; Sherman, 1981).

Lewis (1971) found that the self-concepts of elderly men living in the community were enhanced by reminiscence through positive memories of past pleasures and accomplishments. Pinkus (1970) noted that reminiscence not only can enhance self-esteem but enables the elderly to identify with the past, which can help reinforce a sense of identity for the purposes of sustaining self-continuity (Grunes, 1981). The sense of a continuity of self has been found to be extremely important in helping the "old old" to withstand the trauma and narcissistic assaults involved in institutionalization and further organic deterioration (Tobin, in press).

More specifically, reminiscence can be used as a casework technique to deal with depression by evoking memories of positive self-images that have been decathected in the course of the depression (Liton and Olstein, 1969). It can also be useful in grief work, for it is similar to mourning in that the lost person can be brought to mind, which then allows for further release of emotion (McMahon and Rhudick, 1967). Of course, one has to be aware of possible dangers in the use of reminiscence, for as Butler (1963) noted, panic, guilt, and depression can sometimes occur in the process. Consequently, it is important to assess the content and quality of the client's expressed memories before engaging in systematic use of reminiscence. Such an assessment also has broader uses for both diagnosis and focusing of treatment in that it provides information about the client's self-image, how much stress is being experienced, and the types of relationships being sought (Pinkus, 1970).

There has been a strong emphasis on exploration of the meaning of grief and mourning in this model as a means for developing techniques for dealing with the aged person's reaction to loss. Wasser (1966) called attention to the implications for casework practice of the work of Bowlby (1961), Lindemann (1944), and Bibring (1953). There is insufficient space to go into the actual techniques at this point. The work of Kubler-Ross (1969) and others, which was soon incorporated into this model (Wasser, 1971), is well known and readily accessible to the readers.

It can be surmised from the foregoing that much of the casework using this model deals with depression, particularly reactive depressions resulting from loss and depletion, which takes on added significance when it is recognized that depression is the most common psychiatric problem of the aged (Zarit, 1980).

Another common emotional problem among the elderly is anxiety. Because it is so general a term and emotion, it would be difficult to document that it is more common among the elderly than other age groups. However, the kinds of concerns and fears related to possible further physical, financial, and object losses, together with a concomitant lessening of a sense (internal locus) of control in their lives, has to increase the incidence of dysfunctional anxiety. This can be particularly true for the more vulnerable elderly who might require casework and other services in order to maintain themselves in the community in crisis situations. Crisis intervention will be described as a separate, brief treatment model later in this chapter, but it should be noted that it is very closely related to, if not a part of, this psychodynamic (ego-psychological) model (Parad, 1965; Wasser, 1966). Consequently, dynamic casework handling of anxiety that hampers or prevents effective coping will be covered under "Crisis Intervention."

The second most common psychological disorder after depression among the institutionalized elderly is paranoia (Pfeiffer, 1977). Late-life paranoia is not as apt to manifest itself in delusions involving grandiose persons or plots as in earlier paranoia; the delusions are apt to involve people who have been close to the older persons: family, friends, neighbors, and so on. Of course, para-noid beliefs are more apt to occur in older persons with some significant sensory deficit, particularly hearing and sight. Consequently, how a caseworker handles paranoid ideation and behavior is a most pertinent question in work with the elderly.

There are several ways within this model of handling this problem, but each requires development of trust and strong supportive casework activity within the treatment relationship. Two examples were selected from the treatment literature. One case illustrates the results of two years of intensive casework services with a man in his late 80s who was functioning at a psychotic, paranoid level in a large geriatric center. The worker had weekly half-hour sessions with the client, who was a major source of irritation to other residents and staff with his constant angry accusations and outbursts. The worker allowed herself to be seen by him as an "omnipotent protectress" who would act as advocate for him and manipulate his environment to assure his safety and security. On the basis of this relationship "the patient incorporated into his fragile ego enough discipline so that he could function in a manner acceptable to continued living in the institution" (Ross, 1981, p.108).

Another case example within this model involved some creative use of reminiscence (Liton and Olstein, 1969). Again, the client's paranoid ideas and behaviors created problems with other residents, whom she suspected of trying to harm her, poison her food, and attack her from behind. Since talking about these ideas distressed her greatly, the worker deflected discussion in their casework sessions to recollections of the client's happier past. Her paranoid symptoms were greatly alleviated and she regained some former social abilities with respect to numerous and colorful storytelling. This enhanced her relationship with the other residents and generated positive feedback from them, thereby reducing any environmental reasons for paranoid ideation.

This psychodynamic model has incorporated important new developments over the years and continues to do so (see later notations on cognitive methods under "Crisis Intervention"). Therefore, we can expect that this model will continue to be influential and to contribute heavily to casework practice with the elderly in the future.

The Behavioral Model

This model has not been used as extensively or as long as a specific social-work intervention with the elderly as has the psychodynamic model. However, references in the social-work literature on its use with the elderly have increased markedly since 1975. It is essentially a behavior-modification approach, which was originally called the "sociobehavioral" approach when it was introduced into social work by Edwin J. Thomas (1967). Its origins are in learning theory, and most of the behavior-modification techniques were developed by leading clinical theorists from psychology, such as Albert Bandura (1975), Frederick

Kanfer, and Jeanne Phillips (1970). Since Thomas's 1967 monograph, there has been an increasing number of behavioral texts by social-work educators, including, among others: Fischer and Gochros (1975), Schinke (1981), Schwartz and Goldiamond (1975), and Thomas (1970).

Basically, in this model the caseworker makes planned and systematic use of the principles and techniques of behavior modification so as to decrease undesirable behaviors and increase desired behaviors in the individual. Furthermore, it is seen as a parsimonious approach: "Most of its procedures are derived from three basic perspectives on human learning—the fields of operant learning, respondent learning, and imitative learning" (Fischer, 1978, p.157).

The initial use of behavioral methods in work with the elderly tended to be almost exclusively in institutional settings (Tobin, 1977). It is in such settings, of course, that stimulus-control procedures, contingency management, token economies, and other forms of reward and reinforcement can be put into operation most readily and efficiently. The kinds of target problems identified and worked on initially concerned self-care and activities of daily living involving locomotion, dressing, eating, and continence. The contribution of behavioral methods in dealing with these problems cannot be underestimated, and they have become highly valued additions in institutional settings for the elderly.

One of the first documented social-work efforts to move beyond these problems to more psychosocial concerns was a report on research-based behavioral group work in a home for the aged (Linsk, Howe, and Pinkston, 1975). Using applied behavior analysis, the team devised data-based treatment approaches to encourage more active participation of group members in the home as a way of dealing with the frequent problem of elderly people becoming isolated and uncommunicative in such settings. Observation methods that included reliability measures were developed for the purposes of planning and evaluating the treatment. Results showed a strong relationship between the social worker's use of task-related questions to group members and increased levels of appropriate verbalization by residents in activity groups. Although this study involved a group-work approach, the authors indicated that this type of behavior analysis could appropriately be applied to individualized treatment and evaluation.

This has in fact happened, and the remainder of this section will deal with individualized behavioral-casework services. One example of this is a case in which behavioral contracting was used to reduce the problem behaviors of an 85-year-old male resident of a nursing home (Adams, 1979). The behaviors that were identified target problems included temper tantrums, combativeness, and long episodes of crying. A functional analysis was done in which antecedents, dysfunctional behavior, and consequences were charted and interventions planned. The behaviors to be increased and those to be decreased were written into a contract. A token system was devised that included goods and privileges such as candy, soda, extra television-viewing time, game-room privileges, special field trips to sights and sports events. Verbal reinforcement of positive behaviors was systematically used by staff as well as the worker with positive results.

This case illustrates some well-established behavioral procedures (token systems and verbal reinforcement) to deal with some fairly common behavioral problems in nursing-home settings. What about dealing with problems of a clinically pathological nature, particularly those classified as paranoid? One example of behavioral work with such a problem was described by Cartensen and Fremouw (1981).

This was a case of a 68-year-old woman in a nursing home displaying paranoid behaviors that included hysterical crying because of the belief that she was going to be murdered, probably by poisoning. This situation was potentially life-threatening because it led her to refuse necessary cardiac medication. The individualized treatment program that was designed for her consisted of fourteen weekly counseling sessions in which her verbalizations of positive experiences were rewarded and in which she was asked to keep a daily record of behavior that focused on positive rather than negative events. A training session was also provided to staff members in which they were taught concepts of reinforcement and extinction and how they were to respond to the patient in terms of these principles. They were asked to initiate conversations with the client at times when she was not expressing paranoid concerns. On the basis of a consistent program for staff-client interactions, there was an extinction of frequent paranoid verbalization that in turn served to lessen staff tension and avoidance behavior so that, instead, staff could provide a supportive environment.

These examples of individualized service relate to casework with the elderly in institutional settings, but what represents a more recent development of note is home-based behavioral casework with the elderly (Linsk, Pinkston, and Green, 1982). This approach utilizes family or other involved caretakers who are willing to help, and the focus is on changing the home environment of the elderly person in ways that increase the amount of positive support received. The worker directly teaches these support persons applied behavior analysis. The treatment procedures include prompts, praise, contracting, and instruction geared toward increasing the elderly person's rate of reinforcement and opportunity to receive reinforcement.

A practice illustration of this model from the Elderly Support Project in Chicago, which was designed to demonstrate means of keeping elderly clients in their own homes, was provided by the just cited authors. It was a case of a 69-year-old retired man who was depressed and had a number of health problems including emphysema, tardive dyskinesia, and possible Parkinson's disease. This case therefore represents one behavioral form of work with depression as well as an example of home-based behavioral casework. Most behavioral therapists have linked depression with the amount of social reinforcement available, and in one conceptualization of intervention the assumed weak schedule of reinforcement requires an increase in the amount of positive reinforcement (Lazarus, 1968).

In this case a more reinforcing environment was constructed from simple daily activities that had been identified, specified, and measured according to behavior-analysis procedures for the purposes of treatment and evaluation. This involved specific written contacts, behavioral frequency counts, and review of trends and patterns in graphic form with the client and his wife. Levels of daily activities by the client were targeted as dependent variables, and activities were added serially to his daily functioning while his wife was taught to reinforce him for desired responses such as getting out of bed, cutting down on his smoking, taking daily walks, and so on. The results in this case prompted the authors to conclude that they provided "preliminary support for the use of home-based procedures for treating the impaired elderly" (Linsk, Pinkston, and Green, 1982, p. 231).

It should be noted here that some behavior therapists emphasize the absence of demonstrated social skills as an antecedent condition for the occurrence of depressed behaviors (Lewinsohn, 1976). A major ingredient in treatment therefore is the teaching of social skills so that the client can more effectively evoke the social reinforcements that are necessary to allay the depression. There is, of course, no reason why the two approaches cannot be combined in practice, with the social-skills training complementing the planned social reinforcements.

Having presented behavioral approaches to problems of depression and paranoid behaviors, there is need to consider the other ubiquitous emotional and behavioral problem facing older persons—anxiety. As noted earlier, anxiety can become dysfunctional and incapacitating when it is overwhelming or chronic, and the elderly are apt to be more at risk for the stress, events, and circumstances that can lead to chronic and overwhelming anxiety. The classic behavioral approach to treatment of anxiety has been systematic desensitization, usually in the form proposed by Wolpe (1973). Basically, this technique involves the use of a subjective scale of anxiety or SUDS (subjective units of disturbance —with a value of 0 for absolute calm and 100 SUDS for the most extreme anxiety the person can imagine). Then a hierarchy of anxiety-provoking stimuli or situations is constructed on the basis of the client's assessment of SUDS levels associated with the situations that are of the most focal concern to the client. While this is going on, the client is trained in deep-muscle relaxation on the basis of the empirical fact that one cannot be anxious (which includes muscle tension) while at the same time relaxed. The client then simultaneously maintains the relaxed state and imagines the anxiety-associated stimuli from the hierarchy. When the highest (100 SUDS) stimulus on the scale has been reduced to near 0 by this process, the dysfunctional anxiety associated with the focal problem-stimulus should be extinguished.

While demonstrably effective in dealing with conditioned anxiety of various sorts, it does not fit into the characteristic format of casework practice in its typical settings of family agencies, public-welfare agencies, and social-service departments. The element of rather lengthy and repetitive physical (muscle relaxation) training and practice seems somewhat incompatible with the usual talking therapy" or client-worker dialogue in agency office or client home.

Vattano (1978) proposed stress-management procedures—in addition to systematic desensitization—that can be readily adapted to the usual casework settings. These procedures include relaxation training involving a rather brief muscle-relaxing procedure, empirically tested forms of meditation, and the "relaxation response" technique (Benson, 1975). It is interesting to note in this regard that there has been a proliferation of yoga and meditation classes in many current senior-service-center programs, but the effects of these programs on the lives of the participants have not been properly evaluated.

The virtues of these techniques lie not only in their adaptability to conventional casework practice with the elderly but, more important, that they provide the older person with the tools and techniques for self-management or control. The advantage of *self*-control in contrast to the *external* control of the more conventional environmental, social-reinforcement techniques in behavioral practice is that it can be used with the isolated as well as with other elderly persons living in the community. It can also be used by older persons in institutional settings and by those going through the stressful transition of relocation from community to institution. Self-management techniques also answer, in part, one of the criticisms of certain behavioral approaches in work with the elderly—the problem of too little generalization of therapeutic gains to new situations (Rebok and Hayer, 1977; Tobin, 1977). The fact that a client learns an adaptive response within a specific behaviorally controlled situation does not necessarily lend itself to new problematic situations.

Another new development that has vastly enhanced the range and effectiveness of applied behavioral techniques has been the addition of cognitive techniques. Use of the cognitive capacities of memory, imagination or imagery, logical reasoning, and problem-solving in clients allows them to learn how to develop adaptive responses on their own, so that they can cope with situations that are new or different from those in which situation-specific learning takes place in conventional behavior modification. Thus cognition has been found to be a powerful "mediating variable" in the basic S-R paradigm of behaviorists. These newer cognitive behavioral techniques could just as legitimately be put in this behavioral section of the chapter, for many of the leading contributors to the combined approach are basically behaviorists.

The Cognitive Model

Mahoney and Arnkoff (1978), in a review of the cognitive therapies, identified three major types: rational psychotherapies, coping-skills therapies, and problem-solving therapies. The rational type is most closely identified with Ellis (1962, 1974) and Beck (1976) and usually forms the cognitive core of the other two types of cognitive therapies. It is also the one that is central to most of the social-work literature on the use of cognitive methods in casework (Combs, 1980; Lantz, 1978; Werner, 1965, 1974), including casework with the aged in particular (Sherman, 1979, 1981).

The central idea in the cognitive approach is that human emotion is much more a result of what people think, believe, or tell themselves about a situation or event than the event itself. Ellis built this into a cognitive "ABC theory of emotion" in which A is the *activating event* or situation, B is the *belief* or thoughts about that event, and C is the emotional *consequence* of the thoughts or belief. Thus B is an intervening factor in the experiential process, and if it is an irrational belief (iB) it can lead to irrational and dysfunctional emotional consequences (iC), and the person will experience A as extremely stressful or catastrophic. In fact, Ellis frequently talks about "catastrophic thinking" and notes that irrational beliefs usually contain a "must," an "ought," or a "should" —an implicit absolutistic demand that the person *must* obtain what he or she wants. In other words, what any person might reasonably want—love, acceptance, respect—is irrationally transformed into an absolute *need* or demand, and not receiving it is experienced as traumatic and catastrophic.

In the cognitive approach, the client is taught how to explore the implicit thoughts or self-talk that are associated with the explicit disproportionate and dysfunctional emotions. Then the client identifies the unsubstantiated or irrational elements within the implicit thoughts, and with the guidance of the therapist learns how to dispute them and replace them with rational beliefs (rB). This disputation (D) represents the core activity of the treatment process, and should lead to a new evaluation (E) of the problem situation and the activating event (A). Thus, there is an A-B-C-D-E sequence involved in the total process.

Beck (1976) uses essentially the same approach, and he asks the client to monitor the whole process by identifying "automatic thoughts" or beliefs and the associated emotions on a form called a "Daily Record of Dysfunctional Thoughts," which calls for the following:

1. Describe actual events or thoughts and daydreams of the day leading to unpleasant emotions.
2. Describe the type of emotion (sad, angry) and rate the degree of emotion involved on a scale of 1 to 100.
3. Write down the automatic thought(s) associated with the emotion and rate the degree of belief in the thought on a scale of 1 to 100.
4. Then write a rational response to the irrational automatic thoughts and rate the degree of belief in the rational response (1-100).
5. Rerate the belief in the automatic thought (1-100) and specify and rate the subsequent emotions (1-100).

By the process of identifying and disputing the negative cognitions leading to the negative emotions, the client should be able to gradually decrease the incidence and intensity of those emotions. Clients are given the regular "homework" assignment of monitoring their thoughts and emotions on a continuous basis throughout treatment.

Homework assignments are very much a part of cognitive practice, and clients are encouraged to test and challenge their irrational ideas, beliefs, and fears in real life. The term "cognitive" might belie the rather active type of treatment it often is. It is also one that provides for a great deal of client self-management and control. The basic A-B-C or dysfunctional-thoughts approach is easily and quickly taught and learned, and elderly persons are able to incorporate it into their repertoires quite readily (Sherman, 1981).

The cognitive model, particularly Beck's version, has been most noted for its use in the depressions, where it has some empirical evidence of effectiveness (Rush, Beck, Kovacs, and Holon, 1977; Rush, Khatami, and Beck, 1975; Shaw, 1977). His model posits three specific concepts to explain depression: (1) the cognitive triad, (2) schemas, and (3) cognitive errors or faulty information processing (Beck, Rush, Shaw, and Emery, 1979). The cognitive triad consists first of the client's negative view of self; second, a negative interpretation or construction of her/his experiences; and third, a negative view of the future. These depressive views emerge from a personally unique but relatively stable cognitive pattern called a schema. It is the way the schema processes incoming information that leads to the cognitive errors that are characteristic of depressogenic thinking and feelings.

Therefore, the core of the treatment processes is to have the client "restructure" (repattern) cognitions by continuous use of procedures like the daily analysis of dysfunctional thoughts, together with other techniques. In fact, the term "cognitive restructuring" is a generic term for a number of specific cognitive-behavioral techniques used in different combinations. However, the cognitive review or disputation process is always at the center of these techniques as the mediating treatment variable.

In addition to the disputation or reanalysis of depressogenic thoughts and cognitive errors, certain other techniques are used in treating depression. One of these is called "mastery and pleasure therapy," and is particularly helpful for dealing with the characteristic belief of depressed persons that they never enjoy anything and never will, as well as the belief that they can do nothing with any degree of competence or mastery (Beck et al., 1979). This technique requires that the client keep a daily record of activities and mark down an "M" for every activity during the day that provides a sense of mastery and a "P" for every activity that provides pleasure. For each M or P the client has to rate how much mastery or pleasure is experienced, on a scale from 0 (none) to 5 (a great deal). Almost invariably some activities will provide a modicum of pleasure or mastery, whether a 1 or 2 rating, which provides evidence to dispute the belief that there is absolutely no sense of mastery or pleasure in life.

Another related technique for depression is graded-task assignment, which is called "success therapy" by Beck (1976) because the client is first assigned a simple task that the therapist is sure can be accomplished and is then assigned increasingly difficult tasks. Of course, care has to be exercised so that the tasks are not too difficult, for failure will produce even more feelings of incompetence and worthlessness.

Bibliotherapy is a commonly used technique in cognitive treatment. It involves homework assignments of readings specific to the client's problems and about how the client's dysfunctional cognitions are related to the problems. Obviously, the caseworker has to be sensitive to the client's degree of literacy and potential resistence to a technique as didactic as this. The literature has to be simply, clearly, and directly written to be effective, and it can be quite effective with elderly clients when used in conjunction with other techniques. Beck and Greenberg (1974) prepared a clearly written booklet of this sort, which is routinely provided to their depressed patients at the start of treatment.

An example of the rational form of cognitive therapy associated with Beck and Ellis is provided in the case of Mrs. L, a 69-year-old woman who was referred to Jewish Family Service because of the emotional distress she was experiencing in apparent reaction to her 44-year-old daughter's separation and imminent divorce. The daughter, her only child, lived with her own two daughters, aged 17 and 20, in a city 300 miles away. Mrs. L was very worried and doubtful about her daughter's ability to cope with the separation and the responsibilities of single parenthood. Mrs. L felt that her worries were well founded, but she could not understand the extreme sadness she was feeling along with bouts of increased insomnia, lethargy, and feelings of worthlessness.

In the course of six sessions with the agency caseworker, Mrs. L was asked to monitor the cognitions associated with her negative emotions by using Beck's Daily Record of Dysfunctional Thoughts (Beck et al., 1979, p. 403). In addition, she was asked to read a section of a book (Ellis and Harper, 1975) that provided a list of prevalent irrational beliefs that could possibly help her identify any depressogenic thoughts she might be having that would explain her depressed state. The monitoring of her dysfunctional thoughts revealed a series of automatic thoughts going from immediate situation-specific issues to deeper levels of belief. At the more immediate level she doubted that her daughter could cope with her life after divorce. Mrs. L also recognized that she was disappointed in her daughter but that she was much more disappointed in herself. In fact, she believed she was a bad mother and therefore a failure as a person. So much of her life and identity were wrapped up in being a "good" mother that she was now feeling utterly incompetent and worthless in all respects. Thus it was her irrational belief (iB) of total worthlessness because of perceived failure as a parent that was leading to the irrational consequences (iC) or state of depression after the activating event (A) of her daughter's marital separation.

Mrs. L was given homework assignments involving disputation and continued monitoring of these dysfunctional thoughts and beliefs. In addition, the worker suggested that Mrs. L visit her daughter to check if there was a sound empirical basis for her concerns and beliefs, as well as to offer whatever support she could to her daughter. Mrs. L did make the visit and in the course of it learned that her daughter felt (and actually was) able and competent to cope with the impending divorce. In fact, she was looking forward to it. Therefore, she did not perceive Mrs. L to be a failure as a mother, but rather as a mother who provided her with an emotional foundation and a role model to enable her to cope with this stressful time in her life.

Mrs. L's depressed state was lessening after several sessions with the case-worker, and her symptoms lifted almost completely after her visit to her daughter.

A cognitive technique that can be used to deal with problems of anxiety as well as depression is "cognitive rehearsal" (Beck, 1976). The client is asked to imagine going through some selected activity or situation and to indentify the anticipated obstacles and conflicts, which allows for advance preparation for coping and problem-solving strategies, and enables the client to pinpoint ahead of time the automatic thought(s) that represent obstacle(s) in the situation. This technique serves to allay anticipatory anxiety and depressed cognitions of incompetence and failure.

Other similar cognitive preparatory techniques are "vicariation" or cognitive modeling (Raimy, 1975) and "rational imagery" (Lazarus, 1971). These techniques are often combined with behavioral techniques in a form of cognitive-behavior modification of the coping skills or problem-solving variety (Meichenbaum, 1977). These cognitive behavioral therapies and techniques are proliferating rapidly, and a strong case has been made for their incorporation into mainstream social-work practice (Berlin, 1982; Fischer, 1978).

One of the better known and more influential coping-skills techniques is "systematic rational restructuring" (Goldfried, Decenteco, and Weinberg, 1974). It is similar in almost every respect to the behavioral technique of systematic desensitization in that it includes construction of a hierarchy of anxiety-probing situations, with successful coping at one level a prerequisite for progression to the next. However, it substitutes rational reevaluation in place of muscle relaxation by having the client identify what dysfunctional thoughts are occurring when anxious or depressed and then reevaluating the situation in more rational terms while noting any changes in subjective units of disturbance (SUDS). This technique is a good alternative for older persons who cannot do the muscle-relaxation part of desensitization because of their physical condition. The author has elsewhere described a case of a 74-year-old woman who was in an anxiety state over her physical condition and recent surgery (Sherman, 1981, pp. 122-126). This case included the use of systematic rational restructuring in conjunction with the techniques of rational imagery and "changing attributions" (Mahoney, 1974).

Problem-solving therapy comprises a diverse collection of procedures, including such behavioral ones as assertiveness training, modeling, and positive reinforcement, along with cognitive review and rehearsal (D'Zurilla and Goldfried, 1971). Basically, it trains clients to solve problems in a six-step process: (1) general orientation, (2) defining the situation, (3) identifying positive and neg-ative thoughts about the situation, (4) brainstorming alternative solutions, (5) deciding on the best solution, and (6) practice and implementation of the solu-tion. It has been used by social workers with community-based older persons with generally positive results (Toseland, 1977; Waskel, 1981).

Generally, it is with problems of depression and anxiety related to stress and coping that the cognitive model seems to have the greatest applicability. When it comes to actual organic brain syndromes, loss of cognitive capacities rules out many of the rational-therapy options. Also, in true paranoid thought the delusional systems and distortions rule out a number of cognitive techniques (Werner, 1974). Finally, Emery (1981) has found it necessary to adapt certain procedures, such as the type of diagnostic tests and behavioral task assignments, because of the physical limitations in elderly clients.

The Crisis Intervention Model

The *crisis intervention model* has certain focal concepts that make it particularly applicable for casework with the community-based elderly in both preventive and protective situations.

"Crisis intervention means entering into the life situation of an individual, family, or group to alleviate the impact of a crisis inducing stress in order to help mobilize the resources of those directly affected, as well as those who are in the significant 'socal orbit'," according to Parad (1965, p. 2). Its origins go back to Lindemann's (1944) study of the mourning reactions of the bereaved relatives of victims of the Coconut Grove disaster of 1942 in Boston and to the further development and extension of his concept by Gerald Caplan (1961). Thus, from its very beginnings crisis theory dealt with the trauma of object loss and sharp dislocations in the lives of the bereaved, which of course are problems very pertinent to old age. Again, Erikson's (1963) epigenetic theory contributed with its explication of maturational stages and the potential for crisis at each stage. As noted earlier, ego psychology is very central to it, and a number of social-science concepts dealing with role theory and role transition are also pertinent.

In its simplest terms, "crisis" can be defined as an upset in a steady state, but it must be added that the habitual problem-solving activities are not adequate to the new situation and do not lead rapidly to the previously achieved balanced state (Rapoport, 1965). What usually happens is that a hazardous event creates a problem in the person's life situation, and this event can be conceived of as a loss, a threat, or a challenge. If it represents a threat to basic need or sense of identity, it is met with *anxiety;* if it represents loss or deprivation, it is met with *depression;* but if it represents a challenge it is apt to be met with energetic and purposive problem-solving activities. Thus crisis theory addresses the two most commonly experienced emotional problems of the elderly—anxiety and depression.

One other central concept of crisis theory is the time-limited nature of the crisis state. Caplan (1961) claims that the actual period of crisis lasts from one to six weeks, in which an adequate solution has to be found to restore equilibrium. If it is not found a lower level of functioning and mental health will ensue. This makes it essential that intervention take place quickly and actively, which accounts for the brief-treatment nature of the crisis model (Rapoport, 1970).

Certain patterns of response provide for healthy crisis resolution, and these patterns provide the guidelines for our interventions with the elderly. First, there is a need for cognitive grasp and restructuring as a first step in problem solving, so the role of the caseworker is to help the client identify and isolate the factors (often preconscious and unintegrated) that have led to disruption of functioning. Then, together, worker and client arrive at a formulation of the problem that facilitates cognitive restructuring (Rapoport, 1965), which in itself might provide the kind of problem-solving activity sufficient to reestablish the previously achieved balanced state.

Perlman (1975) has provided an excellent analysis of cognitive functioning in the process of ego adaptation to stress and crisis states that adds significant focal power to the crisis model. In fact, Golan (1978) has identified Perlman's problem-solving model as having contributed directly to the crisis-intervention approach.

The second practice guide is that there needs to be an explicit acceptance by the caseworker of the disordered affect, the irrational and negative attitudes, and the need for the expression and management of feelings on the part of elderly clients. Not only do these behaviors have to be met with empathy and acceptance, but they have to be placed in the rational context of their natural history. This is extremely important for casework with the elderly in order to assure that the affect and responses of the client are not immediately labeled as evidence of senility or organicity. These behaviors should first be viewed as efforts at coping and possible restitution.

The third major guide is the availability and use of interpersonal and institutional resources. The use of formal institutions, agencies, and caretakers has been incorporated in crisis intervention from its inception. So has the recognition and use of significant others, particularly family, for comfort, support, and need-satisfaction. The potential for use of a broader network of human relationships was recognized in the past but not systematically pursued. As far as work with the aged is concerned, the development and availability of mutual support groups has been of major importance (Caplan and Killilea, 1976) as have the self-help groups with more of a social-action orientation (Gartner and Riesmann, 1977; Hess, 1976). In some instances caseworkers have helped to develop informal helping networks in order to initiate helping interaction or to provide for continuity in the informal helping process (Smith, 1975).

All of these happenings bode well for the continued use and further development of the crisis-intervention model for casework service to the elderly. It is also clear that this model can enhance and be enhanced by some of the other models that have already been discussed.

The Task-Centered Model

The *task-centered model* is probably the only one of those covered in this chapter that is truly indigenous to social work, for it was developed and empirically tested in social-agency settings where social work was the host discipline (Epstein, 1980; Reid and Epstein, 1972, 1977; Reid and Shyne, 1969). If it has any theoretical origins, they come out of Perlman's (1957) problem-solving theory of casework, which is also an indigenous social-work-practice theory. At any rate, the task-centered approach has been found to be particularly promising for short-term casework with the aging (Cormican, 1977). Its special strengths as well as certain possible limitations for work with the aged will be noted after a brief recapitulation of the essential features of the model.

Task-centered work normally consists of six to twelve client-worker sessions once or twice a week over a period of two to four months. Assessment is concentrated in the first one or two sessions, with emphasis on exploration and specification of problems, culminating in a problem-reduction program that focuses on certain target problems. The target problem(s) will usually be only one or two, but no more than three in number, so that the client's and the worker's task activities can be concentrated enough for problem-resolution within the brief allotted time.

Next, the client and worker mutually agree upon target-problem priorities, set goals, and specify their respective tasks to be carried out in order to achieve the specified goals. A "task" states a general direction for action, and general tasks can be broken down into operational tasks and subtasks. For example, the target problem for a socially isolated, ambulatory older person in the community might be stated as "lack of sufficient social contact for emotional well-being," in which case the general task will be to substantially increase the number of social contacts within the specified period of service. Specific subtasks of the client might include, sequentially, to inquire about, visit, enroll, and finally attend a local senior service center. To initiate a certain number of contacts per week with friends and neighbors might also be an operational task for the client. The worker's task in this instance might be to provide information about available senior centers or possible social programs, about transportation service if distance is a problem, as well as to provide specific instruction, guidance, or modeling of how the isolated person can initiate these contacts.

There is contracting with the client about the duration, scheduling, and conditions of the intervention. The contract does not have to be written, but it can be if the client wishes. At any rate, the conditions, specification of tasks, and third-party involvements (family members, referring or collaborative agencies, and so on) all have to be mutually and explicitly agreed upon between client and worker. The whole emphasis is to quickly identify and work on the problems that the *client* sees as most pressing.

The actual implementation or problem-solving part of treatment consists of the client carrying out the specified tasks and subtasks while the worker obtains the necessary resources and ancillary services and, if necessary, instructs the client in the skills and actions necessary to accomplish the stipulated tasks. The client's task performance is reviewed and necessary adjustments are made in each session, and at the end there is a review of the overall progress made in alleviating the target problems. If the progress has been sufficient, service is terminated at the contracted time. Certain exceptions of from one to four additional sessions can be made, and there might also be some follow-up at a later date with some monitoring of client task functioning.

In general, the task-centered model is eclectic in nature, drawing upon behavioral, cognitive, and ego-psychological methods and techniques. For example, Epstein (1980) used a five-step variation of the problem-solving therapy noted earlier (D'Zurilla and Goldfried, 1971). Graded-task assignment is used just as in behavioral and cognitive approaches. And, in fact, task-centered and cognitive-behavioral methods can be combined almost in their entirety in work with certain kinds of problems. A case example of this kind of combined use of these two methods was provided by this author in the treatment of a 66-year-old woman with a reactive depression (Sherman, 1981, pp. 127-136).

Golan (1981) notes that the task-centered approach is also well suited for crisis intervention in that its emphasis on quick formulation and systematic work on the most pressing problems of clients fits well into the time trajectory of crisis states. She further notes that it is very appropriate for use during transitional periods, because within its eight-problem typology the model addresses three problems—difficulty in role performance, decision problems, and reactive emotional distress—that can be crucial in transitional situations. For example, a too-frequent problem among elderly couples occurs when one spouse is endangering his or her own health and well-being in maintaining a deteriorating partner at home. This involves a difficulty in role performance for which the caretaking spouse could use help in the form of homecare and other concrete supportive services that the task model was well equipped to provide. The example could also be viewed as a decision problem in that there might be a need to come to a decision about institutional placement of the deteriorating spouse. Finally, it could be a problem of reactive emotional distress in helping the caretaking spouse deal with the fact of loss and institutionalization of the partner.

On the other hand, Golan (1981) sees some problem with the time-limited aspects of the model for some transitional work "where the entire linking interval may cover several months or even years." Of course, this precludes setting in advance a specific number of sessions within a definite span of time. However, this would be true of most short-term models, so the task-centered model is not alone in this. On the other hand, the model does function best as a voluntary service in which the client recognizes a problem and is prepared to work on it. The model could be problematic in protective situations with clients who are negative toward and refuse to see the need for any such service.

With these few limitations, the task-centered model has a great deal to contribute to casework with the elderly. It has not only been found useful in work with the community-based elderly but also for dealing with the psychological problems of the elderly in a long-term residential facility (Dierking, Brown, and

Fortune, 1980). This has led some social-work educators in an MSW program to attempt to develop the task-centered model as an effective base for social work with the elderly by integrating it with gerontological and clinical knowledge and experience (Fortune and Rathbone-McCuan, 1981).

In concluding this section it should be noted that crisis intervention and task-centered are by far the most influential of the brief casework models. There are no other, competing short-term *social-work* approaches that are cohesive enough to be considered models for casework practice with the aged.

FUTURE DIRECTIONS

It must be evident to the reader by now that there is a trend toward convergence and a degree of commonality among the above models of casework. Therefore, one very promising direction for the future lies in the synergistic development and use of these different models in a more integrative manner with the elderly.

If we begin with the fact that in many instances of community casework with the elderly there has been a depletion of tangible, material resources as well as psychosocial resources, a combined task-centered and crisis-intervention approach immediately suggests itself. The task-centered model is particularly well-suited for quick provision of concrete services without "taking over" for the client and thus incurring unnecessary dependency. The crisis model is well equipped for handling the emotional aspects of the situation, of the need for appropriate support based on an assessment of ego functioning, which in turn will indicate the range and limitations of the client's coping capacities. The task-centered model can also provide the kind of structure for rational, sequential coping and problem-solving work required at this stage.

Additionally, some of the stress-management techniques from the behavioral repertoire might be applied if anxiety impinges too much on the client's problem-solving capacities. Also, coping-skills techniques from the cognitive-behavioral repertoire might be taught to the client, according to the demands of the situation (Meichenbaum, 1977). Furthermore, if the brief supportive and problem-solving work of the combined task-centered/crisis-intervention approach is not sufficient to resolve the problem, it might be necessary to provide the elderly client with the more specifically focused problem-solving therapy (D'Zurilla and Goldfried, 1971). This would be particularly appropriate if the client had a functional deficit in systematic problem-solving skills (Goldfried and Goldfried, 1975). When it comes to more extended casework such as the transitional work mentioned by Golan (1981), where issues of role transition, identity, and intrapersonal and interpersonal functioning are prominent, the psychodynamic model appears most appropriate. However, even here the work under that model could be enhanced by some of the cognitive restructuring techniques to bring about necessary changes in self-concept, which is essentially based on a cognitive schema.

The growing application of cognitive, behavioral, and task-centered approaches in casework with the aged may lead in the direction of greater specification of service input and outcome. There might also be a growing use of quantified methods in assessment and evaluation, since these approaches lend themselves to these methods. This certainly has implications for accountability and for empirical testing of the differential effectiveness of treatment approaches.

So far, these projections for the future apply mostly to work with the community-based elderly. In institutional work there will probably not be more direct work by professionally trained workers in terms of the daily living skills of elderly residents, an area which has been enhanced so much by behavioral methods. Such direct behavioral-management services will probably be provided by direct-care staff who will need to be trained by the professionals (Brody, 1977), which could free professionally trained workers for the training of direct-care staff and for planning and consultation with other staff for a more therapeutic and humane milieu. It might also allow the professionals to provide more casework counseling for dealing with the psychological problems of the elderly in long-term-care facilities, as demonstrated by Dierking, Brown, and Fortune (1981). Overall, however, the likelihood is that the professionally trained worker will function more as an "indirect service provider" who performs largely in the role of consultant and of tutor/trainer of direct-service staff and of the BSW associate, as was found in a recent empirical study (Snider, 1981).

IMPLICATIONS FOR TRAINING

A number of educational considerations become immediately apparent in the light of the above directions. To begin with the last point first, it is clear that current MSW curricula, if they wish to take gerontological practice into account, need to accommodate to the fact that social workers in long-term-care facilities do not fit the model of direct-service providers within a department of social service, such as in hospital social work. The new kinds of knowledge and skills future gerontological practitioners in these facilities will need from MSW curricula will be in the areas of consultation and teaching. Experiential learning opportunities in the field would, of course, be an essential ingredient in this.

Another educational implication is inherent in the influx of cognitive, behavioral, and task-centered methods into casework practice with the aged. The sheer numbers and varieties of tested and untested but promising techniques are such that only a fraction can be taught and learned in a two-year MSW curriculum, even in curricula with practice-theoretical orientations that are compatible with them. This suggests the need for additional training opportunities outside the regular curriculum in the form of continuing education workshops and classes and in-service training programs in gerontological practice settings.

Certainly, these techniques should not be offered cafeteria-style in either training programs or in practice. None should be used in the absence of a guiding treatment framework and a sound assessment. Some, especially those using muscle relaxation, should only be used in the light of medical advice because of the greater possibility of physical complications with elderly clients.

There is another important concern about the proliferation and increased use of techniques. It has to do with the kind of professional stance the worker assumes with such a repertoire, which can all too easily become that of technical expert and virtuoso with a bag of "scientific" techniques and procedures, which can lead to inadequate attention to the pervasive social, medical, and economic needs of many elderly individuals. Furthermore, work with the elderly requires a broader view, a life-span perspective, one that "argues that only in gerontological practice are social workers confronted with a person's final destiny and with the true meaning of a person's life" (Monk, 1981, 62). The idea of a social technician or therapist providing casework services to our aged clients is not compatible with the more profound humanistic perspective on aging and work with the aged that is required of us.

REFERENCES

Adams, J. M. (1979). Behavioral contracting: An effective method of intervention with the elderly nursing home patient. *Journal of Gerontological Social Work,* **1**(3), 235-250.

Bandura, A. (1975). *Principles of behavior modification.* New York: Columbia University Press.

Beck, A. T. (1976). *Cognitive therapy and the emotional disorders.* New York: International Universities Press.

Beck, A. T., and Greenberg, R. L. (1974). *Coping with depression.* New York: Institute for Rational Living.

Beck, A. T., Rush, A. J., Shaw, G. F., and Emery, G. (1979). *Cognitive therapy of depression.* New York: Guilford Press.

Benson, H. (1975). *The relaxation response.* New York: William Morrow.

Berger, R., and Piliavin, I. (1976). The effect of casework: A research note. *Social Work,* **21**(3), 205-208.

Berlin, S. B. (1982). Cognitive behavioral interventions for social work practice. *Social Work,* **27**(3), 218-226.

Bibring, E. (1953). The mechanism of depression. In P. Greenacre (Ed.), *Affective disorders.* New York: International Universities Press.

Blenkner, M., Bloom, M., and Nielsen, M. A. (1971). A research and demonstration project of protective services. *Social Casework,* **52**(8), 483-499.

Bowlby, J. (1961). Process of mourning. *International Journal of Psychoanalysis,* **42**, 317-340.

Brody, E. M. (1977). *Long-term care of older people: A practical guide.* New York: Human Sciences Press.

Butler, R. (1963). The life review: An interpretation of reminiscence in the aged. *Psychiatry,* **26**(1), 65-76.

Caplan, G. (1961). *An approach to community mental health.* New York: Grune & Stratton.

Caplan, G., and Killilea, M. (Eds.). (1976). *Support systems and mutual help: Multidisciplinary explorations.* New York: Grune & Stratton.

Cartensen, L. L., and Fremouw, W. J. (1981). The demonstration of a behavioral intervention for late life paranoia. *Gerontologist,* **21**(3), 329-333.

Cath, S. H. Some dynamics of middle and later years. (1963). *Smith College Studies in Social Work,* **33**(2), 97-126.

Combs, T. D. (1980). A cognitive therapy for depression: Theory, techniques, and issues. *Social Casework,* **61**(6), 361-366.

Cormican, E. (1977). Task-centered model for work with the aged. *Social Casework,* **58**(8), 490-494.

Cormican, E. J. (1980). Social work and aging: A review of the literature and how it is changing. *Aging and Human Development,* **11**(4), 251-267.

Dierking, B., Brown, M., and Fortune, A. E. (1980). Task-centered treatment in a residential facility for the elderly: A clinical trial. *Journal of Gerontological Social Work,* **2**(3), 225-240.

D'Zurilla, T., and Goldfried, M. (1971). Problem-solving and behavior modification. *Journal of Abnormal Psychology,* **78**, 107-126.

Ellis, A. (1962). *Reason and emotion in psychotherapy.* Secaucus, N.J.: Citadel Press.

Ellis, A. (1974). *Humanistic psychotherapy: The rational-emotive approach.* New York: McGraw-Hill.

Ellis, A., and Harper, R. A. (1977). *A new guide to rational living.* Englewood Cliffs, N.J.: Prentice-Hall.

Emery, G. (1981). Cognitive therapy with the elderly. In G. Emery, S. D. Holon, and R. C. Bedrosian (Eds.), *New directions in cognitive therapy.* New York: Guilford Press.

Epstein, L. (1980). *Helping people: The task-centered approach.* St. Louis: C. V. Mosby.

Erikson, E. (1963). *Childhood and society* (2nd ed.). New York: Norton.

Fischer, J. (1973). Is casework effective? A review. *Social Work,* **18**(1), 5-20.

Fischer, J. (1978). *Effective casework practice: An eclectic approach.* New York: McGraw-Hill.

Fischer, J. and Gochros, H. L. (1975). *Planned behavior change: Behavior modification in social work.* New York: Free Press.

Fortune, A. E., and Rathbone-McCuan, E. (1981). Education in gerontological social work: Application of the task-centered model. *Journal of Education for Social Work,* **17**(3), 98-105.

Garner, J. D., and Mercer, S. O. (1980). Social work practice in long-term care facilities: Implications of the current model. *Journal of Gerontological Social Work,* **3**(2), 71-77.

Gartner, A., and Riesmann, F. (1977). *Self-help in the human services.* San Francisco: Jossey-Bass.

Golan, N. (1978). *Treatment in crisis situations.* New York: Free Press.

Golan, N. (1981). *Passing through transitions: A guide for practitioners.* New York: Free Press.

Goldberg, E. M., Mortimer, A., and Williams, B. T. (1970). *Helping the aged: A field experiment in social work.* London: George Allen & Univin.

Goldfarb, A. I. (1981). Psychiatry in geriatrics. In S. Steury and M. L. Blank (Eds.), *Readings in psychotherapy with older people.* Washington, D.C.: National Institute of Mental Health.

Goldfried, M. R., Decenteco, E. T., and Weinberg, L. (1974). Systematic rational restructuring as a self-control technique. *Behavior Therapy,* **5**, 247-254.

Goldfried, M., and Goldfried, A. (1975). Cognitive change methods. In F. Kanfer and A. Goldstein (Eds.), *Helping people change.* New York: Pergamon Press.

Grunes, J. M. (1981). Reminiscences, regression, and empathy—a psychotherapeutic approach to the impaired elderly. In S. I. Greenspan and G. H. Pollock (Eds.), *The course of life* (Vol. 3). Washington, D.C.: Government Printing Office.

Hartmann, H. (1958). *Ego psychology and the problem of adaptation.* New York: International Universities Press.

Hess, B. B. (1976). Self-help among the aged. *Social Policy,* **7**, 55-62.

Hollis, F. (1972). *Casework: A psychosocial therapy* (2nd ed.). New York: Random House.

Ingersoll, B., and Goodman, L. (1980). History comes alive: Facilitating reminiscence in a group of institutionalized elderly. *Journal of Gerontological Social Work,* **2**(4), 305-319.

Ingersoll, B., and Silverman, A. (1978). Comparative group psychotherapy for the aged. *Gerontologist,* **18**(2), 201-206.

Kaminsky, M. (1978). Pictures from the past: The use of reminiscence in casework with the elderly, *Journal of Gerontological Social Work,* **1**(1), 19-32.

Kanfer, F. H., and Phillips, J. S. (1970). *Learning foundations of behavior therapy.* New York: Wiley.

Kosberg, J. (1973). The nursing home: A social work paradox. *Social Work,* **18**(2), 104-110.

Kubler-Ross, E. (1969). *On death and dying.* London: Macmillan.

Lantz, J. E. (1978). Cognitive theory and social casework. *Social Work,* **23**(5), 361-366.

Lazarus, A. A. (1968). Learning theory and the treatment of depression. *Behavior Research and Therapy,* **6**, 83-89.

Lazarus, A. A. (1971). *Behavior therapy and beyond.* New York: McGraw-Hill.

Lewis, C. N. (1971). Reminiscing and self-concept in old age. *Journal of Gerontology,* **26**(2), 263-269.

Lewis, M. I., and Butler, R. N. (1974). Life review therapy: Putting memories to work in individual and group psychotherapy. *Geriatrics,* **29**, 165-169, 172-173.

Lewinsohn, P. M. (1976). A behavioral approach to depressions. In R. J. Friedman and M. M. Katz (Eds.), *The psychology of depression: Contemporary theory and research.* New York: Brunner/Mazel.

Lindemann, E. (1944). Symptomatology and management of acute grief. *American Journal of Psychiatry,* **101**, 141-148.

Linsk, N., Howe, M. W., and Pinkston, E. M. (1975). Behavioral group work in a home for the aged. *Social Work,* **20**(6), 454-463.

Linsk, N. L., Pinkston, E. M., and Green, G. R. (1982). Home-based behavioral social work with the elderly. In E. M. Pinkston, J. L. Levitt, G. R. Green, N. L. Linsk, and T. F. Rzepnicki (Eds.), *Effective social work practice: Advanced techniques for behavioral intervention with individuals, families, and institutional staff.* San Francisco: Jossey-Bass.

Lowy, L. (1979). Social work with the aging: *The challenge and promise of the later years.* New York: Harper & Row.

Liton, L., and Olstein, S. C. (1969). Therapeutic aspects of reminiscence, *Social Casework,* **50**(5), 263-266.

Mahoney, M. J. (1974). *Cognition and behavior modification.* Cambridge, Mass: Ballinger.

Mahoney, M. J., and Arnkoff, D. (1978). Cognitive and self-control therapies. In S. L. Garfield and A. E. Bergin (Eds.), *Handbook of psychotherapy and behavior change* (2nd ed.). New York: Wiley.

McMahon, A. W., and Rhudick, P. J. (1967). Reminiscing in the aged. In S. Levin and R. J. Kahana (Eds.), *Psycho-dynamic studies on aging: Creativity, reminiscing, and dying.* New York: International Universities Press.

Meichenbaum, D. (1977). *Cognitive-behavior modification: An integrative approach.* New York: Plenum Press.

Monk, A. (1981). Social work with the aged: Principles of practice. *Social Work,* **26**(1), 61-68.

Nelsen, J. C. (1980). Support: A necessary condition for change. *Social Work,* **25**(5), 388-393.

Parad, H. J. (Ed.). (1965). *Crisis intervention: Selected readings.* New York: Family Service Association of America.

Perlman, H. H. (1957). *Social casework: A problem-solving process.* Chicago: University of Chicago Press.

Perlman, H. H. (1975). In quest of coping. *Social Casework,* **56**(4), 213-225.

Pfeiffer, E. (1977). Psychopathology and social pathology. In J. E. Birren and W. K. Schaie (Eds.), *Handbook of the psychology of aging.* New York: Van Nostrand Reinhold.

Pinkus, A. (1970). Reminiscence in aging and its implications for social work practice. *Social Work,* **15**(3), 47-53.

Raimy, V. (1975). *Misunderstandings of the self.* San Francisco: Jossey-Bass.

Rapoport, L. (1965). The state of crisis: Some theoretical considerations. In H. J. Parad (Ed.), *Crisis intervention: Selected readings.* New York: Family Service Association of America.

Rapoport, L. (1970). Crisis intervention as a model of brief treatment. In R. W. Roberts and R. H. Nee (Eds.), *Theories of social casework.* Chicago: University of Chicago Press.

Rebok, G. W., and Hayer, W. J. (1977). The functional context of elderly behavior. *Gerontologist,* **17**, 27-34.

Reid, W. J. (1978). *The task-centered system.* New York: Columbia University Press.

Reid, W. J., and Epstein, L. (1972). *Task-centered casework.* New York: Columbia University Press.

168   E. Sherman

Reid, W. J., and Epstein, L. (Eds.). (1977). *Task-centered practice.* New York: Columbia University Press.

Reid, W. J., and Shyne, A. (1969). *Brief and extended casework.* New York: Columbia University Press.

Ross, F. (1981). Social work treatment of a paranoid personality in a geriatric institution. In S. Steury and M. L. Blank (Eds.), *Readings in psychotherapy with older people.* Washington, D.C.: National Institute of Mental Health.

Rush, A. J., Beck, A. T., Kovacs, M., and Hollon, S. (1977). Comparative efficacy of cognitive therapy and imipramine in the treatment of depressed outpatients. *Cognitive Therapy and Research,* **1**, 17-37.

Rush, A. J., Khatami, M., and Beck, A. T. (1975). Cognitive and behavioral therapy in chronic depression. *Behavior Therapy,* **6**, 398-404.

Schinke, S. P. (Ed.). (1981). *Behavioral methods in social welfare.* Hawthorn, N.Y.: Aldine.

Schwartz, A., and Goldiamond, J. (1975). *Social casework: A behavioral approach.* New York: Columbia University Press.

Shaw, B. F. (1977). Comparison of cognitive therapy and behavior therapy in the treatment of depression. *Journal of Consulting and Clinical Psychology,* **45**, 543-551.

Sherman, E. (1979). A cognitive approach to direct practice with the aging. *Journal of Gerontological Social Work,* **2**(1), 43-53.

Sherman, E. (1981). *Counseling the aging: An integrative approach.* New York: Free Press.

Smith, S. A. (1975). *Natural systems and the elderly: An unrecognized resource.* Unpublished report of Title III model project grant, School of Social Work, Portland State University.

Snider, L. F. (1981). The role of the qualified social worker in the skilled nursing facility: A unique model of practice. *Journal of Gerontological Social Work,* **4**(2), 31-42.

Thomas, E. J. (Ed.). (1967). *Socio-behavioral approach and application to social work.* New York: Council on Social Work Education.

Thomas, E. J. (1970). Behavioral modification and casework. In R. Roberts and R. Nee (Eds.), *Theories of social casework.* Chicago: University of Chicago Press.

Tobin, S. S. (1977). Old people. In H. Maas (Ed.), *Social service research: Review of studies.* New York: National Association of Social Workers.

Tobin, S. S. (in press). Psychodynamic treatment of the family and the institutionalized individual. In N. E. Miller and G. D. Cohen (Eds.), *Psychodynamic research perspectives on development, psychopathology, and treatment in later life.* New York: International Universities Press.

Toseland, R. (1977). A problem-solving group workshop for older persons. *Social Work,* **22**(4), 323-324.

Turner, F. J. (1978). *Psychosocial therapy.* New York: Free Press, 1978.

Vattano, A. J. (1978). Self-management procedures for coping with stress. *Social Work,* **23**(2), 113-119.

Waskel, S. (1981). The elderly, change, and problem solving. *Journal of Gerontological Social Work,* **3**(4), 77-81.

Wasser, E. (1966). *Creative approaches in casework with the aging.* New York: Family Service Association of America.

Wasser, E. (1971). Protective practice in serving the mentally impaired aged. *Social Casework.* **52**(8), 510-522.

Wasserman, S. L. (1974). Ego-psychology. In F. J. Turner (Ed.), *Social work treatment.* New York: Free Press.

Werner, H. D. (1965). *A rational approach to social casework.* New York: Association Press.

Werner, H. D. (1974). Cognitive theory. In F. J. Turner (Ed.), *Social work treatment.* New York: Free Press.

Wolpe, J. (1973). *The practice of behavior therapy.* New York: Pergamon Press.

Zarit, S. H. (1980). *Aging and mental disorders: Psychological approaches to assessment and treatment.* New York: Free press.

7

Group Work With Older Adults

Margaret E. Hartford, Ph.D.

University of Southern California

For most older adults, group participation has both preventive and therapeutic benefits. From the preventive side, group experiences are particularly valuable for maintaining older people in physical and mental health. Groups may give continuity for social participation that provides a sense of belonging and of being needed. Groups may provide the opportunity to talk out, think about, and express emotion, a chance to be listened to, and an opportunity to receive the caring responses of others. On the other hand many people become incapacitated in old age because life does not make enough demands upon them, and they lack a social structure within which to move and make a contribution. Having left regular employment and been freed of family responsibilities, they may find themselves lacking the role expectations of production and responsibility, the intellectual stimulation, and the personal validation that comes from social interaction. The result is a sense of isolation, even alienation, with a high stress component. A consequence is frequently the physical response of the development of ailments previously fought off by the demands to be productive and responsible. Research shows that inactivity, frustration, and lack of satisfactory experiences make the body more vulnerable to disease and physical disorder.

From the therapeutic standpoint, groups are used extensively for rehabilitation of emotional and physical disorders through opportunities to grow and test out new methods of handling or compensating for lacks or losses. Many older adults with physical impairments are capable of considerable mastery if they have the mental and social stimulation to keep them psychologically involved. Others who have mental impairments resulting from illness may be stimulated to better physical and mental health through contacts with others and through social situations that demand their response, especially when the experiences are guided by a mental health professional. Group participation can provide some of that therapeutic stimulus.

It should be recognized that old age covers a period of approximately thirty years from the 60s to the 90s and that the capacity to participate in group experiences will be related to physical mobility, health, sensory capacities of hearing and sight, and mental and emotional capacity to reach out or respond to more than one person at a time. Therefore generalizations about group use must take into account the particular individual older persons and their capacity for social experiences.

GROUP TYPOLOGY

At the risk of some oversimplification, groups may be divided into two broad types: participant-centered groups (e.g., preparatory, growth and enhancement, support, and therapeutic groups) and task-centered groups (e.g., service and advocacy groups).

Participant-Centered Groups

Preparatory Groups

By preparatory groups is meant those groups that prepare their participants for such major transitions of later years as retirement, movement into institutional living, or other new and usually stressful experiences.

Since some of the problems of aging grow out of the changes of role and status attendant on retirement, preparation for retirement can mitigate the psychological and physical consequences of transition from a lifetime of work. Such preparation requires not only intellectual understanding of one's changed sources of financial support and possible change in legal status but also anticipation and planning for differences in social associations and colleagual relationships. A chance to talk out one's concerns, uncertainties, and anxieties in a group of people facing the same changes may help with the transition. Groups that combine preretirees and others who have already retired may be especially helpful as they set role models for the preretirees and provide a place for those who have retired to talk about their concerns and interests and make a contribution to others.

Retirement homes, nursing homes, and long-term-care facilities often offer groups for the preparation of people anticipating entering these institutions. Older adults facing the necessity of entering a retirement home or life-care facility often express ambivalence or resistance to giving up independent living, even though communal living may be the best arrangement for their continued independence and security. Short-term groups preparing older people and their relatives for entry may ease the trauma usually experienced by people beginning institutional living. Such groups may include long-time residents, new residents, and future residents so that the latter may be oriented to their prospective living arrangements and also establish connections with other residents in advance. Sometimes relatives of potential residents are asked to participate in these groups so that they will gain a better understanding of the demands of residency and the feelings of their relatives about entry.

In using groups for preparatory purposes, care should be taken to ensure maximum group participation and involvement. Too frequently orientation sessions become lectures by a professional to an audience, without the opportunity for the participants to express their concerns or interests. Also, those who have made the transition but who have not resolved some of their own ambivalences or dealt with their grief at loss of status or independence may present a very negative impression that may negate the purpose of the group. Therefore carefully planned group discussions are necessary so that all participants may have an opportunity to use the group experience for growth. While it is important to surface negatives it is also crucial to face the positive and growth aspects so that people are enabled to use the group for preparation and prevention of the breakdown that could result from the tension and anxiety about the change.

It must be recognized at the outset that there are always strengths and weaknesses in the use of the group experience and that professionals who would use groups must have knowledge and skill in the direction of the group process where such leadership is essential.

Growth and Enhancement Groups

Growth and enhancement groups (including clubs and classes) employ such activities as games, crafts, arts, education, discussion, and exercise. Originally the primary offering of community centers, churches, and other social and service institutions, they are now sponsored by a variety of community organizations, including schools, colleges, unions, Y's, public housing projects, retirement communities, and nursing homes. A recent trend is the emergence of "wellness groups" where the emphasis is on physical, mental, social, and emotional well-being of the participants. Programs include exercise, intellectual stimulation, expression of affection, diet and nutrition, relaxation, and creative activity. Many of these groups are self-help groups of seniors who engage professionals as leaders for particular topics.

Two cautions about growth and enhancement groups: First, the group focus should not be on the activity itself but on the activity as a means of intellectual and social stimulation of each individual participant, which is important for the continued intellectual growth and adequate functioning of the elderly members. Second, the group should be structured in an open-ended fashion so that members may enter or leave without disrupting the group's functioning. Group continuity requires planned means for the departure of old members without their feeling guilt or others resenting their leaving. New participants should be able to join so that the group can continue to be nurtured by new ideas and relationships.

Support Groups

Support groups, usually short-term, are effective for older persons at times of crisis or loss such as the death of a spouse, the onset of serious illness, or victimization by crime or abuse. People find solace and understanding among others who have had similar experiences. Sometimes, however, older people with these problems do not wish to be associated with others in similar situations for fear of being stigmatized or isolated. The group leader must move quickly to establish the empathy, cohesiveness, and trust necessary for fruitful exchange. Using the past only to illuminate members' previous coping devices in other crisis situations, support groups tend to focus on the here and now. By sharing their experiences and feelings, group members learn that they are not alone and are able to derive emotional and practical benefits from each other. Many such support groups evolve into long-term self-help groups as the professional leader phases out.

Therapeutic Groups

Therapeutic groups may have either a preventive or remedial objective. For well-functioning older adults, a therapeutic group may contribute to improved coping with stress, frustrations of physical and social aging, and anxiety that, unattended, could lead to depression and physical or emotional breakdown. For frail, dependent, and physically or emotionally ill older adults, therapeutic groups are useful for purposes of diagnosis, treatment, feedback, and support. Therapeutic groups are used in community-service, senior-center, and family-service agencies as well as in psychiatric and medical settings with both inpatients and outpatients.

In analytic group psychotherapy, the therapist—and subsequently group members as they become versed in the method—helps participants to become aware of the sources and meanings of their behavior, feelings, and belief systems. By recalling and reconstructing events and emotions from their past lives, participants gain insight into their current means of adapting and coping and thereby gain increased mastery of their lives. These efforts are complemented by exploration of the participants' behavior in the group both with the therapist and with other group members. Although debate continues as to whether analytic psychotherapy is effective with the elderly, numbers of therapists report varying degrees of success with certain types of patients.

In activity therapy groups, the activity is selected and designed to meet the particular needs and goals of group members. The difference between an activity therapy group and recreation is the therapeutic focus of the former, the use of verbal and nonverbal expression to approach the participants' problems, and the recognition of and deliberate work on the concerns of the participants through the activity. Activity therapy groups have been reported effective in both day-care programs and institutions.

Group music therapy may involve playing instruments, singing, composing, or listening to records. A simple rhythm orchestra, with instruments assigned on the basis of physical need and preference, can stimulate physical movement, improved memory and concentration, release of tensions, improved interpersonal relationships, and heightened personal satisfaction. Group singing also leads to increased socialization, group cohesiveness, and personal contentment. Art is a more individualistic pursuit, but a professional knowledgeable in both art and group processes can use art to therapeutic advantage in a group as a means of stimulating expression, communication, sharing of tools and ideas, and feedback to the participants.

Dramatic group activity is appropriate for elderly people who are well enough physically and emotionally to participate in role playing. Play reading and play writing have been employed with the elderly in many types of settings as a means of surfacing feelings, identifying with characters, and taking the roles of others. Simple role playing, in which the elderly participant enacts previous or current life situations and rehearses alternative roles and functions, is similar to psychodrama, which has been used with elderly patients in institutions, hospitals, and crisis situations as a means of surfacing emotions and exploring ways of coping. Unlike simple role playing, psychodrama probes unconscious defenses or feelings of which the participant has not previously been aware. It is now widely used in family therapy, family members taking each other's roles in order to gain insight into the feelings of others.

Dance therapy, from elementary motions to full-fledged dancing, has been developed as a group activity to assist in nonverbal expression. Interpretive dance steps have been created to help elderly women express their emotions. But even simple motion in response to music is an expressive, collaborative activity that creates a sense of belonging and increased personal satisfaction.

Creative writing—poetry, short stories, essays, plays, song lyrics, autobiography, personal history—can lead to insight and self-awareness, a sense of continuity between past and present, and pride in one's achievement over a long life. Sharing this writing with a group stimulates participants to discover their common linkages to the past. Feedback, support, and encouragement lead to improved social interaction and cohesiveness. As with other groups, of course, the composition of a writing group must be compatible with its goals, and participants needs to be clear about why they are included.

No discussion of therapeutic group work with older adults would be complete without mention of family group therapy and groups for caregivers. It is increasingly recognized that the use of group approaches with multigenerational families is helpful and necessary for older adults and their caregiving relatives. As families come to include several generations, the problem of a widowed, ill, frail, dependent, or economically needful relative can precipitate a family crisis affecting several generations. Evidence suggests that inclusion of the total family group rather than of the elderly or middle-aged members alone leads to a more successful resolution of the problems arising from the presence of the troubled elderly member. Similarly, support groups are helpful for relatives, friends, and other helpers of the frail and dependent elderly, particularly those suffering from Alzheimer's disease, Parkinson's disease, and various other mental and physical disorders. Such groups help caregivers to anticipate the changes they must expect in the ill and degenerating person. They also provide opportunities for support, respite, and catharsis for caregivers. These groups have been of considerable help in warding off the breakdown of caregivers due to the stress of their responsibilities.

In most therapeutic groups, the professional tends to assume a central and managerial role because of the illness, dependency, weakness, or confusion of the members. As participants begin to relate to each other, and as the group begins to take on some form, the worker may take a less central role. Unfortunately, there is a tendency for the old and frail to be made more dependent by the professionals who would help them. Group therapists in particular need to know how to draw upon the strengths of the group participants to reenforce evidence of health and independence. They must make the therapeutic group itself the instrument of help and change, not merely the aggregate in which the professional works with individuals while others look on.

Task-Centered Groups

An important role for older adults is participation in citizen groups involved in the development and operation of senior programs. Many publicly funded senior programs, such as Area Agencies on Aging, senior citizen centers, nutrition programs, and senior multiservice centers are mandated to include older adults on their advisory boards. Retired Senior Volunteers, Foster

Grandparents, Senior Companions, and similar programs involve older adults in important community work. These organizations have a dual focus: first, to manage programs, advise staff, raise funds, and provide services; second, to provide opportunities for involvement and responsibility to older adults. Organizations like the Gray Panthers, the National Council on Aging, and the American Association of Retired Persons have local chapters whose members engage in community action related to the needs of senior citizens.

The group processes in task-centered groups are essentially the same as in other groups except that these groups tend to be more formally structured with elected or appointed leaders, and the focus is more on goal achievement and less on personal gain. While interpersonal relationships and personal development are important by-products of these groups, their primary focus is on the task to be done. Goals are usually clearly stated, and participants are expected to be competent enough to participate effectively. Participants may represent different points of view, sexes, ethnicities, socioeconomic strata, religious faiths, educational attainments, professional or occupational backgrounds, and political affiliations. To be effective, such groups need opportunities to develop cohesion and good working relationships. They also need to have some experiences of success, since success motivates members to invest more in the group. Generally, advisory groups serve on a volunteer basis and therefore need motivation to continue.

Professional workers who facilitate such groups need to understand how to engage participants and make use of their varied talents and capacities. They must be able to serve as moderators to ensure that all points of view are heard. Staff who do not understand group process sometimes attempt to use such groups merely to ratify staff decisions and actions, causing group members to feel demeaned and diminished. Staff who feel competitive and threatened by advisory groups that include retired professionals need to recognize the objectives of such groups.

GROUP PROCESS

The human-services professional who works with groups of older adults must be thoroughly familiar with group process. He/she must appreciate that a group is not a mere collection of people assembled to hear a speaker or to approve some plan or action of the professional. It is a collective with a defined purpose, a distinct identity, clear boundaries, and particular ways of acting. Its development proceeds through well-defined stages. The task of the professional is to facilitate this development of group process to enable the participants to join together to achieve their collective purpose.

Planning

The first important stage is the planning. A well-planned group is more likely to achieve its objectives than one formed haphazardly as circumstances might suggest. The organizers of a group must be clear as to their reasons for favoring the group modality for the population they intend to serve. Eligibility standards for membership should be clearly thought out and defined in advance. When, where, and how frequently the group will meet are other decisions that must be made in advance, at least tentatively.

Convening

When the participants first assemble, some kind of action must take place to help them interact and connect. This may be particularly true for people who feel isolated, ill, disoriented, or anxious, as is often the case with the frail elderly. The convenors of the group must make sure that all the participants meet each other and find some means of connecting through common purpose or concern. Members will want to test themselves in this new situation, to take note of others who are present, and to begin to connect with them. There should be some general review of the purpose of their coming together, some general orientation to place and others.

The degree to which participants become involved witll be related to their physical and mental health and their social capacities. Those who are independent may find the group somewhat encumbering in that they must give up some independence, listen to others, negotiate their positions, and come to shared agreements. Those who are impaired or dependent will rely on the leadership of others and will require assistance in order to respond to the new situation.

Storming

After the initial stage of group formation there often comes a period of resistance or disintegration labeled "storming" by Tuckman. This is a testing period, when members find that the group demands that they share and care more than they expected. It is also a period when leadership emerges and group members compete for power and recognition. Storming may be expressed as overt challenges to the leadership or hostile or argumentative attacks among the members; or it may be expressed by refusal to work or concentrate, by clowning, lateness, or absences. Often inexperienced group leaders misinterpret this storming stage as evidence of failure, poor composition, or the setting of unachievable goals. Actually, groups can grow to a higher level of development if they confront their resistances, talk through their conflicts and discomforts, and get back to work.

Working

When the storming stage has been successfully negotiated, or at least recognized and worked on, the group may move on to a new stage of working toward those purposes for which it was established, or toward new purposes that may have emerged in the storming period. The therapeutic atmosphere may be created, a sense of support established, and activities undertaken or tasks begun to be worked on. This is the longest and most productive period of the group's life.

Terminating

The last stage of the group process is the group's termination. How termination is managed is particularly important for older adults, who must increasingly cope with endings and losses. When the group will end should be clearly established at its start: either after a certain number of sessions, upon the solution of a defined problem, or with the achievement of a set task. Termination should be discussed and planned for several sessions in advance. Opportunities for final spurts of work, for gradual withdrawal from the support of the group, and for summarizing and completing the group's work should be provided. A special event like a party affords a chance for both celebrating the successful completion of a task and for grieving for the end of relationships. In a task group, a review of achievement and a summary session or report to another group may provide a sufficient ending.

CONCLUSION

The use of group methods with older adults began primarily under social-work auspices by workers trained in small-group theory and group-leadership methods. After World War II particularly, group methods were adopted by psychologists, clinical psychologists, psychiatrists, psychiatric and geriatric nurses, recreation workers, occupational therapists, and adult educators, who developed specific techniques for work with groups and have applied those techniques to work with older adults. Nurses, for instance, particularly in geriatric-care facilities, have done some of the original experimentation, teaching, and writing in this field. In California, adult educators under the auspices of local adult schools and community colleges have used remotivation, reality therapy, and reminiscence groups with patients in long-term-care facilities and convalescent homes. Occupational therapists and professionals in such specialties as art therapy, music therapy, dance therapy, or movement therapy are offering groups for older adults within many residential and community settings.

A tremendous body of knowledge is available about groups and therapeutic or social methodologies for their use, as well as about the social and psychological needs of older adults that can be met through appropriate small-group interventions. However, most professionals in the human services receive very little preparation either in gerontology or in group-leadership methods. Apparently, there is still a myth that anyone can lead a group and that one can become an instant gerontologist by reading a book. We are past the time when this type of ignorance in group practice with older adults is acceptable. Furthermore, the potential for harmful effects on the participants precludes inappropriate use of group methods. As professional schools of social work, nursing, gerontology, recreation, occupational therapy, clinical psychology, and medicine/psychiatry upgrade their teaching relative to groups and to social gerontology, professionals will be better prepared for their work. The apparent lack of definitive research on group work with older adults — even of studies of groups where older people are subjects, or textbooks in the methodology of group-work practice with older adults, or examples of work with the older people in the textbooks on group methods — underscores the gap that exists in the education of helping professionals.

The bibliography attached to this chapter gives evidence that considerable use of groups is made in services for older adults. Observations of practice with older adults to improve or support their mental health suggests that a variety of group methods are in general use. What is needed, then, is a more scientific and disciplined use of groups with older adults and their families.

BIBLIOGRAPHY

Abrahams, R. B. (1972). Mutual help for the widowed. *Social Work,* **17**(5), 54-61.

Ackerman, N. W. (1971). The growing edge of family therapy. *Family Process,* **10**(2), 143-156.

Allen, K. S. (1976). A group experience for elderly patients with organic brain syndrome. *Health and Social Work,* **1**(4), 61-69.

Allen, V. (1970). Motivation therapy with the aging geriatric veteran patient. *Military Medicine,* **135**(11), 1007-1010.

Altholz, J., and Doss, A. (1973). Outpatient group therapy with elderly persons. *Gerontologist,* **13**(3:2), 101.

Astle, J., Howsdin, J., and Arquitt, G. E. (1977). *Intergenerational living: A follow-up.* Stillwater: Oklahoma State University Press.

Berger, L. F., and Berger, M. M. (1973). A holistic group approach to psychogeriatric outpatients. *International Journal of Group Psychotherapy,* **23**(4), 432-444.

Berland, D. A., and Poggi, R. L. (1980). Establishing newcomers' groups. In I. M. Burnside (Ed.), *Psychosocial nursing care of the aged* (2nd ed.). New York: McGraw-Hill.

Birkett, D. P., and Boltuch, B. (1973). Remotivation therapy. *Journal of the American Geriatric Society,* **21**(8), 368-371.

Birren, J., and Renner, J. (1977). Research on the psychology of aging: Principles and experimentation. In J. E. Birren and K. W. Schaie (Eds.), *Handbook of the psychology of aging.* New York: Van Nostrand Reinhold.

Blackman, D. K., Howe, M., and Pinkston, E. M. (1976). Increasing participation in social interaction of the institutionalized elderly. *Gerontologist,* **16**(1:1), 69-76.

Boskind, S. (1966). The multi-service center as a community institution for elderly people. In L. Lowy and J. Mosby (Eds.), *Theory and practice of social work with the aging.* Boston: Council on Gerontology, University of Boston.

Brody, E. M. (1979). Aging parents and aging children. In P. K. Ragan (Ed.), *Aging parents*. Los Angeles: Andrus Gerontology Center, University of Southern California.

Brudno, J. J., and Seltzer, H. (1968). Re-socialization therapy through group process with senile patients in a geriatric hospital. *Gerontologist*, **8**(3), 211-214.

Burnside, I. M. (1970). Loss: A constant theme in group work with the aged. *Hospital and Community Psychiatry*, **21**(6), 173-177.

Burnside, I. M. (1971). Long-term group work with hospitalized aged. *Gerontologist*, **11**(3:1), 213-218.

Burnside, I. M. *Working with the elderly: Group process and techniques*. North Scituate, Mass.: Duxbury Press.

Burnside, I. M. (1980). Group work with regressed aged people. In I. M. Burnside (Ed.), *Psychosocial nursing care of the aged* (2nd ed.). New York: McGraw-Hill.

Butler, R. N. (1974). Successful aging. *Mental Hygiene*, **58**(3), 6-12.

Cohen, M. G. (1973). Alternative to institutional care of the aged. *Social Casework*, **54**(8), 447-452.

Conant, R. (1961). *A study for the expansion of the work of the committee on aging*. Boston: United Community Services of Boston.

Conrad, W. K. (1974). A group therapy program with older adults in a high-risk neighborhood setting. *International Journal of Group Psychotherapy*, **24**(3), 358-360.

Coyle, G. L. (1960). Group work in psychiatric settings: Its roots and branches. In *Use of groups in the psychiatric setting*. New York: National Association of Social Workers.

Coyle, G. L. (1962). Concepts relevant to helping the family as a group. *Social Casework*, **43**(7), 347-354.

Craik, F. M. (1977). Age difference in human memory. In J. E. Birren and K. W. Schaie (Eds.), *Handbook of the psychology of aging*. New York: Van Nostrand Reinhold.

de Barry, S. (1981-82). An evaluation of progressive muscle relaxation on stress related symptoms. *International Journal of Aging and Human Development*, **14**(4), 255-269.

Dennis, H. (1978). Remotivation therapy groups. In I. M. Burnside (Ed.), *Working with the elderly: Group process and techniques*. North Scituate, Mass.: Duxbury Press.

Dewdney, I. (1973). An art therapy program for geriatric patients. *American Journal of Art Therapy*, **12**(4), 249-254.

Ebersole, P. (1978). Establishing reminiscing groups. In I. M. Burnside (Ed.), *Working with the elderly: Group process and techniques*. North Scituate, Mass.: Duxbury Press.

Epstein, H. (1964). Developing citizen action through the senior adult program of the Jewish center. In *Proceedings of the national conference on social welfare*. New York: Columbia University Press.

Erickson, R. C., and Scott, M. L. (1977). Clinical memory testing: A review. *Psychological Bulletin*, **84**(6), 1130-1149.

Evans, R. and Jauregay, B. (1981). Group therapy by phone: A cognitive behavior program for visually impaired elderly. *Social Work in Health Care*, **7**(2), 79-80.

Feil, N. W. (1967). Group therapy in a home for the aged. *Gerontologist*, **7**(3), 192-195.

Feil, N. W. (1982). Group work with disoriented nursing home residents. *Social Work with Groups*, **5**(2), 000000.

Franklin, G. S., and Kaufman, K. (1982). Group psychotherapy for elderly female Hispanic outpatients. *Hospital and Community Psychiatry*, **33**(5), 385-387.

Frey, L. A. (Ed.). (1966). *Use of groups in the healthfield*. New York. National Association of Social Workers.

Friedman, S. (1975). The resident welcoming committee: Institutionalized elderly in volunteer services to their peers. *Gerontologist*, **15**(4), 362-367.

Getzel, G. (1983). Group work with kin and friends caring for the elderly. *Social Work with Groups*, **5**(2), 91-102.

Glasser, W. (1965). *Reality therapy*. New York: Harper & Row.

Grauer, H., Betts, D., and Birnbom, F. (1973). Welfare emotions and family therapy in geriatrics. *Journal of the American Geriatrics Society*, **21**(1), 21-24.

Gunn, J. C. (1967). Group psychotherapy on a geriatric ward. *Psychotherapy and Psychosomatics,* **15**(1), 26.

Hahn, J. and Burns, R. K. (1973). Mrs. Richards, a rabbit, and remotivation. *American Journal of Nursing,* **73**(2), 302-305.

Haley, J. (1970-71). Family therapy. *International Journal of Psychiatry,* **9**, 233-242.

Hall, S. (1958). Understanding of developed goals of older adults as an imperative in social group work practice. In *Social work education for better service to the aging,* vol. 2. New York: Council on Social Work Education.

Hartford, M. E. (Ed.). (1964). *Working papers toward a frame of reference for social group work practice.* New York: National Association of Social Workers.

Hartford, M. E. (1971). *Groups in social work.* New York: Columbia University Press.

Hartford, M. E. (1976). Group methods in generic practice. In R. W. Roberts and H. Northern (Eds.), *Theories of social work with groups.* New York: Columbia University Press.

Hartford, M. E. (1978). Groups in the human services: Some facts and fancies. *Social Work with Groups,* **1**(1), 7-13.

Hartford, M. E. (1980). The use of group methods for work with the aged. In J. E. Birren and R. B. Sloane (Eds.), *Handbook of mental health and aging.* Englewood Cliffs, N.J.: Prentice-Hall.

Hartford, M. E., and Parsons, R. (1982a) Groups with relatives of dependent older adults. *Gerontologist,* **22**(3), 394-398.

Hartford, M. E., and Parsons, R. (1982b). Uses of groups with relatives of frail adults. *Social Work with Groups,* **5**(4), 77-89.

Hastorf, A. H. (1965). The reinforcement of individual actions in a group situation. In L. Krasner and L. P. Ullman (Eds.), *Research in behavior modification.* New York: Holt, Rinehart & Winston.

Heap, K. (1983). Purposes in social work with groups. In *Proceedings of the 4th symposium for the advancement of social work with groups.* Toronto: Toronto University.

Hennessey, M. J. (1973). Group work with economically independent aged. In I. M. Burnside (Ed.), *Psychosocial nursing care of the aged.* New York: McGraw-Hill.

Hildebrand, V. (1973). Golden-age 4-H clubs: An expanded concept for the cooperative extension service. *Family Coordinator,* **22**(3), 327-330.

Hochschild, A. R. (1973). Communal life-styles for the old. *Society,* **10**(5), 50-57.

Holmes, T. H., and Matsuda, M. (1974). Life changes and illness susceptibility. In B. S. Dohrenwend and B. P. Dohrenwend (Eds.), *Successful life events.* New York: Wiley.

Ingersoll, B., and Hollenshead, C. (1981). Group work with the deinstitutionalized elderly. *Journal of Gerontological Social Work,* **3**(4), 21-36.

Kilpatrick, A. C. (1968). Conjoint family therapy with geriatric patients. *Journal of the Fort Logan Mental Health Center,* **5**(1), 29-35.

Krauss, I. K. (1981). The psychology of aging. In R. H. Davis (Ed.), *Aging: Prospects and issues* (3rd. ed.). Los Angeles: Andrus Gerontology Center, University of Southern California.

Kubie, S. H., and Landau, G. (1953). *Group work with the aged.* New York: International Universities Press.

Laguer, H. P. (1972). Mechanisms of change in multiple family therapy. In C. J. Sager and H. S. Kaplan (Eds.), *Progress in group and family therapy.* New York: Brunner/Mazel.

Larson, M. K. (1970). A descriptive account of group treatment of older people by a caseworker. *Journal of Geriatric Psychiatry,* **3**(2), 231-240.

Lazarus, L. W. (1976). A program for the elderly at a private psychiatric hospital. *Gerontologist,* **16**(2), 125-131.

Lewis, M. I., and Butler, R. N. (1974). Life-review therapy: Putting memories to work in individual and group psychotherapy. *Geriatrics,* **29**(11), 165-173.

Liederman, P. C. (1967). Music and rhythm group therapy for geriatric patients. *Journal of Music Therapy,* **4**(4), 126-127.

Liederman, P. C., Green, R., and Liederman, V. E. (1967). Outpatient group therapy with geriatric patients. *Geriatrics,* **22**(1), 148-153.

Linsk, N., Howe, M. W., and Pinkston, E. M. (1975). Behavioral group work in a home for the aged. *Social Work*, **20**(6), 454-463.

Lowenthal, M. F. (1977). Toward a sociopsychological theory of change in adulthood and old age. In J. E. Birren and K. W. Schaie (Eds.), *Handbook of the psychology of aging*. New York: Van Nostrand Reinhold.

Lowy, L. (1955). *Adult education and group work*. New York: Whiteside-Morrow.

Lowy, L. (1962). The group in social work with the aged. *Social Work*, **7**(4), 43-50.

Lowy, L. (1967). Roadblocks in group work practice with older people: A framework for analysis. *Gerontologist*, **7**(2), 109-113, 135.

Lowy, L. (1983). Social group work with vulnerable older persons: A theoretical perspective. *Social Work with Groups*, **5**(2), 21-32.

Lowy, L., and Mogey, J. (1966). *Theory and practice in social work with the aging*. Boston: University Council on Gerontology, Boston University.

Maizler, J. S., and Solomon, J. R. (1976). Therapeutic group process with the institutionalized elderly. *Journal of the American Geriatrics Society*, **24**(12), 542-546.

Manis, M. (1955). Social interaction and the self concept. *Journal of Abnormal and Social Psychology*, **51**(3), 362-370.

Maxwell, J. M. (1962). Helping older people through participation. In *Potentials for service through group work in public welfare*. Chicago: American Public Welfare Association.

Mayadas, N. S., and Hink, D. L. (1974). Group work with the aging: An issue for social work education. *Gerontologist*, **14**(5:1), 440-445.

Meredith, G. M., and Amor, C. A. (1976). Indexing the polarization of social groups in a multi-purpose senior center. *Psychological Reports*, **39**(1), 88-90.

Miller, I., and Solomon, R. (1980). The development of group services for the elderly. *Journal of Gerontological Social Work*, **2**(3), 241-257.

National Association of Social Workers. (1963). *Social group work with older people*. New York: National Association of Social Workers.

Nevruz, N., and Hrushka, M. (1969). The influence of unstructured and structured group psychotherapy with geriatric patients on their decision to leave the hospital. *International Journal of Group Psychotherapy*, **19**(1), 72-78.

Rank, B. J. (1963). Content of the group experience in a day center. In *Social group work with older people*. New York: National Association of Social Workers.

Rathbone-McCuan, E., and Levenson, J. (1975). Impact of socialization therapy in a geriatric day-care setting. *Gerontologist*, **15**(4), 338-342.

Reichenfeld, H. F., et al. (1973). Evaluating the effect of activity programs on a geriatric ward. *Gerontologist*, **13**(3:1), 305-310.

Remnet, V. L. (1974). A group program for adaptation to a convalescent hospital. *Gerontologist*, **14**(4), 336-341.

Rosin, A. J. (1975). Group discussions: A therapeutic tool in a chronic diseases hospital, *Geriatrics*, **30**(8), 45-48.

Ross, H. K. (1975). Low-income elderly in inner-city trailer parks. *Psychiatric Annals*, **5**(8), 86-90.

Rossman, I. (1980). Bodily changes with aging. In E. W. Busse and D. G. Blazer (Eds.), *Handbook of geriatric psychiatry*. New York: Van Nostrand Reinhold.

Sainer, J. S., Schwartz, L. L., and Jackson, T. G. (1973). Steps in the development of a comprehensive service delivery system for the elderly. *Gerontologist*, **13**(3:2), 98.

Salter, C. D., and Salter, C. A. (1975). Regression among institutionalized elderly patients following interruption of a therapeutic program. *Gerontologist*, **15**(5:2), 85.

Saul, S. R. (1983). An admissions group in a skilled nursing facility. *Social Work with Groups*, **5**(2), 67-76.

Saul, S. R., and Saul, S. (1974). Group psychotherapy in a proprietary nursing home. *Gerontologist*, **14**(5:1), 446-450.

Schaie, K. W., and Geiwitz, J. (1982). *Adult development and aging*. Boston: Little, Brown.

182   M. E. Hartford

Scott, D., and Crowhurst, J. (1975). Reawakening senses in the elderly. *Canadian Nurse,* **71**(10), 21-22.

Seguin, M. M. (1973). Opportunity for peer socialization in a retirement community. *Gerontologist,* **13**(2), 208-214.

Seguin, M. M., and O'Brien, B. (Eds.). (1976). *Releasing the potential of the older volunteer.* Los Angeles: Andrus Gerontology Center, University of Southern California.

Selye, H. (1974). *Stress without distress.* New York: Harper and Row.

Shapiro, A. (1969). A pilot program in music therapy with residents of a home for the aged. *Gerontologist,* **9**(2), 128-133.

Shapiro, E. (1973). The residents: A study in motivation and productivity among institutionalized octogenarians. *Gerontologist,* **13**(1), 119-124.

Shier, B. R. (1972). Closer communication through interaction in groups of aged persons. *Journal of Jewish Communal Service,* **49**(2), 162-166.

Silvertone, B. (1979). Issues for the middle generation: Responsibility, adjustment, growth. In P. K. Ragan (Ed.), *Aging parents.* Los Angeles: Andrus Gerontology Center, University of Southern California.

Sloan, M. B. (1953). The special contribution of therapeutic group work in a psychiatric setting. *Group,* **15**(4), 11-18, 35.

Stabler, N. (1981). The use of groups in day care centers for older adults. *Social Work with Groups,* **4**(3/4), 49-58.

Stephens, L. R. (Ed.). (1975). *Reality orientation* (rev. ed.). Washington: American Psychiatric Association.

Taulbee, L. R., and Folsom, J. C. (1966). Reality orientation for geriatric patients. *Hospital and Community Psychiatry,* **17**(5), 133-135.

Thralow, J. U., and Watson, C. G. (1974). Remotivation for geriatric patients using elementary school students. *American Journal of Occupational Therapy,* **28**(8), 469-473.

Tine, S. (1960). Generic and specific in social group work with the aging. In *Social work with groups.* New York: National Association of Social Workers.

Toseland, R., Sherman, E., and Bliven, S. (1981). The comparative effectiveness of two group work approaches for the development of mutual support groups among the elderly. *Social Work with Groups,* **4**(1/2), 137-153.

Trela, J. E. (1972). Age structure of voluntary associations and political self-interest among the aged. *Sociological Quarterly,* **13**(2), 244-252.

Tuckman, B. W. (1965). Developmental sequence in small groups. *Psychological Bulletin,* **63**(6), 384-399.

Turbow, S. R. (1975). Geriatric group day care and its effect on independent living: A thirty-six-month assessment. *Gerontologist,* **15**(6), 508-510.

Vickery, F. (1960). *How to work with older people.* Sacramento: California Department of Natural Resources.

Waters, E., Fink, S., and White, B. (1976). Peer group counseling for older people. *Educational Gerontology,* **1**(2), 157-170.

Weiner, M. B., Brok, A. J., and Snadowsky, A. M. (1978). *Working with the aged.* Englewood Cliffs, N.J.: Prentice-Hall.

Williams, E. W. (1972). Patient government on geriatric wards of a state hospital. *Geriatrics,* **27**(2), 70-74.

Wilson, G., and Ryland, G. (1964). The family as a unit of service. In *Proceedings of the national conference of social welfare.* New York: Columbia University Press.

Wiswell, R. (1979). Exercise and stress. In R. H. Davis (Ed.), *Stress and the organization.* Los Angeles: Andrus Gerontology Center, University of Southern California.

Wolff, K. (1967). Comparison of group and individual psychotherapy with geriatric patients. *Diseases of the Nervous System,* **28**(6), 284-286.

Wolk, R. L., and Goldfarb, A. I. (1967). The response to group psychotherapy of aged recent admissions compared with long-term mental hospital patients. *American Journal of Psychiatry,* **123**(10), 1251-1257.

Woods, J. H. (1953). *Helping older people enjoy life.* New York: Harper.

Yalom, I. D., and Terrazas, F. (1968). Group therapy for psychotic elderly patients. *American Journal of Nursing,* **68**(8), 1690-1694.

Zarit, S. H. (1979). Helping an aging patient to cope with memory problems. *Geriatrics,* **34**(4), 82-90.

Zarit, S. H., Cole, K. D., and Guider, R. L. (1981). Memory training strategies and subjective complaints of memory in the aged. *Gerontologist,* **21**(2), 158-164.

Zarit, S. H., and Zarit, J. M. (1982). Families under stress: Interventions for caregivers of senile dementia patients. *Psychotherapy: Theory, Research and Practice,* **19**(4), 461-471.

Ziller, R. C. (1965). Toward a theory of open and closed groups. *Psychological Bulletin,* **64**(3), 164-182.

8

Community Organization

Cynthia Stuen, A. M.

Columbia University

The role of community organization in today's society is taking on new meaning. As America faces an unprecedented demographic trend in the grow-ing proportion of older adults, social problems such as inadequate income, incapacitating illness, deteriorating housing, and lack of access to educational opportunities become overwhelming to social workers. To address these problems, which may disproportionately affect older adults, the people and institutions of a community must first recognize that they are problems of the total community and then work together for change. The effort must be organized with a strategic plan of action. Gerontological social workers are well suited for this task because of their professional values and their knowledge and skill in the area referred to as community organization. Unfortunately, however, not all social workers bring adequate skills to the job (Rothman, 1979).

Community organization focuses on a population needing redress and on the outside forces of the community at large that impact their problem. Community organization is not an end in itself but a process in which a problem is addressed by helping a group of people focus on the issue and enabling them to act on their own behalf.

This chapter is intended to provide information to the person working in the field of community organization with the aged. The literature on community organization is not as fully developed as the direct-practice (casework and groupwork) literature; there is even less literature specific to gerontological practice. However, basic principles can be applied and case illustrations will highlight practice theory.

DEFINITION

Community organization refers to the type of social-work practice that may encompass (1) work with small or large groups with the aim of helping people to express their collective needs, (2) interagency work, and (3) creation of appropriate community structures for the expression and satisfaction of needs through research, planning, and organization. Generally speaking, community organization is characterized by application of the problem-solving process (National Association of Social Workers, 1977). Social advocacy, social action, social planning, and organizing are areas of community organization, the macro social-work method through which the skills of professional social workers can address improvement at the system level of health and human services for older adults. (The term *community work* is often encountered in the British context; both terms will be used interchangeably in this chapter.)

Historically, community organization had its beginning outside the field of social work as grass-roots activities. The term *community* originally connoted a geographical neighborhood; this is now changing to include a broad affiliation — for example, the homeless or the rural elderly.

There has been a controversy over the central purpose of community organization (National Association of Social Workers, 1977). One camp favors the integration/capacity-building purpose, which relies on intergroup work — hence the "relationship focus" of practice. The other camp upholds program development and social reform as the central purposes of community organization and relies on psychoanalytic concepts of practice. This controversy was conveniently settled when NASW's Comittee on Community Organization recognized the diversity of community-organization practice and included equal emphasis on both purposes.

NEED

Demographic Change

Gerontological social work is forecast to be one of the fastest-growing professional fields. A need for 700,000 social workers in this area by the year 1990 has been projected by the NASW, and the *New York Times* has predicted two major themes for jobs in the year 2000: catering to the needs of the elderly and working with computers. The optimistic predictions for gerontological social workers are based on demographic projections that show two population groups growing proportionally faster than the general U.S. population—children in female-headed households and the elderly. The focus here is on the older-adult population and on the variety of needs they express, which are perceived by others in the sectors of health, housing, income, employment, cultural and social services, and education.

It is projected that 45 percent of the older-adult population will be over age 75 by the year 2000 (U.S. Congress, 1980). The over-75 age group is more likely to suffer from multiple chronic diseases and to be increasingly dependent on social and health services. Chronological age is not the only predictor; with increasing health-science advances, populations of younger cohorts may also be dependent on increased social and health resources. It is strategically important to develop at the community level a continuum of care ranging from minimal level of supports to the highest (most skilled) level of care that will allow persons in need to have some choice about where to receive care, thus promoting appropriate utilization of services.

The increased segment of life spent in retirement creates a new leisure role for the elderly, never before experienced. From an economist's point of view, there is a lengthened period of nonproductivity and increased drain on resources; an unfavorable dependency ratio is occurring due to the increase in life expectancy and decrease in the birth rate. Women continue to outlive men on the average by seven to ten years; there is, therefore, a sizable population of women who are usually poorer than their male counterparts. Many of these elderly women are widows, and the role changes experienced with the loss of a spouse present an increased need for social adjustment for the adult. For older black women, the classic triple jeopardy—racism, sexism, and poverty—may often be operative.

Social work in general, and with the elderly as well, has primarily been practiced in urban areas, but rural areas have been gaining the attention of gerontologists. Some of the major concerns of the rural elderly are focused on access issues such as transportation and the availability of various services in their localities. In place of the racial and ethnic differences of urban neighborhoods, rurality brings regional variations in cultures and life styles; rural areas are generally felt to be more heterogeneous than urban environments.

The surge of legislative activity in the mid-1960s that affected the elderly was in response to the recognized needs of this growing population. Community organization emerged as an important social-work method particularly applicable to the development of community-based programs for older adults.

Theories of Aging

Community workers should know the implications of different major theories of aging for understanding and guiding policy decisions and program planning. Disengagement theory, for example (Cumming and Henry, 1961), posits that older adults and society mutually withdraw from one another. This legitimizes an isolationist policy approach toward the elderly. The activity theory (Havighurst and Albrecht, 1953) holds that higher levels of social activity of an older adult will result in higher morale and increased life satisfaction. From a community-organization point of view, this would lead to development of programs to provide social involvement for older adults. The Older Americans Act of 1965 seems to be based on an outlook similar to the activity theory. The developmental theory of Neugarten, Havighurst, and Tobin (1964) says there are life tasks that must be achieved in order to integrate the older-adult role just as there are in other life-cycle stages. This theory prompts a more evolutionary policy approach to program planning.

Another major theory is social exchange, which is built on the assumption that interactions between individuals or collectivities are attempts to maximize rewards while keeping costs at a minimum. It can be useful for the community organizer to understand exchange theory in organizing change activities. A major proposition of the exchange theory is that the interaction between two or more people will probably be continued and positively evaluated if they each see a "profit"—a reward from the interaction (Dowd, 1975). Power is a central concept in exchange, and the power of the aged is diminished by losses in employment, health, social network, and finances. Emerson (1962) delineated four possible strategies to redress the power imbalances:

1. *Withdrawal*—no involvement (which is commensurate with disengagement)
2. *Extension of power*—cultivating new roles in order to obtain new rewards
3. *Emergence of status*—the dependent partner seeks more power through reemergence of status, by a revaluing of a skill possessed by the dependent (older adult) party
4. *Coalition formation*—the less powerful partner seeks alliance with others of similar dependence in hopes of counteracting the more powerful

The last balancing strategy, coalition formation, is perhaps the most popular with community organizers. In work with the elderly, one occasionally observes the coalescing of elderly with younger cohorts in opposition to the middle generation—for example, the Gray Panthers.

It is helpful for community workers to be cognizant of the theoretical views of aging that undergird their assessment of need and hence choice of strategy in working with older persons. However, although a theoretical perspective may be useful for explanatory purposes, no single theory can be used to make judgments about normativity in such a diverse population as older adults.

An understanding of the social, economic, health, and political issues affecting older adults in the community will guide the needs-assessment process and will then lead the professional to the selection of an intervention strategy. Community organization is well suited for many areas of problem-solving relative to older adults, as will be illustrated throughout the chapter.

MODELS OF INTERVENTION

As characterized by Rothman (1979), community organization consists of locality development, social planning, and social action. Locality development (also called community development) is most concerned with capacity building and self-help. Social planning, which emphasizes program-development goals and the use of a problem-solving approach, seems to have arisen along with the growth of the welfare state. Laws and regulatory practice in the social-welfare arena frequently mandate a social-planning process — for example, the Older Americans Act of 1965 and Title XX of the Social Security Act. Social action, which gained much attention in the 1960s, is concerned primarily with organizing disadvantaged groups of the community and looks to promote power shifts and institutional change.

Locality Development

Educational theory is relied on in locality (community) development. It posits that increased interaction focused on knowledge-building in the community will produce change. It is typified by the settlement-house movement in the United States and widely practiced in developing countries. Its major focus is on working with the community to establish common objectives. Development of indigenous leadership and participation through education are key elements (Brager and Specht, 1973).

Participation, primarily voluntaristic, is heavily relied on for locality development. From the tactical point of view of the community organizer, participation is a conditional means to be utilized selectively, depending on selected goals and strategies (Rothman, Erlich, and Teresa, 1981). Federal legislation such as the Older Americans Act promotes citizen involvement in the design of services. Whether this involvement has resulted in significant input or mere tokenism is a subject for further study.

Comparative studies of participation by elderly and nonelderly populations are difficult to locate. The general principles by which to foster participation should guide one's work with the elderly. Social workers must remember the generic principle that people want to both give and receive in order for the relationship (participation) to endure. There are two types of benefits relative to participation, instrumental and expressive (Rothman, Erlich, and Teresa, 1981). Instrumental benefits may be either material, such as obtaining food stamps, or interim-anticipatory, such as getting priority applications for low-rent housing because of age. Expressive benefits are either social-interpersonal or symbolic.

The social-interpersonal benefit recognizes that making new friends and having an opportunity for social interaction is itself rewarding. An award or recognition of participation, usually publicly acknowledged, such as a dinner for recognition of volunteer hours of service, is a symbolic-expressive benefit. The social worker can select the appropriate benefit.

The organizer needs to remember that the path to participation of the elderly individual in community organizing begins with the modest reawakening of the concept that "I count." Match (1970) provides numerous tasks for the community organizer in order to mobilize the entire communtiy, not just individuals. To summarize, the community worker must

1. Foster a focused desire for change at the grass-roots level
2. Identify, involve, and train formal and informal leaders
3. Develop and time change strategies consonant with the capability and culture of the community

Self-help groups gained in popularity through the 1960s, when an anti-institution attitude prevailed, and in the 1970s as service resources began to diminish; these groups are consonant with goals of locality development in many ways. Katz and Bender (1976) define a self-help group as a small, voluntary group established to provide mutual aid in the achievement of a specific purpose.

Older adults and their concerned relatives and care-supporters are represented in the growth phenomenon of self-help groups. Self-help groups meet a variety of needs through provision of information, social/emotional support, and coping strategies useful by others with similar problems.

There is a broad range of types of self-help groups; some require ongoing professional intervention, some require occasional professional support, and some require no professional involvement. There is a continuum of professional support required for self-help groups at different stages of development and with different goals. Pertaining to goals of self-help groups, an extensive review of literature on the role of ideology for such groups is provided by Suler (1984).

A growing number of self-help groups have focused on needs of widowed persons. Although women comprise the bulk of widowed—as high as 75 percent—it is men who appear to suffer more from being widowed (Gartner, 1984, p. 37). Two major studies have reported that widows receiving self-help intervention in widow-to-widow programs adjusted to their bereavement more rapidly than those who did not (Vachon, 1980; Lieberman and Borman, 1981).

Given the growing older-adult population and high likelihood for older women and increasing numbers of men to experience widowhood or widower-hood, gerontological social workers need to be aware of the variety of effective self-help modes available that they can foster as well as the variety of roles they may perform as initiator, consultant, broker, and evaluator.

Self-help groups can provide a valuable interface between the professional bureacracy that delivers the health and human services so vital to older persons and the informal support network of the elderly. Litwak and Meyer (1974) posit that both the formal and informal networks are better able to carry out their respective tasks if there is interdependence rather than complete autonomy. Self-help groups can aid the informal network in negotiating the maze of bureaucratic organizations offering services in the community. Hence the community worker needs to be cognizant of the self-help model and foster it appropriately.

Social Planning

The community-action programs of the 1960s tried to develop indigenous leadership and enhanced participation at the neighborhood level. Social planning involving the elderly was slower to evolve. There are illustrations of effective community organization in the social-planning model. The following case study demonstrates not only the social-planning process but its relationship to community development and social action.

A massive housing project was planned for an urban community with only a token number of units for older persons. Popular opinion held that low priority was given to housing units for the elderly because neighborhood residents were black and their voting records poor. A community organizer worked with the residents for two months gathering facts to support a comprehensive plan to obtain more housing units for the elderly. A number of residents, mostly elderly, canvassed the neighborhood, explained the problem, and asked for a commitment "to come out if ever needed." Keeping the neighborhood network informed of events and progress was a key element of the project. Later, when a voter-registration campaign was undertaken, the mayor offered to visit on only three-days notice. The community developed a statement explaining the demand for more housing units for the elderly and residents again canvassed the neighborhood, reminding residents of their previous commitment to "come out." When the mayor arrived, residents filled the auditorium; the mayor subsequently promised to allocate more housing for the elderly, a promise that was kept. The success of the effort was attributed to the meeting turn-out and to the increased number of registered voters (Corbett, 1970).

This case documents the steps in community organization: identifying a problem, establishing objectives, and building a consensus. The plan developed called for a strategy of door-to-door canvassing in the neighborhood, keeping the constituency informed, and seizing the politically opportune moment to call on the neighborhood for support. A project evaluation showed not only success in the allocation of additional housing units for the elderly but also increased registration of voters, particularly minority elderly. This is akin to Cloward and Piven's (1982) strategy of democratizing the poor that is primarily focused on voter registration.

Although the concept of "contracting" is more commonly used in casework, it is equally important to establish a contract with a community group. It is the responsibility of the community worker to negotiate the timetable, strategies, expected outcomes, and completion or "success" measures.

Program Models

There are three basic models of program implementation that can be put into effect: the decision-making-unit model, the spontaneous-contagion model, and the advocacy model. Practical illustrations of these models from the gerontological field follow.

The decision-making-unit model progresses from participants to a partial target population to decision-making to a general target population. The concern that older adults were not being utilized in volunteer roles prompted a demonstration project known as Serve and Enrich Retirement through Volunteer Experience (SERVE). Participants were elderly persons; the target population was the elderly of Staten Island, New York; the time of the demonstration project was the late 1960s. Upon conclusion of the demonstration project, a decision was made to translate this volunteer program model to the older-adult population nationwide; it became the Retired Senior Volunteer Program (RSVP). This decision-making-unit model is applicable in many program-development arenas; it is a rational approach to planning service programs.

Planning services for minority populations require special attention. The heterogeneity of older adults of different racial and ethnic backgrounds is now accepted by gerontologists, yet policies are made and programs designed and implemented without regard for ethnic and cultural differences. Even when differences are acknowledged, they frequently compare white and nonwhite, or report only black and Hispanic differences. For example, the definition of Hispanic by the U.S. Census includes persons of Spanish, Mexican, Cuban, Puerto Rican, and Central and South American heritages. Manuel and Reid (1982) argue that individual differences in physical (racial) and cultural (ethnic) traits, even within a specific minority group, produce different degrees of identification and minority victimization. Perhaps the social-work ethic of starting where the individual is promotes the best approach for community organizers. Social workers need to recognize and be sensitive to the historical and cultural diversity of older adults.

Certain issues have similarity for minority populations, and income is certainly a major one. The feminization of poverty is a factor for women of all age groups, but most especially for women of ethnic minorities. Health is also a key issue. Minority populations have poorer subjective reporting and functional health status than their white counterparts (Manuel and Berk, 1983).

The 1980 Census report will deliver more information about elderly than ever before (Longino, 1982). Two major improvements in the Census reports are that the age group 65 years and over is not treated as a homogeneous group but is reported in five-year age groups up to the category "75 years and over." The other is a better reporting of the race/ethnicity category. Special subject reports are available from U.S. Census data that provide detailed tabulations on a variety of socioeconomic variables by race and ethnic group.

Caution should be exercised, however, in utilization of Census data on the older population in that it is probable that the data suffer from a greater measure of error and biases than do data for the younger population (Siegel and Taeuber, 1982). Evaluation studies of 1970 Census reports suggest that the undercounting of elderly is high and increases as age among the elderly increases. Coverage was better for whites than for blacks.

Some researchers conclude that minority persons use fewer services proportionally (Bell, 1975; Fujii, 1976; Davis, 1975); others argue that there are no differences or that age acts as a leveler on ethnic variation (Dowd and Bengston, 1978); and still others claim that minorities are favored for services (McCaslin and Calvert, 1975; Cull and Hardy, 1973). The important issue to bear in mind while being sensitive to ethnic and regional variations is that problems faced by older persons are similar across ethnic variations.

In a study of counties with high proportions of minorities, Holmes (1982, p. 397) found:

As the minority population proportion in a county decreases, minorities are less likely to be served.

A minority living in sparsely populated areas is most likely to be overlooked by service providers.

The strongest predictors of the percentage of older minority persons served by an agency are the staffing pattern and location of program offices in the minority neighborhood.

In the area of work and volunteering, Jackson (1978) found that race is irrelevant to retirement after socioeconomic status is controlled. Individuals with low incomes tend to work beyond age 65, and all minority elderly groups have lower incomes than white male and female retirees. The national volunteer programs that provide financial stipends have a high participation of minority elderly (e.g., Foster Grandparents Program, 35 percent; Senior Companions, 44 percent). The Retired Senior Volunteer Program, which provides only travel reimbursement to some volunteer sites, has only a 14 percent minority participation (Keller, 1978). These types of data are important for service planners to understand.

The spontaneous-contagion model occurs when the practitioner sees a need among a target population, develops a program to meet the need, and recruits a pilot population—for example, bag people or homeless persons. The goal is a program that can be replicated elsewhere.

Both of the above models utilize a small group of "converts" to promote the targeted program. These models make broad goals more manageable to implement. They set short-term goals and force the practitioner to think through the entire process on a small scale, to build a support base, and to run on a trial basis with a small group.

Another important model for social workers in gerontological practice is the *advocacy model* that emerged in the 1960s and was made popular by Saul Alinsky. Community organizers of the Alinsky school would "organize organizations" and then try to get the unaffiliated poor to join one of the organizations involved. One case study of Alinsky's work utilized senior centers as a key network.

The Citizens Action Program (CAP) in Chicago began in 1969, originally as the Campaign Against Pollution; when it became concerned with broader issues such as property taxes and consumer issues, the name was changed. By 1973, CAP represented thirty neighborhood associations and fifty senior-citizen centers throughout the city and had succeeded in getting reductions in proposed telephone-rate increases and pharmaceutical prices and a tax-rebate program for the elderly in Illinois (Lancourt, 1979).

Alinsky (1972) considered it critical to utilize an active committee structure staffed by organizers. These were democratic committees with elected memberships. Although Alinsky used the term "radical," extreme measures were not used. Alinsky was a systems-oriented person, interested in making government, landlords, and business more responsive to citizens, which is also the aim of the Gray Panther movement. In a "how-to" organizing manual for older adults prepared by a Gray Panther officer (Bagger, n.d.), the basic recommended reading is Alinsky's *Rules for Radicals*. Advocacy planning, in summary, is that which demands that recipients or consumers of service should be partners in all decisions affecting the operation of such service.

Older adults can and need to be involved in all levels of social planning, implementing, and evaluating through advisory committees, boards, coalitions, councils, and planning teams. The diversity of older-adult participation should be represented; the customary upper middle class, retired professional needs to be balanced with others to reflect the constituency or community at large in which the organizing is taking place.

Legislative Impact on Social Planning

Two major amendments in 1965 to the Social Security Act, namely Title XVIII (Medicare) and XIX (Medicaid), were to have significant impact on older adults. They were written and passed without much involvement of the elderly (Pratt, 1976). By 1970, a power swing away from the elderly and back to the "professionals" was underway. Revenue sharing is illustrative of the original good intentions to allow citizen participation in local planning and fund allocation. It has not proved a successful participatory model, even though Title XX of the Social Security Act provided for training of the elderly to enable them to garner their fair share of funds.

The Older Americans Act of 1965 created an opportunity to turn the tide of "negligible" planning *for* the elderly to planning *with* the elderly. Social movements and planning of services relative to the older-adult population were initially instigated and engineered by interested professionals; the 1973 amendments created an area agency planning network and mandated opportunities for constituent input. Each state has established a state unit on aging to which local Area Agencies on Aging (AAA) channel their inputs. The AAAs are responsible for coordinating existing services and designing future programs for the elderly. Generally, three-year plans that coincide with federal-funding cycles and allocations are developed by each AAA and forwarded to the state unit on aging.

There are now over 700 AAAs across the country mandated to define service priorities and establish comprehensive service systems to improve services to the elderly. AAAs can use their allocation powers to fill gaps in services by contracting for such services, but an AAA has no authority over major system providers—for example, those in the health field that are not directly funded through Older American Act funds. This means that, in order to establish a comprehensive service system, the director and staff of an AAA can operate only by persuasion; they cannot offer any economic incentive for cooperation, nor do they have the capacity to sanction.

Several services mandated by the Older Americans Act require a community-organization perspective—for example, services intended to encourage and assist older persons to use the facilities and services available to them or to assist older persons to obtain adequate housing. Meeting these requirements frequently requires the skills and expertise of a community organizer. Advocacy is a primary skill necessary to identify and gain access to a service or to lobby for its availability. It has been common for advisory bodies of AAAs to be involved in legislative advocacy for the "class of elderly." By the late 1970s, more specific targeting on the high-risk elderly (those with low incomes and members of minority groups) was mandated.

Social Action

Social action, the third category of Rothman's typology of community organization models, is illustrated by a number of social movements. Understanding the history of social movements relative to older adults can be enlightening to the contemporary gerontological social worker planning social activities. The impetus for social movements addressing the needs of the elderly at the turn of the century was provided by the desire for a social-insurance program similar to models already in place in Germany and England. Leaders of various movements advocating pensions for older persons had large followings but were resented by policymakers.

A number of plans were initiated to address the depression economy. Francis Townsend's plan in the 1930s was to pay a pension of $200 per month to each person over age 60. The Ham-and-Eggs Plan proposed by Robert Noble recommended issuance of special scrip that had to be spent by older adults. The Wisconsin Plan, while emphasizing the need for organizations to set aside funds against risk of unemployment, was also concerned with old-age security. The philosophy of dealing with unemployment and the needs of the elderly was promoted by the American Association for Labor Legislation (AALL). Isaac Rubinow, later joined by Abraham Epstein, founded the leading pension-reform organization, the American Association of Old Age Security. This group modeled its recommendations on the European plans and arbitrarily set 65 as the retirement age. All of the movements faded with the passage of the Social Security Act in 1935.

One overriding similarity characterized these early movements. They were all developed and promoted by nonaged charismatic leaders rather than by the elderly themselves. Pratt (1976) concludes that the total lack of elderly constituents in the pension efforts was a critical error and limited their effects. He also speculates that if a more aggressive aging organization had existed, it would have advocated a more comprehensive act and it would not have taken five years to pass the subsequent amendments to Social Security. What these movements did accomplish was to raise the nation's consciousness of the existence and special needs of its aging population.

In the 1940s Ethel Andrus, a retired teacher, founded the National Retired Teachers Association (NRTA), which began offering group insurance to retired teachers. In 1958, the insurance was extended to the American Association of Retired Persons (AARP). Today the combined NRTA-AARP has over 13 million members and provides insurance coverage, preretirement training, and drug and travel discounts. It has also become a major national lobbying group, representing a primarily middle-class group of retirees who tend to be conservative on national issues but still pursue aging rights.

The National Council of Senior Citizens (NCSC) is a national advocacy group with its roots in the fight for health legislation in the early 1960s. Its membership of 3 million comes from organized labor and has a more liberal philosophy than NRTA-AARP. A much smaller organization, based in Washington, D.C., is the National Association of Retired Federal Employees (NARFE). Another mass activist group of uncertain membership size deserves mention—the Gray Panthers, founded by Maggie Kuhn in 1970 and merged in 1973 with one of Ralph Nader's public citizens groups, the Retired Professional Action Group. The Gray Panthers is an activist, universal, citizen-initiated social movement that promotes a basic restructuring of society and in which retirement is seen as a new age of liberation and self-determination. The Gray Panthers, whose official name is Consultation of Older and Younger Adults, seed a coalition of young and old people to explore alternative life-styles, advocate the elimination of ageism, and "radicalize" older persons to assume responsibility for their own lives.

These broad-based advocacy groups provide an opportunity for alliance when community organizers develop change strategies. Depending on the goal of the change effort, involvement of another organization with a similar goal, either at the national or local level, may enhance the prospects for success. Contact with organizations not specifically focused on issues of older adults can also enlarge the base of support—for example, involvement of nonaged disabled persons with the elderly in advocacy efforts for more accessible public transportation.

The Adults Only Movement in Arizona provides an unusual illustrstion of an older-adult social movement. It is theoretically akin to Rose's (1965) subculture theory of aging, which states that older persons have common generational experiences, feel more comfortable with their own peers, and work to self-segregate. Rose felt this trend was supported by an increase in old-age-dominated areas like housing complexes for the elderly and retirement communities.

The Adults Only Movement began in 1973 when a group of elderly were concerned about two minor children living in their adults-only mobile-home subdivision. A court battle resulted in legislation that supported the concept of an adults-only community (Anderson and Anderson, 1978). The movement comprised home and property owners concerned about this one problem. The common background and similar values of the participants provided the basis for effective advocacy. This example, while raising a dilemma for civil libertarians who claim that this type of movement is discriminatory, also presents the social worker with a significant social-policy issue.

The increased interest of the elderly in political activity has been widely observed and encouraged. The elderly and those acting on their behalf recognize the power base they can tap to promote legislation and funding in the constituencies' best interest.

The relationship of political activity and age has fortunately been studied in depth. When voting behavior is studied and socioeconomic status and length of residence in the community are controlled, one finds a gradual increase in political activity over the life span. For overall political participation, a minor decline is seen after the "standard" retirement age of 65. In general, the longer one is exposed to politics the more likely one is to participate (Verba and Nie, 1981).

It is a stereotype that individuals become more conservative as they age. Empirical testing of the relationship of age and conservatism is fraught with methodological problems. Defining "conservatism," for example, has to take into account societal trends toward liberalism or conservatism as well as the aging process per se. Cohort analysis is a much-improved method of documenting how a cohort changes over time when exposed to the same historical influences. Generally, the evidence from this type of research is ambiguous and follows societal trends. Analyzing cohorts over a thirty-year period, Glenn (1974, p. 26) reached two-conclusions:

1. According to almost any constant definition of conservatism, people have typically become less, rather than more, conservative as they have aged in conformity with general societal trends.
2. Cohorts who have aged into and beyond middle age during the past three decades have become more conservative in a relative sense, that is, relative to the total adult population and prevailing definitions of conservatism and liberalism. Paradoxically, people may become more likely to consider themselves conservative by others while, according to a constant definition, they become less conservative.

There has been concern in some sectors that the elderly will become an overwhelmingly powerful voting bloc and will receive an unfair proportion of diminishing resources at the expense of other age groups. Opinion differs, however, on actual voting behavior. Rose (1965) argued that the elderly forsake old alliances and join new age-segregated groups. The NCSC and the NRTA-AARP encourage age-segregated voting, and empirical data supports the claim that this occurs in the area of health care (Weaver, 1976). In contrast, the Townsend Movement, which began in 1933 and introduced a senior-power element into American politics, died out with the passing of the Social Security Act. Binstock and others argue, however, that historically there has not been an elderly voting bloc and that one is not likely to emerge presently (Campbell, 1971; Binstock, 1972).

Community organizers need to be equipped with the knowledge of political-participation behavior of older adults. Whether employing the models of social action, social planning, or locality development, organizers should not minimize the power of an organized interest group of older adults.

MAJOR TYPES OF CHANGE STRATEGIES

Social work deals fundamentally with change. Warren's (1977) typology of change strategies, which acknowledges the relationship between change agents and the targeted system for change, is consonant with social work's definition of change.

The most benign strategy to effect change is *collaboration* where mutually agreed-upon goals of change are carried out through consensus and cooperation. There are three primary methods of collaboration: informal cooperation, coalition building, and the creation of coordinating organizations (Turock, 1983). Informal collaboration relies on person-to-person negotiation between individuals and organizations that know one another and is usually effective for small-scale programs. A coalition is a small group of persons or organizations that share a common objective and come together for a specific purpose. Coalitions are usually convened on an ad-hoc basis and can be useful for educational and sensitization purposes. Insights into rural and urban differences in the formation of coalitions is provided by an evaluation of Operation Independence, a three-year model project of the National Council on Aging in the 1970s.

The purpose of establishing coalitions under Operation Independence was to demonstrate that the quantity and quality of services for vulnerable older adults could be increased through collaborative efforts among local voluntary private and public agencies (National Council on the Aging, 1978). It was found that leaders in some rural communities were reluctant to organize a collaborative effort because they feared there were not enough agencies to make it worthwhile. The opposite was true for urban areas, where leaders feared too much competition. In rural areas, the coalitions' objectives were more limited due to fewer resources; more time was usually spent on the "planning process" and concrete service development was more likely to evolve. In urban areas, geographical boundary setting was necessary before organization of a coalition was manageable. A more formal planning process took place whose emphasis was on coordination of existing services rather than development of new ones.

Churches and farm organizations surfaced as the dominant voluntary organizations in rural areas and were good sources of leadership. In urban areas, prominent agencies in the voluntary sector were looked to automatically to provide such leadership. In both rural and urban environments, the voluntary agencies tended to provide the impetus for coalition formation.

The most sophisticated method of collaboration is the coordinating organization. It is formally established and is usually a legal entity with formal bylaws specifying governance and membership.

The *difference-campaign* strategy is appropriate when there is no consensus but when there is hope for it. A campaign strategy is inaugurated to win support for an objective or idea. Campaign strategies recognize that differences of opinions and values are present. The social worker implementing this type of strategy is in the role of persuader, trying to convert people to look at an issue differently.

The Social Security "crisis" provided an example of campaign strategy. A national organization called Save Our Security (SOS) evolved to address the crisis. It mounted a major campaign urging solution of the fiscal problems of Social Security without benefit cuts. Newsletters, letter-writing, delegations to elected officials, and visits to Congress were tactics utilized in the campaign to win support for identified objectives.

The *contest* strategy, which has as its goal the defeat of the opposition, is appropriate when there is disagreement as to desired outcome and the campaign strategy is deemed ineffective. Strikes, boycotts, sit-ins, and demonstrations are common tactics of this strategy.

The experiences of an elderly activist organization in Cape Cod, Massachusetts, in 1979 illustrate all the strategies just described. In an attempt to gain access to nursing homes that were considered by the elderly to be poorly managed, various change strategies were incrementally applied. First, letter-writing, "befriending" residents and staff through visitation, and educational activities to raise the consciousness of the community about nursing homes were undertaken. Later, one of the contest strategies utilized by older adults was a sit-in, which resulted in the arrest and conviction of the older adults on charges of trespassing (Holmes, 1982).

In selecting a strategy, the purpose of the change effort must be considered, as well as the support base and/or constituencies. For example, if locality (community) development is the goal, a campaign strategy is usually effective in bringing together all significant community groups. Organization of client groups, such as families of Alzheimer patients, to provide education, mutual support, and resource sharing for a group with similar concerns and stresses would best be accomplished by a campaign strategy.

Social action frequently requires a combination of campaign and contest strategies. A class-action suit initiated by spouses of nursing-home residents to allow them more assets to live on in the community is a case in point. This is a legal action against an administrative agency; since it implies more tax dollars to support public programs, it cannot rely on collaborative efforts. Campaign strategies will probably have limited success, so contest strategies may be needed at crucial stages. Civil disobedience, social reform, social movement, bargaining and consensus planning—change efforts all known to the community worker—must be evaluated for feasibility and appropriateness in a particular situation.

At times a practitioner may see his or her role as limited only to facilitation. Morris (1962, p. 168) has suggested: "The exercise of professional leadership requires us to select our goals for action. . . . Our concern with helping others to make up their minds does not excuse us from the obligation of making our own (goals)." In decision making, constituent goals, agency goals, and goals of the professional may be in conflict. It is the role of the social worker to identify the differences and creatively find the path to meet the constituent goals while being cognizant of agency and self-interests. The organizational context sets many boundaries for degrees of involvement for the professional.

ORGANIZATION CONTEXT

Community organization is practiced in many types of settings in both the public and private sectors. Prior to 1935, it was primarily associated with coordinating voluntary agencies such as community chests or health and welfare councils. Since 1935, the federal government's increased role through financial support of programs has meant that most community-organization workers in the field of aging have been in the public sector. The type of interorganizational planning referred to by Perlman and Gurin (1972), in which the role of the social worker is to determine how to organize and allocate resources, is illustrated by the network of Area Agencies on Aging created by the Older Americans Act.

Institutionalized Elderly

Approximately 5 percent of those 65 and over are in a residential-care facility at any given time. However, about 20 percent of the elderly will spend their later years in nursing homes (Litwin, Kaye, and Monk, 1982). This is a significant number of people who come in contact with long-term residential care. Three community-organization strategies are suggested by Litwin and associates for organizing older persons at the residential-care-facility level. These strategies apply to health-care settings of all types; however, macro-level social workers are more prominent in acute-care settings.

Organizing the nursing home from within through residents' councils is one strategy. The pioneering work on establishing such councils was done by Silverstone (1971), who advocated that all residents be involved. As more severely disabled persons are now being admitted, however, questions are raised about the degree of participation and self-governance possible. One possibility is to involve others in the residents' council, particularly outside advocates who could represent the interests of severely disabled.

The second strategy is the nursing-home ombudsman mandated by the Older Americans Act Amendments of 1978. An ombudsman is responsible for responding to resident complaints. Litwin notes that generally the ombudsman is not empowered to change policies and therefore tactics oriented toward consensus rather than contest are appropriate given the lack of authority of the role. The ombudsman is viewed most commonly as an advocate. Few would describe the ombudsman as Berger (1976) does as a militant advocate working to change the balance of power rather than as a spokesperson knowledgeable about the system.

Advocacy for the residents from outside the nursing home is a third strategy applicable to residential facilities. Family and visitors councils and consumer-rights groups of the institutionalized elderly are examples. FRIA (Friends and Relatives of Institutionalized Aged) in New York City orients friends and relatives to the long-term-care system and provides strategies and support for case-by-case interventions. Consumer-rights groups are also flourishing—for example, the Elderly Activist Project in Cape Cod, Citizens for Better Care in Michigan, hotlines for abuse reporting, and the National Citizens' Coalition for Nursing Home Reform, which lobbies for national reform in the long-term-care industry.

A study of ethnic differences regarding patient advocacy services in long-term-care facilities provides insight for gerontological social workers. Black residents were significantly more likely to have heard of the Patient's Bill of Rights than their white counterparts and were more convinced that outsiders were needed to intervene in response to patient grievances. This tendency of greater activism among blacks may reflect the increasing stance of advocacy in the black community carried over to the institution. When complaints or problems arose, blacks were most likely to turn to the nursing staff (52 percent) and then to social workers (17.4 percent) while whites more equally turned to nursing staff (30.3 percent) and social workers (28.9 percent) (Monk and Kaye, 1984, p.9).

The rural elderly as a population group can be characterized as having a double burden—being old and inhabiting a rural environment (Cryns and Monk, 1975). The rural environment poses special problems and hazards relative to elderly who need services and socialization due to geographical expanse and hence lack of proximity to service.

Several characteristics of rural communities are summarized by Wodarski (1983) and are worth noting by gerontological social workers. A major characteristic of rural communities is the higher incidence of poverty in comparison to their urban counterparts. Rural community residents tend to hold more traditional views regarding sex roles, to hold more conservative religious and political views, and to take far greater pride in a "rugged individualism" philosophy. Professional newcomers to rural communities are immediately recognized as new and suspect until they prove otherwise, especially those affiliated with publicly sponsored programs. In the majority of instances, an informal network of control within the rural community performs many of the same functions as its more formalized urban counterpart (Wodarski, 1983, p.6). Community workers need to recognize the power structure and work within it to realize provision of necessary services to clients. Perhaps the greatest challenge to social workers in rural settings is how to deal with the physical isolation of elderly persons due either to geographic location or to lack of access. Transportation or lack of it always seems to surface as a concrete problem for older adults in rural areas.

Rural service-delivery planners can be encouraged that the 1980 Census data includes a one-in-two subsample of the population in rural counties, which will increase the reliability of the data. In addition, the over-65 age group is broken into five-year segments in many of the reports. One area not available to planners from census data is the changing characteristics of older people in a rural county that result from in or out migration patterns (Deimling, 1982; Longino and Bigger, 1982). It is of interest to note that in farming communities, many retired farmers and spouses retire to the nearest local town and hence many small towns are characteristically becoming retirement communities.

Life-Long Learning

Ongoing education is critical so that older adults can remain viable in our high-technology, knowledge-based society. The opportunity to fine-tune current skills, to develop or retool for a second or third career, or merely to acquire knowledge for its own sake is an important element for social planners and policy personnel to bear in mind. The local library, senior centers, community colleges, and universities should address themselves to lifelong learning based on a life-cycle education approach (Turock, 1983). The library, which has a tradition of independent, self-planned, self-directed education, can be tapped appropriately for older adults by community workers focused on preventing the isolation created by lack of knowledge. The National Council on the Aging's Self-Discovery Through the Humanities is a fine illustration, as is the American Association of Retired Persons' Institute of Lifetime Learning, which offers model minicourses in the bimonthly publication *Modern Maturity*.

A Seniors Teaching Seniors model project developed at the Columbia University Brookdale Institue on Aging in New York City promotes a unique learning experience. The program trains seniors to become teachers, leaders, and organizers of educational programs based on their skills and expertise (Stuen, Spencer, and Raines, 1982). The university is an appropriate setting for older-adult learners to be affiliated for learning and sharing purposes. Many older persons grew up in an era when attitudes toward the aged were negative and stereotypes about being old were rampant. Education holds great potential for older adults as well as for the general population and especially for those who serve them.

The educational issues relating to aging are referred to by Johnson (1982) as the three E's: enrichment, expertise, and enlightenment. Enrichment is the reward an older person gains from education; expertise is the capacity to serve the aged; and enlightenment is the education of the public about normal aging. As older persons increase their numbers and their proportion of the general population, they will exert greater influence and hopefully will begin pressing for better educational options.

THE ROLE OF THE COMMUNITY ORGANIZER

There are several generic roles for a community organizer that are particularly relevant to work with older adults. In the role of *enabler*, the worker is directly involved with participants/constituents and his goal is to enable them to realize their potentials. This is a traditional social-work role, based on a residual-practice model and focused on the client-worker relationship. The enabler facilitates local activity in support of the goals of the client group.

The role of *broker* is to assist the participants in locating and accessing various resources. Negotiation skills are called for because there is usually a shortage of services (resources) to meet needs. Creativity is also a useful skill in facing diminished resources. Collective brokerage activity is illustrated by the worker who intervenes, for example, on behalf of all the older-adult residents who need new housing and a variety of other support services to complete relocation from a condemned housing project.

The most confrontational role is the *activist* one. It is a difficult role because it rarely allows a neutral stance on the worker's part and frequently involves partisan situations. The worker often finds himself or herself indentifying with the client group and taking on the cause as his or her own.

Case management became an important role for social workers in guaranteeing access to the service system, particulary after the 1978 amendments to the Older Americans Act. A case manager is defined by Gottesman, Ishizaki, and MacBride (1979) as one who serves as counselor, broker, and advocate. The shift toward case management is a unique change in philosophy toward trying to care for the elderly rather than cure their chronic impairments (Morris, 1977).

The direct-practice worker may be the actual person for the older adult; the community worker is the one who seeks instead to make order out of a chaotic service system, who deals with administrative and funding issues to ensure clients' access to needed services, and who promotes the creation of new or additional services. The development of client pathways through the service maze and documentation procedures—for example, client information systems —is in the purview of the macro social worker. Case management is a good illustration of the interface and symbiotic relationship apparent between micro and macro social-work practice (Monk, 1981).

Engagement in community organization, community development, social action, social advocacy—whatever label is given to the macro approach to social problem-solving with the elderly, there are prescriptive guidelines for action. The first consideration must be examination by the worker or his/her own attitudes toward aging. A gentle reminder for any worker is to exercise caution in stereotyping the population of elderly. Sweeping generalizations about "the elderly" and what they want or need should be avoided. A corollary caution is to avoid being patronizing; even the most sensitive gerontological social worker can be caught saying, "My seniors want. . . ." The older-adult population is extremely heterogeneous, and as the life span increases the aging cohorts will exhibit even greater differences.

Sensitivity to the older-adult constituency in the application of generic roles and strategies is the important element in gerontological practice. An understanding of the unique position in which the elderly are often placed is essential. For example, in addressing the problem of poverty, the organizer needs to ascertain whether the individual was always poor or is recently poor because retirement income has been eroded by inflation. Resistance to dependence will be manifested in any age group; it is more significant for an older person who has spent a lifetime being independent than for a 20-year-old learning independence. Cash poor versus benefit poor is another issue relative to the poverty illustration. Expressed needs versus perceived needs in all situations and by whom are factors to bear in mind.

The elderly possess varied life experiences. Their collective wisdom regarding historical precedents for current activities can be tapped for current applicability. The fact that they have free time available can be advantageous. For the older adult, usually retired, there is no job on the line when activities are undertaken. One's career is not in the making and thus one may be more willing to take risks, speak out, and demonstrate for causes—though less tolerant of elongated processes.

In any organizing effort, individuals are the building blocks. For older persons, the new unrehearsed role of retirement may be traumatic and the thought of community action may be threatening. Approaching community organization in an orderly, incremental way and pacing the activities will usually ensure the program's durability. Negative reactions from the elderly should be viewed positively because they reflect discontent with the status quo and are essential ingredients for promotion of change. This is preferable to the "big bang" approach whereby an organizer steamrolls into a neighborhood, turning the constituents off to further involvement.

Collective action is particularly difficult with a diverse population of older adults. The worker must communicate effectively the commonalities of the issue and the need to coalesce individuals to work together for mutually beneficial goals, sometimes in the face of skeptical reactions from the constituents who feel that the changes are too late for them. The problem to be worked on must be subdivided into realizable goals in order to retain an element of hope. To discuss a five-year strategy with a group of 90-year-olds may not spur the desired commitment to participation.

In any community, the worker needs to recognize the psychosocial fabric and its variety. It is important to seek involvement of all classes and ethnic groups and to build bridges for "different" people to come together and work on a common goal. Working *with*, not *for*, will ensure that the worker is well grounded in community work.

POLICY CONSIDERATIONS AND FUTURE DIRECTIONS

Calhoun (1978) provides historical documentation for two policy options that were open to lawmakers during the 1940s, when it was first recognized that the elderly constituted a growing segment of the population. These two options, material intervention and institutional reform, are relevant today. The New Deal-type programs, of which Social Security is the best example, illustrate material intervention. Institutional reform, which focuses on changing attitudes, was more favored by pioneers in the field of gerontological social work, according to Calhoun. Grace Rubin-Rabson, a geriatric social worker writing in 1948, rejected massive material intervention on behalf of the elderly, favoring instead long-range changes in the social climate designed to improve the position of older citizens. Reformers in the 1940s chose to change the image of older persons on the assumption that improvements in social and economic status would follow.

Senior-citizen movements today similarly tend to champion the institutional-reform option, citing such goals as "promotion of self-esteem in a nonageist society." The objectives of the Older Americans Act also support this option. Social Security is one instance of material reform favored over institutional reform. The Social Security crisis was fostered by partisan political forces and provides a good illustration of how a crisis can be engineered by the media and partisan forces. Derthick's (1979) prediction that when the system had reached maturity improvements in benefits would become increasingly difficult came true in 1982 (Anderson, 1983).

One recurring theme of social policy in macro social work with the aged is the difficulty in establishing a cohesive identity among older persons for social action. Binstock (1972) advocates that the aged need to develop nonelderly identity ties such as with nonaged minority groups. Since the elderly cannot stop consuming essential goods and services, nor have jobs to strike from, they have no leverage, no power, and therefore must join forces with other groups.

Atchley (1972) agrees with Binstock that the elderly as a group are too diverse to provide a singular group identity and cannot therefore make effective pressure groups, but they can be effective in making their plight visible, especially to politicians and the media.

Examination of the Older Americans Act as a case study of how the legally mandated organizational caretaker of the "problems of the aged" promote and perpetuate the aging "enterprise" was carried out by Estes (1979). It is Estes's opinion that the continuation of age-segregated policies assists only the professionals who thrive on jobs in the aging enterprise and that this is a divisive, isolating tragedy for U.S. society. One overall allegation she makes of the Older Americans Act is that it promotes a problem focus in dealing with older persons and hence seeks to improve the individual's adjustment to society rather than promoting long-range structural changes. The basic assumption is that the system to which older adults should adjust is a basically good one (Kuhn, 1978).

The policy decisions adopted in the 1960s to foster separate services for older adults reemerged in a critical debate in the 1980s. There is a backlash view that the elderly have gotten too much at the expense of other needy groups. This debate echoes the social-welfare controversy whether programs should be offered on a universalistic or particularistic basis. A universalistic service orientation advocates that all persons in need, regardless of age, should be served; however, experience with age discrimination in the workplace, Title XX, and community mental-health centers suggests that, unless the elderly are specifically targeted, they will not receive their fair share.

The blame for increasing federal-budget deficits has been placed on the elderly in this backlash era. Analysis of federal spending for older persons reveals that approximately 25 to 30 percent of the total federal budget is now spent on programs directly helping persons 65 and older (U.S. Congress, 1983). Social Security, which accounts for 60 percent of federal outlays for the elderly, is financed by payroll taxes paid by workers and employers. If Social Security is excluded from the unified budget, federal outlays would be less than half of what they now are for older adults. If all partially self-funded programs are excluded from estimates of federal spending, only 4 percent of the federal budget would be devoted to programs for the elderly.

Another tactic of those who claim expenditures for the elderly are "out of control" is to avoid adjusting expenditure figures for inflation. Without this adjustment, a 350-percent increase in expenditures between 1971 and 1982 has been cited. When this figure is adjusted for inflation, however, it is reduced to 3.5 percent a year, which is largely accounted for by the one-time 20-percent increase in Social Security benefits passed in 1972. This increase was passed in response to the 1970 Census data that indicated that 24.5 percent of the nation's elderly were struggling to live on incomes below the poverty level (U.S. Congress, 1983).

The advantage of utilizing the elderly as a focal point for social legislation in the remainder of this century is certainly in their numbers; they are a rapidly increasing segment of the population. Their general popularity in partisan politics and the ethos that supports them as "deserving" is a historical advantage not to be discarded lightly.

The main skill of social workers in community organization is the ability to enable constituents to act on their own behalf. Etzioni (1978) encouraged the mobilization of senior citizens who, with the help of professionals, could systematically refine and expand the senior movement by identifying forces that support reform at the system level. In our industrial society, where mandatory retirement and skill obsolescence have tipped the balance of power in favor of the younger working population, only a well-organized interest group espousing rights of older adults can hope to have an impact.

REFERENCES

Alinsky, S. D. (1972). *Rules for radicals.* New York: Vintage Books.
Anderson, H. (1983. January 24). The Social Security crisis. *Newsweek,* pp. 18-28.
Anderson, W. A., and Anderson, N. D. (1978). The politics of age exclusion: The adults only movement in Arizona. *Gerontologist,* **18**(1), 6-12.
Atchley, R. C. (1972). *The social forces in later life.* Belmont, Calif.: Wadsworth.
Bagger, H. S. (n.d.). *A study program for the elderly and friends of the elderly: An interdisciplinary approach.* New York: Whitney.
Bell, B. D. (1975). Mobile medical care to the elderly: An evaluation. *Gerontologist,* **15**(2), 100-103.
Berger, M. (1976). An orienting perspective on advocacy. In P. A. Kerschner (Ed.), *Advocacy and age: Issues, experiences, strategies.* Los Angeles: Andrus Gerontology Center, University of Southern California.

Binstock, R. H. (1972). Interest-group liberalism and the politics of aging. *Gerontologist,* **12**(3), 265-280.

Brager, G., and Specht, H. (1973). *Community organizing.* New York: Columbia University Press.

Calhoun, R. B. (1978). *In search of the new old: Redefining old age in America, 1945-1970.* New York: Elsevier.

Campbell, A. (1971). Politics through the life cycle. *Gerontologist,* **11**(2), 112-117.

Cloward, R., and Piven, F. F. (1982). A movement strategy to transform the Democratic party. *Ideas for Action,* no. 5, pp. 1-7.

Corbett, F. (1970). Community organization involving the elderly. In S. K. Match (Ed.), *Community organization, planning and resources for the older poor.* Washington: National Council on the Aging.

Cryns, A., and Monk, A. (1975). *The rural aged: An analysis of key providers of services to the elderly.* Albany: State Unviersity of New York at Buffalo.

Cull, J. C., and Hardy, R. E. (Eds.) (1973). *The neglected older Americans.* Springfield, Ill.: Thomas.

Cumming, E., and Henry, W. E. (1961). *Growing old: The process of disengagement.* New York: Basic Books.

Davis, K. (1975). Equal treatment and unequal benefits: The Medicare program. *Milbank Memorial Fund Quarterly,* **53**, 449-488.

Deimling, Gary T. (1982). Macro- and microlevel aging service planning and the 1980 census. *Gerontologist,* **22**(2), 151-152.

Derthick, M. (1979). No more easy votes for Social Security. *Brookings Bulletin,* **16**(4), 1-16.

Dowd, J. J. (1975). Aging as exchange: A preface to theory. *Journal of Gerontology,* **30**(5), 584-594.

Dowd, J., and Bengston, V. (1978). Aging in minority populations: An examination of the double jeopardy hypothesis. *Journal of Gerontology,* **33**(3), 427-436.

Emerson, R. M. (1962). Power-dependence relations. *American Sociological Review,* **27**(1), 31-41.

Estes, C. (1979). *The aging enterprise.* San Francisco: Jossey-Bass.

Etzioni, A. (1978). From Zion to diaspora. *Society,* **15**(4), 92-101.

Fujii, S. M. (1976). Elderly Asian Americans and use of public services. *Social Casework,* **57**, 202-207.

Gartner, A. (1984). Widower self-help groups: A preventive approach. *Social Policy,* **14**(3), 37-38.

Glenn, N. (1974). Age and conservatism. *Annals of the American Academy of Political and Social Science,* **415**, 176-186.

Gottesman, L. E., Ishizaki, B., and MacBride, S. M. (1979). Service management — plan and concept in Pennsylvania. *Gerontologist,* **19**(4), 378-388.

Havighurst, R. J., and Albrecht, R. (1953). *Older people.* New York: Longmans, Green.

Holmes, J. (1982). *The elderly activist handbook.* Hyannis, Mass.: Cape United Elderly.

Jackson, J. J. (1978). Retirement patterns of aged blacks. In E. P. Stanford (Ed.), *Retirement: Concepts and realities.* San Diego: University Center on Aging, San Diego State University.

Johnson, H. (1982). Education in an aging society. *National Forum,* **62**(4), 19-21.

Katz, A. H., and Bender, E. I. (1976). *The strength in us: Self-help groups in the modern world.* New York: New Viewpoints.

Keller, J. B. (1978). Volunteer activities for ethnic minority elderly. In E. P. Stanford (Ed.), *Retirement: Concepts and realities.* San Diego: University Center on Aging, San Diego State University.

Kuhn, M. (1978). Open letter. *Gerontologist,* **18**(5), 422-424.

Lancourt, J. E. (1979). *Confront or concede: The Alinsky citizen-action organizations.* Lexington, Mass.: Lexington Books.

Lieberman, M., and Borman, L. D. (1981). The impact of self-help intervention for widows' mental health. *National Reporter,* **4**, 2-6.

Litwak, E., and Meyer, H. J. (1974). *School, family and neighborhood: The theory and practice of school-community relations.* New York: Columbia University Press.

Litwin, H., Kaye, L., and Monk, A. (1982). Holding the line for the institutionalized elderly: Strategic options for community organizers. *Social Development Issues,* **6**(3), 15-24.

Longino, C. F. (1982). Symposium: Population research for planning and practice. *Gerontologist,* **22**(2), 142-143.

Longino, C. F., and Bigger, J. C. (1982). The impact of population redistribution on service delivery. *Gerontologist,* **22**(2), 153-159.

McCaslin, R., and Calvert, W. R. (1975). Social indicators in black and white: Some ethnic considerations in delivery of service to the elderly. *Journal of Gerontology,* **30**(1), 60-66.

Manuel, R. C., and Berk, M. L. (1983). A look at similarities and differences in older minority populations. *Aging,* no. 330.

Manuel, R. C., and Reid, J. (1982). A comparative demographic profile of the minority and non-minority aged. In R. C. Manuel (Ed.), *Minority aging: Sociological and social psychological issues.* Westport, Conn.: Greenwood Press.

Match, S. K. (Ed.). (1970). *Community organization, planning, and resources and the older poor.* Washington: National Council on the Aging.

Monk, A. (1981). Social work with the aged: Principles of practice. *Social Work,* **26**(1), 61-68.

Monk, A., and Kaye, L. W. (1984). Patient advocacy services in long term care facilities: Ethnic perspectives. *Journal of Long Term Care Administration,* **12**(1), 5-10.

Morris, R. (1962). Community planning for health: The social welfare experience. In *Public health concepts in social work education.* New York: Council on Social Work Education.

Morris, R. (1977). Caring for vs. caring about people. *Social Work,* **22**(5), 353-359.

National Association of Social Workers. (1977). *Encyclopedia of social work* (17th issue), vol. 2. Washington: National Association of Social Workers.

National Council on the Aging. (1978). *The "at risk" elderly: Community service approaches.* Washington: The Council.

Neugarten, B., Havighurst, R. J., and Tobin, S. S. (1964). Personality types in an aged population. In B. L. Neugarten (Ed.), *Personality in middle and late life.* New York: Atherton.

Perlman, R., and Gurin, A. (1972). *Community organization and social planning.* New York: Wiley.

Pratt, H. J. (1976). *The gray lobby.* Chicago: University of Chicago Press.

Rose, A. (1965). The subculture of the aging: A framework for research in social gerontology. In A. M. Rose and W. A. Peterson (Eds.), *Older people and their social world.* Philadelphia: Davis.

Rothman, J. (1979). Three models of community organization practice. In F. M. Cox et al. (Eds.), *Strategies of community organization* (3rd ed.). Itasca, Ill.: Peacock.

Rothman, J., Erlich, J. L., and Teresa, J. G. (1981). *Changing organizations and community programs.* Beverly Hills, Calif.: Sage.

Siegel, J. S., and Taeuber, C. M. (1982). The 1980 census and the elderly: New data available to planners and practitioners. *Gerontologist,* **22**(2), 144-150.

Silverstone, B. M. (1974). *Establishing resident councils.* New York: Federation of Protestant Welfare Agencies.

Stuen, C., Spencer, B. B., and Raines, M. A. (1982). *Seniors teaching seniors: A manual for training older adult teachers.* New York: Brookdale Institute on Aging, Columbia University.

Suler, J. (1984). The role of ideology in self-help groups. *Social Policy,* **14**(3), 29-36.

Turock, B. J. (1983). *Serving the older adult.* New York: Bowker.

U.S. Congress. House. Select Committee on Aging. (1980). *Future directions for aging policy: A human service model.* Washington: Government Printing Office.

U.S. Congress. Senate. Special Committee on Aging. (1983). *Aging reports.* Washington: Government Printing Office.

Vachon, M. L. S. (1980). A controlled study of self-help interventions for widows. *American Journal of Psychiatry,* **37**, 1380-1384.

Verba, S., and Nie, N. (1981). Age and political participation. In R. B. Hudson (Ed.)., *The aging in politics: Process and policy.* Springfield, Ill.: Thomas.

Warren, R. L. (1977). *Social change and human purpose: Toward understanding and action.* Chicago: Rand McNally.

Weaver, J. (1976). The elderly as a political community: The case of national health policy. *Western Political Quarterly,* **29**(4), 610-619.

Wodarski, J. S. (1983). *Rural community mental health practice.* Baltimore: University Park Press.

PART IV
COMMUNITY-BASED SERVICES

9

Services to Families of the Elderly

Mario Tonti, D.S.W.

The Benjamin Rose Institute, Cleveland, Ohio

Barbara Silverstone, D.S.W.

The New York Association for the Blind, New York, N.Y.

BACKGROUND

The solidarity and reciprocity that characterize extended family relationships have been well documented by research findings. Encompassing social contacts and affectional and material exchanges, these relationships have profound meaning for elders, many of whom are segregated from society's formal structures (Bengston and Treas, 1980; Shanas et al., 1968).

The sturdiness of the informal social networks of the elderly is reflected in the care and support given them when illness occurs. A national sample of older persons indicated that in a health crisis 80 to 90 percent of elders with adult children would seek assistance from them if help was needed (Shanas, 1979a, 1979b). Over 80 percent of all homecare is provided to elders by family members, usually the spouse and adult children (U.S. National Center for Health Statistics, 1975).

A 1977 study of a random sample of 1,609 elderly in Cleveland found that the majority were receiving help from family or friends. Transportation and checking were the most frequently provided services, followed by homemaker and coordination assistance. Groceries and food stamps, continuous supervision, nursing care, and general financial help were the least frequently provided services. Family care was costed out and found to exceed the cost or value of services provided by agencies at all levels of impairment (U.S. General Accounting Office 1977a, 1977b).

The most intensive informal caregiving patterns appear to be in those situations where elders are in residence with families. Lang and Brody (1983) found extensive help being given by daughters who lived with their mothers. In a study of mentally and physically impaired elders in residence, Noelker and Poulshock (1982) examined 617 families, half of whom were spouse caregivers and half adult-child caregivers, and found that comprehensive help was being provided for an average of six years. In a study sample of forty nursing-home residents and an equally impaired group of forty-six elders living in the community, the key variable differentiating the two was the presence of spouse and children for the community elders (Brody, Poulshock, and Masciocchi, 1978).

The extent and expense of family services, as well as the meaning of kin relationships to the elderly, has moved the informal network into a position of central consideration by formal service providers. This chapter will summarize the state of the art of social services to families of the elderly, outline the salient issues facing the field, and present a theoretical framework for the further development of services with an emphasis on clinical applications.

The Need and Demand for Formal Services

While family caregiving to impaired elders appears extensive and varied, formal supports assume greater importance as age and degree of frailty increase (Cantor, 1980). One in four elders over 65 enters a nursing home at some point in his/her later years (Kastenbaun and Candy, 1973). Forty-three percent of a sample of 210 families in a 1971 study indicated their difficulty in providing long-term care, and 32 percent reported they would be unable to care for a sick person at home under any circumstances (Litman, 1971). In the GAO study of over 1,600 Cleveland elders, nursing care and continuous supervision comprised a very small percentage of family assistance (U.S. General Accounting Office, 1977a, 1977b).

The research clearly suggests the presence of family stress and dysfunction in relation to caregiving of impaired aged relatives, particularly when there are extensive needs for physical or nursing care and when there is mental disturbance (Hoenig and Hamilton, 1966; Isaacs, 1971; Sanford, 1975). Family stress and dysfunction are manifested by anxiety, depression, role conflict, and physical illness (Gurland et al., 1978; Sainsbury and de Alarcon, 1970). As noted, patterns of caregiving do exist wherein families can manage under trying circumstances (Noelker and Poulshock, 1982). What is not known are the contextual variables that account for some families coping with burden and stress and others "giving up." Needed are longitudinal studies that follow families over time. Zarit, Reever, and Bach-Peterson (1980), in a study of twenty-nine caregivers, noted that the most important factor that seemed to sustain primary family caregivers was help and visitations of other kin. In another cross-sectional study, Noelker and Poulshock (1982) found that the strong dyadic relationship between the primary caregiver (usually a female spouse or daughter) and elder and secondary supports from other kin to be possible mitigating factors.

The obvious burdens and stresses borne by families are not necessarily translated into a perceived need or demand for service, perhaps due to a fear of outside interference or anticipated frustration with bureaucratic processes. Of the 617 families caring for impaired elders in residence, only a small percentage received social-work services or attended a caregiver training or support group, and only 8 percent reported an unmet need for in-home health and personal care. One-fifth complained of difficulty in getting service providers to come to the home and obtaining needed information about available services. Financial need was not mentioned. When the primary caregiver did report a need for help in regard to particular tasks, other kin were usually seen as the source of help (Noelker and Poulshock, 1982). On the other hand, a study of thirty female caregivers reported their needs as relief from some care-providing activities, help in developing management strategies for common problems, and accessible information and referral for service needs (Archbold, 1982).

The quality of family care and the burden and stresses on families must be weighed in determining the need for services. While it has been documented that elders prefer the help of kin, little is known about the degree of skill that families bring to the care of the moderate to severely impaired elder or the extent of abuse. Family members who lived with their elders reported difficulty in caring for the mentally impaired, particularly those exhibiting negative behavior, and in dealing with incontinence and heavy lifting. While 91 percent of the elders who could be interviewed were generally satisified, and stated they preferred to continue their present arrangement, 55 percent complained that the caregivers did too much for them and 30 percent that their relationship with the caregiver made them feel useless (Noelker and Poulshock, 1982). Some of the elders in this population, as with some nursing-home residents, may have been experiencing conditions of "excess disability" or functional loss not justified by their actual physical and mental impairments (Lawton and Brody, 1969). Training of family members who serve as primary caregivers to very impaired elders would appear to be an important unmet need.

The issue of exploitative and aggressive behavior toward helpless frail elders on the part of caregivers has long been recognized in nursing homes. More recently, the focus has broadened to include families and neighbors of elders in the community. Steinmetz (1983) found in a study of seventy-seven families that about 10 percent of the elderly had experienced either threats or acts of violence from their children. Isolated incidents of abuse by family, friends, or neighbors have appeared with increasing frequency, and in some states professionals are required by law to report these situations. Abuse, however, is difficult to document because of the reluctance or inability of elders to complain about their families (Rathbone-McCuan, 1980). Despite this reticence, the need for services to these families is compelling.

It is generally assumed that in the future there will be an increased need and demand for services to elders and their families. A thinning of the family structure appears inevitable as more elders grow very old with fewer children and grandchildren filling the younger generations. As women increasingly join the work force, the number of potential caregivers may diminish. Given their longevity and higher divorce rates, there will be more very old widowed and single women.

While these trends suggest that the burden of long-term care will shift more to the formal system, countervailing forces may offset these expectations. Still unknown are the years of actual frailty that the old will experience. Given predictions of better health and a finite life expectancy, these years may decrease, reducing the caregiving burden for families (Fries and Crapo, 1981). Declining birthrates may free some of the resources of the middle aged for the old.

The future of the informal support system in relation to its frail elders is not clear and thus the quantitative demand for social services by families is difficult to predict. What is clear is that better-informed and vocal families will seek improvements in present types and inadequate levels of services. They will want their specific needs addressed, particularly in caring for mentally impaired elders, and will want to improve their own coping skills. Given advances in clinical research, problematic family situations will be identified and, hopefully, skilled services provided to ameliorate them.

Formal Services Currently Being Provided

Promising developments in services to families are underway. Education, training, respite, and counseling are now being provided to families, and although limited in number and duration, these programs can serve as models for the future.

Nine Administration on Aging model projects have sought to intergrate formal service providers into the daily operations of informal care providers. One of the better known of these programs was the Natural Supports Program of the Community Service Society in New York, which included task-centered casework, support groups, concrete services, and advocacy training (Zimmer, 1983). The findings from these projects were assimilated, and a set of seven implementation guidelines was developed for service providers who wished to expand their programs to the informal support network of the elderly. Among the recommendations was the development of staff expertise in the problems of informal support networks and redefining the term "client" to include the family as well as the elder.

Programs developed at The Benjamin Rose Insititute to serve the frail elderly emphasize helping families to problem solve more effectively in relation to caregiving, supplementing these efforts when necessary with formal services. Of a total caseload of 1,008 elders in 1982, 379 cases were closed. The majority of the closed cases were able to carry on with informal supports, and a six-month follow-up found the majority of elders and families functioning well (Benjamin Rose Institute, 1983).

In another of the few programs providing follow-up data, Meltzer (1982) found a positive correlation between a higher level of need and a higher demand for services in two institutional-respite programs for caregivers in California and New York. Also discovered was an unexpectedly high rate of institutionalization (12 percent) of the respite-care population within one month after use of respite services. These services may have broken down family barriers to insitutionalization or represented one last attempt to avoid institutionalization.

Increased attention by service providers is being given to families of nursing-home residents, in part because they are more vocal but also in recognition of the supplemental services that families can provide and the fact that the segregation of elders from the community does not weaken kin ties (Dobroff and Litwak, 1977; Kirschner, 1979; Safford, 1980; Silverstone, 1978). Smith and Bengtson (1979) found that the emotional quality of family relationships improved following institutionalization, perhaps because the direct burden of caregiving was removed.

Professionals, aware that family need is often not translated into demand for services, have attempted to reach families directly through publications that seek to educate and sensitize them to the aging process and caregiving issues (Cohen and Gans, 1978; Mace and Rabins, 1981; Silverstone and Hyman, 1982). Community-wide education and training programs for families have been undertaken with success in some localities, including the demonstration projects cited above. Support groups for family members caring for Alzheimer's victims have proliferated, mostly supported by local chapters of the Alzheimer's Disease and Related Disorders Association. These and other family groups appear to be successful in offering emotional support and education to families (Cohen and Eisdorfer, 1982).

Unresolved Issues

These developments in services to families of the elderly, few in number and often short-lived, come forth amid a great deal of public and private confusion about the help that should be given to families. This state of affairs is compounded by a lack of longitudinal data about family support and future uncertainties. Opinions about the role of the family seem divided into two camps: one based on the assumption that a strong informal structure is in place and can be tapped further in support of the frail elderly and the other based on the assumption that the informal system, particularly the overburdened family, has been stretched as far as possible and will only weaken in the future (Silverstone, 1983).

The first viewpoint is reflected in efforts to revive relative responsibility laws and to create financial incentives that will encourage family caregiving. It is further argued that an increase in formal services will supplant family efforts. The second viewpoint is reflected in the opinion that nothing further can be expected from the family in the way of support to frail elders now and especially in the future. It is argued that the only course of action is to substantially increase the funding of nursing-home beds and community-based services to serve elders and offer respite to families.

Each of these concerns undoubtedly has some basis in reality, for research findings do suggest a variety of normative family-support patterns. The issues are complex and the policy dilemmas formidable. Study and deliberation are required before irrevocable decisions are made. In the meantime, planners and service providers must respond to current requests for service, and their pragmatic questions, reflecting in part these policy dilemmas, call for tentative answers:

1. What is the appropriate role of the family in regard to its frail elders? What if anything should be expected of families?
2. What is the appropriate role of formal service providers? Will services provided directly to families undermine family support?
3. Given the diversity of family patterns and proclivities of elders, how does the practitioner assess the situation and plan services?
4. Are families capable of performing their tasks more effectively? If so, is outside help appropriate or will it be disruptive?
5. Can and should direct help to families be extended beyond occasional respite services, support groups, and educational efforts? Will this only open the door for more formal services?

A SYSTEMS FRAMEWORK FOR SERVICES TO FAMILIES OF THE ELDERLY

Thus far, we have reviewed the extent and quality of family caregiving to the frail elderly, the burden and stresses involved, and the dilemmas to be resolved and questions answered if services to families are to be developed in a judicious and responsive manner. Called for is a theoretical framework for addressing these issues and questions, rooted in the knowledge generated by gerontological, sociological, and family-systems research and practice in the past several decades. The confluence of these major streams of behavioral-science inquiry offers a rich base upon which to develop services to families of the frail elderly. Given the accepted values of client self-determination and the enhancement of elder and family autonomy, a theoretical framework can be advanced.

Gerontological reserach has established not only the extensiveness and richness of intergenerational relations but has broadened sociological theory as well. The modified extended family took its rightful place alongside the nuclear unit as an important social system (Litwak, 1965; Shanas, 1979a, 1979b; Sussman, 1976). Thus as a system in its own right the modified extended family is regarded as a discrete unit with identifiable, if changing, boundaries yet as an integral part of the larger social structure. Change in any part of the system reverberates on all members of the extended family, which seeks in turn to maintain system equilibrium (Von Bertalanffy, 1966).

From this starting point, the extended-family system with a frail elder must be viewed from two perspectives: first, a look outward at its role and responsibilities in relation to the larger social system, in particular formal services; and second, a view inward to its style of system maintenance and functioning. The consideration of each of these levels and the interplay between them help define our services.

Interface Between the Family and the Formal System

The reliance of frail elders on both the formal system, particularly nursing homes, and on closely knit family units has added to the confusion about the appropriate role of family and formal-service providers. In identifying the primary-group characteristics of the extended-family system, differentiating the tasks it carries out efficiently in contrast to those better carried out by bureaucracies, and underscoring the functions shared by each, Litwak and his associates have helped to unravel this puzzle (Dobrof and Litwak, 1977; Litwak and Szelenyi, 1969).

Because of its capacity for enduring face-to-face relationships, Litwak argues that the family as a primary group can best perform nonuniform tasks, including emotional nurturance, socialization, tension management, and the meeting of the practical needs of its members not requiring a high degree of skill or technology. Its small size, flexibility, and long-standing emotional investment further allow the family to respond appropriately and quickly to the idiosyncratic and unpredictable needs of its members and in situations where a number of contingencies exist. The bureaucracy—including formal services—because of its size, organization, expert resources, can respond more effectively to the uniform predictable needs of persons, to those situations requiring skill and technology, and where economies of large scale are possible.

The theory of shared functions advanced by Litwak suggests that there are numerous occasions when technical knowledge is not appropriate for action because it cannot be brought to bear in time to make a difference. "People with everyday knowledge who have immediate access to each other, who have wide-ranging commitments, and who are devoted to each other may be more effective than those with only technical knowledge" (Dobrof and Litwak, 1977, p.8).

Since primary groups and formal organizations are antithetical structures, the former predicated on noninstrumental affective relations and the latter on rational, hierarchical, and impersonal relations, it is further argued that an optimal distance must be maintained between them. The balance theory of coordination calls for linkages that ensure coordination but maintain sufficient distance to prevent conflict or co-optation (Litwak and Meyer, 1966).

For the frail elderly, both the primary group and the bureaucracy and their shared functions loom in importance. Far more dependent on the environment than in earlier life because of the social and physical depletions of advanced age, frail elders must turn more to their families as well as to formal services. If available, the family, with its unique capacities for emotional sustenance and meeting idiosyncratic and immediate personal needs, becomes indispensable. The complexities and mysteries of aging and impairment, however, require the expertise of the bureaucracy. The extensive use of medical services by the elderly supports this point. By differentiating the tasks best performed by each, the dilemmas facing the service provider can be addressed. Given an optimal distance, family and formal organization can coordinate their efforts without threatening the integrity of the other.

A Model of Service to the Families of the Frail Elderly

Dobrof and Litwak (1977) apply these concepts to the nursing-home setting and emphasize the sharing in the function of caring that should take place between family and staff. The ethical imperative governing intergenerational relations undergirds their formulations with the recommendation that institutions should welcome families as partners, taking into account the tensions in family relationships yet encouraging families to do what they can. Beyond this important consideration, families can perform a host of nonuniform tasks for residents. Citing the inevitable conflict between the needs of staff to achieve economies of scale and to utilize technical expertise and the residents' needs to have their affective, idiosyncratic, and other personal needs handled expeditiously, they stress the need for primary groups to help with the latter tasks and to serve as advocates in nontechnical areas. Linkages are thus required to involve kin in the life of the nursing home, but carefully determined to ensure effective coordination and to resolve the inevitable conflicts that arise between family and staff. Among the linkages they list are outreach workers, volunteer associations, training institutes for kin, and better parking facilities and visiting hours.

The application of the shared-function and balance-coordination theories to the care of elders living in the community setting has important implications for service delivery and planning. Needless to say, a very different set of variables comes into play. The focus of power and control shifts when services are provided in the elder's or family's home. Families and elders have far more say in terms of what tasks will be provided for them by the formal system, and not infrequently services are eschewed out of fear of an encroaching bureaucracy.

Furthermore, families must be organized to cope with the often complex tasks of caregiving and utilization of health and social services. A variety of organizational linkages is required to ensure optimal distance and coordination between the formal and informal long-term-care systems. This latter consideration is of great importance for planning and service-delivery strategies but beyond the scope of this chapter with its emphasis on direct interventions.

Even within the range of direct practice, the theories of shared function and balanced coordination are compelling and provide important underpinnings to our model of service. Referred to as the auxiliary-function model of social-work practice to frail elders and their families, it serves as a guide for determining the appropriate and shifting roles and tasks for the family and service providers and the most effective means of coordination between them (Silverstone and Burack-Weiss, 1983).

Our model of service emanates from the special needs of the frail elder for increased inputs from the environment and the distinctive function that must be carried out to meet these needs. The depletions and chronic impairments of advanced age create a set of emotional and practical needs that call for a relationship with a significant other whose role we have defined as auxiliary in nature: lending support for as long and only as long as needed. The tasks associated with the auxiliary role include noninstrumental ones such as emotional support, socialization, and instrumental efforts on behalf of the frail elder, including money management, coordination and supervision of services, and advocacy.

The family, if available, usually fills the auxiliary role. Its primary-group characteristics best equip it for these purposes. When there is no family or the family, for lack of expertise or resources, cannot totally fill the auxiliary role, then it becomes a shared one with the formal system. Examples of the latter situation would be professional counseling of a mentally impaired or depressed elder or complex case-management tasks, both requiring expertise. The auxiliary role may also be temporarily shared as the social worker directly helps the family organize itself in a more functional manner. The worker can be an important linkage between the formal and informal systems working to maintain the integrity and improve the autonomous fuctioning of the family but also bringing to bear the resources and knowledge of the formal system so critical to the care of the aged. These direct interventions will comprise the remainder of this chapter. A look inward and an understanding of the family as a system is first required, for this perspective will determine the nature of our interventive strategies.

The Functioning of the Elder Family System

For the family with a frail elder living in the community, organizational and problem-solving skills are required to perform the auxiliary role. Boundaries and roles may have to be altered, tasks defined, information gathered, and decisions made. The dynamics involved in the maintenance of the family system as changes occur must also be considered. These processes are not only affected by changes in the elder but can profoundly affect the family's behavior toward the elder as dependency increases. They may, in some situations, become the target for therapeutic change.

Attention was first drawn to these processes by family-systems theorists who, in trying to understand the etiology of childhood schizophrenia, delinquency, and other conditions, looked beyond explanations of individual pathology to the functioning of the family. Broadly, three different schools of thought evolved. Concerned with the family life of the inner-city ghetto, Minuchin (1967, 1974) focused on the structural issues of boundaries and tasks. He viewed the key to family functioning as the ability of the family to maintain clear boundaries between subsystems and to perform the roles designated by the subsystems. In families with excessively rigid boundaries, the therapeutic emphasis is on creating more flexibility and diversity in the family system.

A second cluster of interests centered on family-system maintenance. Patterns of family communication were seen as regulating tension among family members, thereby maintaining the equilibrium in dysfunctional families. The need to maintain equilibrum was seen as so intense that it could produce a schizophrenic member as a scapegoat through a communication process labeled the "double bind process" (Bateson et al., 1956). These theories expanded to encompass other issues in understanding how families maintain their balance (Satir, 1967) and how therapists can effectively alter this balance to create change (Haley, 1973).

Bowen (1978) developed a historical family-systems perspective, focusing on the transgenerational etiology of dysfunctional families. In his model, parental anxiety was transmitted across generational lines, "triangulating" the child between husband and wife in an effort to maintain a comfortable distance between the couple. Each family has its own level of tension or comfort with distance or "level of differentiation." Change comes through reconnecting family members to their families of origin, thus altering the tension level and enabling the client and his/her family to modify their current relationship.

The common themes underlying these approaches is that the family is engaged in two ongoing processes. The first is to perform the work necessary to ensure the well-being of all family members. These primary tasks include concrete efforts, such as working, cooking, and cleaning, and affective responses such as loving, caring, and providing support. The second process that taps family energies is the maintenance of a level of *system tension* necessary to provide a familiar and comfortable environment in which to perform the primary tasks. Equally important to the family's level of optimal tension, which can vary greatly, is the family's capacity to tolerate changes or variations in its tension level, an ability that determines the family's capacity to cope with new situations and to engage in new behavior.

Although these systems concepts claim to describe universal family functioning, most of the work of family-systems theorists and practitioners was directed toward the younger family with children. Exceptions include the work of Boszormenyi-Nagy and Spark (1973), who utilized the concept of a "family ledger" composed of a multigenerational system of debits and credits that can accumulate over generations and lead to a "chain of displaced retributions," in turn creating dysfunctional family functioning. This concept helps to explain the "injustice collecting" undertaken by families at the expense of their elders and the level of expectations that elders have for their families. An intervention approach would bring these debits to the family's awareness in a manner that allows the family to forgive and forget the past "crimes" of any member.

Another formulation of the issues of the family in later life was developed by Froma Walsh (Carter and Orfanidis, 1980). Utilizing a developmental perspective, Walsh discusses social tasks and transitions normally encountered during the later phase of family life, including the launching of the last child, retirement, widowhood, grandparenting, illness, and dependency. The success of the family in adjusting to these changes is in part dependent on the previous coping ability established by the family and in part by the "cross generational interplay of life cycle issues." In any family, the individual life tasks of the different members may or may not be in synchronization, affecting the capacity of family members to be available for each other. The author cites three major clinical issues for the therapist working with families in later life: first, that somatic complaints that elders often present may mask family stress; second, the need to consider relationships beyond the elder's household or the elder's own claim of "no family"; and third, the need to consider the elder when younger family members present themselves for treatment.

A Clinical Model for the Elder Family System

Integrating the concepts of family-systems theorists and those who have examined the developmental tasks facing the older family, Tonti (1983) has reformulated their contributions to address the unique features of the extended-family system with a frail member. Table 9-1 displays the key concepts and interventions relevant to the older family.

The older family differs from the younger family primarily in the life tasks that must be negotiated when frailty strikes. The direction of family activity shifts from expanding outward to drawing inward. Whereas autonomy and accomplishment are the hallmarks of family activity as the family grows through the early and middle years, the emphasis appropriately shifts as families pass through the middle to later years. The need for autonomy becomes mixed with a need for support as dependency inevitably grows in importance in the elder's life. The primary tasks of the family increase to include mourning the elder's losses, responding to the elder's increased emotional and concrete needs, and planning for caregiving.

Table 9-1. Key Concepts and Interventions Relative to the Older Family

Family System Concept	Aged System	Intervention
(1) Family boundary: Defines the membership of the "family" and marks the relationship between people inside the family.	Time and distance may change the constituency of the family. Nonfamily members may be included, while relatives who are not involved may be excluded.	(a) Extending the boundary —may need to include alienated family or include friends or neighbors in more involved roles with the elder. (b) Strengthening boundaries —creating space between people where overinvolvement has created problems of burnout, use of respite programs, day care, etc. (c) Clarifying boundaries—by setting up contracts and discussing obligations and commitments of family members to elder and vise versa.
(2) Tasks: The work the family needs to perform.	Dealing with losses, chronic illness, societal pressures.	(a) Identification (b) Provide information and education about aging tasks. (c) Help prioritize tasks. (d) Help identify blocks to task performance. (e) Restructure tasks as transactional events important for everyone.
(3) Tension level/homeostasis: The level of tension at which the family feels most comfortable and will work to maintain.	Tension may be increased due to fragility of the elder and the anxiety that the frailty creates in the family.	(a) Educating family about process they are involved in. (b) Involving others to relieve tension through support: (1) Home health aides (2) Social workers (c) Problem-solving around tension creating issues. (d) Supporting family to make clear choices as to how they wish to care for their elder.
(4) Reverberation: Anything that affects one member affects entire system.	Tendency to try to isolate elder from rest of family to reduce and control reverberation.	(a) Make tendency explicit. (b) Speak for elder if necessary. (c) Support reactions of others to elder's statements. (d) Open channels of communication.

(5) Equifinality: There are many ways to change a system.	The elder's losses and frailty often make change through the elder most difficult and least desirable.	(a) Help other family members to change to support elder. (b) Involve other systems. (c) Change other systems that maintain the elder's current functioning.
(6) Triangulation/scape-goating: Utilization of a person to avoid other family issues, usually highly emotional ones.	Increased propensity to focus on an elder in family.	(a) Refocus attacks by redefining issues from elder to family. (b) Help family member to share responsibilities. (c) Introduction of others, i.e., home health aides. (d) Impose restraints to prevent abuse.
(7) Double binds: Trapping of individuals in family through distortions of communications.	Powerful message can have severe effect on elder.	(a) Clarifying messages sent and received. (b) Reframing negative responses and resistance to positive actions. (c) Separating individuals in the family.

As the elder grows more dependent upon others and increasingly vulnerable to acute and chronic illness, the situation inevitably requires greater family involvement, thus shifting the tension level. The increase in family primary tasks, concern over the elder's condition, struggle over the elder's autonomy, the family need for control, and other factors will alter the tension level.

The altered tension level and the reverberations brought to the family system by the changes of late life will activate mechanisms of systems maintenance that will either benefit or detract from the well-being of family and elder. Not infrequently elders are scapegoated and emotionally isolated as the family struggles to cope with loss. Overinvolved children may triangulate an elder as a way of avoiding other personal issues in their lives. The inordinate energies that families devote to systems maintenance may detract from effective problem-solving and performing the auxiliary role for an elder.

The boundaries for older families are more difficult to identify than for younger ones. Geographical distance and differentiating life experiences can redefine "family" for elders. The definition of family may often need to include friends living in proximity to the elder and exclude blood relations who have not had contact with the elder for a long time. A useful guideline in establishing "who is in the family" is to determine who is affected by events in the life of the elder and who is touched by reverberations within the system considered part of the family. It may be necessary to go beyond the elder's own definitions, which may be too limiting or exclusive.

These theoretical perspectives—viewing the family system in terms of its auxiliary role vis-à-vis the frail elder in the larger system and looking inward at the family unit, its problem-solving capacities, and the dynamics involved in systems maintenance—offer a framework for the service provider and beginning answers to the questions raised earlier. The role of the family is determined by its primary-group characteristics: its capacity for face-to-face enduring affective relationships with a history of reciprocity and its flexible responsiveness to the idiosyncratic and auxiliary needs of its elders. Our values dictate that families are self-determining in terms of their role in relation to their frail elders, for these characteristics cannot be externally imposed but rather emanate from deep-rooted filial commitments and capacities for growth and change.

The role of the formal service provider is to share in or substitute for these primary-group tasks if they are not carried out by the family and to provide expert help where dictated either by the condition of the elder or by the internal problems of the family. Flexibly and appropriately provided, services provided by the formal system blend with the cultural and individual characteristics of families, maintaining an appropriate distance that utilizes sparingly the resources of the service provider and enhances the family's role and that of other informal supports. The following section offers a beginning application of these theoretical notions. This framework is broad enough, yet sufficiently specific to the needs of the older family, so that continuing and varied practice hypotheses can be generated and tested and, in turn, can enrich family-systems theory.

PRACTICE APPLICATIONS

Those service providers most likely to come face to face with families of the elderly are hospital social workers and discharge planners, case managers and other community workers providing home-based services, and nursing-home social workers. An increasing number of social workers in private practice are serving older families. Often these encounters are at times of crisis, but families are increasingly seeking help before a serious problem arises. Assessment and planning form the baseline for services, which can include clinical interventions aimed at altering the functioning of the family unit.

Assessment and Planning

Assessment and planning, the cornerstones of professional practice, are integral components of the problem-solving process undertaken by families. When change occurs, families ideally gather as much information as possible to identify the problem, its causes, and possible solutions. Internal resources for coping with the problem are measured and external resources garnered if necessary. In the best of circumstances, all family members affected are involved, communication lines are kept open, various options are considered, and a plan is arrived at that is acceptable to all. Families, including elders, at times need help with this process, particularly in light of the medical complexities and unknown factors associated with old age. Consultation with health-related disciplines is essential, but usually it is the social worker who helps the family put all the pieces together and arrive at a course of action.

The professionally bound study, assessment, and plan and concomitant family problem-solving efforts around the frailty of an elder have been spelled out elsewhere (Silverstone and Burack-Weiss, 1983, chap. 2; Tonti, 1983, chap. 10). Those family variables that need to be explicated and the range of planning options open to the service provider are given further consideration here. A systems approach to the older family described earlier offers a suitable framework. To be identified and evaluated are family boundaries, the tasks the family can perform, and the family's mechanisms for systems maintenance.

Family Boundaries

The network of kin relations (and in some cases nonblood relations) who can serve as potential resources for the elder requires examination. When the family itself seeks help, boundaries are more readily identifiable. When the elder seeks help he or she may minimize family involvement out of a concern for burdening the children or a wish to remain independent or because of alienation from the family. Careful exploration is in order. With a little encouragement and knowledge, and with the elder's consent, family helping ties may be reestablished. It is at this juncture that value issues come to the fore with self-determination of elder and family respected.

Mr. Peters, who lived alone in a hotel, had been referred by the manager because of the 83-year-old man's obvious deterioration. The worker sought to determine if there were any relatives, and after offering reassurance that none would be contacted without Mr. Peters's permission, learned of a niece who lived in a nearby city. At a later time when he felt more comfortable with the worker, Mr. Peters permitted her to contact the niece, who was relieved and pleased to learn of the whereabouts of her uncle.

For families already involved, constricted boundaries should also be questioned. Ready and able family members kept on the periphery of the events surrounding an elder's frailty may be willing to offer help.

Mrs. Gerard was frantic about the burden her mother's condition was placing upon her and her husband, and resentful that her siblings had refused to help out. Further exploration revealed that a brother and sister, at first willing to help, felt unable to cope with Mrs. Gerard's angry behavior and kept their distance.

Our knowledge and theory point to extensive kin interest and concern for elders. Boundaries must be tested and identified. In situations where the care of the primary caregiver seems all-encompassing, support from other kin might be mobilized to perform indirect tasks.

Affective and Instrumental Tasks

The capacity of the family to perform *affective* and *instrumental tasks*—to fill the auxiliary role—must be assessed. The increased needs of the elder along these dimensions present new challenges to the family system. Families ready and able to serve the elder in a variety of concrete tasks may have difficulty in communicating or may be unable to respond empathically to the elder's losses. By the same token, nurturing, empathic families may lack the skills to negotiate a complex service system or to perform nursing tasks. The subjectivity and protectiveness that stand them in good stead as loving kin may render them less effective in case management and technical tasks. Time-limited help and training may enhance the family's capabilities, or long-term sharing of the auxiliary role may be required.

The identification of the broadest possible range of informal supports and the tasks the family can and cannot perform outlines the *plan* of care for an elder. The gaps suggest the role of the formal service provider, who may share in the auxiliary role or seek other programs and service providers to do so.

After meeting with the Smith family—two daughters, their husbands, and children—it became clear that a variety of different tasks if not all could be performed by the family. With a better understanding of the needs of the 85-year-old mother who required help with shopping, housekeeping, and money management, these tasks were divided between the adults and teenagers. The elder herself felt capable of coordinating family efforts, but found both her daughters' anxiety so great that she could not confide in them. The worker arranged for a day program for the elder where she might be able to develop supportive friendships.

The whole range of long-term services to the frail elderly come into play in planning with the family—homecare, day programs, respite beds, and meals on wheels. These services indeed offer relief and support and can supplement on an ongoing basis the efforts of the family. Direct interventions by the social worker in these situations are time-limited, at least until the elder's condition changes. Assessment and planning with the family are often straightforward, with the needs of the elder and the available resources for performing auxiliary tasks identified, and family and elder linked to supplemental services. The assessment, however, may uncover problems in family functioning that interfere with planning and caregiving. They may simply be related to a lack of family resources, requiring that the auxiliary role be shared, or to intolerable levels of family tension and problems in systems maintenance. The aforementioned Smith family, taken a step further, is a case in point.

The daughters' anxiety over their mother's aging created such stress for them that they continued to isolate the mother emotionally although providing her with concrete services. Their need to maintain family equilibrium in this way seemed entrenched, and the worker decided to remain involved monitoring Mrs. Smith's participation in the day program and meeting occasionally with the whole family. At a later time the death of a son-in-law who had been ill with cancer led to a closer relationship with the mother, who was no longer scapegoated in a difficult family situation.

Clinical Interventions

Clinical interventions may be a required part of a service plan for the family if intolerable levels of family tension interfere with an elder's care or the performance of the auxiliary role. Day programs, in-home services, and rehabilitation programs that may be essential for the elder will also have to be weighed in terms of their implications for the family. A rehabilitation program for an elder, for example, requires family support and encouragement. If the risks involved create too much tension for the family system, the therapy will fail. Here direct intervention with the family is an important preliminary step, and ongoing counseling may be necessary.

Families may directly seek help with the anxiety and stress they are experiencing, but the need for help in these situations is often locked into a request for a concrete service. Usually help is sought at some point along a continuum reflecting the elder's condition and involving different living arrangements: at an early stage, when the family or elder becomes aware of the problems of frailty; at a middle stage, when the elder or spouse is incorporated more closely into the family; and at a late stage, when intensive care is provided or arranged for the declining elder. Each of the stages presents different challenges depending on the elder's living situation.

Clinical interventions may be required at these junctures — overlapping with the processes of assessment and planning — directed toward adjusting the level of family tension to meet the auxiliary needs of the frail elder and the family. Family group meetings are a preferred vehicle for such clinical interventions, including the elder if not too impaired. Family communication and problem-solving strategies are opened for review, and the worker can actively participate in realigning family interactions that lead to tension. Meetings with one family member, the elder alone, or with dyads are also appropriate in certain circumstances, particularly in those instances where a large family meeting reinforces dysfunctional patterns. These differential approaches will be discussed in conjunction with the challenges presented by different levels of frailty and family living situations.

Whether the elder's needs for support and help are minor or major—in the early or advanced stages of frailty—family members seeking help are usually responding to an intolerable level of tension that they cannot resolve alone. Not infrequently this difficulty is due to disagreements with the elder over the safety of living arrangements, the elder's wish to remain alone and relatively independent, or the amount of protection and care needed. The adjustment of family tension becomes a primary therapeutic tool for creating a better congruence between the needs of the elder and the needs of other members of the family.

Families that have difficulty with the level of tension generated by an elder who lives alone will either engage in denial of the elder's age and condition, responding by offering little help (a diffuse response), or become overinvolved, rushing into the elder's life and causing the elder to submit to the family's wishes or sometimes creating greater distance from the elder.

Mrs. Dangler was angry at her daughter and had refused to see her or talk to her for several months. The daughter, Mrs. Dixon, also felt confused and angry. She explained to the social worker that all she was trying to do was to protect her mother, who had become ill and needed some care. When her mother recovered, Mrs. Dixon continued to urge that a move from her apartment into a protective living situation was now really essential. This discussion escalated into an argument, with Mrs. Dangler finally refusing to talk to her daughter. The social worker arranged several meetings alone with the daughter, whose heightened anxiety appeared related to the mother's condition and recovery, which she did not understand. With clarification and sensitization to the mother's need for independent living, she felt better able, particularly with the worker's support, to "risk" her mother's living alone. The daughter was then able to reengage her mother at a less conflictual level.

When the elder's situation requires some active changes in his or her life and in the lives of family members, the family tension level can again shift. Usually, the struggle for control escalates. The elder's role in exacerbating family tension must also be examined. Frequent anxious phone calls from elder to children can reverberate throughout the family. A useful intervention that can help adjust the tension level is to help the family and elder devise a mutually acceptable prearranged schedule for visits and phone calls.

When the elder can no longer live alone without active intervention from family, friends, and social-service providers, the issue of the elder's autonomy becomes paramount, and boundaries of the family extend to encompass the life of the elder. Family boundaries may be flexible, allowing adult children to move in and assist the elder and then retreat when appropriate, tolerating the risks involved. In other situations clear decisions regarding the elder's ability to live independently may not be possible, or the family may not be able to tolerate the tension, particularly where geographical distance is involved. Meetings with the whole family, walking them step-by-step through an assessment of the living situation and the tasks to be performed, can reduce anxiety, help to avoid triangulation and scapegoating of the elder, and prepare the family for future changes.

Helping the Family with Frail Elder in Residence

The family's decision to have a parent or elder live with them is a normative pattern of family caregiving. This solution to the elder's loneliness, physical decline, or economic need can be fraught with problems, however. Systems-boundary issues are paramount. Nuclear families must create space for their parent. The elder must give up his or her own home and, thus, a part of his or her own life when moving into the children's home. Both parties will probably feel a combined sense of relief and anger: the relief resulting from a lowering of family tension as the security of the elder is assured and as certain problems are solved; the anger resulting from the loss of both privacy and a sense of personal control.

For the most part, elders and children decide to live together far in advance of marked dependency on the part of the elder. If the aging parent has always lived with a child, widowhood usually precipitates such a move. A strong relationship between an elder and a primary caregiver can sustain caregiving into stages of severe impairment. In some circumstances, an illness or sudden decline will precipitate such a decision. At whatever stage of frailty the elder joins the family residence, the overriding motivation of families is that "we have no alternative." Moving in is, therefore, an adjustment process for all concerned since the decision is usually considered to be predetermined and negative or ambivalent feelings are suppressed. Families and elders often feel trapped by circumstances, and expressions of doubt are seen as enhancing the feeling of entrapment.

The family's tasks, when the elder has entered the home, revolve around establishing routine and territoriality. Decisions need to be made about tasks and responsibilities that are appropriate to the elder's level of health. A flexible family can appreciate the elder's assistance in cooking (on occasion) and providing child care for an evening or weekend. Mutually, the family and elder will recognize each other's right to privacy and their own life. Less flexible families may need a more clearly spelled out schedule of responsibilities. Professional intervention may be required to enable effective communication of familial expectations.

When the elder is mildly impaired, issues of territoriality are uppermost. The failing competencies of the elder and the need to master familiar tasks can be misunderstood by family and viewed as competitve and "taking over." For the very impaired elder living in a child's home, different problems occur. During this stage the elder's care needs predominate. No longer can the elder care for himself or herself or contribute to the family in an active way, a situation requiring the family to divert resources to caregiving for many hours of the day. The tasks for the family at this stage are to reorganize family activities, particularly those of a primary caregiver, around the needs of the elder. Intervention aimed at increasing kin support for the primary caregiver is indicated. Without a primary, committed caregiver, the ability of the family to maintain a frail individual will be more limited. In these situations the social worker will share the auxiliary role with family members aiding in the coordinate services and thereby helping to maintain a tolerable level of tension.

Mr. James was 83 years old and was living with his granddaughter Janet, her husband Tom, and their small son. Mr. James's children had all died, and the only alternatives were for the granddaughter to take him in or for him to enter a nursing home. The granddaughter wanted to take care of her grandfather, but he needed a great deal of attention since he was bedridden and had a catheter. To make matters more difficult, the granddaughter had a part-time job. The social worker called into the situation quickly realized that there were no other available resources beyond the granddaughter and her family, although Mr. James did have a moderate income of his own that he preferred to use for in-home supportive services rather than go to a nursing home. The worker discussed a plan with the family of having a home-health aide come into the home for a few hours Monday through Friday to provide personal care under the supervision of a nurse. While the granddaughter felt this sufficiently enhanced her ability to provide care for her grandfather, her husband wanted reassurance from the worker that additional help and support would be available if the situation changed. The worker was able to allay his anxiety about being trapped by pointing out this situation.

In this instance, the social worker complemented the capacity of the family to care within a framework based on open communication between the elder, the agency, and the family. The possibility of the elder being scapegoated or emotionally isolated was also prevented.

Helping the Family with the Nursing-Home Decision

The decision to place an elder in a nursing home is a time of crisis for most families regardless of how they view such a course of action. Family tension is usually heightened by the misgivings of the family, and if it becomes intolerable is not infrequently acted out at a later time. Family group interventions are invaluable at such a time, encouraging a problem-solving approach whereby all options can be weighed and the resources of the family and wishes of the elder considered. Full participation of all involved brings the family more closely together at a time when it feels its boundaries are dissolving.

Social-work attention is also needed in the case of those families who are precipitous about nursing-home placement or where the refusal of the family to consider placement is detrimental to the elder or family. Premature placement is often the result of the family's inability to risk the elder's continuing residence in the community. What may be an acceptable level of tension for some families is intolerable for others because of their fear that something will happen to the elder. In order to lower the tension level, these families have to feel in control. They perceive nursing-home placement as a means of providing this control. In this case, as in many situations, the family's tension may increase the likelihood of premature placement. In response to the tension level, the elder may experience concern about angering or being a burden to the family. Unexpressed, these fears may also contribute to an inappropriate decision.

A much more difficult dilemma for social workers is working with a family that refuses to consider or act upon placement of an elder since much value is placed on preventing institutionalization. This dilemma notwithstanding, there are valid and compelling situations in which placement in a nursing home is the treatment of choice. Most frequently, these situations occur when elders' needs can no longer be met at home because of the skilled treatment or the amount of care required or when there is family abuse. When the family does not move toward placement, social-work intervention may be necessary.

Often involved in these circumstances is an "enmeshed family," a dyadic relationship in which a husband and wife, or daughter and mother, have built their lives around one another to such an extent that the thought of living alone is intolerable. In these cases, the care providers will sacrifice themselves or the elder to maintain the union.

Mable Johnson, age 81, widowed for twenty-five years, lived with her daughter Irene, 55. The mother and daughter had always lived together since Irene had never married and were an angry, inseparable pair. They rarely went out, and their only entertainment was their constant disagreements. Mrs. Johnson was suffering from several disabling chronic illnesses as well as periods of mental confusion. When a hospital social worker referred Mrs. Johnson to an agency for homecare services, the two agreed, but only with the clear understanding that Mrs. Johnson was not going into a nursing home. The living conditions, the elder's physical condition, and the health and life of the daughter suggested that Mrs. Johnson would be better off in a nursing home, but both Mrs. Johnson and her daughter refused to consider the option and the social worker accepted their decision.

This type of situation can, of course, change at any moment. The caregiving daughter can become ill or the elder deteriorate to the point where the daughter is no longer able to deny the illness. The social worker, understanding that the family balance is tenuous, should take a position of wait and see with the family.

Another reason for resistance to placement by a family is based on a financial rather than emotional dependency. In these situations, the elder is kept at home because his or her money, whether large amounts from savings or a pension or a small Social Security check, is deemed more important to the family than is the health of the elder. If abuse is involved, legal action may be required.

A family that can make a clear, appropriate placement decision, with the elder's involvement if possible, will suffer less guilt and have more energy available for the elder after admission. They will, in essence, extend family boundaries into the nursing home. The feelings that this decision can arouse in families can also erect a barrier between elder and family. If feelings are too strong and the family cannot live with its decision, family members may inadvertently isolate the elder by not visiting, or they may project their feelings onto the nursing home staff. The elder may contribute to this destructive process by fanning the negative feelings of the family or by acting out in the nursing home.

Kirschner (1982) identifies the challenge to the social worker in the nursing home as one of facilitating a shift away from interactions within the family to transactions between the family and the nursing home. The triangulation among elder, family, and institution can be avoided by programs that involve the social worker early in the placement and adjustment process.

Helping the Family with Emotional/Behavioral Problems in the Elder

Families will often seek help with emotional and behavioral problems of elders. Regardless of the degree of the elder's organic impairment, certain behaviors are understood within the context of the family system. Frequently exhibited emotional and behavioral problems of elders can be redefined as family-systems issues and can then be treated as such. This section will examine some specific emotional and behavioral problems that occur in the aged and appropriate family-systems interventions.

Hoarding, Collection, Paranoid-like Behavior

For elders who are experiencing losses in their social lives as well as in their functioning, there is a very clear need to reestablish a sense of control and mastery over the environment. These elders have few options and few areas in their own lives that they can control. Collecting and hoarding becomes, for them, a substitute control mechanism for mastery of their social lives. They will collect anything and everything and, in so doing, will often produce health and safety hazards for themselves and their families. Elders who resort to this type of behavior may also demonstrate paranoid-like feelings about their collections. The paranoid symptoms can be interpreted as the failure of this hoarding behavior to effectively maintain a sense of control. Unable to tolerate the helpless feelings brought about by their losses, the elders project them onto others.

A secondary gain from hoarding is that it focuses the family's attention on the elder. This shift, however, also creates tension, and the resulting triangulation can further isolate the elder. The family will often spend considerable time and energy trying to convince an elder of the inappropriateness of her or his behavior and feelings. Families seem especially drawn to the upsetting emotions of their elder, possibly because they feel their rational explanations should be able to unweave the paranoid web that the elder has woven. How many families have organized efforts to clean up apartment and house only to be met with an enraged elder or to find two weeks later that the elder had successfully recreated the messy, cluttered environment? The family's attempts at logic and restoration often lead to frustration with the elder and increased tension. The family places the elder in a double bind by telling him or her that they care but do not give the elder what he or she really wants: the freedom to make his or her own choices.

To successfully intervene in such a system, a social worker must recognize the paranoid and hoarding behavior as an authentic attempt on the part of the elder to regain a sense of control in his or her social environment. In a family system where members tend to distance themselves from one another, the elder might go to considerable lengths to involve the family in a way that will produce a sense of control. Armed with this insight, the social worker must establish a pattern of family contacts and interventions that will move the family in the direction of empathic interchanges and away from ones concerned with control.

Mrs. Jenkins, age 73, had been complaining to her four children that people were breaking into her apartment and stealing things. Mrs. Jenkins had a history of collecting and hoarding anything she could lay her hands on, and the family had just recently moved her from her own home into a lovely apartment. They feared that the collecting and paranoid behavior were beginning again and that they would soon be back where they started. At a family group session, the worker assessed the family as concerned but unwilling to deal with the issues Mrs. Jenkins was raising, except on a practical and logical level. The worker reinterpreted Mrs. Jenkins's statements of being robbed as expressions of loss. The family tone changed, and the children were able to deal directly with their relationships with their mother and with each other. The tasks assigned at the end of the session were for the children to call their mother on a specific schedule and for Mrs. Jenkins to become involved in group activities within the building. This was the beginning of a series of family sessions, all with the theme of empathizing and meeting needs. Once the sessions began, Mrs. Jenkins's suspiciousness diminished as did her hoarding behavior. What did come to the fore was much more direct anger at her family, which was then handled in the sessions.

This example illustrates the value of understanding the paranoid, hoarding complex in terms of its family-maintenance function. Once the family can be persuaded to cease the fighting that encourages the behavior, they can be helped to reengage the elder in dealing with more authentic emotional issues.

Resistance in the Elder

The need for control and security by the elder can produce suspiciousness and other behaviors that appear irrational and even destructive to the elder. While these behaviors can be understood as an elder's attempt to exercise control over his or her social and physical environment, they are often viewed by family members, friends, or professionals as resistance, and they usually produce a great deal of anger and frustration in the care provider and a great deal of pain and isolation in the elder. Such behaviors include refusal to follow procedures (not taking prescribed medications), engaging in self-destructive behavior (drinking, smoking), or refusing to move to a better or different environment. Whatever the form of "resistance," it has the following traits: it usually keeps the elder involved in familiar routines or surroundings; it involves others who wish to change the routine or the environment; and it involves a situation where the elder has sufficient power to remain in control. As has been discussed, the elder who is experiencing losses and feels insecure will often value that which is familiar. The conflict begins when the familiar or known is regarded as less beneficial or even destructive by caring others. The struggle will have great meaning for the elder if it is one in which he or she can exercise power, usually by doing nothing or by stubbornly resisting change.

A family may become upset, irate, and disturbed by a mother who refuses to leave her "unsatisfactory" (in the family's eyes) housing, give up her pets, or take her pills. The social worker's task is to understand the meaning this resistance has for the elder and the family and to intervene to transform the family's battle against the resistance of the elder into an alliance with the elder. This alliance needs to be built in such a way as to provide the elder with a sense of control over the situation and can be accomplished through clarifying the available options and the consequences for both the elder and the family. If the worker can help the family to support the right of the elder to make difficult, even destructive choices, then the elder will no longer need to feel a sense of control over the family or the professional and can look at the choices more appropriately.

Mrs. Barry, age 82, had taken to her bed, against the orders of her doctor and the wishes of her daughter, Madeline. The more the doctor or her daughter pleaded or demanded that Mrs. Barry get out of bed and walk around, the more she resisted. It was clear to the worker that Mrs. Barry was not depressed and that she had plenty of available energy. This became evident when her daughter tried, unsuccessfully, to physically pull her out of bed. It was after this episode that the social worker was contacted. Mrs. Barry quickly sized up the worker as another opponent to be defeated and, as the joint session with the elder and her daughter began, announced that she wouldn't be moved. The worker stated that she didn't blame Mrs. Barry for not wanting to get out of bed and praised her tenacity. The worker then discussed with the daughter her fears of her mother giving up and wasting away. The daughter explained that her brother had given her orders to get mom up, which also added to her frustration. She felt trapped between her mother and her brother. The worker suggested that she really could do nothing if her mother wanted to stay in bed and that she should have her brother call her mother so that the two of them could deal with each other directly. The worker then helped the daughter see, with the mother's assistance, that mom had the right to stay in bed if she wanted. Once the daughter "gave up" and the worker clearly aligned herself with the elder, Mrs. Barry began to discuss the ramifications "if" she decided to get out of bed.

The worker, by joining with the elder in her resistance, was able to relieve the daughter of her overly developed sense of responsibility and her need to control. In this way the worker was able to help the mother lower her guard and make new choices. In addition, the worker was able to break up the triangulation of the daughter by the son and mother that was also preventing this family from making constructive decisions. After several sessions the family made considerable progress in allowing both mother and daughter more freedom.

The Alcoholic Elder

Alcoholism that is identified by the family as a problem does not disappear with advance age. Those alcoholics who live into their 60s and 70s present unique and different problems for their families and for those responsible for working with them. It is important to understand that the family dynamics of alcoholism are such that the aged individual who drinks is supported in his or her drinking by loved ones and, in many cases, by agencies and institutions that provide care for the individual. Family members may support the drinking by purchasing alcohol for the elder if he or she cannot get to a store. Tacit approval of the problem can also be seen in the resignation and acceptance of the drinking as a long-standing pattern that renders the caregivers helpless. While the drinking is a problem for the family, it is less painful than dealing with intense interpersonal issues. The alcoholic's behavior is reinforced by his or her successful manipulation of family and professionals. This manipulative skill is often very difficult for anyone, including social workers, to resist. It is because of this skill and the unwitting cooperation of friends, family, and professional that the elderly alcoholic system becomes a very difficult one in which to effect change.

In order to create change in such systems, the worker must intervene with all involved, including other professionals to eliminate the support for the drinking. The family must be helped to see how their actions actually promote the drinking. Contracts outlining family tasks that can aid the elder in changing this self-destructive behavior are helpful. With these elements in place, the worker and family can confront the elder directly and clarify the available options, which may include an alcoholism treatment program, hospitalization, or nursing-home placement, depending on the health needs of the elder. The elder will resist these efforts by pleading and attempting to manipulate not only the family but the worker and other elements of the system. The success of the intervention will depend on the worker's ability to maintain system cohesion in support of the elder's change.

By understanding the family and other system roles in alcoholism, the social worker can effect change. Sometimes the change will focus on the family and will not initially or directly affect the drinking. Such support to the family needs to be maintained so they remain committed to their new role with the elder.

There are other situations in which elders, because of physical decline, lack of opportunity to obtain alcohol, or personal growth, suddenly and spontaneously stop drinking. These individuals, though free from the current physical effects of alcohol, maintain the manipulative and disruptive patterns of behavior that evolved during a lifetime of drinking. With such individuals the family must be supported to allow the elder to gain access to the family. The elder in turn must be taught to interact with family members through means other than deception and manipulation.

Mr. Torres had been drinking all of his adult life. At age 67, bedridden and sick, he stopped even trying to get alcohol. He needed care and angrily called his children, whom he had not seen for years, to come and help him. The result was that they refused to even visit their father. The social worker became involved and suggested a meeting with the two brothers and one sister. During the meeting, a great deal of anger toward Mr. Torres came to the fore. His crimes against their deceased mother and themselves were stated over and over again. When the family cooled down, the worker wondered if any of them could risk becoming reinvolved with their father. The daughter felt that since she had struggled successfully with her own husband's drinking problems she could be available to her father on a limited basis, but she added, "He cannot live with me." The family then softened and discussed the safeguards they would need to recreate relationships with their father. Slowly, with the worker actively helping Mr. Torres to change his behavior and communications with his family, he was able to rejoin them.

Helping Families with Mentally Impaired Elders

Of all the frail elder's conditions that trouble the family, none is more frightening and confusing than mental impairment and the confusion, loss of memory, or bizarre behavior that accompanies it. A painful emotional issue for the family is the powerful sense of loss they feel when the elder they have known does not know them. In helping the families of elders where progressive mental impairment has been established by definitive diagnosis, the worker can intervene on several levels. Nursing-home placement, day programs, family support, and training groups are but a few courses of action.

Clinical interventions with the family may also be important and would focus on reconnecting the elder to the family regardless of how profound the impairment, helping to mitigate the sense of loss for both elder and fmaily, and reducing their level of anxiety. The use of nonverbal communications can be particularly effective, and the worker can serve as a model for the family (Bartol, 1979).

Mrs. Towers, age 92, was living with her sister. She had almost no long- or short-term memory and was confused as to time, place, and person. The family meeting was being held to discuss placement plans for Mrs. Towers. Present were Mrs. Towers's sister and her only son and his wife. After a brief initial discussion of Mrs. Towers's condition and the need for placement, the worker took Mrs. Towers's hands and gently tried to make contact with her. He was partially and briefly successful in doing so and, when he turned to face the family, found everyone in tears. They discussed the fact that they had not thought to try to reach Mrs. Towers since the diagnosis was so pessimistic. The worker discussed how Mrs. Towers was, and would continue to be, a family member and would have an effect on them as they would on her. This seemed to reduce some of the anxiety and guilt that the family was feeling about placing Mrs. Towers, for they now felt they could maintain some contact with her.

CONCLUDING REMARKS

Our chapter has offered a systems model of services to the families of the frail elderly that addresses the dilemmas and issues facing service providers at this time of demographic and social change. It is predicated first on linkages between the formal and informal support systems wherein appropriate tasks are performed and shared by each in response to the changing and phase-specific auxiliary needs of the elder; and, second, on the systems-maintenance dynamics of families that can enhance or detract from their performance of all or part of the auxiliary role. This model of social work services to families is often time-limited, focusing on flexible linkages that support the autonomy and self-determination of the family as well as the elder and a sharing of tasks only as long as is necessary. Families may function on their own, receive a modicum of concrete services, or become involved in respite or support programs for long-term relief. Changes in the family system—its boundaries, tasks, and maintenance mechanisms—brought about by clinical interventions can strengthen both the family and its support of the frail elder.

Direct practice with the families of the elderly present unique challenges to the service provider. There are the exhilaration and difficulties endemic to pioneering efforts with new client populations. There is also the necessity for professional self-discipline in an area of human behavior where the social mores are uncertain. With no consensually agreed upon "right way" in which filial responsibility to an aging parent can be operationalized, and with various family patterns of caregiving, practitioners must be careful not to apply their own familial standards to those of their client.

Another caveat is in order. That families of elders can be helped is clear to us. That the benefits resulting from this help will relieve the formal service system remains to be seen. Many elders have no children. It is hypothesized that a greater investment of services to families in the earlier stages of frailty—education, training, assessment, planning, and clinical interventions—will strengthen the family for the period of long-term care. A fairer distribution of limited resources seems possible; what is certain is a better quality of life for the frail and impaired elderly clients and their families.

REFERENCES

Archbold, P. G. (1982). All-consuming activity: The family as care-giver. *Generations,* **7**(2), 12-13, 40.
Bartol, M. A. (1979). Nonverbal communication in patients with Alzheimer's disease. *Journal of Gerontological Nursing,* **5**(4), 21-31.
Bateson, G., Jackson, D. D., Haley, J. and Weakland, J. (1956). Toward a theory of schizophrenia. *Behavioral Science* **1**(4), 251-264.
Bengtson, V. L., and Treas, J. (1980). The changing family context of mental health and aging. In J. E. Birren and R. B. Sloane (Eds.), *Handbook of mental health and aging.* Englewood Cliffs, N.J.: Prentice-Hall.
Benjamin Rose Institute (1983). *Quarterly report of costs and services, January-March, 1983.* Cleveland: Benjamin Rose Institute.
Boszormenyi-Nagy, I., and Spark, G. M. (1973). *Invisible loyalties: Reciprocity in intergenerational family therapy.* Hagerstown, Md.: Harper & Row.

Bowen, M. (1978). *Family therapy in clinical practice.* New York: Aronson.
Brody, S. J., Poulshock, S. W., and Masciocchi, C. F. (1978). The family caring unit: A major consideration in the long-term support system. *Gerontologist,* **18**(6), 556-561.
Cantor, M. H. (1980). The informal support system: Its relevance in the lives of the elderly. In E. F. Borgatta and N. G. McCluskey (Eds.), *Aging and society: Current research and policy perspectives.* Beverly Hills: Sage.
Carter, E. A., and Orfanidis, M. M. (Eds.) (1980). *The family life cycle.* New York: Gardner Press.
Cohen, D., and Eisdorfer, C. (1982). *Family handbook on Alzheimer's disease.* New York: Health Advancement Services.
Cohen, S. Z., and Gans, B. M. (1978). *The other generation gap: The middle-aged and their aging parents.* Chicago: Association Press/Follett.
Dobrof, R., and Litwak, E. (1977). *Maintenance of family ties of long-term care patients: Theory and guide to practice.* Rockville, Md.: U.S. Department of Health, Education, and Welfare.
Fries, J. F., and Crapo, L. M. (1981). *Vitality and aging: Implications of the rectangular curve.* San Francisco: Freeman.
Gurland, B., et al. (1978). Personal time dependency in the elderly of New York City: Findings from the U.S.-U.K. cross-national geriatric community study. In Community Council of Greater New York, *Dependency in the elderly in New York City: Policy and service implications of the U.S.-U.K. cross-national geriatric community study.* New York: The Council.
Haley, J. (1973). *Uncommon therapy: The psychiatric technique of Milton H. Erickson.* New York: Norton.
Hoenig, J., and Hamilton, M. (1966). Elderly psychiatric patients and the burden on the household. *Psychiatria et Neurologia* **152**, 281-293.
Isaacs, B. (1971). Geriatric patients; Do their families care? *British Medical Journal,* **4**, 282-286.
Kastenbaum, R., and Candy, S. E. (1973). The 4% fallacy: A methodological and empirical critique of extended care facility population statistics. *International Journal of Aging and Human Development,* **4**(1), 15-21.
Kirschner, C. (1979). The aging family in crisis: A problem in living. *Social Casework,* **60**(4), 209-216.
Kirschner, C. (1982). Institutions and the family: Overcoming inevitable problems. *Generations* **7**(2), 10-11.
Lang, A. M., and Brody, E. M. (1983). Characteristics of middle-aged daughters and help to their elderly mothers. *Journal of Marriage and the Family,* **45**(1), 193-202.
Lawton, M. P., and Brody, E. M. (1969). Assessment of older people: Self-maintaining and instrumental activities of daily living. *Gerontologist* **9**(3), 179-186.
Litman, T. J. (1971). Health care and the family: A three-generational analysis. *Medical Care,* **9**(1), 67-81.
Litwak, E. (1965). Extended kin relations in an industrial democratic society. In E. Shanas and G. F. Streib (Eds.), *Social structure and the family: Generational relations.* Englewood Cliffs, N.J.: Prentice-Hall.
Litwak, E., and Meyer, H. J. (1966). A balance theory of coordination between bureaucratic organizations and community primary groups. *Administrative Science Quarterly,* **11**(1), 31-58.
Litwak, E., and Szelenyi, I. (1969). Primary group structures and their functions: Kin, neighbors, and friends. *American Sociological Review,* **34**(4), 465-481.
Mace, N. L., and Rabins, P. V. (1981). *The 36-hour day.* Baltimore: Johns Hopkins University Press.
Meltzer, J. W. (1982). *Respite care: An emerging family support service.* Washington: Center for the Study of Social Policy.
Minuchin, S. (1974). *Families and family therapy.* Cambridge: Harvard University Press.
Minuchin, S., et al. (1967). *Families of the slums; An exploration of their structure and treatment.* New York: Basic Books.
Noelker, L. S., Poulshock, S. W. (1982). The effects on families of caring for impaired elderly in residence. *Final report to the Administration of Aging.* Cleveland: Benjamin Rose Institute.
Rathbone-McCuan, E. (1980). Elderly victims of family violence and neglect. *Social Casework* **61**(5), 296-304.

Safford, F. (1980). A program for families of the mentally impaired elderly. *Gerontologist,* **20**(6), 656-660.

Sainsbury, P., and de Alcaron, J. G. (1970). The effects of community care on the family and the geriatric patient. *Journal of Geriatric Psychiatry* **4**(1), 23-41.

Sanford, J. R. (1975). Tolerance of debility in elderly dependents by supporters at home: Its significance for hospital practice. *British Medical Journal,* **3**, 471-473.

Satir, V. M. (1967). *Conjoint family therapy: A guide to theory and technique* (rev. ed.). Palo Alto, Calif.: Science and Behavior Books.

Shanas, E. (1979a). Social myth as hypothesis: The case of the family relations of old people. *Gerontologist* **19**(1), 3-9.

Shanas, E. (1979b). The family as a social support system in old age. *Gerontologist,* **19**(2), 169-174.

Shanas, E., et al. (1968). *Old people in three industrial societies.* New York: Atherton.

Silverstone, B. (1978). The family is here to stay. *Journal of Nursing Administration,* **8**(5), 47-51.

Silverstone, B. (1983). *Informal social support systems for the frail elderly.* Paper presented at the National Research Council/Institute of Medicine Committee on an Aging Society, National Academy of Sciences, Washington.

Silverstone, B., and Burack-Weiss, A. (1983). *Social work practice with the frail elderly and their families: The auxiliary function model.* Springfield, Ill.: Thomas.

Silverstone, B., and Hyman, H. K. (1982). *You and your aging parent.* New York: Pantheon.

Smith, K. F., and Bengtson, V. L. (1979). Positive consequences of institutionalization: Solidarity between elderly parents and their middle-aged children. *Gerontologist* **19**(5), 438-447.

Steinmetz, S. K. (1983). Dependency, stress and violence between middle-aged caregivers and their elderly parents. In J. I. Kosberg (Ed.), *Abuse and maltreatment of the elderly: Causes and interventions.* Boston: John Wright.

Sussman, M. B. (1976). The family life of old people. In R. H. Binstock and E. Shanas (Eds.), *Handbook of aging and the social sciences.* New York: Van Nostrand Reinhold.

Tonti, M. (1983). Working with families. In B. Silverstone and A. Burack-Weiss, *Social work practice with the frail elderly and their families: The auxiliary function model.* Springfield, Ill.: Thomas.

U.S. General Accounting Office. (1977a). *Home health—the need for a national policy to better provide for the elderly.* Report to the Congress by the Comptroller General of the United States. Washington: U.S. General Accounting Office.

U.S. General Accounting Office. (1977b). *The well-being of older people in Cleveland, Ohio.* Report to the Congress by the Comptroller General of the United States. Washington: U.S. General Accounting Office.

U.S. National Center for Health Statistics (1975). *Vital statistics of the United States: 1973 life tables.* Rockville, Md.: U.S. Department of Health, Education, and Welfare.

Von Bertalanffy, L. (1966). General systems theory and psychiatry. In S. Arieti (Ed.), *American handbook of psychiatry,* vol. 3. New York: Basic Books.

Zarit, S. H., Reever, K. E., and Bach-Peterson, J. (1980). Relatives of the impaired elderly: Correlates of feelings of burden. *Gerontologist,* **20**(6), 649-655.

Zimmer, A. H. (1983). Community care of the aged: The natural supports program. In G. Getzel and J. Mellor (Eds.), *Gerontological social work practice in long-term care.* New York: Haworth.

10

Counseling Widows and Elderly Women

Phyllis R. Silverman, Ph.D.

*Massachusetts General Hospital, Institute of Health Professions
Boston, Mass.*

In this paper I discuss the problems not only of newly widowed older women but of women who have been widowed for some time and who, as they get older, are affected anew by their single status. I suggest that the most effective helping modality to facilitate coping with their loss may be through mutual-help exchanges and organizations. I describe this help, why it is effective, and how professionals can involve themselves in programs of this sort.

Elderly women are the largest growing population in this country. They are for the most part poor. The median income for women over 65 is $4000. This declines as the women get older. According to the 1980 U.S. Census, two-thirds of women 75 and over are widowed and only 50 percent of women 65 and over are married. Contrary to popular conception, most women are widowed in their fifties and live another fifteen to twenty years alone. Most men who are widowed remarry; few women do, and those who do are likely to survive their second husband as well. Women are twice as likely to live alone as men, 35 percent compared to 14 percent (Rathbone-McCuan and Hashimi, 1982).

If we define elderly as over 65, we see this period as one of increasing risk for women to become poor and to live alone. Aging for them is not associated with increased security and tranquility but with profound change in a direction that may involve "learning to live without." Not only may they be widowed and face living alone for the first time, but they may retire from meaningful work or develop chronic illnesses that limit their mobility and independence. Loss and change are the hallmarks of the elderly. They may experience more transitional situations during their later years than ever before in their adult lives.

On the other hand, Peter Marris (1978-79) observed that the elderly may, in fact, be better able to manage change than younger people. Youths do not have the benefit of experience to aid them in meeting new situations. They may by nature, in spite of any facade to the contrary, be very conservative. In contrast, the elderly, who have managed over a lifetime, can see events in perspective and in context may have more resources to manage change and be better able to cope successfully. Block, Davidson, and Grambs (1981) suggest that women may be better equipped to deal with change than men, since they generally experience more change over their life cycle. This is not to suggest that older women will know what to do in every situation. In facing new and sometimes stressful situations, they seem to be more predisposed to learn how to cope. Age itself does not imply reluctance or inability to grow and change.

THE TRANSITION TO WIDOWHOOD

When a woman is widowed she faces two experiences. One relates to the intense feelings of grief and mourning that reflect the pain she feels as a result of her husband's death. The other relates to the need to redefine herself and her social space in view of the fact that the role of wife is no longer available to her. (Silverman and Cooperband, 1975). Traditionally, the period of bereavement is thought of in terms of the grief that follows the death of a loved one. For the widow this explains only part of what she experiences. The role of wife was usually central to the way she lived her life and the way she saw herself in relationship to the rest of the world. Her sense of self was reflected in her relationship to her husband; she was accustomed to sharing her life with him on an intimate daily basis, which was an important consideration in her friendship network as well. While she may still feel related to this man after he dies, it is no longer possible to relate to him and interact with him on a daily basis. In her older years, she may find herself with inadequate financial resources and in a situation where she has to build a new life for herself. Furthermore, although she may have experienced other losses, these losses may not serve her well as a model for coping with widowhood. In addition, this is the first generation of elderly to benefit from changes in patterns of morbidity. They may grow quite old before experiencing the death of a family member. We cannot assume that they have relevant experience, and, with the declining death rate, patterns of mourning are no longer clearly articulated.

Loss is always associated with change (Marris, 1974; Silverman, 1981), and bereavement can be characterized as a time of transition. This transition has three aspects to it: (1) a disequilibrating event or series of events occur; (2) a role change is involved; and (3) this change takes place over time. The work of the transition can be divided into three phases (Bowlby, 1961; Tyhurst, 1958). During *impact*, the first stage, the individual is numb or dazed. There is a strong sense of disbelief that the death has occurred regardless of the age of the widow. She continues to act in many ways as her husband's wife. The second stage, *recoil*, is characterized by a growing recognition of the reality of the change and by a growing frustration and tension that results from the widow's inability to continue to live as if no change has taken place. Finally, an *accommodation* is achieved when the individaul finds a new direction and in part assumes a new identity (Silverman, 1966, 1981). Any help offered would then have to facilitate change to help the widow move through the stages of transition so that she develops a new and meaningful way of living and a new sense of self in this changed context.

Since people do not recover from grief but are changed by it, we must recognize that to some extent there is no closure. New dilemmas associated with being a widow can develop at a later time. For example, for women who have been widowed for some time such a new problem may develop related to their now facing old age alone. If they worked, they may now have to retire. If they are now ill, their aloneness is a heavy burden. These new stresses may reawaken their grief and they may realize that they need to negotiate anew their current situation. Silverman (1983) found that women who never married did not mind their aloneness when they retired, while the widow found it very difficult. Lipman and Longinop (1982) found that always-single women did not perceive their isolation in terms of loneliness but as an extension of their lives when young. Difficulties arose for them when changes of old age made a single life less viable. The widow of some years not only suffers when the single life is no longer possible but, even if she has learned to give up the role of wife and has developed a new identity, she may face the crisis of her widowhood over again at this time.

Although elderly women today share the common problem of widowhood, with the loneliness, limited financial resources, and increasing frailty the longer they live, they are by no means a homogeneous population. They differ in their experiences of marriage, in the opportunities available to them throughout their life cycles, in the ways in which they manage their lives, and in the ways they look at themselves as women. For example, women over 80 today were not required to go to school, and the literacy rate is low in this population. Historically, none of the elderly women were raised to plan for their own retirements. In many instances, they were expected to be "ladies," to be cared for by their husbands or their families. Their lives revolved around the caretaking roles of wife, mother, or daughter. Their roles as money managers, as workers outside the home, was deprecated by themselves as well as by others, in spite of any real skills they may have had in these areas. While many worked outside the home, they did so to supplement family income, not to find personal satisfaction. Many of these women were first-generation immigrants who did not speak English at home.

They bridged two cultures, and their energies were spent in building an economically secure base for themselves and their children. While they were the first generation to have the vote, if they were married they had no standing before the law. Their identities were merged with those of their husbands. On the whole they tend to defer to the expert and the authority and to be very self-effacing. They do not always appreciate the wealth of experience they possess. Bart (1975) reminds us that some of these women were activists as well as competent professionals. All of these factors will affect how a woman copes. What is critical is that they all lost an important relationship that by its nature framed their identity and how they lived their lives. They will differ in the resources they have for rebuilding their lives and in the amount of help they need. Future generations of widows may differ in the skills they have for coping since their sense of self may be more adequate as a result of the women's movement, although the pain of grief and the need to change may be no less real.

What factors make a difference for the widowed in how they deal with the stress? The critical variables that relate to high morale and a sense of well-being for elderly widows are a stable social network, few life changes, and only time-related health deterioration (Heyman and Gianturco, 1973). Social network can mean different things to different people. Several studies have found that childless widows are more depressed than those with children. Studies of living arrangements do not support the idea that living with family is less isolating than living alone. Life in her children's home in a dependent role may be very isolating and demoralizing for the widow (Silverman and Cooperband 1975). Gore and Eckenrode (1981) note that the context of relationships makes an important difference in the degree of support experienced by the participants. Arling (1976) found that family members, especially children, did little to elevate morale, while friendship-neighboring was clearly related to less loneliness and worry and a feeling of usefulness and individual respect in the community. Widows who rejected the grandmother role and who reported frequent telephone calls or other daily conversations with friends did better. In this context the availability, by phone, of children was helpful.

Gubrium (1975) studied the role of siblings in the lives of older people. Many people grow closer as they age. For the never-married woman, relationships not only with siblings but with the siblings' children may be essential parts of her network. For the childless widow, nieces and nephews play equally critical roles in her extended network.

Recent studies of the psychology of women (Gilligan, 1982; Miller, 1976; Silverman, 1981) have begun to look at the meaning of attachments and affiliations to a woman's identity. A woman's identity seems to grow out of her involvement with others. Her sense of self is organized primarily around her ability to make and then maintain affiliations and relationships. This is especially true for older women. If relationships with others are indeed central to her sense

244 P. R. Silverman

of well-being, it may be essential for her to develop new relationships, to let go of the past and develop a new self, before she can fully mourn. These observations may account, in part, for why widows do better who are involved in reciprocating relationships and further support the value of mutual-help groups. In the latter, they find new opportunities for relationships that can serve to bridge the gap between the past and the future (Silverman, 1972, 1982a), and in this context to develop a new sense of self.

In summary, the ability to be involved in a meaningful, stable, intimate relationship based on common interests and life styles seems to make a difference in how older widows live their lives. However, limited financial resources and increasing infirmity can prevent them from acheiving these goals. Rathbone-McCuan and Hashimi (1982) note that one of the consequences of poverty for these older women is that they cannot afford the expenses of social involvement. Atchley (1975) found that among working-class women widowhood was associated with lower automobile use, lower social participation, and higher anxiety and loneliness. Many widows suffered from contrasting their past abundance with their current isolation. Abrahams and Patterson (1978-79) noted that those elderly who were able to be involved in mutual helping situations had improved mental-health status. Regardless of how infirm an individual might be, she needed to feel that she could reciprocate. This may account for the value of help from friends rather than from children. There need to be opportunities for mutuality and interdependence rather than the single-dimensional dependence that often occurs in professional relationships or with children who want to "take care of their parents." These findings support the value of mutual-help efforts as the vehicle for providing assistance at times of stress. The assistance has to link the women into a new friendship network where they can help and be helped, and where they may need to learn for the first time to define themselves in a role other than wife or mother.

CHARACTERISTICS OF MUTUAL HELP GROUPS

When people come together in some formal way to find or exchange solutions to common problems, they form mutual-help groups. Such groups are highly specialized "agencies" that generally focus on a single issue that their constituents have in common. They become organizations when the groups regularize their practices and formalize membership. In these voluntary organizations, members control the resources of the groups as well as plan and carry out programs. They develop their own governing mechanisms and often take on characteristics of what is known as a club. Each organization develops its own techniques for helping members. There are a wide range of services offered by mutual-help organizations: outreach, small discussion groups, one-on-one helping, newsletters, public education, and advocacy as well as social activites (Silverman, 1980).

Helpers in these programs are themselves members of the groups and are involved in reciprocal and mutual relationships with those they help; thus I use the term *mutual help* rather than *self-help*. People who are recipients of service can become helpers in turn. The help offered is based on people's experience coping with the problem rather than on the training or education the helper may have. The focus of help is on promoting well-being in situations where people are adapting to change. The groups help by providing information to their members about the transition they are living through, perspective on their feelings, and an understanding of the tasks they must complete to make an accommodation. The helpers are role models providing people with hope and direction for what they can accomplish. Helpers also legitimate feelings so that the newly widowed, for example, do not feel as if they are the only ones in the world with these feelings and therefore unique and perhaps damaged. People feel cared about and know that they can reciprocate. Those who aspire to become helpers in turn can do so. Gartner and Riessman (1977) speak of the "helper principle," the person in difficulty helped by helping others.

Differences Between the Two Systems

Mutual-help groups and professional organizations differ in many ways, although both share the common goal of promoting the well-being of their constituents and both occasionally have the same people as members and clients. Nonetheless, there are real differences in values and organizational structure between the two systems. Serious tensions develop when the professional does not understand these differences and how they can affect practice in each system (Silverman, 1982a).

One critical difference between the two organizations is in who qualifies to become a helper in each system. Help in an agency setting is offered only by someone who is trained and has credentials to qualify for licensing. Professionals stress the technical superiority of their knowledge and skill, thus justifying the exercise of professional authority with clients. Professionals feel that credentials are essential in order for people to be helpers to anyone experiencing serious personal difficulties. Mutual-help groups, in contrast, value experiential knowledge and do not require credentials for people to qualify as helpers except to demonstrate their capacity to cope well with their problems and to be able and willing to share their experience with others (Borkman, 1976), and as noted above the beneficiary is not restricted to that role but can and does become a helper in turn. To allow for this type of mobility in the organization, its structure has to be fluid. The organizational structure in professional organizations is generally bureaucratic; staff typically relate in a hierarchical order, with each position regulated by specific rights and duties, including that of client, patient, or beneficiary.

A further difference between the two systems is in their view of the nature of help. Mutual-help groups reward people for changing their behavior. The emphasis is on the ability to function effectively within the constraints of their problem. The nature of the help provided by mutual-help groups is sometimes judged by professionals to be superficial. The implication is that "real" help must involve restructuring of the personality. In addition, the professional often sees continued participation in the mutual-help groups as an indication of dependence rather than as a demonstration of new-found strength. Further, professionals traditionally value objectivity and detachment and are uncomfortable with the level of personal involvement exhibited by members of such groups. Mutual-help groups are really a separate helping system with its own values and helping style.

Why Mutual Help?

In considering the problems of the elderly, human-service providers often reserve for themselves the right to decide the nature of people's problems and the kind of help they need. They see troubled people as potential clients, focusing on their problems and deficits and looking for areas that can be remediated by counseling. The implication is that with proper treatment they can be cured. Borkman (1982) calls this approach to practice another form of "ageism." The elderly are stereotyped as frail and ineffectual; lifetimes of learning and experience are ignored. Patterson and Abrahams (1982) suggest that an ecological approach be taken to planning services for the elderly. They propose looking at the broad sweep of needs people have to see how they interact to cause difficulties. It would be impossible, for example, to think of counseling as the main service if there is not enough money for rent or food. Helping programs for elderly women need to consider their mobility and ability to engage in activities that would "repeople" their network.

Practitioners often see the response to stressors as a product of inadequate functioning, perhaps over a lifetime. They sometimes overlook the fact that the stress may be appropriate under the circumstances and intrinsic to the situation. Many times feelings and behavior are normal or expected in light of the difficulty with which the individual is dealing. For example, a transient depression may be appropriate in the bereaved. It may be important to learn to accept these feelings rather than to try to mediate them, to make them go away. For example, people are not cured of grief, they are changed by it, and this change may take up to two years to be accomplished. There is no recovery, there is an accommodation. The capacity to accommodate may have more to do with opportunities for social support and the nature of this support than with any prior functioning of the individual.

It is also important to consider what it means to ask for and accept help, that is, to be a beneficiary of service. Most older women who are struggling to maintain their independence do not readily assume the role of client, a role often associated with dependence and with public acknowledgment that they are deviant or defective. The current generation of elderly are not predisposed to bring their personal problems to mental-health professionals. They often accept their pain as appropriate and bear it alone. They sometimes suffer unnecessarily before they voluntarily ask for assistance. Often it is the children, who are uncomfortable with their mother's grief and want to hasten her "recovery," who make the referral.

Providers often talk of the elderly as too independent and unwilling to participate in service programs or, in contrast, too dependent. Many programs that require women to become clients in order to participate inadvertently foster dependency or turn people off. They provide little opportunity for women to plan for themselves and to decide what they can do for themselves and what other services they need. In housing for the elderly and in communal dining, for example, the elderly become passive, sometimes complaining recipients. When the opportunity is available for them to become involved they do so with imagination and energy. Professionals need to learn to appreciate the basic competency of most people, and they need to give up control of all the resources.

In contrast, in a mutual-help program, problems are not defined as illness or as consequences of some deficit in the individual's ability. Instead, they are seen as appropriate reactions that anyone suffering from that condition or in that type of situation would experience. Their feelings are legitimated and they are no longer alone with them.

Many women (Kuhn, 1977-78) are developing, at their own initiative, new guidelines for how to live as an older person in the late twentieth century. They are learning what supports they need to maintain viable lives and in so doing are participating in developing new social institutions to meet the needs they cannot meet by themselves or with each other. Mutual-help groups like the Gray Panthers represent such new institutions where participants maintain control over the resources and decide what help is appropriate. This is one reason why mutual-help groups are an effective helping modality for elderly women and why they are growing in number.

Another reason why mutual-help groups may be most helpful relates to their ability to respond to the needs women have during a period of transition. The goal of intervention during a transition would be to facilitate a woman's coping and to promote competency, thereby preventing the development of any disabling emotional problems. Such problems often follow inadequate or maladaptive coping causing the individual not to make the change associated with a transition (Silverman, 1982b). Often, if a woman is facing a situation for the first time, she may have little or no experience and few resources to use in developing a coping strategy. She may need to learn how to cope. Appropriate help would provide her with learning opportunities. What are the conditions under which such learning can take place? White (1974) identified the following needs for individuals in stress or transition; information about the problem; awareness of alternative ways of coping; and a supportive environment that enhances their sense of competence and ability to act on their own behalf.

Help, therefore, for people dealing with a transition may involve creating learning opportunities, with a curriculum developing an effective coping strategy. Bandura (1977), Gartner and Riessman (1977), Silverman (1970), and Leiberman and Videka (1983) found that learning is facilitated when the teachers are peers who have been through the experience. Ingersoll and Silverman (1978) found that the most important aspect of participating in a group-therapy program for the elderly, as reported by the participants, was the opportunity to interact and share with peers. These conditions are met in a mutual-help experience such as described above in a mutual-help organization where members plan and implement service programs for themselves and each other. All teaching is done by peers who are peers sometimes only because they have lived through the same problems (Silverman, 1980).

A study of affiliation patterns in the elderly found them most likely to participate in voluntary programs such as are sponsored by church groups or councils for aging (Cutler, 1976), which may be a consequence of their having control of the resources in these programs. They come not as clients or patients but as members. These church groups and other voluntary associations, like mutual-help groups, provide learning environments that are supportive and caring and in which the women have control.

Immediately after a death occurs the new widow may not be interested in affiliating with a mutual-help group. In the first stage of transition, she does not yet see herself as a widow. She needs to reach a point where she accepts this designation as appropriate to herself. This occurs in the recoil phase. Part of the tension in this period is caused by her awareness that she can no longer live as wife. At this point she is ready to meet another widow. However, the very awareness of the existence of an organization may be helpful to her in letting the numbness lift. This knowledge that there are other widows who have survived and are now involved in helping others provides some of the support she needs to move on (Silverman, 1981).

MUTUAL HELP PROGRAMS FOR THE ELDERLY

Mutual-help programs for the newly widowed are developing throughout the country. They are sponsored by the American Association of Retired Persons, councils on aging, YWCAs, churches and synagogues, mental health associations, hospices, and hospitals. Typically they are known as Widow-to-Widow Programs or Widowed Persons Service. THEOS (They Help Each Other Spiritually) is a religiously oriented organization with chapters around the country. Some are free-standing corporations. Mutual-help groups have been most successful when they focus on specific transitions rather than on an age group. Borkman (1982), in a survey of participation by the elderly in mutual-help groups, found that the elderly were integrated into groups for specific problems — alcoholism, diabetes, cancer, and so forth. Therefore, for the most part, programs for the widowed focus on the needs of the widowed of all ages. The elderly join because they have the specific problem of bereavement in common with the others, but their age is not the critical factor during the period of acute bereavement. Groups tend to become more age-specific as the widowed build friendship networks and adapt their lives to their single status. The older women no longer focus on work as a coping strategy, and their social interests tend to be different. Younger women may see their involvement in mutual-help programs as temporary, as part of the process of learning to cope and adapt. Older women seem to become involved in the group as an extended friendship network. Programs sponsored by councils on aging usually limit their services to people over 65 and use the extensive community programs for the elderly, such as those sponsored by the councils on aging, as resources to engage their members in more extended activities. For example, in Arlington, Massachusetts, the Widow-to-Widow Program encourages people to come to hot-lunch programs so they will not have to eat alone. When the widows are ready, the are encouraged to come to the drop-in center for senior citizens. The widowed helper serves as a link between other services and the newly widowed (Silverman and Cooperband, 1975).

Older widows who retire may join a widowed social group, where if they want to talk about their reawakened grief they will find ready listeners. They may now have time to become helpers in a mutual-help program and to share their experiences with the newly widowed, as one strategy for dealing with retirement.

These programs provide a range of services, as noted earlier (Silverman, 1980, 1981). Many groups have outreach components. Experienced members call on the newly widowed in their community to tell them about their program and to offer to visit if the widow would like. Names of the newly widowed are obtained from obituary columns or through funeral directors. The newly widowed report that they are too disorganized to know where to turn for help, and this offer of friendship and assistance from someone who has been there is very meaningful. Acceptance rates vary, depending on the length of time a program exists in a community, from 30 percent to 80 percent (Silverman, 1974, 1981; Silverman and Cooperband, 1975; Vachon et al., 1980). For those widows who will want a visit, as well as for members who are interested, education and informational meetings are held at least once a month. Other groups have small group-discussion meetings just for the newly widowed. They can arrange groups on specific topics of interest — for example, managing money, helping grown children with their grief, dating, and so forth. One-to-one contact is sometimes carried on over the phone over several months before people meet. Most groups have newsletters. Widow groups have become involved in advocacy or public education to a very limited extent. However, more and more of the members are appearing on panels at professional meetings, invited by professionals who are beginnning to appreciate experiential knowledge (Borkman, 1976) and the value of learning from the widowed.

THE ROLE OF THE PROFESSIONAL

Human-services professionals can interact with mutual-help groups and organizations for the widowed in at least four ways: (1) making referrals, (2) serving on advisory committees, (3) consulting with an existing group, and (4) helping to develop a new group (Silverman, 1978).

To make a referral, the worker simply needs to know the name of the group, the type of work it does, and how to link the client with the group (Gartner and Riessman, 1980). Before a worker should initiate other types of interaction, several factors need to be considered: (1) What kind of help does the group need? (2) Does the professional have the knowledge needed to solve the group's problem? (3) Are there differences between the group and the worker that would make their relationship problematic? The remainder of this chapter will focus on the professional role as consultant to a mutual-help program.

The Professional as Consultant

Consultation is a professional activity that in its simplest sense refers to a process by which an expert attempts to help a less knowledgeable consultee solve a problem (Rapoport, 1963). For the most part, when a social worker consults with another agency or organization, this organization has very similar values and similar organizational structure. Techniques for consultation have been developed between parallel organizations (Kadushin, 1977). There may be some difficulty in using this approach when dealing with fluid and changing organizations, as exemplified by mutual-help groups. A consultant may need to develop a different model for relating to this system.

Regardless of the setting and the model used, there are certain givens in every consultant-consultee interaction: (1) the consultant becomes involved by invitation, (2) the relationship between consultant and consultee is that of colleagues, (3) a consultant must appreciate that the client has a value system of his or her own by which his or her own work is judged and how to achieve its goals, (4) the consultant cannot tell the consultee how to integrate the additional information he or she provides into the consultee's system, (5) the consultant, as a temporary or transient member of the consultee's system, has no responsibility to see that his or her ideas are carried out, and can be dismissed at any time. Thus, the consultant gives information and advice, but is without power to act in the system.

There are at least two constituent groups in a mutual-help organization with whom a consultant may be asked to consult: the leadership and those members who are designated as helpers. However, since membership changes, it is not always possible to develop an ongoing relationship with a stable group. In addition, since the settings for most groups are very informal, it is often difficult to establish a clear delineation of roles. A consultant who regularly comes to meetings could be asked to help serve coffee, to share personal experiences and feelings about a subject under discussion, or to work with an ad-hoc committee. A consultant, therefore, must have a good deal of flexibility to match his or her activity with the uneven rhythm of the organization.

Types of Help That Groups Need

Most mutual-help organizations are small with limited memberships and are constantly struggling to maintain themselves. They seem to have similar problems for which they seek help. They ask for help in developing and maintaining leadership and in developing procedures for involving members in the work of the organization. They sometimes have difficulty in defining their goals and in implementing the range of helping efforts for which they see the need. They sometimes seek advice in how to reach out to new members and in publicizing their work. In order to get things done, they tend to let one or two people carry the burden of the organization. Some groups feel self-conscious when interacting with professionals, not appreciating the value of their own work. This is especially true for the current generation of elderly, who tend to defer to professionals as authorities. A small minority of elderly activists and people with education beyond high school may have more sense of their own worth and ability and have an awareness of how to collaborate with other systems. Most elderly, however, need to learn something about the professional system and the real limitations of professional knowledge. For many, their current volunteer activity may be their first experience in a community organization.

Knowledge Base

A clinical worker needs to consider the applicability of his knowledge base and related skills to work effectively with these organizations. Clinical skills for working with individuals or groups in therapeutic relationships are not necessarily helpful when dealing with organizational and programmatic issues. Rather than an understanding of personality theories, the worker needs an understanding of organizational theory, of the working of voluntary organizations and clubs drawing from the practice area of social group work, not group therapy (Alissi, 1980, Bernstein, 1976).

The professional who does not understand the value of experiential knowledge, who does not allow for the inadequacies of his professional knowledge, and who does not understand the fluidity of the organizational structure of mutual-help groups runs the risk of being at the very least ineffectual and, in the extreme, disruptive. If a worker finds that his or her own value system or knowledge base makes it difficult to accept those of the mutual-help organization asking for help, he or she should not accept such an assignment (Silverman, 1978).

What the Consultant Can Do

The consultant can do many things with a group. The primary function in all of these roles is to link a group in need with available resources. The consultant can do this by actually putting groups in touch with each other to work together on common problems. These groups are not always dealing with the same problem. One may have already solved a problem the other is now facing. They may not be aware of each other's need or expertise, and the professional becomes the linking agent. This type of linking is very useful for groups trying to solve organizational problems (Silverman, 1982a).

A second way the professional can function as consultant is to meet regularly with members of a group to help them develop additional skills. For example, in outreach programs, helpers need to learn to be comfortable visiting or calling someone they do not know. A professional consultant, especially for a first generation of helpers, can help plan an orientation program (Silverman, 1980). As part of this program he or she can guide the helpers in conceptualizing their own experience that will be useful to other widows. The professional can lead a discussion on creative listening, teach people about community resources, and help the group decide what to do if they visit someone with a major mental illness. In new Widow-to-Widow programs, the outreach group may ask a professional, in addition to the orientation, to consult with them at least once a month to review their outreach efforts. They need to develop experience in visiting, and the professional can help them see their successes and learn from their failures. Often, as some visitors gain experience, they can assume this role for their groups, with the professional being available by phone if they see a situation that may require additional help.

When programs develop group activities, the members may not be comfortable leading discussion groups. Professionals are often asked to teach members how to plan and implement programs and how to facilitate groups.

The problem for many professionals is to learn to step back and let members take over as they are ready. Good consultants in many ways should work themselves out of a job. They should leave the widowed with a new sense of competence and an appreciation of what they can do for themselves and others. They will be capable of developing new pools of helpers. The concept of provider and consumer may be set aside, as people work together to find ways of adapting effectively to change.

REFERENCES

Abrahams, R. B., and Patterson, R. D. (1978-79). Psychological distress among the community elderly: Prevalence, characteristics and implications for service. *International Journal of Aging and Human Development,* **9**(1), 1-18.

Alissi, A. S. (Ed.). (1980). *Perspectives on social group work practice: A book of readings.* New York: Free Press.

Arling, G. (1976). The elderly widow and her family, neighbors and friends. *Journal of Marriage and the Family,* **38**(3), 757-768.

Atchley, R. C. (1975). Dimensions of widowhood in later life. *Gerontologist,* **15**(2), 176-178.

Bandura, A. (1977). *Social learning theory.* Englewood Cliffs, N.J.: Prentice-Hall.

Bart, P. B. (1975). The emotional and social status of the older woman. In P. B. Bart et al., *No longer young: The older woman in America.* Ann Arbor: Institute of Gerontology, University of Michigan-Wayne State University.

Bernstein, S. (Ed.). (1976). *Explorations in group work: Essays in theory and practice.* Boston: Charles River Books.

Block, M. R., Davidson, J. L., and Grambs, J. D. (1981). *Women over forty: Visions and realities.* New York: Springer.

Borkman, T. (1976). Experiential knowledge: A new concept for the analysis of self-help groups. *Social Service Review,* **50**(3), 445-456.

Borkman, T. (1982). Where are older persons in mutual self-help groups? In A. Kolkner and P. Ahmed (Eds.), *Aging.* New York: Elsevier Biomedical.

Bowlby, J. (1961). Process of mourning. *International Journal of Psychoanalysis,* **42**, 329.

Cutler, S. J. (1976). Membership in different types of voluntary associations and psychological well-being. *Gerontologist,* **16**(4), 335-339.

Gartner, A. (1977). *Self help in the human services.* San Francisco: Jossey-Bass.

Gartner, A., and Riessman, F. (1977). *Help: A working guide to self-help groups.* New York: New Viewpoints.

Gilligan, C. (1982). *In a different voice: Psychological theory and women's development.* Cambridge: Harvard University Press.

Gore, S., and Eckenrode, J. (1981). Stressful events and social supports: The significance of context. In B. Gottlieb (Ed.), *Social networks and social support in community mental health.* Beverly Hills: Sage.

Gubrium, J. F. (1975). Being single in old age. *International Journal of Aging and Human Development,* **6**(1), 29-41.

Heyman, D. K., and Gianturco, D. T. (1973). Long-term adaptation by the elderly to bereavement. *Journal of Gerontology,* **28**(3), 359-362.

Ingersoll, B., and Silverman, A. (1978). Comparative group psychotherapy for the aged. *Gerontologist,* **18**(2), 201-206.

Kadushin, A. (1977). *Consultation in social work.* New York: Columbia University Press.

Kuhn, M. E. (1977-78). Learning by living. *International Journal of Aging and Human Development,* **8**(4), 359-365.

254   P. R. Silverman

Lieberman, M., and Videka, L. (1983). *Mutual help for the widowed.* Paper presented at the annual meeting of the American Orthopsychiatry Association, Boston.

Lipman, A., and Longinop, C. (1982). *The wife, the widow, and the old maid: Support network differentials of older women.* Paper presented at the 33rd Annual Scientific Meeting of the Gerontological Society of America, San Diego.

Marris, P. (1974). *Loss and change.* New York: Pantheon Books.

Marris, P. (1978-79). Conservatism, innovation and old age. *International Journal of Aging and Human Development,* **9**(2), 127-135.

Miller, J. B. (1976). *Toward a new psychology of women.* Boston: Beacon Press.

Patterson, R. D., and Abrahams, R. B. (1982). Providing services to the elderly. In H. C. Shulberg and M. Killilae (Eds.), *The modern practice of community mental health.* San Francisco: Jossey-Bass.

Rapoport, R. (1963). *Consultation in social work practice.* New York: National Association of Social Workers.

Rathbone-McCuan, E., and Hashimi, J. (1982). *Isolated elders: Health and social intervention.* Rockville, Md.: Aspen Systems.

Silverman, P. R. (1966). Services for the widowed during the period of bereavement. In National Conference on Social Welfare, *Social work practice.* New York: Columbia University Press.

Silverman, P. R. (1970). The widow as a caregiver in a program of preventive intervention with other widows. *Mental Hygiene,* **54**(4), 540-547.

Silverman, P. R. (1972). Widowhood and preventive intervention. *Family Coordinator,* **21**(1), 95-102.

Silverman, P. R. (1974). Anticipatory grief from the perspective of widowhood. In B. Schoenberg et al. (Eds.), *Anticipatory grief.* New York: Columbia University Press.

Silverman, P. R. (1978). *Mutual help groups: A guide for mental health workers.* Rockville, Md.: National Institute of Mental Health.

Silverman, P. R. (1980). *Mutual help groups: Organization and development.* Beverly Hills: Sage.

Silverman, P. R. (1981). *Helping women cope with grief.* Beverly Hills: Sage.

Silverman, P. R. (1982a). The mental health consultant as a linking agent. In D. Biegel and A. Naparstek (Eds.), *Community support systems and mental health.* New York: Springer.

Silverman, P. R. (1982b). Transitions and models of intervention. *Annals of the American Academy of Political and Social Science,* **464**, 174-187.

Silverman, P. R. (1983). *Self study, widows' society.* Unpublished report, Boston.

Silverman, P. R., and Cooperband, A. (1975). On widowhood: Mutual help and the elderly widow. *Journal of Geriatric Psychiatry,* **8**(1), 9-27.

Tyhurst, J. S. (1958). The role of transition states—including disasters—in mental illness. In *Symposium on preventive and social psychiatry.* Washington: Government Printing Office.

Vachon, M. L. S., et al. (1980). A controlled study of self-help intervention for widows. *American Journal of Psychiatry,* **137**(11), 1380-1384.

White, R. W. (1974). Strategies of adaptation: An attempt at systematic description. In G. V. Coelho, D. A. Hamburg, and J. E. Adams (Eds.), *Coping and adaptation.* New York: Basic Books.

11

Outpatient Mental-Health Services

Miriam Teplitz, C.S.W.
Peninsula Counseling Center, Woodmere, N.Y.

Outpatient mental-health services for the elderly are most effective when delivered by a specialized unit of a functioning community mental-health center (CMHC). Whether community based or hospital based, a CMHC has the personnel and other resources to undertake this task. Moreover, it will already have knowledge of a potential client population. Within the caseload of patients already in treatment in a CMHC (in marital, individual, family, or parent and child therapy), there will be evidence of a disturbed or distressed grandparent generation contributing to the pathology of the younger generation. This elderly generation is often neglected and untreated.

In a recent survey among twenty psychotherapists at the author's agency, the untreated problems of the grandparent generation included: paranoia, manic-depressive psychosis, schizophrenia, alcoholism, and blurring of generational boundaries; obsessive-compulsive, narcissistic, and borderline personality disorders; emotional deprivation; sociopathology; chronic depression; senile dementia; hypochondriasis; phobic, dependent personalities; drug abuse; accident proneness; marital dysfunction; learning disabilities; chronic mental illness due to organic brain dysfunction or stroke; and extremes of withdrawal and closeness. The most frequent pathology was severe depression. The dependency demands of the depressed elderly were experienced by family members as intolerable, which resulted in anger and often in neglect of the difficult aged person.

THE CLIENT POPULATION

The client population of an outpatient mental-health unit serving the elderly will comprise (1) independent elderly living in housing projects or attending senior centers; (2) institutionalized elderly in nursing homes, adult homes, and health-related facilities; (3) homebound elderly recently discharged from general hospitals; (4) elderly patients recently discharged from psychiatric hospitals; and (5) the functioning elderly scattered in the community.

The Elderly in Housing Projects and Senior Centers

The elderly found in these locations are usually ambulatory, maintaining independent life-styles, and open to socialization. The mental-health unit should assign a professional social worker to act as liaison between its service and the housing projects and senior centers to communicate information about the services available from the unit, to lead discussion groups (e.g., on later-life problems), to familiarize the elderly with mental-health issues, and simply to become a familiar person to the elderly in these locations by adhering to regularly scheduled on-site visits.

Mrs. A, widowed, aged 78, recently moved to the housing project. Her neighbor persuaded her to join the senior center. Mrs. A had enjoyed club activities throughout her life and viewed this new opportunity as a way to connect to her past pleasures. Initially she interacted with the senior center members. Then she began to withdraw, keeping to herself, sitting alone. The social worker from the community mental-health clinic, assigned to identify aged with mental-health needs, observed her withdrawal and made contact with her. Each week the social worker deepened the contact by communication, sharing lunch hours, expressing interest in Mrs. A's background. One day, Mrs. A was waiting for the social worker and requested a "private talk," during which she was able to share her depressed reaction to what she perceived as abandonment by her daughter, who did not invite her to live with her. Fearful of further abandonment, she internalized her anger. The social worker, whose trustworthiness Mrs. A had experienced in a benign setting, could now be utilized to help her with her depression. She began treatment at the CMHC.

The Elderly in Nursing Homes, Adult Homes, and Health-Related Facilities

The American Psychiatric Association has called attention to the fact that, although half of all nursing-home patients suffer from mental impairment, mental-health services are generally lacking. The association of a CMHC with a nursing home or other facility is complicated by accountability requirements connected with Medicaid and Medicare reimbursement. When this problem has been worked out with the appropriate governmental authority, it should be possible to establish a referral agreement with the management of the facility to provide psychiatric services when indicated, despite the fact that the residents are not living independently. Referrals would come from the facility's administration. Since these are medical health-care facilities, the referral would have to be initiated by the attending physician. When psychotropic medication is indicated, the outpatient unit's psychiatrist would supervise medication; when psychotherapy is indicated, the unit's social worker should be part of the team of specialists attending to the health-care needs of the institutionalized elderly.

Mr. B, aged 72, widowed, children out of state, had a stroke that left him unable to walk, confined to a wheelchair. He could no longer remain in his apartment and was placed in a health-related facility. His cognitive functioning and ability to communicate were intact. The aides were concerned because he had no appetite, was losing weight, stayed in his room, and cried whenever someone tried to talk to him. They alerted the physician, who was concerned about Mr. B's depressed state. The physician ordered a psychiatric evaluation from the CMHC psychiatrist. The psychiatrist interviewed Mr. B in his room and prescribed medication. He then referred Mr. B to the agency's social workers for ongoing treatment. This assignment began immediately on site in the health-related facility, enabling Mr. B to mourn the loss of his home and mobility.

The Elderly Discharged from General Hospitals

These elderly people are usually recuperating from heart problems, arthritis, broken limbs, ulcers or surgery and require skilled nursing care. The physician generally refers such cases to the Visiting Nurse Association, and the referral for clinical social worker would generally come from the nurse, who recognizes a depressed patient, a disorganized spouse, or a chaotic family unit. The social worker attending to a homebound patient works within the regulations of the Visiting Nurse Association.

Mrs. C, aged 82, was discharged back to her home after several weeks in the hospital with a broken hip. She was able to walk, haltingly, with a walker. Her husband, accustomed to being served by his wife, refused to recognize the extent of her limitations and placed unrealistic demands on her. Mrs. C tried to please but was unable to perform her daily activities as she had in the past. Mr. C responded with impatience. The Visiting Nurse Association had been ordered by Mrs. C's physician to provide physical and occupational therapy. A home health aide was assigned for three hours a day. Mr. C was uncooperative. Mrs. C developed pain, found it difficult to hold onto the small gains she had made in the hospital. She became depressed and stopped walking. The nurse referred her for psychiatric evaluation and counseling. The social worker met Mr. and Mrs. C and prepared them for the psychiatrist's visit. Mr. C was encouraged to be part of the process. The social worker was present when the psychiatrist came. This reduced the couple's anxiety. The psychiatrist prescribed antidepressants to Mrs. C, clarified to Mr. C her limitations, and recommended that the social worker see them conjointly on a weekly basis to work out a new plan for better functioning. Mrs. C began walking once more.

The Elderly Discharged from Psychiatric Hospitals

Service to this population requires planning in advance of discharge with hospital personnel, the patient and his family, and other community agencies (e.g., Meals on Wheels, church, home-health care, volunteer friendly visiting) that will be involved in the aftercare of the patient. This ensures the social worker's access to clinical information, liaison among the agencies involved, and continuity of care. Appropriate feedback to the hospital on the patient's progress in outpatient care is also advisable.

Mrs. D, aged 79, widowed, became delusional after her husband died. She boarded with one child after another. The family brought her to the special unit for the elderly at the CMHC. She was found to be severely depressed, requiring immediate hospitalization. The social worker arranged for her admission and helped the responsible adult child through the admission procedures. She spoke to the charge nurse and arranged a conference with the treating psychiatrist. They agreed that the plan to maintain contact with the patient and family during hospitalization would enhance treatment and provide an air of confidence in the continuity of care. As the patient recovered within the hospital setting, a plan was initiated for the patient to maintain residence with her oldest daughter, who had been persuading her to live with her initially. Aftercare involved supervision of the psychotropic medication that had stabilized Mrs. D in the hospital as well as individual psychotherapy to help her with her bereavement. When she was ready, group therapy to increase her socialization would be recommended.

The Functional Elderly Scattered in the Community

This group, with no visible problems, should nevertheless be informed of the availability of mental-health services through the CMHC. The group can be reached by informational flyers in supermarkets, libraries, and the offices of geriatric physicians. Health screenings and mental-health fairs will keep this group in touch with a community resource they can turn to at a time of need.

Mrs. E, aged 72, widowed, was very active in the community. She golfed and hiked extensively. Philanthropic activities filled her days. She did not consider herself a "senior citizen" and enjoyed the friendship of women who were younger. One day, as she returned from the supermarket, she was mugged in her driveway. She became fearful of going out alone and began to withdraw. Her friends suggested she seek help. She remembered seeing a brochure at the library. A friend delivered this to her. Mrs. E called the CMHC and asked for an appointment. The social worker spent several sessions in Mrs. E's home, helping her to become more trusting of the environment so she could again venture out to the clinic and then to her former community activities.

OPERATIONS

The Initial Contact

The initial contact with the agency is usually made by phone and most often by someone other than the potential client. When, however, the elderly person initiates the contact, the phone call should be delegated to a staff person sensitive to the hesitant elderly client, who may be reluctant to answer many questions over the phone or whose anxiety level may prevent concentration on the questions, resulting in increased anxiety and withdrawal. Phone contact should be kept to a minimum, the staff person requesting only a brief articulation of the problem and the caller's name, address, and phone number.

While most mental-health agencies have staff social workers who do the "intake" interview, this policy is not advisable with the elderly. In dealing with the agency, elderly people need a sense of continuity from the beginning. It is confusing and unproductive for them to tell their story to two different therapists. The clients' first contact should allow them to become familiar with the person who will be helping them, to present themselves with much of their defense structure shored up, and to report what they feel safe with. The clients need time to react to the social worker, to assess and clarify what treatment will be like. Developing relationships should not be interrupted.

For this reason, the social worker who responds to the initial request for help should be the one who will conduct the treatment. Data collection begins when this social worker makes the first phone contact with the potential client, the referring source, or some collateral contact. When the social worker's first contact is with the potential client, the social worker should:

1. Make few information demands on the potential client
2. Understand how much orientation around the first visit the client can tolerate
3. Be sensitive to the anxiety level of the client
4. Establish confidence in the applicant that he or she has chosen a nonthreatening approach to dealing with the present crisis

When the social worker's initial contact is with someone other than the client, it is important to ascertain:

1. The referring person's relationship to and knowledge of the client
2. The reason for the referral
3. What triggered the referral at this particular time
4. The reason the patient did not initiate contact himself
5. If the patient is aware of the referral
6. If the patient is prepared for the contact
7. If the referral source wants follow-up contact

When the patient's preparation for contact has not been addressed by the referring source, it is important to help the referring person prepare the patient for the initial interview. If the elderly person is resistant or confused about the role of the social worker, it may be advisable to set the first appointment with the family in order to clarify problematic issues in preparing the patient. This meeting will often reveal family dynamics, information about the mental status of the client, potential areas of difficulty, and the client's potential level of motivation.

When the patient has been appropriately prepared, the nature of the first interview should be clarified:

1. Will it be at the agency?
2. Will the patient be seen alone or with a family member?
3. Will the patient's home be more conducive to a lower level of stress?
4. Will a home-health aide be present?
5. What about privacy?

The well-functioning aged person who has safe transportation and someone to accompany him or her will usually be ready to come to the agency. The client sees it as "going to the doctor." The aged person, however, has little tolerance for added hurdles. When transportation becomes a hassle, or when the client has no relative to accompany him or her and is fearful of unfamiliar surroundings, a first appointment in the home may be advisable. It will provide the social worker with knowlege of the client in the client's familiar setting. It will also demonstrate the social worker's understanding of the special needs of the client, who is struggling to survive the onslaught of so many changes and who is fearful of his diminished competence.

The Assessment Interview

The initial assessment of the aged client may require several interviews, depending upon the complexity of the situation. It begins with the client's or collateral's definition of the problem that brought this aged person or family to the CMHC. Areas to be covered are:

1. What is the problem?
2. What motivated the client or collateral to request help at this particular time? This should be attended to in as much detail as possible. What happened today? Yesterday? Before the phone call? At the time of the phone call? What was the referral process?
3. What expectations does the client or collateral have in bringing the problem to the agency?
4. Orientation of the client or collateral about the agency role and the nature of the assessment period
5. Time for questions

Since the aged need more time in reporting, this initial assessment is conducted with appreciation of the client's slower pace, cognitive functioning, heightened anxiety, and lack of familiarity with the agency setting. The method will differ when the family is the client.

A full medical history and report of the aged client's present physical state is required at this time. Since every aged person presents some evidence of physical deterioration, this data will determine the precision of the clinical psychiatric diagnosis. The gathering of this data from the aged person or from the family enhances the development of the relationship between the client and the social worker. It starts with a familiar area, the client's physical condition. This encourages the aged person to see the social worker as a helping person, interested in all his or her complaints, asking questions for which the client has available answers. It affords an opportunity for the worker to observe the client's behavior, to detect anxiety, to be alerted to possible overmedication, to assess cognitive functioning, and to evaluate the client's support system with little resistance from the client, who views this kind of probing as appropriate and nonthreatening.

The source of accurate medical data is the elderly client's physician. During this initial assessment period, contact with the physician is made by phone or letter after the client has signed the required form for release of information. In presenting this form to be signed, the social worker can observe the client's level of stress. Does the client hesitate? Does the client feel stigmatized and unwilling to share this experience with the physician? Is there motor difficulty in the process of signing his or her name? Does the client understand what is being asked of him or her? If thought processes are slowed, how long and at what point does understanding and implementation occur? Who takes over for the confused client?

Mrs. F, aged 72, married, experienced increasing anxiety attacks during which she had spots before her eyes. She claimed her physician had checked her out and had suggested counseling because she had chronic high blood pressure. She "walked in" to the mental-health clinic and was given an immediate appointment. During the first interview she decribed her medical history in detail. As the interview progressed, her speech became slurred. Her answers were not relevant to the questions. The social worker became suspicious and handed her the medical form to sign. The client could not judge the distance between herself and the form. She lacked the coordination to sign her name. The worker calmly led the client back to her chair and called a staff psychiatrist to the interview room. The client was having a stroke and required immediate hospitalization.

In the collection of medical data, it is important to obtain complete, specific information about all the prescription drugs the client has taken in the recent past for chronic physical or mental disorders: the time, reason, event, and physician prescribing the medication. All over-the-counter drugs should also be noted. It helps if the client brings all these medications to the interview. Since drugs interact with each other and cause side effects that may account for some mood disorders, this information will influence the diagnosis. The collection of this information gives the social worker an opportunity to observe the client's reliability in taking medication and his need for supervision. It will also reveal possible areas of medication abuse or uncoordinated medical treatment.

Psychiatric Evaluation

The assessment interviews and the medical history provided by the client's physician may suggest the advisability of a psychiatric evaluation. A psychiatric evaluation is indicated when the client presents:

1. History of depression
2. Presence of clinical depression
3. History of suicidal thoughts, gestures, or suicide in the family
4. Presence of suicidal ideation
5. Severe anxiety attacks
6. Phobic disorders
7. Preoccupation with somatic distress
8. Disabling personality disorders
9. Hallucinations
10. Thought disorders
11. Disorientation in time, place, or person
12. Inability to respond appropriately to questions
13. Marked psychomotor agitation or retardation
14. Incoherent speech
15. Severe memory loss and confusion
16. Bizarre behavior
17. Preoccupation with death
18. Drug and/or alcohol abuse
19. Disabling chronic illness
20. Overmedication
21. Paranoia creating severe social functioning impairment
22. Headaches
23. Neurological symptoms
24. Weight loss
25. Insomnia
26. Other somatic symptoms

Elderly persons may equate going to a psychiatrist with being "crazy" or "being put away." It may be advisable, therefore, to use a less threatening label such as "physician," "specialist," or "geriatric doctor" in combination with the word "psychiatrist." The social worker should describe to the aged client or the family the purpose of the psychiatric consultation, its nature, and its value for the client's treatment. The worker should also prepare for the psychiatrist a written summary of the reasons for the referral, including the client's presenting problems and symptoms, all medical data, and medications currently prescribed. Specific questions may be included, such as the need for psychotropic medications or hospitalizations, the extent of suicidal risk, whether the disorder is treatable and the recommended treatment. When schedules permit, and depending upon the staff psychiatrist's orientation, the presence of the social worker at the psychiatric evaluation is strongly recommended. This ensures continuity of care, has positive transferential ingredients, and provides an additional reassurance and security regarding findings and recommendations.

After the psychiatric evaluation, the social worker should confer with the psychiatrist to clarify findings and recommendations and to decide if psychological testing for undetermined organic impairment is indicated. Psychotropic medication prescribed by the psychiatrist requires ongoing monitoring by the psychiatrist or the agency's medical staff. The client's personal physician should also be informed of any psychotropic medication to ensure coordination of all medical aspects of the client's treatment.

Feedback to the aged client and family is the responsibility of the social worker. Using guidance, support, reassurance, clarification, and persuasion, the social worker helps the client and family to integrate this important element of the assessment and to implement the psychiatrist's recommendations.

When the Client Presents Risk of Suicide

When the client in the course of the assessment presents a history of suicidal gestures or attempts, a family history that includes suicide, current episodes of suicidal gestures, attempts, threats, or ideation — especially when coupled with feelings of powerlessness, hopelessness, absence of self-esteem, isolation, multiple bereavements, and alcoholism — the social worker should recognize a high risk of suicide. Suicide rates for white, isolated, and alcoholic men increase dramatically as the person ages. Retirement, chronic disability, marginal income, changes of life-style, and isolated residence — particularly in deteriorating neighborhoods — are factors that contribute to suicide.

Interventions should be swift and frequent in cases of high suicide risk. They should include:

1. Immediate psychiatric evaluation
2. Possible hospitalization
3. Contact with family or other supports (There is a confidentiality issue here, but an angry client protesting a breach of confidentiality is preferable to a dead client whose confidentiality was protected.)
4. Intensive and frequent contact of the aged client with his support system
5. Placement of the client on the agency's "high risk" list, with follow-up dictated by agency procedures

All or some of these interventions during the crisis stage of acute depression may reduce the client's feelings of abandonment and loss of meaning in life. The severely depressed and suicidal aged client is not available to psychotherapy until the acute stage has passed. The nurturing, therapeutic interventions of the social worker significantly help the client and his or her family through this period of stress.

When the Client Must Be Hospitalized

When psychiatric evaluation indicates the advisability of hospitalization, the social worker can ensure continuity of care by:

1. Preparing the client and/or the family for implementation of the psychiatrist's recommendation
2. Preparing the appropriate hospital personnel for the patient's admission (The inpatient psychiatric ward of a local general hospital is preferable to a state hospital if the patient's stay will be short.)
3. If no collateral contact is available, accompanying the client to the hospital to reduce fears of the unknown and fantasies of abandonment
4. Establishing a contact person on the patient's floor to monitor treatment, progress, and discharge planning.
5. Visiting the patient when possible
6. Coordinating discharge plans with hospital and family

When the Family Is the Client

When working with the elderly, it is often the adult child who will be in treatment. Aged parents may have reached a level of mental deterioration at which they can no longer be candidates for psychotherapy, and their physical conditions may preclude the use of psychotropic medications. The physical and emotional demands resulting from their condition may cause severe stress to the caring adult children.

The rage of middle-aged adult children caught in "parent caring" when they had looked forward to relief from the responsibilities of raising children or had planned their own retirement may affect their ability to provide adequate care for the aged parent. The presence of the aged parent in the home may disturb the marital balance, while their placement in custodial care may trigger disabling guilt. When adult children are in their late 50s or early 60s, they are struggling with their own aging process and find in the aged parent a prophecy of what life has in store for them. This may become so threatening that it results in withdrawal from the aged parent and unintentional emotional neglect. In coming to the agency, adult children implicitly ask the agency to share their burden of responsibility. Expectations may be unrealistic. They may expect the therapist to return the parent to the parent's former level of functioning, or to become a surrogate child to the parent, or to resolve long-standing parent-child conflicts. In such situations, a thorough assessment of the aged parent and of the interactions with the adult child is necessary, through direct contact whenever possible. The best place for this is in the setting where the aged person lives. This conjoint assessment will identify the primary client in situations where this is not clear. When the family member is in treatment around the problems presented by the parent, the aged parent's needs can be addressed through the support, guidance, and working through of conflicts on the part of the adult child. This will correct some misconceptions about the parent's limitations on the part of the adult child and keep the treatment focused on the aged person's objective needs as well as on the dilemmas of "parent caring."

Mrs. G, aged 59, applied to the agency for help with her mother, aged 86, who rarely went out and watched TV all day. Mrs. G was fearful that "mother would become a vegetable." Her mother did not feel she needed help and was unreceptive to social work intervention. The daughter accepted a visit from the social worker to her home to meet her mother, who could not grasp the nature of the social work role. During this conjoint interview it became clear that the mother had always lived quietly, with few social needs, and had enjoyed radio soap operas as she enjoyed those on TV today. It was her daughter who was struggling with her own fears of losing her mother and of her own aging process. The daughter entered treatment for herself to learn to accept her mother's limitations and to acknowledge the developmental tasks of becoming 60.

When the aged parent's disorder has been diagnosed as "senile dementia" or Alzheimer's disease, interventions with the family are crucial for all concerned. An irreversible disease of the cerebral tissue, Alzheimer's accounts for a high percentage of all individuals with progressive cognitive failure occurring during late adult stages of life. Depression can complicate this mysterious and complex disease. It requires close supervision of the patient, extending from sporadic care in the initial stages to custodial care when the patient has lost all capacity for self-care. The problems encountered by the family include:

1. Management of the patient
2. High cost of long-term care in the home or an institution
3. Legal concerns with estate issues
4. Support for family members coping with the ill relative

SERVICES

Psychotherapy

Stereotyping of the aged person as one who has lost the cognitive functioning needed for addressing his or her problems has contributed to the negative appraisal of the usefulness of psychotherapy with the aged. Experience, however, suggests that psychotherapy brings a very special dimension into the life of the aged person. It provides a nurturing relationship with positive transferential benefits. When the focus of treatment remains on the present difficulty, using the past to understand the present; when the therapist enlists the strengths of the aged person to actively participate in the treatment and underscores preservation of his identity; when the client gains control over as much of his or her environment as reality permits and addresses the issue of adaptation to stressful circumstances—then the prognosis for a positive therapeutic experience is optimistic.

The aged require much support from a therapist, including active involvement in the therapy session. A passive, nonparticipating therapist withholds the stimulus of interaction so necessary to the aged person whose opportunities for being listened to and responded to are limited.

The tendency of society is to negate, talk down to, or infantilize the aged. To counter this, the therapist concentrates on an "eyeball-to-eyeball, adult-to-adult" approach. The age or sex of the therapist need not affect the outcome. A mature young woman in her 20s, who understands and conveys respect to the aged, will achieve a positive transference as well as an older, fatherly man. What counts is the respect and trust within the therapy session and the clarification, support, and guidance geared to the level of functioning, both cognitive and emotional, of the aged client.

The key issue for the aged person is dependency compounded by severe loss. When a personality disorder precludes the possibility of insight as a means of change, the therapeutic task is to strengthen aged persons' support systems to compensate for their loss. These clients usually feel that without the lost "other" they can no longer function, that abandonment has been total. They are frightened because the person or situation that held them together is gone. Unable to manage their lives, they place outrageous demands on their family or therapist to magically rescue them from their abandonment.

Treatment of such deeply entrenched dependency acknowledges and helps aged clients to accept their feelings of helplessness and explores appropriate compensatory resources in order to decrease panic. The therapist allows the transfer of dependency, with clear boundaries, to himself or herself. When therapists can accept the vital role they play and can set appropriate boundaries without guilt as the dependent aged person pulls them into their dependency needs, they gratify needs for affection and protection. Feelings of safety return.

The other end of the dependency continuum is the aged person who, in a hypomanic way, places value on independence, viewing the input of family or agency as an assault on the ego. This person feels that he or she has lost control, that he or she is a burden. When there is a narcissistic or compulsive personality component, the issue of control often interferes with necessary protection as the aged person deteriorates. Dependency is unacceptable since pseudoindependence has been masking dependency throughout his or her life. Panic is conveyed through his or her lack of experience and negative attitude toward asking for help of any kind.

The aged matron who has been a "do-it-yourself" person all her life, unconsciously manipulating others through guilt to attend to her dependency needs with no awareness of that dependency, presents as an agitated, depressed client, furious with disappointment that those to whom she "gave" of herself have let her down. This aged client struggles to control the relationship with the therapist, tries to defeat the therapist, displays her ambivalent nature whenever connection on an emotional level is experienced in treatment. This client will benefit when the therapist joins the resistance, reinforces those ego strengths that enable this client to maintain as much control as possible, elicits solutions to problems *from* the client, and delegates responsibility for suggestions, recommendations, and maneuvers to the aged person. The therapist helps in the problem-solving aspect by cognitively guiding the client along the route he or she has selected. The dependency needs of this client are gratified within the subtleties of the transference as the therapist listens and engages in a nondirective way. The client will reach out for affection, maintaining her image of herself as a wise, giving grandmother or aunt. When this act of affection is reciprocated by the therapist, it provides a needed experience of the touch and warmth of another human being.

It is important for the social worker to prepare the client for what will happen in therapy and to clarify the role of the psychiatrist or clinical social worker as part of the treatment team. In this way the social worker reduces the client's fear of the unknown. By encouraging questions from the client the social worker permits fears and concerns to be verbalized. The patient gains control over this new environment and feels less threatened. For the aged person who has had little contact with psychotherapy, this orientation can be critical to the success of treatment.

Mrs. H, aged 79, widowed, lived alone for fifteen years in a deteriorating neighborhood. She had an only child, Mrs. I, who worried about her safety. Mrs. I had a stable marriage; the relationship between Mrs. H and her son-in-law had always been that of a son. He was her financial adviser. When Mrs. H was mugged returning from the supermarket, Mr. and Mrs. I decided that it was time for her to move. Mrs. H was reluctant. She had moved to her present home when she was married. Her daughter pressured her, selling her the idea that she would be closer geographically to them and that there would be frequent contact. Mrs. H yielded. An apartment was rented ten minutes away from the only family Mrs. H had.

In the process of moving, Mr. I, the son-in-law, continued in his role of financial adviser. He sold the house, converted the money to a more manageable and growth-producing medium, and established bank accounts in several places.

Mrs. H moved expecting her daughter and family to gratify her emotional needs. As she settled into her new environment, with its unfamiliar setting, she realized that her daughter and family were not available to her as she had fantasized. She felt abandoned, hurt, and furious. She couldn't comprehend their behavior. Her agitation increased. She became intrusive, presenting herself daily, interrupting the activity of her grandchildren, demanded to be taken care of. Her daughter, attempting to control the deteriorating relationship, withdrew. Her son-in-law distanced himself. Mrs. H felt she was in an enemy camp.

Mrs. H looked for reasons to explain what was happening. She decided that her son-in-law had an ulterior motive, had been planning to steal her money all along and had in fact stolen everything. This explained the family pressure on her to move. She decided that the doctor who had treated her injury after the mugging was a partner in the plan to steal her money, that the medicine he gave her was to control her mind so she wouldn't object. As she came to these conclusions, Mrs. H became more agitated, more paranoid, more depressed. Every contact was pulled into this delusional system. Her behavior became bizarre.

Mrs. H had been attending a senior center. The social worker had established a relationship with her. She brought her paranoid complaints to the social worker, who had already observed her increased agitation. Through a difficult process, Mrs. H accepted psychiatric treatment. She actively mourned the loss of her home and realized the extent of her disappointment due to unrealistic expectations of her only child. Psychotherapy in combination with psychotropic medication reduced her anxiety, making her more comfortable and lessening her fatigue. Family sessions provided the opportunity for her to convey her needs and for the family to comfort her by cementing the relationship in appropriate ways. Her paranoia was considerably reduced. The family learned to diagnose her mental status and need for their interventions. When her agitation increased paranoid projections, they learned the kind of family activity that would reduce her symptoms and allow for clear-cut boundaries between aged parent and children. Mrs. H made an adequate adjustment.

Reminiscence Therapy

Aged people bring their problems to the social worker-therapist at a point in time when they have lost connection with their past. They see themselves as narcissistically wounded in their appearance, as having lost usefulness and status. They fear that the therapist is as uninterested in their history as their family appears to be when they fail to listen to stories about their childhoods or their days of success.

When the therapist uses reminiscence as a therapeutic tool to understand the present difficulty, to solidify and preserve the self-identity that the aged person is losing contact with, he or she provides gratification and solace to the narcissistic needs of the aged person. Memory is selective, preserving a sense of significance. In reminiscence therapy, the past is brought to the surface through the emotional set of the present. The past is secured for the patient in a way that meets the client's needs. It provides an opportunity to express conflicts without rekindling them, to accept guilt and unrealized goals, to maintain connection with irreversible losses, preserving the idealized version of the valued person as a justification for the degree of bereavement and pride in the past relationship.

In reminiscence, pictures, creative memorabilia such as crafts, original poems, letters—any objects that the patient might offer to bring to the session—provide that special dimension within the therapeutic relationship. This allows for sharing stories from the past to be valued by the sharing, protecting, interested, status-endowed therapist. The patient feels important. Self-esteem rises, suffering is relieved, and the patient is perhaps closer to a higher level of adaptation to change.

Bereavement

Bereavement requires special attention. The aged patient may have experienced multiple losses of significant persons. The very old may have lost children, siblings, and friends as well as spouses. Parents will have died at least twenty years before.

Grieving and mourning are ever present in the feeling states of the elderly. The most common reaction is depression. To detect the presence of mourning in the depression of the aged person and to assess whether the mourning is within a normal, appropriate range or whether it is pathological in its severity and duration, data of recent and past losses are essential. These data are evaluated together with an assessment of how this grieving person has adapted to other losses throughout his or her life. What were his or her strengths in coping with losses? How long did he or she take to recover? Is there a history of depression related to losses of significant others?

Grief affords an opportunity to make a loving relationship with the lost person and to relate more lovingly to the world. When the patient is able to disengage from the representation of the dead through grief, to form a loving relationship with this lost person, and to move on in adjusting to life without that presence, the patient's depression is a reaction to grief. But when the loss creates disruptive disorganization and when the mourner exhibits pathological guilt, hopes that the dead will come back to life, and dreads that this might happen, the therapist can differentiate between reactive depression and pathological grieving.

Group Therapy

Group therapy is highly beneficial for the depressed elderly client. Since depression results from the loss of social supports, it is important to help aged clients to compensate through connection with new sources of socialization. The therapeutic goal is to relieve their isolation, not to keep them isolated with their therapists.

Two group modalities in particular can enhance the life of the elderly patient. One is a therapy group for depressed older adults, kept small (a maximum of ten members) and open-ended so clinicians can refer elderly patients to the group as needed, either as the treatment of choice or in combination with individual therapy. Unlike group therapy for other age groups, the focus here is not on behavioral change or the resolution of conflicts but on socialization, which remains the key issue for the elderly. All forms of creativity, fun, and nurturing are employed to lessen the elderly patient's feelings of abandonment. In such a group patients achieve a measure of control over their lives in the face of multiple losses. It strengthens characteristic defenses that enabled them to cope with their crises. It does not burden them with new tasks but reinforces ego strengths and narcissistic needs by valuing their history and their sorrow.

The second modality is the formal, organized senior center. Elderly patients should be introduced to a senior center only if they have a history of successful group experience and have achieved a level of functioning that will be further enhanced by the senior center. There are many aged people for whom a senior center is contraindicated. The clinician must be careful that the client will experience connection rather than failure or loss of control.

Referral to a senior center should not terminate therapy but rather be a part of the therapeutic program to reconnect the client to new areas of socialization. Therapy is terminated only when the client is fully integrated into the new activity. When he or she shows some pleasure, and presents sufficient evidence of a higher level of adaptation, contact can be spaced and eventually terminated.

Self-Help Groups

Self-help groups can provide support, guidance, and education to persons caring for elderly relatives, particularly those who are ill, handicapped, or mentally impaired. By sharing their common experiences, such persons learn from each other, adapt better to their disorganizing situations, and lessen the stress and despair under which they live.

An agency seeking to provide this service may begin with outreach to the community to locate people experiencing difficulty in caring for elderly relatives. Potential group members are carefully screened by the professional group leader to make sure that the group and not individual counseling is the appropriate modality for them. At an orientation meeting, the group leader negotiates meeting arrangements, fees, and goals. The leader and the members then contract for a limited number of group meetings under his or her professional guidance. Five to eight sessions are generally acceptable to most members. By limiting his or her participation to a small number of meetings, the professional underlines the self-nature of the group. After the contracted number of meetings, the professional worker withdraws; members may continue to meet under their own leaders, preserving telephone contact and supportive networking among themselves.

The Homebound

The disabled, homebound elderly are often neglected by the mental-health system. They are cut off from the outside community, their contacts limited to the few people in their immediate environment or to the telephone. Most of this population remains hidden. It is only through outside referral or a call of desperation that the barrier is broken.

Yet the homebound or institutionalized elderly deserve the same opportunity for treatment as those who present themselves at agency doors. The social worker who visits a homebound or institutionalized client establishes a relationship with a person who has lost almost all control over his life space. The first step, therefore, is to allow the client significant input in determining the time and place of the home sessions. Provision for privacy must be made with others who may be present in the home, such as home-health aides or family members. The consistency of these arrangements symbolically establishes office and appointment wherever the sessions are held.

The role of the social worker will need to be clarified and reclarified, since the elderly patient may be unfamiliar with the social-work function and confused to see the social worker in the home. Since isolation intensifies the mental impairment of the elderly, the visits of the social worker can be supplemented by visits from an emotionally nourishing volunteer.

Countertransference is likely to occur as a result of meeting disabled elderly patients in their homes or institutions. The clinician must guard against tendencies to avoid this group of clients or to convey a distancing attitude because of the intensity of the disabilities. Supervisors must attend to "burnout" issues that arise in these circumstances.

Termination

The elderly client who achieves an improved level of adaptation presents a dilemma to the social worker. With a younger client, termination is indicated when the goals of treatment have been reached. But the supportive, nurturing professional has become a focus of the dependency needs of the elderly client. Termination of the relationship might be experienced as another loss at a time in the patient's life when there may not be enough significant others to compensate.

To resolve this dilemma, the social worker should consider:

1. The client-worker relationship (does its ending represent another death?)
2. The aged person's level of functioning
3. The need for "maintenance therapy," spaced, consistent contact to monitor functioning and prevent premature deterioration or regression
4. The aged person's support system
5. The aged person's opportunities for social and cognitive stimulation

Review of these considerations may indicate the need for the elderly person to become an "ongoing client" of the agency, with the agency recognizing the appropriateness of the client's dependency and functioning as a surrogate family to the abandoned, orphaned client. The social worker now coordinates all aspects of service to the elderly client, employing volunteers, senior-center attendance, medical scrutiny, direct services, etc. Several individuals may now be involved in the treatment plan, but the social worker remains the consistent, dependable "other," providing reassurance to the isolated aged person that further abandonment will not occur.

Mrs. J, aged 84, lost her husband three years ago. She had been in treatment for a reactive depression that was separate from her progressive mental impairment of confusion, memory loss, and disorientation. As her depression lifted, it became clear that she would need placement unless some plan for ongoing monitoring of her functioning was established. She had no living relatives. In her lucid moments she adamantly opposed any relocation from the home she had lived in for over fifty years. She reminisced constantly and displayed evidence of transferring the role of the protective husband to the caring social worker who had sustained her at her time of loss. It was clear that the social worker remained her sole line to the community and her sole representative of the protecting person. Her functioning on all levels was questionable. A volunteer to visit, a part-time home health aide, and regular health screening is maintaining this aged lady in her home. "Her" social worker visits briefly twice a week, gets feedback from the team caring for the lady, troubleshoots when a crisis is predictable, and supplies the presence of a trusted, dependable, protective person who understands and supports. Mrs. J is in "maintenance therapy." No termination is planned.

BIBLIOGRAPHY

Berkman, B. G., and Rehr, H. (1972). Social needs of the hospitalized elderly: A classification. *Social Work* **17**(4), 80-88.

Busse, E. W. (1981). Therapy of mental illness in late life. In S. H. Arieti and K. H. Brodie (Eds.), *American handbook of psychiatry* (2nd ed.), vol. 7, *Advances and new directions*. New York: Basic Books.

Busse, E. W., and Blazer, D. G. (Eds.) (1980). *Handbook of geriatric psychiatry.* New York: Van Nostrand Reinhold.

Busse, E. W., and Pfeiffer, E. (Eds.) (1973). *Mental illness in later life.* Washington: American Psychiatric Association.

Busse, E. W., and Pfeiffer, E. (Eds.) (1977). *Behavior and adaptation in late life* (2nd ed.). Boston: Little, Brown.

Butler, R. N., and Lewis, M. I. (1982). *Aging and mental health: Positive psychological and bio-medical approaches* (3rd ed.). St. Louis: Mosby.

Carp, F. M., and Carp, A. (1981). Mental health characteristics and acceptance-rejection of old age. *American Journal of Orthopsychiatry,* **51**(2), 230-241.

Cassem, N. H. (1978). Treating the person confronting death. In A. M. Nicholi, Jr. (Ed.), *The Harvard Guide to Modern Psychiatry.* Cambridge: Harvard University Press.

Gatz, M., et al. (1980). The mental health system and the older adult. In L. W. Poon (Ed.), *Aging in the 1980s.* Washington: American Psychological Association.

Gershon, S., and Herman, S. P. (1982). The differential diagnosis of dementia. *Journal of the American Geriatrics Society,* **30**(11), S58.

Gitelson, M. (1975). The emotional problems of elderly people. In W. C. Sze (Ed.), *Human life cycle.* New York: J. Aronson.

Glassman, M. (1980). Misdiagnosis of senile dementia: Denial of care to the elderly. *Social Work* **25**(4), 288-292.

Gray, B., and Isaacs, B. (1979). *Care of the elderly mentally infirm.* New York: Tavistock.

Gwyther, L. P. (1982). Caregiver self-help groups: Roles for professionals. *Generations* **7**(1), 37-38.

Kahana, R. J. (1980). Psychotherapy with the elderly. In T. B. Karasu and L. Bellak (Eds.), *Specialized techniques in individual psychotherapy.* New York: Brunner/Mazel.

Kosberg, J. J. (1973). The nursing home: A social work paradox. *Social Work,* **18**(2), 104-110.

Langsley, D. (1980). Community psychiatry. In H. Kaplan, A. Freedman, and B. Sadoch (Eds.), *Comprehensive textbook of psychiatry* (3rd ed.). Baltimore: Williams & Wilkins.

Levin, S., and Kahana, R. J. (Eds.) (1967). *Psychodynamic studies on aging: Creativity, reminiscing, and dying.* New York: International Universities Press.

Mace, N. L., and Rabins, P. V. (1982). *The 36-hour day.* Baltimore: John Hopkins University Press.

Margulies, A., and Havens, L. L. (1981). The initial encounter: What to do first? *American Journal of Psychiatry,* **138**(4), 421-428.

Miller, M. B. (1979). *Current issues in clinical geriatrics.* New York: Tiresias Press.

Neugarten, B. L. (1979). Time, age, and the life cycle. *American Journal of Psychiatry,* **136**(7), 887-894.

Perrotta, P., and Meacham, J. A. (1981-82). Can a reminiscing intervention alter depression and self-esteem? *International Journal of Aging and Human Development,* **14**(1), 23-30.

Pincus, A. (1967). Toward a developmental view of aging for social work. *Social Work,* **12**(3), 33-41.

Reifler, B. V., et al. (1982). Five-year experience of a community outreach program for the elderly. *American Journal of Psychiatry,* **139**(2), 220-223.

Rosow, I. (1973). The social context of the aging self. *Gerontologist* **13**(1), 82-87.

Rothblum, E. D., et al. (1982). Issues in clinical trials with the depressed elderly. *Journal of the American Geriatrics Society,* **30**(11), 694-699.

Schneck, M. K., et al. (1982). Overview of current concepts of Alzheimer's disease. *American Journal of Psychiatry,* **139**(2), 165-173.

Schram, S., and Hurley, R. (1977). Title XX and the elderly. *Social Work,* **22**(2), 95-102.

Schwartz, M. D., and Karasu, T. B. (1980). Psychotherapy with dying patients. In T. B. Karasu and L. Bellak (Eds.), *Specialized techniques in individual psychotherapy.* New York: Brunner/Mazel.

Shader, R. I. (Ed.) (1975). *Manual of psychiatric therapeutics.* Boston: Little, Brown.

Silverstone, B., and Hyman, H. K. (1977). *You and your aging parent.* New York: Pantheon Books.

Simos, B. G. (1973). Adult children and their aging parents. *Social Work,* **18**(3), 78-85.

Volkan, V. D., and Josephthal, D. (1980). The treatment of established pathological mourners. In T. B. Karasu and L. Bellak (Eds.), *Specialized techniques in individual psychotherapy.* New York: Brunner/Mazel.

Watzlawick, P., and Coyne, J. C. (1980). Depression following stroke: Brief, problem-focused family treatment. *Family Process,* **19**(1), 13-18.

Zarit, S. H. (1980). *Aging and mental disorders: Psychological approaches to assessment and treatment.* New York: Free Press.

12

Multipurpose Senior Centers

Louis Lowy, Ph.D.

Boston University, Boston, Mass.

The multipurpose senior center is a community facility in which older people come together to fulfill many of their social, physical, and intellectual needs. The center can help expand their interests, tap their potentials, and develop their talents.

The center is also a bridge linking the senior community to the community at large. It is a bridge over which people and ideas, services, and resources can flow back and forth to the benefit of the entire community and which offers older people opportunities to create a special community of their own without isolating themselves from the larger community.

DEFINITION AND HISTORY

A multiservice senior center provides a single setting in which older people can take part in social activities as well as have access to essential services. A broad spectrum of activities and services is available at or through centers to those who come to the center as well as to the homebound through outreach. These activities and services include: nutrition, health, employment, transportation, social work and other supportive services, education, creative arts, recreation and leadership, and volunteer opportunities. They are provided through a center's paid and volunteer staff, through social and community agencies that use the center as a base to provide their services, through service linkages and referrals to other agencies, and through outreach to older community residents unable to attend the center. Senior centers also serve as community resources for information on aging, for training professional and lay leadership, and for developing new approaches to aging programs.

"Since time began, people have come together with others of their own age to exchange experiences common to their particular life stage, to shake their heads over or wonder at the generations younger or older than they are, to solve the problems of the world as seen from their vantage point" (NCOA, 1962). The history of centers for older people begins in 1943 when the William Hodson Community Center was established in New York City by its welfare department. The idea of a center arose among social workers who noticed how desperately their older clients sought communication to escape the loneliness and isolation of their lives. At first the city merely provided the space, some refreshments, and games and then left the 350 or so original participants to fend for themselves. The hope was that somehow a program would develop; eventually it did, under the leadership of Harry Levine and Gertrude Landau. Subsequently the Sirovitch Center opened on Second Avenue in New York City to serve the older population in that neighborhood.

The next centers were established in San Francisco and in Menlo Park, California. Though each served a different type of community, both centers came to play an important role in the daily lives of the older people they served. The San Francisco Senior Center opened in 1947 as a result of the efforts of many community organizations. Though focused more on recreation and education than the Hodson Center, its programs were similarly supervised by professional staff, some detailed from various city agencies. Little House was designed to meet the needs of middle-class elderly in Menlo Park. This center was also sponsored by community agencies. Its distinctive feature was that most of its program was designed and directed by the elderly themselves. Among the center services was a referral agency that furnished the members with the locations of places and people to contact when problems arose. In Bridgeport, Connecticut, a multiservice "leisure lounge" was developed in 1951 for late-middle-aged and older people to offer cultural, educational, and social-support programs.

During the following thirty years the concept of a multiservice senior center was adopted by an ever-increasing number of communities across the country. The resulting growth can be seen in the following figures: in 1961, 218 centers were identified as operating; by 1965 the number had grown to 404; the National Council on the Aging's (NCOA) first directory, published in 1966, listed 360 centers; by 1969, another 754 centers had been founded, bringing the total to 1,058; that same year, Anderson's major study on senior centers identified well over 1,000 centers; in 1970 NCOA's second directory listed 1,200 centers; from 1970 until 1973 another 1,169 centers were founded, and in 1974 NCOA identified 2,362 centers in its directory (NISC, 1974); in 1977 the Administration on Aging (AoA) estimated that there were 3,600 operational centers, and currently NCOA states that over 8,000 such centers are in operation.

Accompanying this growth in numbers was a diversification and consolidation of the internal structure of centers. Different models of center organization emerged. Interest groups were formed to create better voices for advocacy and research, and information programs developed to fill the increasing demands for data and evaluation. A perusal of the early literature on senior centers reveals the enthusiasm as well as the ad-hoc nature of then-current practices.

A concrete measure of the internal differentiation can be found in the growing organization of the field. In 1959 the first state association (Ohio Association of Centers for Senior Citizens) was formed; it was soon followed by associations in other states. At present most states and many regions and communities have their own organizations, providing representation of and communication within the center field. At the national level this evolution is equally noticeable: in 1962 an exploratory conference on senior centers was held, and, from 1964 on, the Annual Conference on Senior Centers got larger each year. Accompanying this trend was the establishment in 1963 of a National Institute of Senior Centers (NISC) as a permanent arm of the NCOA. In the following year the NISC Delegate Council was formed to widen the input structure from the centers representing various regions.

NEED FOR MULTISERVICE CENTERS

The rapid growth of the aging population has created a demand for societal responses and mechanisms to deal with the differential needs of older people, be they biological, physical, economical, social, cultural, political, or spiritual. In the past fifteen years we have witnessed the emergence of federal, state, and local social policies, as well as programs that address some of the needs of a heterogeneous aging population to varying degrees. Three White House conferences have brought together older and younger people and have led to an exchange of ideas culminating in a number of recommendations on how to shape and design our social policies on aging.

At the 1981 White House Conference the following statement was adopted by delegates:

Over the years, senior centers have demonstrated their ability to enhance the physical, social and emotional well-being of large numbers of older persons. Senior centers are an essential part of the community's continuum of care. The senior center is a community focal point which services the elderly with dignity and respect, supports their capacity to grow and develop and facilitates their continued involvement in the community. There must be support for senior centers at all levels of government as well as in the private sector (White House Conference on Aging, 1982, vol. 3, p. 128).

Whether a senior center is needed in a community depends upon answers to these two questions: (1) Are the services that it offers needed by older persons? (2) Are these services currently available from other providers? At a national-policy level, the issues of whether senior centers as a whole are a needed institution cannot presently be answered by specific criteria but only by indirect impressions.

Originally senior centers were established in response to grass-roots, local initiatives in different communities. The expansion of the numbers of senior centers across the nation established their growing popularity, and their service record nationally indicates that senior centers are in demand and are being used. The experience of visiting a "good" senior center leaves many observers with quite a strong impression of their value. Indicators such as these can often be found in congressional hearings as the reason for a policymaker's endorsement of senior centers.

For example, during one of these hearings, one Senator opened his statement by recalling, "It's usually heart warming to visit a center; sociability and good works abound." Another cited the membership size of the NISC as evidence that "Senior centers are now fulfilling a vital role for members and communities in all parts of the nation." Another felt that "The growth in number of such centers testifies to their increasing popularity and should be seen as a 'grass-roots' response to a clearly identifiable need." And others stressed the role of senior centers in the aging network of services and programs, and their capacity to become an "effective means of delivering social and other services to participants" (U.S. Congress, 1978).

These observations are not direct measures of the need for senior centers, yet, in the absence of more accurate measures, they are a legitimate alternative. If for decades more and more people have been coming to senior centers, and if the number of such centers—even before availability of any federal funds—has been steadily growing, a senior center must possess significant utility to make both communities and center participants feel their efforts are worthwhile.

How many centers are needed? What kind of centers are needed? How shall centers be financed? How many centers should there be per 100,000 citizens? What does the average cost of operating a center amount to?

Looking closely at demographic data (number, education, income, and residence patterns of senior citizens) will yield an estimate of the number of centers needed during the next decades and also their approximate cost. Another approach to estimating the need for senior centers is based on the concept of target population, that is, the number and characteristics of people in a community or neighborhood that a senior center should serve. Here an assumption is made that the people to be served are in need of center services. The target population for most senior centers includes all the people over age 60 living in a particular geographic area. While a community institution should be accessible and open to all community residents, the just mentioned standard of target grouping is all-encompassing. The group of people it purports to want to serve is equal to the maximum conceivable number. Clearly, no center could actually serve all the elderly in a geographic area, nor is it desirable that it should. A good number of elderly have neither wish nor need to be served by any center or social agency.

Another method of defining need is based on the number and characteristics of people who are already attending a center. To obtain a national estimate of need for senior centers, we can see how many people in a given community are attending a center and extrapolate this ratio. The average center reports over 500 older adults participating in program activities per month. If this statistic includes duplicated counts, the actual number of persons attending is likely to be smaller. If we contrast this figure with the average total population of a community (around 360,000, approximately 11 percent of whom are elderly), we see that the proportion of people actually served is quite small. Center staffs estimate that they serve about 30 percent of the elderly in their geographic areas. With well over two-thirds of the national sample having daily attendance numbers of less than 75 persons, this staff estimate is either overly optimistic or reflects a minimal level of service.

Although actual attendance figures at a multiservice senior center reflect both the supply and the demand for services, the just quoted figures may be taken as a rough indicator of need. According to national census figures, in 1983 there were about 26 million people 65 or older. If we assume that roughly one-third could utilize center services, this yields a possible service population of 8.6 million. The number of older people actually served at the present time is estimated to be approximately 8 million in approximately 8,000 centers. This averages 1,000 service recipients per center. If we project into the immediate future, the need for centers would increase. By the year 2000 it is estimated that there will be over 32 million people over 65 and, therefore, over 10 million potential center users.

This estimate can be improved by recognizing that, even in communities that already have senior centers, not all people who would like to attend are actually able to do so. Therefore, attendance records probably understate the need. To reflect this need more accurately, we would want to add the number of nonusers who are interested in senior centers. According to the Harris data, almost 22 percent of those not currently attending a senior center would like to (Louis Harris and Associates, 1981). Nationally, this group may comprise about 7 million people, a figure somewhat larger than the one extrapolated purely from attendance figures. Based on these calculations, roughly 11,000 senior centers would be needed during the next decade. Whether these centers would be leased, purchased, or constructed, the establishment of such centers would require appreciable dollar outlays. Since it seems rather unlikely that the entire amount of money required to bring the country to these standards of service will actually be made available, another strategy is to forego the goal of broad national-center availability in favor of developing a few model centers to illustrate the role senior centers could play in a properly developed aging-service network.

This was the approach chosen in the aborted AoA initiative of 1977. In each state a minimum of two multipurpose senior centers were to be established that could meet professional guidelines as to range and volume of delivered services. In an environment of limited resources, such a selective approach does make sense but only if combined with a planning approach that calls for a nationwide inventory and assessment of the senior centers within each AoA Title III area, in order to determine a priority listing as to which communities are most in need of expansion or the establishment of a senior center.

PARTICIPATION IN CENTERS

For a number of years now, research findings have begun to attest to the multiple needs of the elderly. Sensory deterioration, self-concept decline, role changes, reduction of social reinforcement, income drop, growing isolation, physical infirmity, and external/internal stereotypes of aging—to name but a few—are cited as reasons for the special service needs of the elderly. It has been assumed that attendance at senior centers will meet some of these needs.

Actual comparison of user with nonuser profiles disproves some of these assumptions: no relationship between income and center attendance was found in several studies. In the NCOA sample, three-fourths of the users versus about one-half of the nonusers were retired. This probably indicates that center attendance is related to loss of the work role and increase in leisure time among the young old (Anderson, 1969; NCOA, 1972; NISC, 1974).

One might expect that older and generally needier people would join the centers. Again the data have not supported this assumption. The one factor that does distinguish members from nonmembers across a variety of studies is health. Indeed, health emerges as the key factor in predicting both service need and center utilization. It is the nonusers who are much more likely to have serious health problems. In the NCOA study, for instance, 22 percent of nonusers versus 13 percent of users had difficulty walking or climbing. Nonusers were also much more likely to rate their health prolbems as very serious. This is not to say that center members enjoy perfect health but that, of the two groups, nonusers have more serious health problems.

It is further suggested that older persons' decreasing social supports, their sense of isolation and loneliness, are major reasons for joining a center. For those isolated from meaningful social opportunities and detached from supportive relations, age-graded social clubs may provide relief from loneliness, while for those active in a variety of roles such groups may offer little attraction. Marital status shows little difference between members and nonmembers, although NCOA reports that more users are widowed, which supports the results of earlier studies that have viewed loss of a spouse as a major reason for center attendance.

And yet several other factors weigh against the social-isolation hypothesis.

The vast majority of respondents in the NCOA study, irrespective of center attendance, did not view loneliness as a problem. In fact, studies have indicated that center participants enjoy good social relations and friendships. It is difficult to say to what degree social contacts and friendships preceded center attendance or resulted from it (Hanssen et al., 1978; Trela and Simmons, 1971).

A different view holds that people don't join senior centers because they need to overcome loneliness and isolation but because they simply want to join. Since joining is viewed as continuation of a lifelong pattern of organizational membership, this perspective suggests that people who join a senior center are more likely to belong also to other social groups (Adams, 1971; Graney, 1975; Storey, 1962; Tuckman, 1967).

A related explanation of center attendance stresses people's life-styles and preference patterns. Studies have found that senior-center members enjoy recreation, socializing, and organizational participation to a greater degree than nonmembers. They do not care for passive activities but like to go places and do active things. Nonusers, on the other hand, are more likely to spend time at home, caring for a family member or "just doing nothing."

Finally, let us turn to the variable that has been used as an outcome measure in almost every study of senior centers—life satisfaction. The findings here are varied. Taietz (1976), for example, found no difference at all between the users and nonusers in his sample; Hanssen (1978) reported that senior-center users were less depressed than those who didn't attend; and the NCOA (1972) study indicated that users showed a slightly greater degree of life satisfaction than nonusers.

Conspicuously absent as participants in multiservice centers are minority elderly, unless such centers are specifically geared to black, Hispanic, or other nonwhite populations. Ethnically oriented programs address special white-ethnic groups, notably Jews (via Jewish community centers) or Italian, Irish, and Polish elderly in areas where they are demographically concentrated. While centers make attempts to conduct activities across ethnic or racial boundaries, there is still an absence of ethnically and racially integrated program activities. Senior centers reflect pretty much the state of affairs in the United States of the 1980s. More than a decade ago, Vickery (1972) argued that minority elderly were hard to reach mainly because they often reside in poor neighborhoods.

While lack of access may prevent their involvement, some aged subgroups, such as the black elderly, have shown a desire to be involved in senior centers. National data indicate that two in five blacks aged 55 and over do not currently attend senior centers but would like to. Lack of facilities and transportation are cited as the main inhibiting factors (Ralston, 1982).

To adequately serve minority elderly, it is necessary to explore different models. One senior-center model that has been implemented in some areas is the "neighborhood senior center." The neighborhood senior center is decentralized; it is located within the neighborhood to be served and incorporates programs that reflect the local, personal needs of the elderly. While there is hardly any literature concerning the effectiveness of the neighborhood senior center, several authors have suggested that neighborhood-based services are essential to take into account the heterogeneity and ethnicity of the aged population and to attract nonwhite elderly as participants.

In a study exploring the impact of the neighborhood senior center on the black elderly by determining their perceptions of senior centers (Ralston, 1982), three groups of black elderly were interviewed: attenders of a neighborhood senior center, nonattenders in the same community, and nonattenders in a comparable community without a neighborhood senior center. A twenty-nine-item interview schedule was constructed that determined awareness of senior-center activities and services. Significant differences were found among the three groups, with the attenders and nonattenders in the same community having the highest levels of awareness of senior-center activities and services. Age, sex, and marital status were not found to influence perception of senior centers. These findings suggest that the neighborhood senior center needs to be further examined as a model for serving minority elderly.

The most frequently given reason for attendance at a center is the wish to meet others. Over half the sample in the NCOA study indicated that they came because the center provided them with opportunities for use of leisure time. These responses match with the view of centers as places for recreation and socializing, and most center users report that they have friends both inside and outside the center. This is the major reason why people are initially motivated to attend a center. Once they begin to come more regularly, their experience during the visit itself has an influence on why they come back.

In the NCOA study, members indicated identification with "their center." About two-thirds reported that they preferred "their" center to other similar ones, and over one-third said they would just stay home if their center closed instead of seeking out another one. Furthermore, feelings of loyalty to the center director were pronounced.

Groups of nonusers who have been studied fall into two categories: those who don't attend a center but would like to and those who don't wish to come at all. The chief reason for nonattendance given by the former is lack of a nearby facility, whereas the latter say they are just not interested, too busy with other activities or too sick to attend. Lack of a facility is a response given frequently by elderly in rural areas where fewer senior centers are available. But even within cities geographic distance and accessibility are key predictors of attendance.

A profile of a typical center user in the 1980s would describe her as a lower- to middle-middle-class white woman in her late 60s or early 70s, socially oriented and not given to feelings of depression. She might not be perfectly healthy, but she is not greatly functionally impaired. She prefers going out and doing things with other people to staying around home working or resting. She belongs to several clubs or organizations and has friends in and out of the center. She is a low- to middle-income person, has some high-school education, and is interested in the world around her. To what extent this profile will change depends on the efforts of new initiatives to address the needs of minority, vulnerable, and frail elderly.

To summarize, senior-center participation can be viewed as an outgrowth of life-style and activity preference. Some people enjoy active group experiences more than others. Some people are more socially outgoing than others. When these people become older, the senior center becomes one setting in which they can fulfill many of their needs and wishes. But the location of centers in neighborhoods and access to them does have an influence on the actual as well as potential use by all elderly, particularly the minority aged.

THE PROGRAM OF THE SENIOR CENTER

What are the program goals of a multiservice senior center? Based on Morris Cohen's testimony before the U.S. Senate Special Committee on Aging in 1978, the following can be cited as major center goals:

For the individual, senior centers are to provide opportunities for:

1. Meaningful individual and group relationships
2. Learning new skills for personal enrichment in the arts, languages, music, dramatics, nature, sports and games, dance, and crafts
3. Being useful and helpful to others through volunteer community service
4. Assisting a person to maintain physical strength
5. Promoting mental health through the use and development of creative abilities
6. Developing a valued role in society
7. Helping the individual to keep informed about changes in the community and the world
8. Developing an individual's group-leadership skills and personal effectiveness in dealing with others
9. Information and consultation on personal problems

For the family, senior centers are to offer opportunities for:

1. Developing new skills and experiences to share with family members
2. Helping older persons to be less dependent on family for activity and interests and appropriately dependent on family relationships for emotional support
3. Helping people continue to contribute to the family's emotional well-being

For the community, senior centers are to offer opportunities for:

1. Helping older people to remain in the community by assisting them to maintain their emotional well-being
2. Helping the community to be aware of the needs of its older citizens, pointing up gaps and needed services
3. Providing a resource of volunteer manpower from among the membership for public and private nonprofit community agencies and organizations

Achieving these goals requires that a center's program be integrated and woven into the community fabric.

Lowy (1974) categorizes center programs into four groupings:

1. Direct services to older people
2. Services offered to and through other institutions
3. Community action with and on behalf of older people
4. Training, consultation, and research activity

Direct services include: recreation-educational programs (arts and crafts, nature, science/outdoor life, drama, physical activity, music, dance, games, social activities such as parties, literary activities, exercises, hobby/special interests, speakers, lectures, movies, forums, etc.); social services (information; counseling and referral; protective services that are preventive, supportive, and therapeutic; friendly visiting; homemakers; telephone reassurance; day care; group work; etc.); nutrition services (congregate meals programs, meals on wheels, nutritional and dietary information); and respite care to relieve caretaking family members.

Services offered to and through other institutions, such as hospitals, housing projects, nursing homes, and rehabilitation centers, include: bringing together existing institutions for the delivery of services to older persons and setting up and arranging for homecare programs with appropriate community institutions and agencies.

Community action, transportation, and advocacy include: planning for community projects and programs, coordinating facilities and making them accessible to older people near places where they reside, identifying new needs and new problems as well as representing the interests of older people as a group (e.g., at public hearings) through advocacy and setting up legislative information services.

Training, consultation, and research include: training volunteers and part-time staff for a variety of functions, consulting to community agencies and institutions related to needs and problems of the elderly, and serving as centers for research on needs and problems of older people in our society.

"A Senior Center should serve as a community facility to provide services on a coordinated, continuous, and comprehensive basis and thereby reduce fragmentation to a minimum. Such a Center would be able to deliver services where they are needed and when they are needed" (Lowy, 1974, p. 8).

Another way of classifying services has been adopted by the NISC:

1. Individual services: counseling/referral, employment, health maintenance and screening, services for the homebound, transportation
2. Group services: recreation, nutrition, education, social group work
3. Community services: social services provided by older persons to community institutions, social action, and advocacy

Data collected by NISC/NCOA showed that most multipurpose senior centers offer at least three basic services: education, recreation, and information and referral/counseling. Presently most provide, in addition, volunteer opportunities and health and social services. Averaging across all types of senior group programs, the most frequently offered services are recreation (especially arts and crafts), information and referral (especially for health), participant and outreach counseling (mostly in areas of health), and education. Recreational activities (arts, crafts, games, and movies) are not only frequently offered but also draw very large attendances. Information and referral services are also much used. The largest turnout, however, is generated by nutritional programs on the premises. In 1979, 50 percent of all centers were serving hot lunches on five or more days each week. An additional 15 percent were serving lunches between one and four times per week. These figures have increased significantly due to increased availability of public funds under Title III-C of the Older Americans act. In addition to meals served at the center, almost a third of the centers report that they offer meals-on-wheels programs to homebound per-sons in the community. Membership on governing groups, although offered by most centers, shows a markedly low use. Self-governance has declined since the 1960s and early 1970s. Now most senior-center members are not active in any governance activity and rely on staff to govern and operate centers, which is a serious problem since leadership development is a major objective of senior-center programming.

The degree to which senior centers are linked with the community's service network is illustrated by the fact that most centers report contacts with local or county agencies, welfare departments, and local Social Security offices. Com-munity health and welfare organizations are also seen as two-way contact points; for referral and communication and as information and service resources for communitywide programs for the elderly. Centers assist other community agencies, cooperate in joint service delivery, or convene meetings of aging groups. Many centers provide training opportunities for college and graduate students and for agency personnel.

Institutions most often contacted by senior-center members are nursing homes, schools, and colleges. Outreach services are offered in over half the centers. Outreach is one of the methods most often used by centers to let the community, especially older residents, know about its programs. Other frequently used publicity channels include newspapers, newsletters, and posters. Television, radio spots, and community bulletins are also widely utilized.

PROGRAMS FOR IMPAIRED OLDER PERSONS

A recent study (NISC, 1980) found that 84 percent of the 8,000 centers nationwide are serving at-risk/frail, physically or mentally impaired, and chronically ill older people in some form or another. Since many center programs are oriented to recognize individual needs, they enhance the continuity of care for at-risk older people through coordination of services with community agencies and thereby facilitate access to a broad spectrum of health and social services. Strategies designed by senior centers to help at-risk older persons include encouraging self-help and mutual support, promoting integration of frail older adults with their more able peers, and drawing at-risk individuals into program planning and decision making.

Centers, sporadically but increasingly, offer respite care to families; integrate the visually and hearing-impaired into group programs; link day-care clients to senior centers; reach out to the homebound and nursing-home patients; provide information, education, and support programs for families; and expand opportunities for access to services for the mentally impaired.

Training programs sponsored by centers, often in concert with colleges, offer guidance to practitioners on serving and integrating the frail and impaired older person into the center's group program. The overall purpose of such training is to provide knowledge and skills required to meet special needs and to develop and strengthen linkages between center programs and other community-based service providers.

To what extent further inclusion of at-risk elderly will affect the attitudes, feelings, and participation of the "well elderly"—who have been the mainstays of the centers—and how such an integration of two groups of the elderly population on the health continuum will reshape the goals, purposes, operation, and organization of the centers is at this time an unknown. Will the center become another competing institution in the aging network mainly oriented to serving the vulnerable, or will it maintain its original quality with a potential for the future as was expressed in the early 1970s:

A Senior Center must become a core-institution (in the sociological sense of the term) which is truly identified and visible as an indigenous facility of the elderly. Children have their schools, young and middle-aged adults have their institutions, whether in the world of work or in the world of leisure. Somehow, older people have become excluded from most of them and their world has become identified as the Nursing Home and the Old Folks' Home. The Senior Center can indeed become a community institution for all the older people whether "needy" or not. It is identified with well-ness and not with debility. This can be enhanced by linking it with younger people through joint projects which have meaning to old and young. Youth would work with the elderly on their own "home ground" and they in turn could reciprocate by working with young people on their "home ground." Thus a base for identity would be established and intergenerational communication would be facilitated. This may lead to opportunities to develop new roles and a new status for the elderly simply by being aged in their own right. A Center can become a springboard for learning new roles such as making a contribution in new service roles such as home-health aides, foster grandparents, friendly visitors, and tutors to children, to name a few. Needed by our society, such roles can raise the status of the elderly on their own terms and would lead to the establishment of new relationships with the community. Instead of isolation and alienation, a sense of belonging would result because older people have a stake in the community again, which would be manifested to them by community acceptance (Lowy, 1974, p. 9).

In such a community institution older people can be hosts rather than guests and, thereby, achieve a more equitable symmetry in negotiating their status with the nonelderly.

SOME MAJOR CHARACTERISTICS OF SENIOR CENTERS TODAY

Size and Location

Since there is no rigorous definition of a senior center, and since there are a great variety of senior group programs (many of them represent small local initiatives) and no registration or licensing standards are in force, one should not be surprised if neither an exact number of senior centers nor detailed characteristics about them are known. As of 1982, NISC claimed that an estimated 8 million older persons were being served in 8,000 centers throughout the country. Over half of all senior group programs are located in cities. In suburbs, senior clubs are far more prevalent than multipurpose senior centers, whereas in rural areas multipurpose senior centers predominate.

Finances and Facilities

Over half the senior centers are funded by public funds, while less than a fifth rely exclusively on private dollars. The remaining numbers receive funds from both public and private sources, a trend that is likely to increase despite present economic and social-policy directions.

The average center budget expanded from $17,652 in 1968 to $50,000 in 1974, and by 1982 it had exceeded $90,000. These figures do not include in-kind contributions, which in some instances may represent a significant portion of a center's resources.

As the senior center is often the single most visible institution for a community's older residents, and as the type of facility greatly determines programming possibilities, the type of facility in which senior centers are located is of considerable importance: a fourth of all centers operate out of their own facility; approximately a fifth operate from churches or synagogues; a third are located in recreation centers or local- or county-government facilities; approximately 10 percent meet in community centers of nonprofit organizations; and another 10 percent in Housing Authority buildings; and about 5 percent meet in private, commercial facilities.

As to the condition and appropriateness of these facilities, half of center facilities were renovated, presumably with the needs of senior members in mind. However, over a third of all centers operate in old buildings that have not been altered. On the other hand, a fourth of all present centers are located in new buildings, and roughly two-thirds are single-level facilities, eliminating the architectural barrier of stair climbing.

While facilities thus range from large, modern, well-designed centers to modest two- or three-room storefronts, several problems are shared by most of them. Two out of three centers are too small to function properly, which leads to all rooms being continually in use, often for purposes for which they were not designed. An important shortcoming is the frequency with which centers fail to provide adequate facilities for handicapped members. Parking ramps and bathrooms are often inadequate for members confined to wheelchairs. Even when accessibility has been assured, often the locations of phones, fountains, towel dispensers, and elevator call buttons are inconvenient. These physical shortcomings have a negative impact on a center's capacity to provide adequate services for vulnerable and handicapped elderly. With the advent of increasing numbers of at-risk ederly center members, concern about physical shortcomings of facilities will mount significantly.

Staffing

Staffing is perhaps the single most important organizational parameter. The nature, the atmosphere, indeed the very success of a senior center is in large measure dependent on the size, attitudes, competence, skills, dedication, and creativity of its staff.

The average center staff is small. As many as a fourth of all multipurpose senior centers did not have a single full-time, paid staff person in 1975. Another third had only one full-time staff person, and about a fifth of the centers had a full-time staff of four or more. Many centers rely on volunteers and staff from other agencies for part of their regular programming. Also, over half of all centers are part of a larger network of multiple sites with personnel and services distributed throughout, so that the staff at any given site represents only a portion of the available manpower.

Although many centers have their staffs provide all services offered at the site, those that have time-sharing arrangements with other agencies concentrate their own activities mostly on information and referral, arts and crafts, and

288   L. Lowy

recreation. They are unlikely to provide educational programs, home-delivered meals, or health, legal, employment, and library services that require special skills. Staff from other agencies are utilized to provide these services.

Volunteers (including members) in many centers contribute substantially to the program. Center participant volunteers usually assist with serving meals and with arts and recreation activities; community volunteers generally help with delivering meals to people's homes and with conducting educational programs.

The educational level of center directors is diverse. According to 1975 data, most had at least some college experience and approximately a fifth had attended graduate schools, chiefly schools of social work; a fourth had no post-high-school training. One explanation for the small size of many center staffs and their modest educational levels can be found in the low salaries; only a fourth of all center directors received salaries over $20,000 in 1980.

Seminars, on-the-job training, and paid attendance at professional meetings are offered by about half of all centers, whereas paid tuition for attending institutes and workshops has markedly decreased in recent years.

Representative Centers

The following brief profiles describe three typical multiservice centers of varying size and type:

H Center is open five days a week and offers a variety of social, educational, and physical activities. The center has bowling lanes and a swimming pool. Its members assist the staff with all the programs, including the therapeutic swim program for Stroke Club members.

P Center was built with capital improvement funds in 1967 on an eighteen-hole golf course. The center has lawn bowling, tennis, and shuffleboard courts. P Center organized one of the first summer camping programs for seniors and has both men's and women's choruses. It is the home of Senior Adults, Inc., publishers of News since 1968, and the home of an extensive travel program serving more than its 3,000 members. Numerous other activities are offered during the hours of operation each week. Programs are funded by public and private sources, including federal, state, county, and city agencies, the board of education, as well as United Way, unions, churches, and schools. The center includes special programs for the physically and mentally handicapped.

E Retiree Center serves a rural community, using a converted residence. Volunteers (there is no paid staff) oversee the center's operation. Open five days a week, it provides recreation and social services and is funded through the municipality as a special project of state government.

The organization chart in Figure 12-1 illustrates the structure of a typical multipurpose senior center.

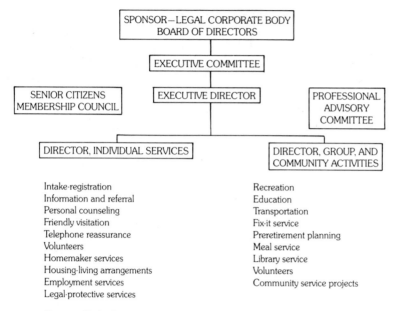

Figure 12-1. Organization Chart of a Typical Multipurpose Senior Center

STANDARDS FOR MULTISERVICE SENIOR CENTERS

For many years the NISC has sought to develop standards for senior centers. In 1975 the AoA of the U.S. Department of Health, Education and Welfare provided funds to the NCOA to develop program guidelines and standards of practice for senior centers.

The need for standards was documented by the findings of a two-year comprehensive national study of community-based senior group programs. The findings supported the senior center's function as a focal point for services, providing opportunities for older persons and serving as a community resource for all age groups. It also revealed that there were no evaluation criteria or even clear definitions for senior-center programs. While some senior-center programs were the focal point for a community's concern for its older citizens, others were functioning in a limited manner and not serving segments of the older population who could benefit from a more adequate center program. While some of the weaknesses revealed in the study could be attributed to limited resources, there was evidence that they were also related in important ways to an inadequate understanding of good center practices and sound administration.

A Standards and Guidelines Steering Committee and five subcommittees of the NCOA developed guidelines and standards in areas related to management, operation, programming, facility, and community relations. These subcommittees were made up of recognized authorities reflecting not only the serveral professions and disciplines that underlie center programming and operations, but also the diversity of facilities that function as or sponsor senior centers.

In addition to providing general information input, center directors and others related to centers participated in pilot testing of the standards and the self-assessment instrument developed by the committee, reviewed the guidelines, and made recommendations regarding their dissemination and utilization. The resultant standards are contained in NISC (1978).

Senior-Center Philosophy

Through the years, the senior-center field has evolved a philosophy that provides a perspective concerning the place of a senior center in the community's network of human services and an associated value orientation about older persons. Whereas other organizations and groups focus their attention upon health, housing, economic stability, and other more limited aspects of the older person's existence, a senior center has a commitment to all aspects of living, its program providing opportunities and alternatives for enhancing the quality of life of the later years. "The Senior-Center Philosophy" appears in NISC (1978, p. 5):

A senior center seeks to create an atmosphere that acknowledges the value of human life, individually and collectively, and affirms the dignity and self-worth of the older adult. This atmosphere provides for the reaffirmation of creative potential, the power of decision making, the skills of coping and defending, the warmth of caring, sharing, giving, and supporting. The uniqueness of the senior center stems from its total concern for older people and its concern for the total older person. In an atmosphere of wellness, it develops strengths and encourages independence, while building interdependence and supporting unavoidable dependencies. It works *with* older persons, not *for* them, enabling and facilitating their decisions and actions, and in so doing creates and supports a sense of community that further enables older persons to continue their involvement with and contribution to the larger community.

The philosophy of the senior-center movement is based on the premises that aging is a normal developmental process; that human beings need peers with whom they can interact and who are available as a source of encouragement and support; and that adults have the right to have a voice in determining matters in which they have a vital interest.

In accordance with these premises and on the basis of experience, the senior-center field adheres to the following beliefs:

Older people are individuals and adults with ambitions, capabilities and creative capacities.

They are capable of continued growth and development.

They, like all people, need both access to sources of information and help for personal and family problems and the opportunity to learn from individuals coping with similar experiences.

They have a right to make choices and to be part of decision-making processes.

Senior center staffs are obliged to create and maintain a climate of respect, trust, and support, and to provide opportunities for older people to exercise their skills and to develop their potential as experienced adults within the context of the whole community to which they belong and to which they bring their wisdom, experience and insight.

As senior centers evolve and adapt to meet the changing needs and interests of older persons, so the philosophy will continue to evolve until positive images of age have become a general perception of reality and senior centers are regarded as a regular community facility serving the older population. Then senior centers will truly be "social utilities," as freely available and generally supported as libraries, parks, and beaches.

Senior Center Principles

The standards are organized into nine sections, each enunciating a basic principle: purpose, organization, community relations, program, administration and personnel, fiscal management, records and reports, facility, and evaluation (NISC, 1978, p. 17).

I. Purpose—A senior center shall have a written statement of its purposes consistent with the Senior Center Philosophy and a written statement of its goals based on its purposes and on the needs and interests of older people in its service area. These statements shall be used to govern the character and direction of its operation and program.

Major subject areas include: philosophy, goals, and program objectives and their uses.

II. Organization—A senior center shall be organized to create effective relationships among the participants, staff, governing body and the community in order to achieve its purposes and goals.

This section deals with legal sanctions; documents related to the constitution and bylaws of the center; information about the organizational structure, role, functioning and composition, and responsibilities of the governing and advisory body; and involvement of the membership in governance.

III. Community Relations—A senior center shall form cooperative arrangements with community agencies and organizations in order to serve as a focal point for older people to obtain access to comprehensive services. A center shall be a source of public information, community education, advocacy and opportunities for community involvement of older people.

Linkages with community, involvement of other agencies of the aging network, coordination and planning mechanisms, and creation of volunteer and employment opportunities are part of this section.

IV. Program—A senior center shall provide a broad range of group and individual activities and services designed to respond to the interrelated needs and interests of older people in its service area.

This section addresses the way in which the needs of older persons are taken into consideration in program planning, in the setting of priorities, and in the operation of activities and services. It looks at program scope, diversity, atmosphere, accessibility, outreach efforts, engagement and participation by members, quality of program, and use of staff.

V. Administration and Personnel—A senior center shall have clear administrative and personnel policies and procedures that contribute to the effective management of its operation. It shall be staffed by qualified, paid and volunteer personnel, capable of implementing its program.

The deployment of personnel, staffing patterns and responsibilities, job descriptions, personnel policies and practices, staff development programs, use of volunteers in relation to nonvolunteers, interaction of staff, and emergency arrangements are included in this section.

VI. Fiscal Management—A senior center shall practice sound fiscal planning, management, record keeping and reporting.

Securing of financial resources, fiscal planning and reporting, risk, protection (insurance), fiscal management and purchasing procedures as well as inventory control belong in this section.

VII. Records and Reports—A senior center shall keep complete records required to operate, plan and review its program. It shall regularly prepare and circulate reports to inform its board, its participants, staff, sponsors, funders and the general public about its operation and program.

To what extent participant records and reports related to programs, and administrative records and reports related to operations, are kept is at the heart of the maintenance of confidentiality and necessitates appropriate safeguards.

VIII. Facility—A senior center shall make use of appropriate facilities for its program. Such facilities shall be designed, located, constructed or renovated and equipped so as to promote effective access to and conduct of its program and to provide for the health, safety and comfort of participants, staff and public.

Responsibilities for building, grounds, and equipment and assurance of physical comfort, safety, and quality is the concern of this part of the assessment and planning guide.

IX. Evaluation—A senior center shall have adequate arrangements to monitor, evaluate and report on its operation and program.

A senior center shall have or be part of an evaluation system that will assist it to determine the extent to which the center is achieving its purposes, goals, and objectives, is truly meeting the needs and interests of its participants, and is efficient and effective in the operation of the center and its program.

The formal and informal evaluation arrangements, the basic elements of an evaluation system, and its sources and results to be used and disseminated are the essential aspects of this criterion.

Based on these criteria, a "self-assessment instrument" has been developed (NISC, 1979). The emphasis is on self-assessment and not on accreditation, though the idea of accrediting centers has been entertained by the NCOA for some time. So far no concrete plans have emerged that would place an accreditation function in the hands of NCOA or any other organization. Standard-setting and upgrading center quality is predicated upon voluntary compliance rather than upon mandatory review.

Whether the advent of these standards and the use of the self-assessment instrument has contributed to a more uniform quality of practice of center operations is as yet unknown. The practice principles guiding each of these nine sections are criteria not only to assess prevailing standards of a multiservice center but also serve as prescriptive tools to plan and operate such a facility. The self-assessment instrument can assist a center in a number of ways:

(1) It can help assess the extent to which a senior center's policies, procedures, and program conform to the standards of good practice.

(2) It can help a center systematically prepare and plan responses appropriate to growth in the program, changes in the demographic composition of older people in the community, and changes in available resources.

(3) Through its use, a center can systematically collect information about its operation and program, showing how each component of the center is interrelated.

(4) It can help recognize areas where further training and technical assistance may be needed to improve a center's operation and program.

(5) Its use can promote the development of skills related to planning, evaluation, and program development and provide opportunities for all those involved in the process to exchange ideas about a center.

SOCIAL WORK AND SENIOR CENTERS

Historically, social work has played a significant role in the creation, design, and operation of senior centers. Names associated with the center movement such as Landau, Mathiason, Levine, Eckstein, Maxwell, Lowy, Tarrell, Cohen, Schreiber, Marks, and Dobroff attest to this fact. And social workers have continued to play an important part in the provision and administration of a variety of services to older persons in and through multiservice centers as part of gerontological social work. Social action to bring about changes on the community level, and human growth and development through group participation on the individual and family levels, have been the twin focuses of social work and the senior-center movement.

Social workers have assumed major functional responsibility for counseling, information/referral, and case-management functions. Techniques of psycho-social support, crisis intervention, problem identification, assessment and resolution are essential ingredients of many direct-service programs offered in or through a senior center. The role of case manager as a link to other services calls for social-work competencies.

Self-help and mutual-support groups rely on the skills of social workers to get them started and to be available as consultants and backup persons. Advocacy functions demand community organization skills that are made accessible and available in a variety of ways. Social workers also conduct training programs (in-service or orientation) for staff, volunteers, and board members, and frequently offer supervision to staff members (paid and volunteer) and students in field training.

Senior centers have a diversity of staffing patterns; this is reflected in the use and distribution of social workers. Although centers are not an exclusive domain of social-work activity, social workers are engaged in planning and providing services as well as in mangagement functions at many centers. The inclusion of at-risk elderly as a result of the implementation of the NISC study has led to an increased infusion of social workers as well as other mental-health professional into the staffing patterns of senior centers.

THEORETICAL BASES OF SENIOR CENTERS

Senior centers base their efforts on a philosophy of human growth. A humanistic belief in the creative potential of people emphasizes that older people are individuals in their own right. They are adults with capabilities, creative capacities, and aspirations. They have the capacity for continuing development. They may need access to information and services. They may need help for personal or family problems. They may need opportunities to learn from individuals coping with similar experiences. Yet most of all, they may need support for being themselves to affirm their identity in dignity and with respect. These beliefs bear unmistakable resemblance to the humanistic psychology of Maslow and the therapeutic theory of Rogers.

Most centers prefer an activity rather than a disengagement view of aging. They believe that aging is a natural part of life and that adults have a right to make their own life choices. One major assumption of centers is that human beings need peers for interaction and support. Senior-center staff are expected to create an atmosphere that acknowledges the value of human life and affirms the self-worth of the older person through projecting an attitude of respect, trust, and mutual support. To help older people actualize their potential, centers provide opportunities for decision making, service to others, and creative activity. To support ego maintenance, opportunities for exercising coping skills are combined with interpersonal support and warmth. The concern for vulnerable older people and their needs and problems requires further theoretical articulation that has not yet occurred.

Two conceptual models of senior centers can be contrasted: the "social agency model," which views the senior center as a collection of programs designed to meet the needs of the elderly and predicts that the poor and disengaged are the most likely candidates for participation in senior centers; and the "voluntary association model," which views the senior center as a joinable community group and predicts that those elderly will join who are more actively involved in voluntary associations and who manifest a stronger interest in the community (Taietz, 1976).

Senior centers fulfill a useful function under either model. But if center representatives wish to stand by the social-agency model, intervention efforts can be directed to more isolated or at-risk target groups with attendent consequences for membership, program, and image.

PUBLIC POLICY

Since senior centers have been, for the most part, born out of local initiative and are supported by local governments, private nonprofit organizations, or civic units, they have developed their own priorities and their own place in the community and will continue even without federal money. In the early 1960s there were attempts to support the growth of senior centers with federal funds. In 1964, for instance, Congressman Claude Pepper introduced H.R. 4055 and H.R. 4056. In the same year the Smothers-Mills Bill (H.R. 5840, S. 1357) proposed to secure funding for both the construction and operation of senior centers. No action was taken then.

The Older Americans Act

In 1965 the Senate considered a bill entitled the Senior Citizens Community Planning and Service Act of 1965 that would have covered 50 percent of center construction costs. The House then considered a more comprehensive bill (H.R. 4409), the Senior Activity Centers and Community Service Act of 1965, which would have supported both construction and operational expenses. The act that finally passed both houses and was signed by the President was the Older Americans Act of 1965. It contained no separate title for senior center funds, but Title IV was devoted to "Research and Development Projects," and it specified in Section 401(2) that the Commissioner on Aging could provide funds for the purpose of "developing or demonstrating new approaches, techniques, and methods (including the use of multipurpose activity centers) which hold promise of substantial contribution toward wholesome and meaningful living for older persons." Yet the same act also stated explicitly that, with respect to the extablishment of new programs or expansion of existing programs with Title III funds, "... no costs of construction, other than for minor alterations and repairs, shall be included in such establishment or expansion." Thus senior-center applications were limited to the relatively smaller funds in Title IV.

In 1972 a major revision of the Older Americans Act provided an explicit title for senior centers. This bill was pocket vetoed by President Nixon. However, in the following year the 1973 amendments to the Older Americans Act (P.L. 93-29) resulted in a major revision of the entire Act. These amendments (incorporated mainly in the revised Title III) overshadowed the incorporation of another new title called Multipurpose Senior Centers, known as Title V.

The purpose of Title V was "to provide a focal point in communities for the development and delivery of social services and nutritional services designed primarily for older persons." The strategy through which this purpose was to be achieved consisted of making available grant or contract funds to pay up to 75 percent of the costs of acquiring, altering, or renovating existing facilities to serve as multipurpose senior centers. The title vested authority for application approval and fund disbursement directly in the Commissioner on Aging.

With the 1978 amendments to the Older Americans Act, another overhaul took place. Title III was expanded by consolidating the social services, nutrition, and multipurpose-center provisions of the act and thereby eliminated Title V. (Since 1978, the Senior Community-Service Employment Program has been Title V). Funding for multi-service centers was now included as part of funding for supportive social services and congregate and home-delivery nutrition services. Through grants to states, which award monies to Area Agencies on Aging for community planning, these funds are used in accordance with a state-approved area-agency plan.

Since the amendments of 1978 require the development of specified services (states are to spend at least 50 percent of social services on three categories: access, in-home, and legal services), senior centers have found it necessary to develop such specified services in order to qualify for federal funding. The impact of federal dollars on the goals, directions, and programming of senior centers is quite evident.

Reauthorization of the Older Americans Act was passed by Congress in the fall of 1981, and again in the fall of 1984. The Act retains language to continue separate authorizations under Title III, as under the 1978 amendments. Senior centers have to compete with other Title III programs for funding; this means a loss of identity for them with attendent consequences for goals, programs, membership composition, and philsophy as well as organizational context. Only during 1977 and 1978 were separate funds for senior centers appropriated ($20 million and $40 million, respectively). Now centers have to compete again for funds via budgets of Title III and other federal programs besides the Older Americans Act. Both the Nixon and Ford administrations argued that no money should be authorized for Title V, since there already existed sufficient other programs (e.g., under the Housing and Community Development Act of 1974) that could fund senior centers. A look at the record of the Department of Housing and Urban Development indicates that the overall impact of grants made by this department has been small: few dollars actually reached senior centers. In times of inflation and local tax revolts, many communities have difficulties financing even their basic services (school, fire department, criminal justice system), and the proportion of federal tax receipts continues to decrease. That is why senior centers find it increasingly difficult to compete effectively for a share of the shrinking dollar base. When they are successful, it is primarily for those activities that are "fundable" under the federal guidelines.

When President Reagan signed the Older Americans Act Amendments of 1984, he created a new Title VII, "Personal Health Education and Training Programs for Older Individuals," for discretionary grants and contracts with institutions of higher education to design health education and training programs for replication in multipurpose senior centers. It is too early to tell how this new title will affect the role of senior centers in the health education field, especially since no money was appropriated for the program in fiscal year 1984-85.

In addition, funds from nongovernmental sources continue to be sought by NCOA as well as by individual senior centers. Service contract agreements with federal programs, matching funding from private foundations, and creative fund-raising activities are the fiscal underpinnings of multiservice centers today.

Policy Issues and Future Directions

At least three major policy issues can be identified dealing with program membership and functional emphasis.

1. Program emphasis: education/recreation vs. treatment

Senior centers started as places for older people to gather for enjoyment and relaxation. As the multiple needs of older people became more apparent, however, social and health services began to be offered along with recreational activities in many centers. In these budget-conscious times, paying millions of dollars for "fun and games" is seen by many as frivolous. In a climate of inflation, tax revolts, and curtailment of social programs as against expansion of military programs, the federal government has taken the position that its resources must address the most basic needs of the most destitute elderly, "the truly needy." Senior-center advocates support offering more services because their location in a senior center makes them more acceptable to the elderly client. But to "help impaired older persons maintain independent living" requires a major shift in program focus and staffing patterns.

Faced with such a shift, many members of a center may feel alarmed and even resentful. While it is true that, as an expression of concern at the national-policy level, senior citizens strongly support the goal of independent community living, this does not mean that members of a local senior center would support having their facility turn into a major health-service institution.

And what will distinguish a senior center from another type of social/health service agency in competition for scarce resources? How will the vision of a center as an indigenous social-host institution for the well older person fare?

2. Membership emphasis: mainstream vs. impaired elderly?

Since senior centers started as a grass-roots movement in local communities, they were initiated by and designed for people with fairly adequate economic resources. As a result, current data reflect underrepresentation of the less economically privileged and the minority elderly.

With increased federal involvement and new grass-roots awareness in senior centers, the emphasis on serving low-income and minority elderly at a center now serving white, middle-class people can be increased. But the federal commitment to minorities—old or young—has considerably abated in the 1980s, and establishing new centers in areas where minority members reside so far achieves only program availability, not integration of different-background elders.

Another issue concerns the elderly's health status. The new emphasis on attracting "at-risk older persons" will invariably bring about not only shifts in service and program directions but also lead to new membership compositions. Will membership status become client status, and will a "social utility" become a "case-service" facility?

3. Functional emphasis: direct services vs. coordination

Since 1973, state and area agencies have been viewed by the AoA as the cornerstone of the aging network. Senior centers had emerged long before the Older Americans Act, at a time when the aged were first discovered as a group with special service needs. Indeed, many of what we now consider aging services can be said to have originated around senior centers. During the past thirty years, senior centers have become in many communities the symbol of services to the aged, the outward and visible focus for the community's concern for its elderly residents. As such, centers are already involved in or informed about many aspects of community activities that would be of interest to their members. Centers do perform direct program *and* coordinating functions.

With the advent and maturation of state and area agencies, the relationship of senior centers to the aging network needs further study and analysis. Generally, centers will acknowledge the area agencies as the central planning and administrative agencies. In return, they want to be acknowledged as the community focal point for aging services. In this model a community would have two focal aging institutions: the area agency would be responsible for fund administration and area-wide planning; the senior center would be the delivery site for these services and programs. Developments so far have not supported the practical implementation of such a model. Despite the intent of Title III to coordinate various social, nutrition, and senior-center services within their planning and service areas, such coordination was not very successful, and fragmentation is still the order of the day. Given the political and economic climate of the 1980s, centers are unlikely to become major coordinating mechanisms; in fact, they will more likely move more and more toward direct-service provisions and, if any coordinating takes place at all, leave this to state and area agencies or councils on aging. The rejection of the 1977 AoA's Multiservice Senior Centers Initiative, introduced by then Commissioner Arthur Flemming, to designate centers as focal points for meeting needs of the elderly in a community in 1978, made the trend quite clear. This does not suggest that individual centers in individual communities may not fulfill some coordinating functions.

Future Options

At this juncture of our social policy, a number of major questions must be addressed and research must be undertaken to bring data to bear on the process of social-policy shaping.

1. What are the demographic trends in specific states, areas, and communities? Who are the most likely target groups for senior centers? Will we move toward a family orientation and eventually toward a family policy?
2. What are the political trends in the field of aging? How will aging policy be shaped following the 1981 White House Conference on Aging, and how will this policy affect senior centers?
3. What are the economic trends affecting the social, health, and educational priorities in the United States? How will these trends influence income, health, housing, and social-service policy and their implementation in the aging network? What will be the place of centers in this network within the context of supply-side economics?
4. What are the sociocultural trends in our society and how will the high-technology revolution affect not only the social and cultural macrostructure but also the microstructure of four-generation families and their individual members? Will senior centers be able to respond to newly

emerging needs, problems, and crises? Will they become instrumental in designing programs that serve the differential needs and aspirations of a heterogenous aging population and the "sandwich generation"? Will they become "host" institutions, with identities of their own, as socio-cultural centers for older people and serve as "guests" for others? Will they be hammer or anvil, leaders or followers, in the redesign of social institutions to respond to demographic, political, economic, and socio-cultural changes.

Penetrating analytical thinking will produce more refined and differentiated questions, which, in turn, must be examined and studied. A research strategy that concentrates on such an agenda is likely to yield answers not only for the future role of multiservice senior centers, but also for the population as a whole.

REFERENCES AND BIBLIOGRAPHY

Adams, D. L. (1971). Correlates of satisfaction among the elderly. *Gerontologist*, **11**(4), 64-68.

Anderson, N. (1969). *Senior centers: Information from a nationwide survey.* Minneapolis: American Rehabilitation Foundation.

Conrad, W. R. Jr., and Glenn, W. E. (1976). *The effective voluntary board of directors: What it is and how it works.* Chicago: Swallow Press.

Gelwicks, L. E. (1975). The older person's relation to the environment: The effects of transportation. In E. J. Cantilli and Schmelzer (Eds.), *Transportation and aging: Selected issues.* Washington: Government Printing Office.

Graney, M. J. (1975). Happiness and social participation in aging. *Journal of Gerontology*, **30**(6), 701-706.

Hanssen, A. M., et al. (1978). Correlates of senior center participation. *Gerontologist*, **18**(2), 193-199.

Jacobs, B. (Ed.). (1974). *Social action: Expanding role for senior centers.* Washington: National Council on the Aging.

Jacobs, B. (1976). *Working with the impaired elderly.* Washington: National Council on the Aging.

Jacobs, B., Lindsley, P., and Feil, M. (1976). *A guide to intergenerational programming.* Washington: National Institute of Senior Centers, National Council on the Aging.

Jordan, J. J. (1975). *Senior center facilities: An architect's evaluation of building design, equipment and furnishings.* Washington: National Institute of Senior Centers, National Council on the Aging.

Jordan, J. J. (1978). *Senior center design: An architect's discussion of facility planning.* Washington: National Institute of Senior Centers, National Council on the Aging.

Kubie, S. H., and Landau, G. (1953). *Group work with the aged.* New York: International Universities Press.

Leanse, J., Tiven, M., and Robb, T. B. (1977). *Senior center operation: A guide to operation and management.* Washington: National Institute of Senior Centers, National Council on the Aging.

Louis Harris and Associates. (1981). *The myth and reality of aging in America.* Washington National Council on the Aging.

Lowy, L. (1955). *Adult education and groupwork.* New York: Whiteside/Morrow.

Lowy, L. (1974). The senior center—A major community facility today and tomorrow. *Perspective on Aging.* **3**(2), 5-9.

Lowy, L. (1979). *Social work with the aging.* New York: Harper & Row (2nd ed., Longman, 1985).

Maxwell, J. (1973). *Centers for older people.* Washington: National Council on the Aging.

National Council on the Aging. (1962). *Centers for older people: Guide for programs and facilities.* New York: The Council.

National Council on the Aging. (1972). *The multi-purpose senior center: A model community action program.* Washington: The Council.

National Council on the Aging. (1978). *Fact book on aging: A profile of America's older population.* Washington: The Council.

National Institute of Senior Centers. (1974). *Directory of senior centers and clubs.* Washington: National Council on the Aging.

National Institute of Senior Centers. (1975). *Senior centers: Report of senior group programs in America.* Washington: National Council on the Aging.

National Institute of Senior Centers. (1978). *Senior center standards: Guidelines for practice.* Washington: National Council on the Aging.

National Institute of Senior Centers. (1979). *Senior center standards: Self-assessment workbook.* Washington: National Council on the Aging.

National Institute of Senior Centers. (1980). *Senior centers and the at-risk older person: A project report.* Washington: National Institute of Senior Centers, National Council on the Aging.

Ralston, P. A. (1982). Perception of senior centers by the black elderly: A comparative study. *Journal of Gerontological Social Work, 4*(3/4), 127-137.

Storey, R. T. (1962). Who attends a senior activity center? A comparison of Little House members with non-members in the same community. *Gerontologist, 2*(4), 216-222.

Taietz, P. (1976). Two conceptual models of the senior center. *Journal of Gerontology, 31*(2), 219-222.

Trela, J. E., and Simmons, L. W. (1971). Health and other factors affecting membership and attrition in a senior center. *Journal of Gerontology, 26*(1), 46-51.

Tuckman, J. (1967). Factors related to attendance in a center for older people. *Journal of the American Geriatrics Society, 15*(5), 474-479.

U.S. Congress. Senate. Special Committee on Aging. (1978). *Senior centers and the Older Americans Act.* Washington: Government Printing Office.

Vickery, F. E. (1972). *Creative programming for older adults: A leadership training guide.* New York: Association Press.

Weiss, C. H. (Ed.). (1972). *Evaluating action programs.* Boston: Allyn & Bacon.

White House Conference on Aging. (1982). *Final report: The 1981 White House Conference on Aging.* 3 vols. Washington: The Conference.

Author's Note: The author wishes to acknowledge helpful ideas contributed by the work of W. Maulen, Chicago, Ill., in his studies of senior centers.

13

Services to Older and Retired Workers

Judith Wineman, M.S.W., C.S.W.

International Ladies' Garment Workers' Union, New York

The provision of social services by trade unions antedates the large and complex social-service bureaucracy we know today. In recent years, the parallel interests of unions and employers have given rise to a rapidly expanding field of industrial social work under private auspices, such as unions. Fifty or sixty years ago, these "parallel interests" were nowhere to be found. Trade unions were young and struggling for recognition. The concept of people working together meant people helping each other, too. The union representative whose initial task was to help members with job-related issues soon became the basis of "social unionism," the belief that the union is a way of life rather than an economic organization whose sole purpose is to improve wages and working conditions.

The trade unions' commitment to their retired members stems from this philosophy of social unionism. This chapter describes union retiree service programs with particular reference to the International Ladies' Garment Workers' Union (ILGWU), the Amalgamated Clothing and Textile Workers' Union (ACTWU), and District 65 of the United Automobile Workers (UAW). The members of these unions have not participated in the trend toward early retirement characteristic of the U.S. labor force as a whole that is due in part to the institution of private pension plans that supplement workers' Social Security benefits. In the steel and auto industries (at least until the difficult times for these industries in the late 1970s) a major retirement period was between ages 60 and

62. In the public employee unions—police, fire, and government—the trend has been toward even earlier retirement—for example, between the ages of 50 and 55.

The workers described in this chapter are at the opposite end of the scale in terms of skills and wages. For example, there has never been a mandatory retirement age in the women's apparel industry. The major incentive to retire is eligibility for full Social Security benefits at age 65. Pensions in the industry are low, and the seasonal nature of the work builds in a certain amount of "forced unemployment" over a person's work history that may delay eligibility for a full pension. The retired workers served by the ILGWU, ACTWU, and District 65 are therefore older and, in most cases, retired from industries that are themselves rapidly aging: apparel, textile, and light manufacturing. The population is overwhelmingly female, part of the huge immigrant wave of the first quarter of the twentieth century. They are multilingual, multiethnic, multiracial: Jews, Italians, Irish, Hispanics, blacks. They worked as sewing-machine operators, weavers, milliners, shipping clerks, and packers. Their wages were low and their work often seasonal.

Many of these people view social work as charity for poor people; the image of "welfare worker" still often attaches to the name social worker. Furthermore, they perceive the social-agency system as alien and difficult to negotiate. By contrast, the social services provided by their unions are familiar, the system is negotiable, and access is assured. Many elderly retirees will not accept service unless it is from their union because to do so would (in their eyes) mean accepting charity. Retired union members feel they have earned their right to union services. They paid dues and struggled to make their unions strong. The unions, in turn, promote this concept and take pride in their relationship to retired workers. Unions mandate services to retired workers in recognition that their responsibilities to them do not end with retirement. Retired workers are encouraged to turn for services to their unions first, and unions are committed to serving their retired members from within the organization. Union retiree departments are not mere referral systems.

Services to retired workers may be the agenda of the unions's social-service department but these services are not the main priority of the union. "The world of work is an adversarial setting where the parallel interests of the individual and those of the organization may not be readily apparent" (Akabas and Kurzman, 1982). It is essential for social workers practicing in union settings to understand the structure and functions of the union and the background of its members. Visiting a "shop" (the work site), for example, enables the social worker to catch a glimpse of the worker's life before retirement and thus to establish valuable reference points for future interaction. Reading the union constitution will help the social worker understand the union's complex organizational hierarchy: the election process for officers and staff, the nomenclature of adminstrative units, the responsibilities of elected officials to their constituencies, and the rights and benefits of the members themselves. Effective delivery of social services to retired union members depends upon social workers in these settings broadening their knowledge of both the "nontraditional" auspices in which they work and the industry in which their clients have spent nearly a lifetime.

TYPES OF SERVICES

Direct Services

Direct services to union retirees include (1) one-time services such as completion of an application form for a union benefit; (2) longer-term, often task-centered casework involving more than one presenting problem; and (3) long-term service continuing over several years. Wherever possible, the union expects its social workers to resolve retirees' problems "in house." When referral to a community agency like a hospital or nursing home is necessary, the union social worker coordinates and monitors the delivery of these external services.

The services requested of their unions by retirees involve transportation (assistance to shopping, doctors' offices, banks); counseling (for individual and family problems); legal problems (wills, estates); union and government benefits (applications, appeals); medical and hospital bills (assistance with Medicare, Medicaid, and health-insurance claims); homecare arrangements; nursing-home placement (for retirees or family members); housing (help in relocating, landlord/tenant issues); and crime (victim compensation, safety courses). The actual provision of services is affected by the size of the retiree population and the priorities of the union. For example, a request by a District 65 retiree for transportation from the borough of Queens to the union dental clinic in Manhattan would be handled by the dispatch of a van maintained specifically for such purposes. For the much larger ILGWU, the provision of actual transportation would not be cost-effective; instead, their retiree service department would provide a companion to assist the retiree on public transportation.

Mrs. B, a 92-year-old retired garment worker, lives alone in a decaying inner-city neighborhood. She has vision and hearing impairments, and an operation on her knee two years ago has greatly restricted her mobility. Mrs. B has no family nearby. She has a brother overseas and two nieces, to whom she is closest, in her native country in the West Indies.

Mrs. B initially came into contact with her union retiree services program through her participation in a union-sponsored retiree club. At one club meeting she approached the social worker who was present that day to speak about a new health insurance benefit for retirees. Mrs. B wanted to apply for food stamps. The social worker and Mrs. B arranged for a meeting later in the week at the retiree services office to give Mrs. B time to gather the necessary documents. While completing the food stamp application, the social worker noticed that Mrs. B's rent seemed abnormally high. An appeal for a city-sponsored rent abatement was initiated.

Mrs. B came to see the social worker regularly over a period of about six months after the initial consultation. She was very depressed over her inability to secure visas for her two nieces in the West

Indies to come to the United States. She wanted her relatives to live with her in New York but, although they were eager to do so, a complex and already long-standing problem with the immigration authorities had developed. Mrs. B asked the social worker for help in bringing her nieces to America. The social worker turned first to the union legal department for assistance in securing an attorney if necessary. The social worker also contacted a local agency specializing in immigration problems. This task, which unfolded over a period of two years, ultimately involved city and state agencies, Mrs. B's congressman, the office of the union president, and religious agencies as well as an immigration attorney and the U.S. Department of State. Mrs. B's nieces were finally able to visit their aunt but have not yet been permitted to remain permanently in the United States.

The social worker also helped Mrs. B with linkage to a neighborhood nutrition center and with appeals for new housing and energy assistance from the city, and she supplied a union para-professional to visit Mrs. B at home regularly to assist her with light shopping and transportation to doctors.

Retiree Clubs

Retiree clubs are another way in which unions preserve their ties with retired members. For the retirees, the clubs are important sources of support, socialization, and leisure, educational, and political activities. For the unions, they provide forums by means of which the unions can readily communicate with retirees on issues of concern to them and also mobilize the retirees' efforts on issues of concern to the union.

Retiree service departments serve the clubs in a number of ways. They often provide technical assistance in beginning a new club — site selection, fund raising (often from union sources), mailings to potential members, and program development. Union social workers may assist the clubs in arranging events and in some cases accompany groups on outings. They often address clubs, bringing information about union and government benefits and receiving feedback from members about the effectiveness of union retiree programs. They also make use of these opportunities to reach out to retirees who may need the direct services provided by the retiree service department.

Their numbers and locations will of course determine how retirees are organized. When retirees are widely scattered, a club may meet at a central union office. When retirees are concentrated in a particular community, community-based clubs are appropriate. Community-based clubs are desirable for their potential for heightened involvement in community affairs and greater networking with community agencies.

District 65 holds meetings in areas of heavy retiree concentration, both to publicize the programs offered at its headquarters in downtown Manhattan and to recruit volunteers for its home-visiting program. Social-work students are then assigned to organize retirees into community self-help networks. Large international unions may have clusters of retirees living in areas quite removed from any union activity. The ILGWU, with international headquarters in New York City and one of its regional offices in Chicago, has a retiree club in the upper peninsula of Michigan.

In response to the extremely heavy concentration of retirees in the New York City area, the ILGWU in 1981 formed an Association of Retiree Clubs to bring together representatives of all its retiree clubs in New York State. The association meets monthly to act as a clearinghouse for benefit, educational, leisure, and cultural information; to coordinate political action on labor and aging issues; and to train club leaders. ILGWU social workers staff the association's committees, write its monthly newsletter, and provide technical support for such association activities as voter-registration drives.

Political Action

Union retirees may be mobilized for political action on two fronts: issues of primary concern to the aged (e.g., Medicare) and issues of concern to the labor movement (e.g., trade agreements with foreign nations). These areas may overlap (e.g., Social Security concerns), and the mutual interests of active and retired workers will be the force behind political action.

Preliminary to political action must be education. Staff social workers may address gatherings of retirees, the retiree club being the natural vehicle through which to begin the educational process. Their purpose at these gatherings is to describe the issue at hand and to elicit retirees' initial impressions and concerns relative to the issue.

Political action is not unfamiliar to retired trade unionists. Through their years as active workers, members responded to as well as initiated calls to political action on behalf of their union. Social workers who represent and service retirees must be particularly sensitive to their impressions. Likewise, the resultant action should reflect a balance between the social workers' agenda and those impressions and concerns. One may explain an entire legislative campaign only to have a retiree ask why he or she should care in the first place. Clear, nontechnical language in presentation is critical to motivate retirees to take action. Social-work training provides outreach and community organizing skills that can be readily transferred to political action with retiree groups.

The education process may include the development of "fact sheets" and "action guides" for retirees and their organizations. Fact sheets can look like glossaries—they help to visually sort out technical terms and concepts. They are perhaps most useful when kept separated from action guides. Their purpose is to supplement materials presented orally or in newsletters and union newspapers when an issue is exceptionally complex or critical.

Action guides tell retirees what to do. The following is an outline workers may find helpful in developing this sort of literature.

1. A concise statement of the issue at hand. If more than one issue requires action, separate pieces should be used. Example: "Reduced fare trans-

portation is in jeopardy. Those of you 65 and older may now obtain an I.D. card free of charge to use our local transportation facilities. The county wants to charge you for this card, payable on a yearly basis."

2. Explain why retirees should be for or against the issue. Example: "This charge will impose undue hardship on you, our retired members living on fixed incomes."
3. Recommended action. Example: "We must oppose this charge and take action immediately. Write to your county legislators. Tell them . . . "Here a short sample letter can be inserted. Long letters are not necessary; it's what is being said and the signature that has an impact.
4. The social worker's (or department's) name, phone, and address so retirees can obtain additional information.

Letter-writing campaigns may be most effective when explained and carried out simultaneously. Retiree clubs often have on hand paper, envelopes, stamps, and legislators' addresses. The social worker may address the club on an issue, distribute sample letters, and then help club members with their letters.

To better acquaint a target group with the legislative process at different levels of government, workshops may be held in which union staff and outside experts participate. Our hypothetical transportation issue might justify a workshop at which county legislators and retirees discuss the problem as each group sees it. The goal of preventing the imposition of a fare increase may be better achieved by the retirees themselves, not the union staff, describing their concerns.

Retraining and Employment

The Labor Force Participation of Older Workers

Four out of every ten workers 55 and older say they would prefer to continue working part-time after retirement (Sheppard and Mantovani, 1982). In 1982, 20 percent of older employed men and women were employed part-time on a voluntary basis, while only 10 percent of workers aged 20 to 54 were employed in this manner.

The 1981 Harris Poll for the National Council on Aging (on which the Sheppard study was based) concluded that the preference for part-time work, particularly in the same field as prior to retirement, was even more marked among those aged 55 to 64 (79 percent) and among those 65 and older (73 percent). Schulz (1980) noted that almost all older workers who work part-time do so by preference to supplement income. In addition, he offered three other reasons why older workers prefer to work part-time: (1) health concerns limit full-time employment; (2) the individual is participating in a phased retirement program; (3) the individual may "want more leisure but still value[s] highly the various social and monetary benefits arising from some amount of labor force attachment."

Thus, the Harris report noted: "The American labor market, and employers in particular, should anticipate extended participation of older workers in the world of work." The Work in America Institute (1980) went beyond the "anticipatory references" of the Harris report to set out minimal guidelines for options to extend labor-force participation (pp. 3-4):

Employers should introduce and continue programs, where practicable, to provide new options for employees such as job sharing, part-time jobs, job redesign, new work schedules, phased retirement.

The reemployment of retired workers offers an opportunity that may benefit both workers and the organization. Therefore, management and unions should try to resolve the problems that presently prevent retired employees from returning to work on a full-time, part-time, or temporary basis, where practicable.

Areas in which these retirees can benefit the company [or industry] include (1) contributing to the needs of the organizations, (2) filling in for employees on vacation or leave, (3) assisting the organization during peak work loads, and (4) assisting in training present employees.

Before we examine the possible role of unions, and of social workers employed by unions, in developing training and employment programs for older and retired workers to facilitate reentry into the labor force, we must look at what motivates people to retire, to leave the work force in the first place. Subsequently, we must look at why those who have left the work force seek to return.

"The decision to retire is one of the major job-related *choices* people make and, once made, is usually not reversed. Among the factors affecting this decision are: health limitations, retirement income sources, the state of the economy and the demand for older workers" (Rivlin, 1982). Yet what happens if the decision to retire is *not* voluntary? Health-related concerns are most often cited by Social Security studies as the reason for increasingly early retirement. The second major reason for early or "forced" retirement that these studies cite, however, is layoff or discontinuance of jobs. Among the workers in the unions described in this chapter the realities of unemployment too often displace well-laid plans for a secure and voluntary retirement.

As workers reach their late 40s and early 50s, joblessness increases. The duration of unemployment is also greater for older workers. Kirkland (1982, p.12) states:

Once unemployed, the older worker runs the greatest risk of being without work for long periods of time. Official statistics do not include labor force "drop outs." Millions of older men and women have withdrawn from the labor force unwillingly because they simply could not find jobs and eventually gave up looking for them.

Long-term unemployment of older workers erodes savings earmarked for retirement. If and when these workers return to their original jobs, pension benefits may have been irreversibly reduced.

There are many disincentives, from an employer's point of view, to the hiring of older workers. (Kirkland reminds us that unions are rarely involved in the hiring of *any* new employees.) For example, hiring older workers adds costs to health and welfare benefit packages because older people use more health-care services. The 1982 changes in the Medicare program have only exacerbated this particular situation (although, at this writing, full regulations have not yet been issued by the Department of Health and Human Services) by requiring employers to provide their regular health-insurance package for workers 65-69 should the worker so desire. In this case, Medicare becomes the secondary payor (or supplemental insurer) instead of the primary insurer as is generally the case for individuals over 65. Thus the employer has a disincentive to hire an older worker because the employer and not the government could be responsible for providing the bulk of that individual's health benefits.

Studies have shown that older workers seem to be less willing (or able?) to shift from looking for one type of work to looking for another. Finally, the skills developed by the current pools of older workers in labor-intensive industries such as auto, steel, apparel, and textiles are not readily transferable to today's "high tech" marketplace.

Many questions arise as to the role unions can or should take in the retraining and employment of older workers: Should unions establish training programs for workers 55-65 still on the job or—particularly in the industries described here—should they focus on employed workers in the same age group? Should unions develop reentry programs for already retired workers 65 and over? Is reemployment in the same industry they formerly worked in a realistic or suitable goal for older unemployed or retired workers? Should unions seek to train their workers for entry into other industries? Is it fair to younger workers when jobs are scarce in labor-intensive industries to introduce added competition for the same few jobs? Finally, what are the psychological realities relevant to these age groups and the lack of employment? Have the already retired done so voluntarily and made the necessary adjustments away from full-time employment? Can they cope with many added hours a day without a routine or regular schedule? Have their relationships with spouse and family become tense and strained? Haven't the unemployed been forced, unprepared, into a traumatic and vulnerable state and shouldn't their unions, therefore, attend to these unprecedented stresses before those of the retired group?

Organized labor has been active both nationally and locally in responding to the needs of the unemployed and the older worker. Congressional action has resulted from labor advocacy in the areas of extended unemployment benefits and health care for the unemployed. Local unions have conducted seminars on stress and family problems arising from both short- and long-term unemployment. District 65 and the ILGWU have begun such programs under the auspices of their Member Assistance or Personal Service units. These units are, for the most part, distinct from programs in the same union that offer services to retired members (i.e., unless a worker is actually receiving a pension check, the afore-mentioned programs and *not* retiree service departments will be responsible for the delivery of services).

When possible, collective-bargaining agreements have also included the concerns of older workers. They have sought to provide, for example, stronger seniority systems in an effort to protect older workers from arbitrary layoffs caused by economic instabilities or changing technology.

Friendly Visiting as an Employment Program

Social workers in union retiree service programs will often be required to develop retraining or employment programs for *retired* workers 65 and older. A model program of this sort is the ILGWU's Friendly Visiting Program established in 1967.

The ILGWU Friendly Visiting Program employs retired garment workers in the service of their fellow retirees. Friendly visitors (FVs) are trained by the professional social-work staff of the union's retiree service department to assist retired members with support, guidance, companionship, and in an advocacy capacity with matters such as benefit-application procedures, nursing-home placement, and linkage to community resources such as health clinics and nutrition programs.

FVs meet every three weeks for two hours with their supervisors. Small groups of five or six FVs meet together following individual supervision to share information and discuss cases. Social workers are responsible for overall supervision of FV cases and for assuring FVs of current and comprehensive information on procedures, case handling, and government, community, and union benefits.

The essence of the FV contact with a retiree is the home visit. (Regular phone contact is also maintained.) Each time a FV meets with a retiree (appointments are arranged in advance), he/she must fill out a report sheet describing the visit. FVs must be able to supply the following information for each contact:

1. Does the retiree live alone or with spouse, family?
2. How does the retiree manage? Can the retiree do his or her own cooking, shopping, cleaning?
3. Does the retiree have Medicare Parts A and B? Does the retiree have supplemental health insurance to Medicare?
4. Does the retiree qualify for a city rent abatement?
5. Does the retiree know about: reduced fare benefits; neighborhood senior centers; union retiree clubs; union drug, eyeglass, health clinic benefits; other community services; direct deposit of Social Security and other benefit checks?

These reports are the basis for the supervisory session between the social worker and FV. Follow-up is conducted by both social worker and FV in many cases where a retiree requires sustained, coordinated services. Almost all direct services of the retiree service department are delivered through this collaborative model. Friendly visiting is a preventive service. The program does not wait until a retiree asks for a visit or is ill and in need of help. The program mandates that each new retiree be visited within the first year of retirement. Case histories illustrate the value of this program:

A widowed retiree mourning the death of her only daughter is comforted by the FV's shared experience of a similar loss.

A retiree is crippled with arthritis and struggling to use crutches. The FV suggests she consult her doctor for a walker, accompanies the retiree to her doctor's office, and assists with the purchase of the walker, which the retiree receives in two weeks.

A retiree living comfortably with his daughter is desperately lonely for friends from the "old days." The FV introduces the retiree to the retiree club in his union local.

FVs are paid at the prevailing minimum wage and are entitled to specific sick and vacation benefits arranged through their employer, the union. Expenses such as transportation, postage, and telephone calls are reimbursed. A FV may set his or her own work schedule, but each month he/she will receive an "assignment" of twenty or thirty retirees to be visited. FVs work in their own neighborhoods, where they are familiar with helping networks available to older persons.

A friendly visiting program developed and sponsored by a union enables retirees to reenter the world of work through involvement with their own union and their contemporaries from the shop. Dressmakers, cutters, and pressers are retrained in a battery of new skills. With retiree numbers increasing, unions and their service departments can provide a dual service with the establishment of a friendly visiting program: training and employment for one, outreach to many.

Employment in Retiree Service Departments

Union retiree service departments may also directly employ retired workers as part-time clerical and support staff. These individuals may be retired union staff as well as members. Tasks may include secretarial work, reception, computer operation (for which the retiree would be trained), and special projects such as developing recreational programs or a pilot project for housekeeping assistance under the direction of a professional social worker.

The incorporation of retirees as staff in retiree service departments is a natural outgrowth of a philosophy that unions have held for years: to build the organization through the ranks, from within. There should be no question of appropriateness or age discrimination or turf struggles in the employment of retirees in union service departments. Retired trade unionists have organizing skills. The protection of their rights as active workers depended on their abilities both to initiate and to respond collectively to a call for action. The hiring of retirees as staff in union service departments offers an exemplary model for the training and employment of older and retired workers in less "age related" sectors of the economy.

Employment Outside the Union

What is the role of the social worker in helping retired workers to find employment outside of the union? The focus here shifts, of necessity, to that of information specialist and technical adviser. The social worker must ask: What skills and strengths do retirees already have? Can they be retooled and, if so, how?

Employment agencies and services in both the public and private sectors geared specifically to older workers are rare at best. Hiring and training practices remain tainted by stereotypes of the elderly as lacking the motivation and skills to cope with modern technology. Intervention is necessary, therefore, to promote elderly workers in a more realistic light, to move away from generalizations such as those stated above. This is not an easy task in a society that is geared to the image of the perpetual "Pepsi generation."

Sheppard (1971) noted that society and its organizations (family, school, church, etc.) does little to prepare its members for "multi-careers prior to entry into the labor force." He further stated: "Our popular mentality . . . is dominated by the single career concept, the notion that an individual should have a single lifetime occupational role-identity." We even have stereotypes that say: Blue-collar workers don't have careers, they have jobs! Our increasingly specialized professionalization allows this label to be attached only to the white-collar world. However, the labor force is graying, and increased longevity and better health should force a revision of this damaging type-casting.

In the area of employment, social workers' strategies should be to help clients set new goals for second careers: Can on-site training programs be set up? For example, if a computer system is available, will training retirees to use it facilitate their reentry into the labor force outside the protective auspice of the union? Can those interested be evaluated and referred to community-sponsored training and employment programs? Economic contingencies, in both the public and private sectors, will impact heavily on social workers' abilities to advocate retraining programs for older workers. A union's agenda, for example, may place a higher priority on retraining younger workers, especially if unemployment is high. Does this then conflict with the social workers' mandate to service retirees? Once again, the questions and dilemmas are many. Constant reevaluation is necessary if retirees wishing to reenter the labor force are to be offered services by their unions.

Postretirement Programs

Although postretirement programs are infrequent at this time, the notion may become better accepted in view of the trend toward early retirement and the increased longevity of American workers. Preretirement programs are designed to help workers anticipate and plan for life in retirement. A postretirement program (a single seminar may be enough) offers additional help from the vantage point of six months or a year after retirement. One's outlook and thus the assistance required may be vastly different once the transition from work to retirement has been completed.

The union social worker conducting a postretirement program asks: "What is it like now that you have retired?" The social worker encourages exploration of that "state" from several perspectives: What is the retiree's relationship with family now that he or she has retired? How, if at all, have roles changed? How does a retiree feel about himself or herself in the midst of all these changes? Has the retiree noticed changes in attitude as the first year of retirement progresses? Aging stereotypes must be carefully discussed and worked through.

A postretirement program can also be a refresher course on company and union benefits, health insurance, and community services. The focus here is on specific coping strategies so that if a particular service is required the retiree will know where, how, and when to apply. Retirees will probably have been exposed to this information at their preretirement programs, but the postretirement program gives the social worker a chance to review this material and also to update it. Distribution of packets of information on Social Security, Medicare, senior discounts, and community resources is particularly important at this time.

Postretirement programs can encourage retirees to remain active and to do so through their union, reconnecting them to the union through retiree clubs, classes, and social services. "Reconnection" serves two purposes: For the retiree, it increases options for activities, usually at little or no cost. For the social worker, it enhances the credibility of the retiree service department by assuring retirees' utilization of available union services.

Finally, postretirement programs provide a good opportunity to evaluate the union's own preretirement program. Through observation, discussion, and written evaluations with postretirement attendees, service providers can gauge the strengths and weaknesses of their preretirement programs.

POLICY

The union-retiree and older-worker programs reviewed in this chapter fall within the private sector. That is, the unions are private entities, and the workers they represent are not engaged in city, state, county, or federal-government jobs.

Unions mandate and, for the most part, fund their retiree services. Shortly after its inception in 1967, the ILGWU Retiree Service Department received a state grant to underwrite a portion of its program. Although unions continue to solicit government funding for a variety of projects, basic funding is provided by the unions themselves. For example, UAW retirees voluntarily contribute one dollar from their monthly pension checks toward the support of retiree programs. District 65 retirees pay dues to a retiree local. The ILGWU offers yearly contributions to its retiree clubs.

On the other hand, public social-welfare policies impact broadly on the delivery of retiree services, and union social workers must be knowledgeable about both the theory and the application of these policies in order to provide quality service to their constituents.

Unions and their workers are highly politicized. Labor legislation is the direct result of the struggles of workers and their representatives for government recognition and protection. The social worker's task will as often be to "translate" for a client the implications of a certain public policy (e.g., a change in Medicare reimbursement regulations) as it will be to alert the organization to that policy's importance to retirees. Similarly, social workers must be ready to relate current union legislative goals to retirees, frequently in the quest for retiree support and assistance. Social workers may use their knowledge of policy to bridge what seems to be a rapidly widening gulf between the perceptions of active and retired members of their respective interests. The 1981-82 Social Security crisis is illustrative of this gulf, since it was often viewed solely as an "old persons" issue.

The intent of this section is to increase the social worker's awareness of public social-welfare policy as it affects their roles as service providers. Detailed descriptions of programs such as Social Security and Title V can be found in handbooks published by the government. Unlike specific legislation mandating home-health care or legal services, for example, public policy on services to older workers can only begin to be described by a review of particular acts and regulations.

Social Security

The Social Security Act of 1935 recognized, for the first time, a compact between government and the citizenry to provide for income adequacy in old age. The original intent of the Act was to provide for a "floor of protection" for workers in retirement. Workers began paying into the Social Security System in the form of a payroll deduction (FICA) in 1937. The first benefit check was issued in 1940. Congress added benefits for survivors and dependents in 1939, and disabled workers became eligible for benefits in 1956.

The 1978 *Social Security Handbook* describes the program as one that has the "basic objectives of providing for the material needs of individuals and families, protecting aged and disabled persons against the expenses of illnesses that could otherwise exhaust their savings, keeping families together, and giving children the opportunity to grow up in health and security." Programs under the Social Security Administration include Retirement Benefits, Disability and Survivors Benefits, Medicare, and Supplemental Security Income.

Approximately 36 million persons in the United States in 1982 were receiving monthly Social Security checks. These were primarily retired workers (but also the disabled and survivors of deceased workers). Social-Security retirement benefits are available to workers retiring as early as 62, although at reduced levels. Full Social Security benefits are available at age 65. For each year that an individual over 65 works and does not collect Social Security, the benefit may be increased (3 percent a year in 1983).

Workers contribute to Social Security through payroll tax deductions (6.7 percent in 1983). Employers pay an equal tax for employees. Work performed in a covered employment (almost all American workers are covered by Social Security) is "credited" to an individual's work record for eventual eligibility for Social Security benefits. Thus the concept that Social Security is an earned right.

Social Security credit is measured in what is known as "quarters of coverage." A worker's actual benefit is figured by means of a complex formula reflecting actual earnings and adjustments for national changes in average wages. Workers with high incomes receive higher benefits. On the average, benefits equal 42 percent of earnings just before retirement. Examples of maximum monthly benefits in 1983 were $709 for an individual retiring at age 65 and $526 for one retiring at age 62. The average monthly payment for an individual who retired with full benefits at age 65 in 1983 was $406. Social Security benefits are adjusted for inflation.

Eligibility for Social Security benefits is limited by an earnings test. In 1983 retired persons aged 65 to 70 drawing Social Security benefits could earn up to $6,600 ($4,920 for persons under 65) before losing $1 in benefits for each $2 of additional earnings. Until the 1983 amendments to the Social Security Act, all Social Security income was tax free. The 1983 amendments placed a threshold on nontaxable income of $32,000 yearly for a couple and $25,000 yearly for an individual.

In considering Social Secuity, special attention must be paid to the situation of women, particularly in view of the fact that most of the constituency of the union retiree programs discussed in this chapter are women. These women are most likely to be single. In 1980, 67 percent of all single women 72 and over were almost totally dependent on Social Security for income. Therefore problems of elderly female retirees stemming from income inadequacy are frequent concerns of union social workers. They must often assist these clients in negotiating the Social Security bureaucracy on matters ranging from lost checks to retrieval of benefits. Other benefits such as rent exemptions, energy assistance, and food stamps may have to be obtained for clients with low Social Security benefits. Applications for Supplemental Security Income (SSI) may also be necessary. (SSI, although administered by the Social Security Administration, is not financed by payroll taxes and is not therefore a part of the Social Security system. It was designed to provide a minimum monthly income to needy individuals 65 and over or blind or disabled. An individual must have limited income and assets to qualify.)

Medicare

Medicare is Title XVIII of the Social Security Act, passed in 1965. Parts A and B of the Title mandate hospital and medical insurance, respectively. Medicare is available to most individuals over 65 and in some cases to persons under this age. Administration of Medicare is assigned to the Department of Health and Human Services. The Health Care Financing Administration (HCFA) is the agency within that department with jurisdiction over Medicare.

Medicare Part A (hospital insurance) covers inpatient hospital care. The Medicare beneficiary is responsible for the payment of a deductible, since Medicare is not designed to cover 100 percent of health-care costs for the elderly. Supplemental insurance policies—"medigap" plans—are available from private insurance carriers to assist in payment of health-care costs not covered by Medicare.

An individual should apply for Medicare three months before his or her sixty-fifth birthday, whether or not he or she intends to retire at that time and begin collecting Social Security benefits.

Medicare Part B (medical insurance) helps to pay for doctors' services, outpatient care, and home-health care. Part B requires both a monthly premium (deducted from the beneficiary's Social Security check) and a yearly deductible that must be satisfied before Medicare will begin reimbursement.

Medicare reimbursement rates are based on 80 percent of the "reasonable and customary" charges for health-care services. Beneficiaries are responsible for the remaining 20 percent plus whatever difference exists between the doctor's actual charge and the amount approved by Medicare for reimbursement.

Part B coverage is optional, and, if a retiree does not have the insurance, enrollment in the plan is open only from January 1 to March 31 each year. Coverage does not actually begin until July 1.

Union social workers are often called upon to help clients negotiate the Medicare and related health-care service systems. If a beneficiary is not satisfied with a decision on a claim, social workers should be cognizant of the Medicare appeals process and be able to take the client through it (or seek assistance from trained advocates in fair-hearing procedures).

Title V of the Older Americans Act

Title V of the Older Americans Act of 1965 (Section 502) authorizes the establishment of programs for part-time community-service employment of low-income individuals 55 years of age or older with "poor employment prospects," including, for example, the unskilled and women. Employment sites include hospitals, day-care centers, and nutrition and energy projects.

The Administration on Aging contracts with agencies and organizations for the delivery of training to workers and for employment. In 1982, the Title V budget of $277 million provided an estimated 54,000 jobs. Also in 1982, the Congressional Budget Office reported that two-thirds of the participants in Title V programs were female, more than half were 65 or older, and the average hourly wage was $3.50.

Union social workers should be aware of these opportunities when assisting appropriate clients to reenter the labor force. Davis (1980), however, describes Title V as a "quasi-employment program which emphasizes income transfer to the eligible elderly poor participants as much or more so than it does mainline employment. It lacks the training, job development and appropriation essential for an employment program."

Employee Retirement Income Security Act (ERISA)

ERISA, passed in 1974, was the culmination of a decade of legislative work in the area of pension reform. Its basic intent was to set minimum standards for pension-rights protection. It applied to all pension and welfare plans in existence on September 24, 1974 and those established thereafter. ERISA's impact was felt nationwide in almost every private pension plan since it required a step-by-step reevaluation of pension funding, finance, and administration.

After ten years, the complexities of the Act are still being sorted out by legislators, economists, and pension experts. Seemingly minute variations in plans from company to company or union to union may have significant consequences in application.

ERISA has played a major role in establishing and redefining minimum vesting requirements for pension eligibility. Schulz (1980) defines vesting as "the provision [of a pension plan] that gives a [plan] participant the right to receive an accrued benefit at a designated age regardless of whether the employee is still employed at that time. Thus, vesting removes the obligation of the participant to remain in the pension plan until the date of early or normal retirement." As an example of the application of vesting to pension rights, consider the union member who, in order to qualify for a full pension, needed twenty years of employment covered under the plan. Before ERISA, if the worker left the industry or retired with only fifteen years, all contributions to the plan in his or her name would have been lost and the pension forfeited. ERISA set up requirements for all pension plans to provide minimum vested benefits based on at least one of three options for benefit accrual. Schulz notes that by far the most prevalent plan is one that provides for vesting of 100 percent of accrued benefits after ten years of service. Thus our hypothetical union member above would, under ERISA, be eligible for a pension reflecting his/her fifteen years of service. Suppose seven of those fifteen years had been spent as a sewing-machine operator in one factory and eight as an operator in another. Would that influence eligiblity for a vested pension? In the garment industry the answer would be no, because of the "portability" of pension rights for garment workers. Portability is "a type of vesting mechanism that allows employees to take their pension credits with them when they change jobs" (Schulz, 1980). Although in theory portability should reduce erosion of benefits for workers who change jobs, "the administrative, financial, and actuarial complexities of setting up such arrangements have discouraged any significant action in this area" (Schulz, 1980, p.134) and thus the positive effects of portability on workers have been minimal thus far.

Age Discrimination in Employment Act (ADEA)

ADEA was originally passed in 1967 and amended as of January 1, 1979. In its 1967 form it focused on age discrimination against employees between 40 and 65 only (thereby defining an older worker as one 40 or older!). The 1978 amendments made it illegal for a nonfederal employer to force workers to retire before the age of 70. ADEA applies to most work sites with more than twenty employees.

ADEA represented a major step toward a national policy on older workers. Yet stereotypes of older persons' ability to perform on the job, their perceived health concerns, and the notion of increased costs of their employment persists some fifteen years after enactment. Realistically, of course, the major thrust of ADEA should be to combat mandatory retirement as a form of age discrimination. Kingson (1982) summarizes the potential impact of ADEA in relation to current retirement trends as follows:

Faced with projections for increased pension costs, longer life spans, and future declines in the number of younger workers relative to older workers, there is a clear need to begin to readjust our expectations concerning retirement age. The passage of this legislation [the 1978 Amendments to ADEA] may well be the beginning of the legitimization of later retirement (or, to put it another way, the beginning of the delegitimization of early retirement).

The expected broad impact of the 1978 amendments to ADEA has not materialized. (Several state legislatures have been far more progressive in enacting statutes abolishing mandatory retirement, among them California and Florida.) This is attributed in the literature to several factors, including: stereotypical attitudes that older workers are recalcitrant, untrainable, and unreliable; high rates of unemployment, and preference for younger workers when jobs become available; and weak administration and enforcement procedures of the Act. (Originally administered by the Department of Labor, ADEA is now under the jurisdiction of the Equal Opportunity Employment Commission.)

Union social workers will not find their primary role to be the enforcement of ADEA. This is the domain of a government agency. However, when working with clients who have recently lost jobs and are seeking new ones, social workers should be aware of the existence of ADEA and be able to help clients negotiate its systems.

THE FUTURE OF RETIREE SERVICES

In the spring of 1983 the AFL-CIO established a new committee of its Executive Council known as the Committee for Retiree Affairs. A similar committee had been established some twenty-five years earlier under the late AFL-CIO president George Meany, but its success had been negligible. Why would the AFL-CIO reestablish such a committee now?

Demographics has much to do with the answer. In the past twenty-five years, the number of people 65 and over in the United States has increased by more than two-thirds, from some 16 million to well over 26 million. Since the 1981 White House Conference on Aging, the "senior lobby" has become recognized as a potent political force. Social Security became a major election issue in 1982 because older Americans made their concerns felt.

The growing ranks of the elderly include thousands of retired trade unionists. Thus the establishment of a Committee on Retiree Affairs signifies organized labor's recognition both of its continued responsibility for these retired workers and of the contributions these retired workers can make to the labor movement. Organized labor can speak out on issues of concern to its retirees: Social Security, Medicare, housing. In turn, retirees can assist organized labor with its social, educational, and political agenda. Active and retired workers can work together for their mutual interests.

In times of limited financial resources, some unions may regard retiree social services as luxuries they can no longer afford. Social workers in union retiree service departments are in a position to help retirees prove their value to the union as a whole. A legislative education program in a retiree club can enable retirees to help the union lobby a bill to protect strikers; a "foster grandparent" type of program in which retirees spend time with children of active workers in a city where day-care programs are costly and scarce will help the union to take care of its own. It is in the continuing interests of retirees, active workers, organized labor, and social workers in industrial settings that such options for reciprocity be well explored.

REFERENCES AND BIBLIOGRAPHY

Akabas, S. H. (1977). Labor: Social policy and human services. In *Encyclopedia of social work* (17th ed.). Washington: National Association of Social Workers.
Akabas, S. H. and Kurzman, P. A. (Eds.). (1982). *Work, workers and work organizations: A view from social work*. Englewood Cliffs, N.J.: Prentice-Hall.
Akabas, S. H., Kurzman, P. A., and Kolben, N. S. (Eds.). (1979). *Labor and industrial settings: Sites for social work practice*. New York: Columbia University/Hunter College/Council on Social Work Education.
Amalgamated Clothing and Textile Workers Union. (1982). *Social services: Department profile* (2nd ed.). New York: The Union.
Brodsky, J., and Robinson, W. (1981). Current employment programs: NCOA/TVA senior energy counselor program. *Aging and Work*, **4**(1), 58-60.
Burkhauser, R. V., and Tolley, G. S. (1978). Older Americans and market work. *Gerontologist*, **18**(5), 449-453.
Clague, E., Palli, B., and Kramer, L. (1971). *The aging worker and the union*. New York: Praeger.
Copperman, L. F., and Rappaport, A. M. (1980). Pension and welfare benefits for older workers: The preliminary impact of the ADEA amendments. *Aging and Work*, **3**(2), 75-87.
Davis, T. F. (1980). Toward a national policy on older workers. *Aging*, nos. 313-314, pp. 12-19.
District 65. (1982). *Programs for retired members*. New York: The Union.
Doctors, S. I., et al. (1980). Older worker employment services. *Aging and Work*, **3**(4), 229-237.
International Ladies' Garment Workers' Union. (1971). *After a life of labor*. New York: The Union.
International Ladies' Garment Workers' Union. (1982). *Retiree service department*. New York: The Union.
Keizer, J., and Habib, M. (1980). Working in a labor union to reach retirees. *Social Casework*, **61**(3), 180-183.
Kieffer, J. A., and Fleming, A. S. (1980). Older Americans: An untapped resource. *Aging*, nos. 313-314, pp. 2-11.
Kingson, E. R., (1982). Current retirement trends. In M. H. Morrison (Ed.), *Economics of aging: The future of retirement*. New York: Van Nostrand Reinhold.
Kirkland, L. (1982). Employing the older worker: A labor perspective. *Generations*, **6**(4), 12-13.
Korn, R. (1976). *A union and its retired workers: A case study of the UAW*. Ithaca, N.Y.: New York State School of Industrial and Labor Relations, Cornell University.
Kurzman, P. A., and Akabas, S. H. (1981). Industrial social work as an arena for practice. *Social Work*, **26**(1), 52-60.
Louis Harris and Associates. (1981). *Aging in the eighties: America in transition*. Washington: National Council on the Aging.
Meier, E. L. (1980). New ERISA agency considered and pension issues of women and minorities. *Aging and Work*, **3**(2), 135-139.
Morrison, M. H. (1982). Economics of the older worker: A national perspective. *Generations*, **6**(4), 18-19, 65.
Morrison, M. H. (Ed.). (1982). *Economics of aging: The future of retirement*. New York: Van Nostrand Reinhold.
Rivlin, A. (1982). *Work and retirement: Options for continued employment of older workers*. Washington: Congressional Budget Office.

Schulz, J. H. (1980). *The economics of aging* (2nd ed.). Belmont, Calif.: Wadsworth.

Sheppard, H. L. (1971). *New perspectives on older workers.* Kalamazoo, Mich.: Upjohn Institute for Employment Research.

Sheppard, H. L., and Mantovani, R. E. (1982). *Part-time employment after retirement.* Washington: National Council on the Aging.

Social work and the workplace. (1982). *Practice Digest,* **5**(2).

Stein, L. (Ed.). (1977). *Out of the sweatshop: The struggle for industrial democracy.* New York: Quadrangle/New York Times.

U.S. Administration on Aging. (1970). *Older Americans Act of 1965, as amended.* Washington: Government Printing Office.

U.S. Department of Health, Education, and Welfare. (1979). *Social security handbook* (6th ed.). Washington: Government Printing Office.

U.S. Department of Health and Human Services. (1982). *Your medicare handbook.* Washington: Government Printing Office.

Weiner, H. J., Akabas, S. H., and Sommer, J. J. (1973). *Mental health care in the world of work.* New York: Association Press.

Work in America Institute. (1980). *The future of older workers in America.* Scarsdale, N.Y.: The Institute.

14

Preretirement Planning Programs

Abraham Monk, Ph.D.

Columbia University

Retirement marks the transition from productive maturity to a nonoccupational status in later life. It is the focal point that triggers a confrontation with aging and its concomitant economic and social deficits. With mandatory retirement already sanctioned as a major national policy in the United States, the current forecast is that by the year 2000 there will be nearly 32 million persons 65 and over with an average of fifteen to twenty years of retirement living (U.S. Congress, 1981). Will their transition into retirement be a stressful one, marred by anxiety and uncertainty, or will they find meaningful opportunities for growth and even improve the quality of their lives? Much will depend on the extent of "anticipatory socialization," a conscious and systematic preparation that these prospective retirees have undertaken in midlife or in the years that precede their impending retirement.

Studies have shown that most workers today do not plan for their retirement, although almost all workers perceive a need to plan. Unfortunately, most do not know how to proceed and generally spend their time worrying rather than engaging in realistic planning efforts. It is estimated that only about 10 percent of the labor force have actually gone through programs aimed at helping them prepare for their retirement.

Preretirement planning programs have emerged only during the last twenty-five years and remain, for the most part, in their experimental stages. Federal legislation fostered their implementation about ten years ago with the 1973 amendments to Title III of the Older Americans Act. A variety of programs for retirement preparation were launched during the last decade by a new professional cadre of preretirement counselors. The main objective of their efforts usually consists of providing information and planning skills that will enable individuals to make adequate choices concerning their postretirement lives. The program content invariably includes financial planning, health maintenance, nutrition, changing roles and attitudes, volunteer roles, leisure-time activities, and housing alternatives. Most focus only on tangible "nuts and bolts" issues. A few venture into more sensitive psychological concerns.

As preparation for retirement is being recognized as a legitimate public priority, there is reason to wonder whether the programs that resulted from pioneer efforts of the 1960s and 1970s are suited to the needs of the swelling ranks of retirees of the 1980s and 1990s. What features of the present "first generation" preretirement programs have worked and should be continued in the future? Which ones will have to be discarded? What new directions should future programs follow in terms of format, auspices, and content? What will be their central themes? How will they account for emerging realities such as inflationary pressures, postponement of the retirement age, high unemployment rates, loss of confidence in the Social Security system, and rapid occupational obsolescence? What role will corporate employers and unions play in the sponsorship, design, and implementation of such programs? As these questions are answered, the very nature of a "second generation" of preretirement programs more responsive to the 30 million retirees of the 1990s may begin to unfold.

The economic recession of the early 1980s has forced, however, many industrial and service firms to cut expenditures for nonessentials. This category includes, in some instances, the provision of preretirement planning programs. Some employers are searching for new approaches that do not become financially burdensome. Social workers entering this field of service are confronted with two central questions:

1. Do preretirement preparation programs actually work? What service do they render?
2. What shape will these programs adopt in the next generation, and how can they become attractive to cost-conscious sponsors?

Before these questions are answered, it is befitting to observe the field at large. A review of the literature and its main issues will provide the proper perspective to this critical service.

THE RETIREMENT SYSTEM IN TRANSITION

Retirement has become an established institution in modern societies for those nearing the age of 65. The right of older people to continue working if they so desire, irrespective of overall manpower, mobility, or efficiency considerations, is being advocated, however, at a time when large numbers of workers opt to retire *before* the 65-year age limit. Furthermore, the proportion of early retirees receiving Social Security benefits has grown during the 1970s at a rate of 2 percent per year. To determine what percentage of people eligible for retirement would choose to continue working or return to the work force, Motley (1978) examined the Social Security Administration's retirement history data base. Findings indicated that more than 13 percent of retirees were likely or able to return to work, while 50 percent were found unable or unwilling to do so. Motley suggested that no great change in retirement rates would occur with the elimination of mandatory retirement or amendments to the Social Security earnings test. It is conceivable, however, that, given the upward shift in occupational structure and education, older workers may delay retirement to sustain higher standards of living to which they have grown accustomed.

While policymakers speculate about the age at which American workers will opt to retire, it is a fact that more people than ever are retiring today. A three-fold retirement pattern is likely to evolve: first, the present trend toward early retirement (ages 60 to 62) will continue as larger numbers of workers begin drawing income supports from private pensions; second, conventional retirement at 65 will probably attract occupationally stable and financially cautious workers; and, third, late retirement at 70 will probably appeal to healthy, achievement-oriented older workers.

Regardless of the option selected, retirees can expect to spend an increasing number of years in retirement. As stated by Greenough and King (1977), in 1935 a male retiree of 65 could expect to live about thirteen years in retirement. Today, the life expectancy of a male aged 65 is eighteen years. Moreover, the labor-force participation of older workers has been steadily declining over the past twenty-five years. It reached a low of 19.1 percent in 1980 for men 65 and over, compared to 27 percent ten years earlier. It is worth mentioning that working older women held their ground during the same period, but they constituted a small minority of their cohort (U.S. Congress, 1981). True, this trend may slow down given the experience of double-digit inflation and the recent postponement of the mandatory retirement age, but it is doubtful that it will be reversed in light of both chronic high unemployment rates and scarce opportunities for older workers to remain employed, let alone be rehired.

Older workers' preference for some form of part-time or flexible employment clashes with employers' entrenched rationalizations for upholding mandatory retirement. Employers insist that productivity declines with age and that it would be difficult and costly to assess each worker's productivity on a case-by-case basis. It is therefore administratively more practical to institute a universal system of retirement that does not get bogged down in suits and appeals connected with charges of age discrimination. There are also intergenerational arguments, including the need to promote younger workers and union-negotiated seniority systems that explicitly require a point of termination or retirement.

In any event, our labor practices and social policies currently discourage gradual transitions from work to retirement, or cycles of departures and reentries of varying intensity and duration. They sanction instead the drastic separation of the two.

THE NEED TO PLAN

The retirement transition usually involves a loss of income, an alteration of familial and social relationships, increased leisure time, and, for many, the loss of status and of meaning derived from one's work. Each of these areas, when unforeseen or unplanned for, can create obstacles to a successful adjustment.

Sheldon, McEwan, and Ryser (1975) have identified lack of preparation for retirement as a major obstacle to its success. Such preparation, they suggest, should include the development of financial and social alternatives to employment, the anticipation of change, and the planning of a response to that change that will lead to a positive accommodation to one's newly developed life-style.

The extent to which planning for retirement is altogether feasible was questioned, however, by Schulz (1980), who stated that the individual preparing for retirement cannot establish with certainty when he will die, what his basic retirement needs will be, nor what life-style he will ultimately prefer for that period. Moreover, he cannot anticipate the future rate of inflation, which may depreciate the value of those retirement assets that do not adjust fully and reduce the buying power of income from those assets. Ultimately, he cannot predict the rate of economic growth, which is likely to affect his economic position relative to that of the wage-earning population. Preretirement planning programs are called for, however, to help the potential retiree shape expectations and spell out realistic personal goals, not to engage in guesswork about future events. Yet the majority of people do not plan prior to their retirement. Pyron and Manion (1970) reported that nearly two-thirds of respondents (employees and retirees) in a major study had made almost no plans for meeting their financial needs in retirement and almost three-fourths had made no plans for care and maintenance of health.

Ossofsky (1980) reported that a survey of the nation's largest corporations revealed a heightened awareness among corporate leaders of the grave financial ramifications of inflation for retirees. There is also an increasing sense of corporate responsibility for the welfare of older workers and an interest in developing retirement planning programs. Retirement programs, however, remain the exception rather than the rule among survey participants. The absence of programs can be attributed to their low priority status and the lack of personnel to implement them. Respondents agreed that the responsibility for planning should be shared by the individual and the employer.

Although many workers perceive a need to plan, according to Kasschau (1974), many do not know how to proceed and often spend their time worrying rather than engaging in appropriate planning efforts. Studies conducted with retirees by Louis Harris and Associates (1975) indicate that the majority regret not having planned more effectively, especially in the financial area.

THEORETICAL PERSPECTIVE

Retirement constitutes for some the advent of a leisured life-style, the reward for long years of work and a liberation from boring and draining employment. For others, it is a painful transition because it terminates status-enhancing roles without replacing them adequately. Moreover, it demotes most individuals to standards of living far below those they were used to most of their lives. Both views concur, however, that anticipatory socialization can facilitate an adaptation to the impending transition. Anticipatory socialization, in the form of pre-retirement planning, thus serves to reorient the individual and to give continuity to a series of role positions. It softens the abruptness of change and makes the future more manageable. Cumming and Henry (1961), postulating that retirement is part of the natural and universal process of disengagement, gave advocates of the first perspective their long-awaited theoretical justification. Disengagement is a social process that occurs even in the absence of a psychological urge to sever ties from society. It serves to functionally minimize the disruptive consequences of the ultimate disengagement—death—and, in all circumstances, it is the basic prerequisite for "successful" aging, here conceived as a stage when society no longer places obligatory demands on the individual and the individual responds by withdrawing from dominant, producing roles. Rosow (1973) did not agree with the alleged naturalness of the disengagement process and viewed the cessation of the work role as affecting the person's sense of self-esteem. "The process of role loss," he stated, "steadily eats away at these crucial elements of social personality and converts what is to what was. . . . If the social self consists of roles, then role loss erodes self-conceptions and sacrifices social identity" (p. 83). Through every other stage of the life cycle, individuals have managed to cope with crises and develop ways to substitute and even improve upon the losses they experienced. Retirement, however, constitutes entrance into a stage devoid of socially prescribed roles. It throws individuals into a limbo of rolelessness. Lacking any sense of purpose, many retirees feel, as Rosow added, "oppressively useless and futile."

The notion that retirement is a "stressor" that negatively impinges upon the central component of the person's identity was challenged by Streib (1958), who discovered that the alleged psychological trauma was not as profound as had been assumed and could be caused by other factors besides retirement. Personal circumstances such as poor health and low socioeconomic status may depress the morale of the older worker more than retirement itself. Simpson and McKinney (1966) similarly found that the adjustment patterns that evolve after retirement depend heavily on previous lifelong coping behaviors and the kind of work from which the individual retires.

Theoretical interpretations have expanded into a more diversified array of conceptual systems, and preretirement programs based on their premises have followed course. While often similar in structure or content, programs differ in their underlying philosophical orientations. Monk (1977) identified five theoretical models of preretirement planning programs. The first four models correspond to Schein's (1980) four sets of images of man: rational-economic; social; humanistic; and complex. The fifth model centers on crisis theory. The following is a summary of these five models:

1. The *rational-economic* model assumes that economic self-interest and, therefore, work-oriented values are the bases of all human motivation. Life after retirement must therefore involve a rechanneling of the achievement motive into hobbies and voluntarism. The focus of programs founded on this premise is to help prospective retirees remain active and seek rewards in civic or community oriented volunteer roles.

2. The *social* model identifies man's need to belong and to be accepted by others as the major human motivator, more important than financial motives. Programs that reflect the social perspective rely primarily on group peer support. The content of such programs emphasizes:
   a. *Role flexibility* or the capacity to take on new life roles which were not typical of the middle years.
   b. *Interpersonal competence.* Group dynamics, sensitivity training, encounter groups, and transactional analysis are emphasized in some programs to promote better self-awareness, communication skills, and the ability to handle conflict, ambiguity, and dissidence in human interaction.

3. The *humanistic-existential* model assumes that man primarily strives for meaning in life and that pride and self-esteem are enhanced when creative capacities are developed. It sees retirement as an opportunity for human liberation through increasing self-awareness and encouraging individual growth and self-exploration of one's potential. This humanist trend seeks to promote the concept of "lifelong learning," continued personal growth, and self-renewal.

4. The *complex-systemic* model starts from the premise that man is a complicated and highly variable system. Each individual is unique in terms of interests, concerns, and motivational patterns. Variance exists not only between people but also within the individual at different points in his/her life. Therefore, in order to fully appreciate these personal differences, individualized preretirement counseling must be provided, rather than any kind of standardized program. This includes case

diagnosis, planning, and the provision of information based on an assessment of each person's situation and needs.

5. The *crisis model* is not independent of the four preceding archetypes, since there is a crisis component in each of them. All programs must contend with emotional turmoil, anxiety, and fear. This model emphasizes that retirement is a loss that must be grieved. The ego sustains an injury as a result of this loss which creates a high risk of depressive reactions in retiring workers. Programs are therefore designed to foster a life-review process including the recognition of the succcesses one has achieved as well as one's strengths and assets. Preparation for grief work and reconciliation with impending losses are primary goals.

These five models do not represent strict or pure categories. Many programs incorporate features or attributes of more than one model. However, they identify trends and central ideas within the new and growing field of preretirement and life planning.

THE PROVISION OF SERVICES

The designation "retirement preparation programs" refers, according to Olson (1981), to "formally organized interventions so that an employee . . . can gain information about, and begin to prepare for his or her impending retirement." Olson inventories the various names given to such programs: preretirement assistance, preretirement counseling, preretirement planning, preretirement education, etc. Of more recent vintage, however, are broader, euphemistic labels such as "life transitions counseling," "life-long learning," "life planning," "personal growth," etc.

The designing and implementation of such programs was initially the province of education specialists. Counseling personnel, industrial psychologists, and social workers made subsequent claims of competence and expertise and by and large succeeded in validating them over a couple of decades of trial and error. Most programs are offered by private corporations and public employers as an employee benefit. It is not unusual, however, for unions to fill the vacuum. More recently, community colleges, continuing-education programs, public libraries, senior-citizen organizations, life-insurance companies, savings and loan associations, chambers of commerce, and Area Agencies on Aging have assumed a share of the task. It is virtually impossible to establish which is a better or more successful sponsor as each may be appealing to a different constituency.

More than twenty years ago Wermel and Beideman (1961) alerted us that most programs are "limited" in scope because the information they provide does not exceed pension and Social Security benefits. Only a few are "comprehensive" — that is, include housing, health, legal, and leisure issues and even some psychological concerns. The picture may now have been reversed, a recent survey by Research and Forecasts (1980) indicating a substantial trend toward increasing comprehensiveness.

However, preretirement planning programs have consisted for the most part of an employer's providing last-minute, one-shot presentations of the company's pension program. Corporate or management initiatives have often been motivated by a desire to encourage employees to utilize early-retirement options and to improve the corporate image, or by the belief that such programs would enhance worker morale and thereby increase productivity. Glamser and DeJong (1975) found the effectiveness of these programs to be relatively minimal. As case examples reported by the *50 Plus* retirement newsletter of comprehensive programs, it is worth mentioning one started by the Westinghouse Electric Corporation of Pittsburgh in 1980. This program consists of seven weekly, two-hour sessions covering the following topics: Planning for Your Successful Retirement; Your Home; Health; The Law; Leisure; Money; and The Company's Benefits. It recruits resource speakers from the community and usually includes ten to fifteen couples in each seminar. The program offered by the International Minerals and Chemical Corporation of Northbrook, Illinois, is structurally similar but the sessions are lengthier, up to three hours. It is occasionally offered in the evening, preceded by dinner, and includes, as an incentive, a special-education-assistance bonus of $500 for pursuing hobbies or specialized training.

Fitzpatrick (1980) reported that the National Council on Aging had developed a program structured for middle-aged workers ranging from blue-collar employees to middle-level executives. The program included eight planning areas: life-style planning, financial planning, new careers in retirement, leisure time, health, personal relationships, living arrangements, and community services.

Several prototypes of comprehensive preretirement planning programs have been developed by the Center for the Study of Aging and Human Development at Duke University (1977). One is a short version designed for use when time and resources are limited. Two expanded versions have also been developed, one for the blue-collar employee of average resources and one for the executive or professional employee. The expanded version for the first of these two potential consumer groups includes eight formal sessions and one or more unstructured sessions. There is a full-time coordinator and counselor available to participants for individual counseling between sessions. The program emphasizes the financial and legal aspects of retirement, since it is anticipated that employees may have significantly less income during retirement. The eight sessions of the program cover: the challenge of later maturity; company benefits for retirees; Social Security and Medicare benefits; planning retirement budgets, savings, and investments; legal problems facing retirees; physical and mental health; family relations; choosing a place to live; earning extra income; using leisure time; and participating in a social and planning session and a series of special-interest groups.

Consultants and audio-visual materials were used to stimulate discussions in group sessions. Another feature suggested by the Duke staff is the formation of special committees of participants who research special problems that may arise during the program. The recommended group size is from twenty to thirty-nine participants, including spouses. Group homogeneity is recommended for enhanced participation.

The specifics of this model are flexible enough to allow for adaptation in the many different settings of business and industry and for variation in such participant factors as age, marital status, socioeconomic status, etc.

THE EVALUATION OF PROGRAM EFFECTIVENESS

Almost simultaneously with the design and implementation of program models, preretirement counselors pondered whether their initiatives actually accomplished their stated objectives. Initial evaluation efforts have shown some promising results. Mack (1958) evaluated a preretirement program through the use of preprogram and postprogram questionnaires and concluded that the questionnaires were useful in that participants developed more positive attitudes toward retirement and increased the amount of retirement planning. Charles (1971) studied workers who participated in preretirement planning at the Drake University Pre-Retirement Planning Center and found that there was an increase in awareness and involvement in many aspects of retirement — financial concerns, health, life-styles, etc. The National Council on the Aging (1973) surveyed participants before and after a retirement preparation program given by United Airlines and concluded that participants had a more positive attitude toward retirement as well as possessing more accurate information about its various aspects. Greene et al. (1969) reported after a survey of eight companies that participation in preretirement programs aided in the adjustment of retirees. Favorable results involved measures of overall life adjustment and better subjective ratings of health and income. Companies without programs were used as control groups.

Ash (1966) also compared those who completed a course in preretirement planning with a comparable group of retirees who were not involved in such a program. The experimental group was more favorably disposed toward post-retirement life. Three years after retirement, the group members retained a higher sense of purposefulness compared to the control group.

Overall, the evidence to date suggests that preretirement preparation programs are helpful to the preretiree in planning activities and in easing the transition from work to retirement. Relationships have been established between exposure to programs and succcessful retirement factors (e.g., acceptance of retirement transition, sound financial plans, realistic view of retirement, disbelief in the stereotypes and myths of retirement, retirement activities, good health, etc.). However, it is important to mention the possibility of selective bias in research findings. As Kasschau (1974), Monk (1977), Heidbreder (1972), and others have suggested, those who are most likely to experience problems in retirement are the least likely to plan for it, while those who do participate in planning may already be mindful and positively inclined toward retirement. For instance, Heidbreder studied factors in the retirement of blue- and white-collar workers and reported that poorly adjusted retirees were twice as likely to have engaged in little or no planning.

Comparative program evaluations are beginning to shed some light on the controversies surrounding the relative effectiveness of various program models. Kasschau has delineated programs in terms of "planning" functions and the "counseling-adjustment" approach. In view of the fact that the majority of people arrive at retirement without realistic plans, the "planning" perspective seeks to help one develop reasonable expectations about retirement life and to anticipate and prepare for income loss. Since adjustment is correlated with health and income, the ideal program should emphasize the planning function. Kasschau suggests that counseling programs based on the view of retirement as a transition crisis are successful in promoting planning.

Many programs emphasize group processes, human growth, and conscious-ness-raising approaches as instructional strategies as opposed to the more traditional methods of instruction. Bolton (1976), at the University of Nebraska, evaluated a humanistic program entitled Planning and the Third Age. He reported that 74 percent of the participants thought the program was useful and 94 percent were favorably disposed to the humanistic (affective) group processes. Glamser and DeJong (1975) compared a group-discussion model to an individual-briefing model using an experimental control-group research design. The group-discussion method was reported more effective in increasing knowledge of retirement issues. Participants felt better prepared for retirement, were less uncertain about the future, and showed significant increases in the number of preparation activities undertaken. The individual-briefing program was relatively ineffective, suggesting the need for comprehensiveness in pre-retirement program design. Boyack and Tiberi (1975) reported the findings of the first phase of a project comparing three approaches: a group-counseling model; a lecture-discussion model; and an information-media model. The following results were cited:

1. There were significant differences between each program and the control group in regard to attitudes, behavior, and information growth.
2. The group-counseling approach indicated the greatest degree of positive change on attitudinal and behavior variables.
3. The lecture-discussion approach indicated the greatest degree of change in information-growth variables.

4. The information-media approach indicated the greatest degree of change in one financial-information variable.

Thus research to date on techniques and program formats implies that a variety of methods are effective on different outcome measures related to the major objective of preretirement planning.

ROLE OF THE SOCIAL WORKER COUNSELOR

Social workers involved in preretirement counseling usually perform three major tasks:

1. *Developmental.* This consists of "selling" the idea of preretirement preparation, of generating self-awareness and involving as many people as possible, and of assuring that these programs are offered on a continuing basis in a variety of settings. The organizational task is manifold and ranges from planning and implementation through the evaluative stage.
2. *Educational.* The transition into retirement implies an adjustment to new life conditions. Retirees need to discover where they can find satisfaction for their needs, interests, and expectations. Assessing the person's personal needs, determining the most suitable and gratifying sources, and facilitating the connection with such services resembles the information, referral, and monitoring functions of classical case management. The role- and skills-learning process operating at the retiree's end makes the task indistinguishable from adult-education models.
3. *Therapeutic.* When the impending transition is negatively experienced and the person harbors unrealistic expectations, the ensuing conflict may require therapeutic assistance. It may lead to a better sense of self-awareness and a new sense of direction like the one he/she possibly experienced in past work roles. As stated by Schlossberg, Troll, and Leibowitz (1978), it is the responsibility of the therapist "to help clients regain a sense of control by pointing out to them expanded alternatives, by offering them guidance in narrowing down options, and by making them aware of existing resources."

In a more schematic fashion, the range of social work tasks may be outlined as follows:

1. *Developmental*
   a. *Research.* Surveying workers' needs and interests and problem form-

ulation. Inventorying benefits, entitlements, and resources. Implementing a process and impact evaluation.

  b. *Organization and Planning.* Negotiating auspices and support for the program. Securing staff, speakers, and consultants. Designing the format and course content. Training volunteers or professional staff. Developing training content, evaluative instruments, and advertising materials. Reaching out to potential participants and promoting program objectives.

2. *Educational.* Gathering information about participants. Obtaining sources of information and negotiating consultative participation from major sources (pension administrators, health-insurance administrators, Social Security officials, etc.). Delivering course content in lecture format, group discussions, and individual tutoring sessions. Referring participants to specialized sources and monitoring the linkage process. Eliciting feedback.

3. *Therapeutic.*
  a. *Individual:* Casework counseling; individual assessment; crisis intervention; problem solving annd setting of life goals.
  b. *Group:* Resocialization; problem solving, task-oriented and self-help groups.

Many of the tasks in reference are generic requirements of any information and referral service, but no other aging-related service may require such a vast arsenal of information sources. Social workers delivering preretirement training and counseling must become aware of the potential inputs of

Area Agencies on Aging
Social Security Administration
Consumer protection agencies
Adult- and continuing-education programs
Life-insurance companies
Investment consultants and estate planners
Bank trust officers
Tax attorneys
Health-insurance carriers
Interstate service commissions
State real-estate commissions
Better Business Bureaus
Transportation departments and public transit authorities
Internal Revenue Service
Local bar associations
Local bank managers
Crime and fire-protection agencies
Health maintenance organizations

State lawyers referral services
Legal-aid services for the elderly
Local hospitals
Nutrition programs for the aged
Physical-fitness programs
Blindness, arthritis, heart, cancer, and Alzheimer's disease prevention
   organizations
Franchise organizations
Departments of Commerce
National Park Service and Forest Service
National Center for Voluntary Action
Service Corps for Retired Executives
Multiservice senior centers
Utility companies
Chambers of Commerce
Private employment agencies
University extension and career-training programs
Recreation programs
Self-help organizations
Veterans Administration and veterans organizations
Homecare services

The list, obviously, is a partial one and keeps expanding. Preretirement counselors cannot be expected to master in detail what each of these resources offers, but they should know how and whom to turn to for the pertinent information on a one-time basis or even for a continuous advisory relationship.

Similarly, it cannot be assumed that they know the couple of hundred pieces of federal legislation with direct bearing on the aged. There are five major legislative statutes, however, with direct relevance to retirement preparation that they ought to become specifically acquainted with:

1. The Social Security Act of 1935, which created the very institution of retirement through a social-insurance and intergenerational transfer mechanism of income maintenance
2. The 1965 amendments to the Social Security Act (Title XVIII—Medicare) sanctioning health insurance based only on an age-eligibility criterion
3. The 1973 amendments to the Older Americans Act, authorizing the design and sponsorship of preretirement programs
4. The Employee Retirement Income Security Act of 1974 (ERISA), regulating pension practices
5. The Age Discrimination in Employment Amendments of 1978 (ADEA) changing the compulsory retirement age from age 65 to age 70 for most private sector employees

ASSESSMENT

Assessing preretirees' needs also transcends the generic psychosocial inventories of the social-work profession and requires additional fine tuning and in-depth exploration in the following areas:

Age, race, sex.

Marital status. Length of marriage, onset of widowhood, presence of children and extent and quality of interaction with them, presence of living elderly parents and responsibilities toward them

Educational advancement. Educational level reached, continuing-education record, retraining and updating occupational skills, initiation and possible completion of a second career

Health status. Onset of chronic conditions, functional ability and history of work-related disabilities, health maintenance, prevention and fitness practices

Housing and interregional move. Status of possible home ownership, equity, outstanding debts, condition of house and extent of needed repairs, local taxes, access to services, amenities, and possible employment; future housing and regional preference, incidence of climate on health, and proximity to relatives and friends

Labor-force participation. Career patterns, job security, and advancement prospects if remaining in the labor force; labor-force demand in present occupational sector

Financial resources and assets. Savings, Social Security credits, and vesting in private pension plans; estate planning

Use of time. Leisure interests, skills, hobbies, physical activities, and cultural interests

Social participation. Volunteer experience and community participation; networks of same cohort friends and intergenerational involvement

Life goals. Formulation of postretirement objectives based on personal interests and a realistic appraisal of available resources

IMPLEMENTING THE PROGRAMS

The actual presentation of the instructional material in lecture, group, or tutorial fashion is usually based on fairly standardized and professionally reliable guidelines and handbooks, issued by specialized organizations, universities, and private corporations. The most widely used are those published by the American Association of Retired Persons through its division called Action for Independent Maturity (AIM), the National Council on Aging, the Industrial Relations Center of the University of Chicago, the University of Michigan, the Ethel Percy Andrus Gerontology Center of the University of Southern California, and Duke University. The International Society of Pre-Retirement Planners — a membership organization of individual counselors, designers of packaged programs, and corporate providers — acts as a clearinghouse of most ready-made instruction resources.

Because none of the instructional kits are tailor-made for the needs of a specific group of learners, social workers must make proper adaptations, combine elements of several such programs, and experiment and invest their ingenuity in innovative departures. The instructional series of meetings is, however, only the first stage. It serves to create awareness, but it must be followed by problem-solving tasks in a collaborative group atmosphere. It is ultimately intended that participants will feel stimulated to actually formulate a set of objectives, a plan, and begin working toward its implementation. On occasions, the plan will be tested in a group situation through role playing, simulations, and self-analysis. In a more realistic sense, the implementation phase will be a lengthy one, during which the social worker, possibly in conjunction with the group, will provide feedback and encouragement and assist in the reexamination of the objectives and in acquiring the necessary skills for their realization. To this end, preretirement counselors are often inspired by the andragogical method (Ingalls and Arceri, 1972). Andragogy is defined as the art of leading adult learning. Learners are committed to a process of self-diagnosis in a facilitative group environment and learn a problem-solving orientation. Individuals go through a sequence that includes:

1. *Needs assessment.* Identification of personal lags and problems that require resolution.
2. *Competency model building.* Inventorying the person's potential abilities and actual preferences, identifying the actual gap between the two and what may be required to overcome the gap. The gist of the method consists precisely in working on that gap, between what the person can do and what he or she wishes to do.
3. *Decision-making model.* Individual reeducation starts from the above-mentioned gap and assumes the form of a commitment, a sense of purpose with a definition of priorities or a rearrangement of existing priorities. The trainer assists in creating a learning climate, provides clarification, helps discerning between realistic and unrealistic aspirations, encourages mutuality, and acts as a consultant in the formulation of personal measurable objectives.

FUTURE DIRECTIONS

Programs presently in operation have obvious weaknesses. Most fear touching upon psychological issues because they regard that as an intrusion into the private lives of the participants. They tend to begin too late, when retirement is practically around the corner. Few really venture into painful concomitants of old age such as disability, widowhood, and death. Finally, most programs are too short, covering, at best, eight sessions of one to two hours each, and little attention is given to reinforcing previously acquired skills.

The future character of preretirement counseling programs will depend on the sequencing patterns between work, leisure, and education. Work, according to Hirschorn (1977, 1979), is undergoing a change from the fixed linear pattern of schooling and job scheduling of classical industrialism to a more flexible or cyclical pattern of interspersing work and education. It will also include a more subtle interpenetration of work requirements and personal life-styles. Initial symptoms of the transition are in early retirement, alienation from job ladders, more restlessness and career switching in middle life, more flexible time schedules, and dual careers in families that need to be coordinated. New organizational forms are emerging in the more advanced sector of the economy, based on temporary, task-centered teams, like "throw away" organizations rather than fixed job hierarchies.

Programs will then be geared to facilitating gradual retirements and periodical reentries to occupational roles. It is possible that present-type programs will give way to "life planning," "second-careers programs," planning for life transitions throughout the life span, or more specific forms of leisure education. "Second-career" programs, however, are too often euphemisms for volunteer recruitment. At times, they capitalize on the retiree's technical experience and seek suitable assignments in the service sector like the Second Careers Volunteer Program of New York and the Los Angeles Second Careers Program reported by Shackman (1980).

However, there are hardly any employment programs directed to older workers. As reported by Root and Zarrugh (1982), the few in operation are targeted to specific categories of workers and tend to exclude unskilled blue-collar workers. Sheppard and Mantovani (1982) found pervasive interest in post-retirement, part-time employment precisely among Hispanics, blacks, women, and low-income older workers. Both studies suggest that planning for post-retirement employment should occur prior to retirement and that proper incentives must be offered to employers to generate work opportunities. Coberly, Bentsen, and Klinger (1983) list such possible incentives: hiring subsidies, tax credits of up to 50 percent on the first $6,000 of an employee's first year's wages, training subsidies, Social Security waivers, tax credit for health-insurance costs, and placement and screening services. In a study of a *Fortune* 500 sample and smaller southern California companies, they found a positive disposition to hire older workers if such inducements were sanctioned by public policy. Long-range initiatives tend to underscore the policy inadequacies in current retirement practices and advocate the provision of partial retirement options in public-pension systems, abolition of work disincentive provisions in Social-

Security benefits, and tax incentives for experimenting with retirement options such as shorter work weeks, sabbaticals, extended vacation periods, part-time employment, job sharing, educational leaves, phased retirement, "flextime" systems, etc.

Many of the above initiatives remain, for the moment, in a hypothetical stage. It is not known how effectively they would respond to the challenge of demographic trends, economic realities, and personal value aspirations of the emerging adult cohorts. Increasing life expectancy and escalating costs of Social Security have already resulted in the gradual postponement of the mandatory retirement age.

In the more immediate future, there is moderate evidence of increasing employer concern with employee retirement preparation. Siegel and Rives (1980) found that most companies responding to their survey agreed that improvements are needed in existing programs and recommended, among others, expanding program content, exploring topics in greater depth, reducing the size of the groups of trainees, individualizing counseling sessions, and including more retirees as resource persons. Putting into effect such changes will require a variety of formats and better-trained, full-time professionals. It all results in greater costs. Yet not all employers are willing to bear such costs, nor are workers going out of their way to demand the provision of preretirement counseling as an employment benefit. Employers may eventually realize that such programs enhance workers' morale and may lead to higher productivity. Workers, in turn, may ultimately find that they increase their life options. At the end, advocates of preretirement programs will have to demonstrate that, by designing new retirement life patterns, they can prevent or postpone many of the costly problems of old age. It is possible that only then will society commit itself to a steadfast sponsorship of preretirement preparation programs.

REFERENCES

Ash, P. (1966). Pre-retirement counseling. *Gerontologist,* **6**(2), 97-99, 127-128.

Bolton, C. R. (1976). Humanistic instructional strategies and retirement education programming. *Gerontologist,* **16**(6), 550-555.

Boyack, V. L., and Tiberi, D. M. (1975). *A study of pre-retirement education.* Paper presented at the 28th Annual Meeting of the Gerontological Society, Louisville.

Charles, D. C. (1971). Effect of participation in a pre-retirement program. *Gerontologist,* **11**(1:1), 24-28.

Coberly, S., Bentsen, E., and Klinger, L. (1983). *Incentives for hiring older workers in the private sector: A feasibility study.* Los Angeles: Andrus Gerontology Center, University of Southern California.

Cumming, E., and Henry, W. E. (1961). *Growing old: The process of disengagement.* New York: Basic Books.

Duke University. (1977). Center for the Study of Aging and Human Development. *Duke University pre-retirement planning program.* Durham, N.C.: The Center.

Fitzpatrick, E. W. (1980). An introduction to NCOA's retirement planning program. *Aging and Work.* **3**(1), 20-26.

Glamser, F. D., and DeJong, G. F. (1975). The efficacy of pre-retirement preparation programs for industrial workers. *Journal of Gerontology.* **30**(5), 595-600.

Greene, M. R., Pyron, H. C., Manion, U. V., and Winklevoss, H. (1969). *Pre-retirement counseling, retirement adjustment, and the older employee.* Unpublished manuscript. University of Oregon Graduate School of Management.

Greenough, W. C., and King, F. P. (1977). Is normal retirement at age 65 obsolete? *Pension World.* **13**(6), 35-36.

Heidbreder, E. M. (1972). Factors in retirement adjustment: White-collar/blue-collar experience. *Industrial Gerontology.* no. 12, 69-79.

Hirschhorn, L. (1977). Social policy and the life cycle: A developmental perspective. *Social Service Review.* **51**(3), 434-450.

Hirschhorn, L. (1979). Post-industrial life: A US perspective. *Futures.* **11**(4), 287-298.

Ingalls, J. D., and Arceri, J. M. (1972). *A trainers guide to andragogy.* Washington: U.S. Social and Rehabilitation Service.

Kasschau, P. L. (1974). Reevaluating the need for retirement preparation programs. *Industrial Gerontology.* **1**(1), 42-59.

Louis Harris and Associates. (1975). *The myth and reality of aging in America.* Washington: National Council on the Aging.

Mack, M. J. (1958). An evaluation of a retirement-planning program. *Journal of Gerontology.* **13**(2), 198-202.

Monk, A. (1977). *Pre-retirement planning models: Social work inputs and applications.* Paper presented at the 5th Professional Symposium of the National Association of Social Workers, San Diego.

Motley, D. K. (1978). Availability of retired persons for work: Findings from the retirement history study. *Social Security Bulletin,* **41**(4), 18-29.

National Council on the Aging. (1973). *Preparation for retirement: A comparison of pre- and post-tests.* Washington: The Council.

Olson, S. K. (1981). Current status of corporate retirement preparation programs. *Aging and Work,* **4**(3), 175-187.

Ossofsky, J. (1980). Retirement preparation: Growing corporate involvement. *Aging and Work,* **3**(1), 14-17.

Pyron, H. C., and Manion, U. V. (1970). The company, the individual, and the decision to retire. *Industrial Gerontology.* no. 4, 1-11.

Research & Forecasts, Inc. (1980). Retirement preparation: Growing corporate involvement. *Aging and Work,* **3**(1), 1-13.

Root, S., Lawrence, and Zarrugh, L. H. (1982). *Innovative employment practices for older Americans.* Paper prepared for the National Commission for Employment Policy.

Rosow, I. (1973). The social context of the aging self. *Gerontologist,* **13**(1), 82-87.

Schein, E. H. (1980). *Organizational psychology* (3rd ed.). Englewood Cliffs, N.J.: Prentice-Hall.

Schlossberg, N. K., Troll, L., and Leibowitz, Z. (1978). *Perspectives on counseling adults: Issues and skills.* Monterey, Calif.: Brooks/Cole.

Schulz, J. H. (1980). *The economics of aging* (2nd ed.). Belmont, Calif.: Wadsworth.

Shackman, D. (1980). Second career volunteer program. *Sharing,* **4**(6), 5-6.

Sheldon, A., McEwan, P. J. M., and Ryser, C. P. (1975). *Retirement: Patterns and predictions.* Rockville, Md.: National Institute of Mental Health.

Sheppard, H. L., and Mantovani, R. E. (1982). *Part-time employment after retirement.* Washington: National Council on the Aging.

Siegel, S. R., and Rives, J. M. (1980). Preretirement programs within service firms: Existing and planned programs. *Aging and Work,* **3**(3), 183-191.

Simpson, I. H., and McKinney, J. C. (Eds.). (1966). *Social aspects of aging.* Durham, N.C.: Duke University Press.

Streib, G. F. (1958). Family patterns in retirement. *Journal of Social Issues,* **14**(2), 46-60.

U.S. Congress. House. Select Committee on Aging. (1981). *Abolishing mandatory retirement: Implications for America and Social Security of eliminating age discrimination in employment.* Washington: Government Printing Office.

Wermel, M. T., and Beideman, G. M. (1961). *Retirement preparation programs: A study of company responsibilities.* Pasadena, Calif.: Industrial Relations Section, California Institute of Technology.

15

Legal Services

Julia C. Spring, M.S.W., J.D.

Columbia University

Nancy A. Hufnagle, M.S.W., J.D., L.L.M.

Shanley and Fisher, P.C.

The "graying" of the American population has had effects on the need for legal services to the elderly that are greater than the actual population changes themselves. One effect has been an increasing number of persons who—because of problems in mobility, access, finances, communication, or comprehension—are unable to avail themselves of legal help for the problems adults of all ages have. The same population has additional legal problems because of its statistically greater vulnerability to fraud and abuse. But most important, for the infirm and firm elderly alike, a whole new area of legal problems has emerged because of the reliance of the middle-class elderly on Social Security and Medicare and of the elderly poor and near-poor on SSI, Medicaid, food stamps, and other government income and in-kind entitlement programs. A large body of substantive law, as well as law regarding the administration of these programs, has developed. Because there is no constitutional right to many of these benefits, and because there are strong cost-containment pressures in these programs, many programs for the elderly have become adversarial despite their beneficial intent. Thus even clearly entitled elderly clients must have assistance for mere initial access to those government benefits. As Nathanson (1982) summarizes it:

More than any other group, the elderly depend upon complex public and private institutions for their daily subsistence. Therefore, their legal problems frequently relate to the policies and actions of government agencies and private corporations, both of which often present themselves as bureaucratic mazes.

Superimposed upon the lives of the low-income (and especially the lives of the frail) elderly is a vast array of complex statutory, regulatory and decisional law. Their shelter may be provided or secured under federal and state public and subsidized housing laws, and zoning laws. Their health is often dependent upon Medicare, Medicaid, laws regulating nursing homes, and laws relating to the advertisement of prescription drugs. Their nutrition is often secured by the food stamp program and nutrition programs established by other federal laws. The source of their income may be Social Security, Supplemental Security Income, civil service or railroad retirement programs or private pensions. Their dignity, personal freedom and control of property are subject to the vagueness of the laws of guardianship, conservatorship and involuntary commitment.

Since they enter into contracts, own property, and have family relations, the elderly also have many of the same legal concerns as the rest of the population.

However, as front-line gerontological-services agency workers know well, this upsurge in legal needs of the elderly has not been matched by an upsurge in legal services. On the contrary, the political and cost-containment pressures that have made access to government entitlement programs more difficult have also made access to legal services more difficult. In addition, historically the law of government entitlements is "welfare" law and as such is not a crucial domain of private lawyers who earn their livings from client fees, nor of the law schools that train them. An attempt on the part of the American Bar Association since the mid-1970s to activate the private bar to provide more free and low-cost legal assistance to the elderly has been only partly successful (ABA Commission, 1981a). Among government-funded legal services, those of the Legal Service Corporation (LSC) are for the poor of all ages and cannot serve those whose income and resources fall above certain amounts; in fact, proportionately fewer of the poor elderly than of other age groups are served by LSC grantees. Additional legal services for those 60 and over have taken up only some of the slack since being funded under the Older Americans Act in 1975. Furthermore, AOA statistics indicate that the number of elderly served by both programs decreased in 1982 from 1981, due to political and economic pressures to limit government-paid legal assistance for the poor and elderly (U.S. Administration on Aging, 1982).

OBTAINING LEGAL ASSISTANCE

The Role of Social Work in Linking the Elderly Client to Legal Services

Given the many areas (listed in Appendix 15-1) where the elderly need legal assistance, and the fact that the elderly remain legally underserved, the gerontological social worker has a particularly important role both in facilitating referrals to available legal resources and in using other means to resolve legal problems when possible.

Social workers are uniquely qualified to serve as links between elderly clients and legal professionals. Social workers have a commitment, held by no other profession, to their clients' overall ability to cope with life and whatever problems life may present. Whatever the treatment approach, the social worker's role is to recognize psychological or environmental barriers—including legal ones—to effective functioning and to assist the client in overcoming these barriers. Further, gerontological social workers are frequently the clients' primary social contacts since many elderly clients served by social agencies are isolated: institutionalized in medical or nursing facilities; homebound for psychological, physical, or environmental reasons; impaired in communication ability. This commitment to, and contact with, the elderly client can be used to help the client overcome threshold difficulties in asserting legal rights—depression, mistrust of lawyers, often-realistic fears of futility or reprisal in "fighting city hall" (Bernstein, 1980). The social worker's ability to help a client overcome such fears and hesitations is as important when the underlying source of the problem is legal as in any other area.

To do so, the worker may have to put aside his or her own reluctance to deal with the legal system and lawyers. Clients and workers share the general societal perception of lawyers as inadequately responsive to human concerns and therefore not to be sought out except in acute and specific instances—for example, an imminent eviction. In addition, social workers and lawyers tend to draw rigid boundaries separating legal problems from social or emotional problems (Ehrlich and Ehrlich, 1979). Just as lawyers are often unwilling to recognize or deal with the emotional aspects of a legal concern, so too social workers often do not recognize the legal dimensions of a client's problem. This difference is exacerbated by the fact that in practice it is usually social workers who must adapt to the language and patterns of the higher-status professions— medicine as well as law—in order to secure the services that their clients need (Foster and Pearman, 1978).

In summary, gerontological social workers must recognize both their ability and their responsibility to deal with the legal concerns of the elderly. Geron- tological service agencies also must recognize this responsibility and provide front-line workers with the time, training, and other supports to perform this technical and time-consuming work. The social worker's role in regard to legal problems is the same problem-solving role as always: providing objective information about rights, remedies, and resources; activating the elderly client by working through the client's anxieties and fears that interfere with getting help; and assisting the referral or outside resource—the lawyer—in understanding the client's problem.

Identifying Legal Issues and Deciding Whether Referral to a Lawyer is Necessary

In order to decide whether or not legal referral is required, the gerontological social worker must have basic information about the function of law, specific substantive areas of law relevant to the elderly, and due-process concepts (Jankovic and Green, 1981; Miller, 1980).

Law in our society is intended to structure the behavior of citizens toward one another and between the government and individuals by providing a set of rules generally regarded as mandatory. The law involves both rights and responsibilities. The fact that something is called a "right" does not mean it's a *legal* right unless a court or a legislative body has assigned reciprocal rights and responsibilities on the topic. The "human right" not to be hungry, for example, is much broader than the legal right to food in congregate feeding programs or to food stamps.

However, the fact that a problem is identified as "legal" does not automatically mean a lawyer is needed or that a lawsuit is involved. In fact, whenever a client asks what can be expected in the way of health-care coverage or income supplement from the government, he/she is raising a legal concern — for example, what rights under the law does this client have? Thus every social worker in a specialized area is wise to become conversant with the law regarding that area, as well as with the structure of the legal and court system (Brieland and Lemmon, 1977; Landsman, McWherter, and Pfeffer, 1977). While no social worker — and no lawyer — can possibly master all substantive areas of law affecting the elderly, he/she should be aware of the general areas in which laws have been enacted (Appendix 15-1).

Two specific problems should be noted about learning the law in a particular subject area. First, a general manual or handbook such as those listed in the Bibliography may become outdated at any time; one small change in a statute (passed by a legislature) or a regulation (put into effect by an executive agency) may make it inapplicable to a particular client's situation. Lawyers usually use "reporter" (subscription) services to keep up-to-date on the law; a worker without such resources must always check out with those who have them whether the general law stated in a manual or handbook is still in effect. Second and similarly, many laws vary from one geographical area to another; a federal law (Social Security, SSI, Medicare) will generally be uniform across the country, while a law that has federal and state components (Medicaid, taxes) or is entirely state (mental health, guardianship) varies from state to state. Appendix 15-1 also lists the primary source — federal and/or state — of many substantive legal areas relevant to the elderly.

In addition, there are procedural aspects of law that cut across the different substantive areas — analogous to the processes of working for and with social-work clients that cut across the particular problems that are being addressed. Most of the procedural laws regulating government action are defined by federal and state statute and regulation; in addition, they must conform to constitutional "due process" principles (Dickson, 1976; Stone, 1978). As one of the most fundamental constitutional concepts, due process in the government-entitlement context refers to "what process is due" at all stages of the government's interaction with a person who applies for or receives an entitlement. The process due starts with the requirement that the government accept the application of every person who wishes to receive a benefit. The government must then determine whether or not that person is eligible and give the individual written notice and an opportunity for a hearing to contest a finding of ineligibility. Similarly, once a person is receiving a benefit, the government may decide that he/she no longer qualifies — and may ultimately reduce or discontinue benefits — but only after notice and an opportunity for a hearing at which the individual may present his/her side of the story.

Although specific procedural safeguards vary depending on the context, in essence due process is a requirement that the government be "fundamentally fair" in its dealings with an individual by informing him/her of its proposed actions and the reasons for those actions, and letting the person tell an impartial decision-maker of reasons for disagreement with that action. It does not stop the final action if legally justified — eviction, termination of benefits — but it protects the client from arbitrary or premature action. A worker with the elderly may well find that his/her intuitive reaction to whether an elderly client has been treated fairly comports with due-process requirements. Thus a client may come in with a letter stating that Medicaid recertification has been denied because the client failed to document eligibility. The client says he gave the agency everything asked for, but that he didn't know he had to submit those papers by a certain date or the application would be rejected. If the worker's reaction is "That's not fair, how can they do that — they didn't even give him a chance to comply," he/she would be focusing on exactly the right legal issue.

With a basic knowledge of procedural concepts and substantive areas of law relevant to the elderly, a worker is prepared to identify legal problems of the elderly. It is crucial to note that the questioning necessary for a potential legal referral should be keyed as closely as possible to the specific legal issues involved (Binder and Price, 1977; Shaffer, 1976). Thus, for example, a social worker might need to question an elderly client about her living arrangements for a possible challenge to an SSI reduction after she has moved in with her sister. Although the social worker would usually focus on whether or not the elderly sisters are adapting to life together, in the SSI context the concern would be to determine whether the client is paying her share of the rent in order to establish legally that she is still entitled to maximum "living alone" benefits. Such specific, legal-issue fact-finding is crucial either for referral of a client to a lawyer or fo representation of the client by a nonlawyer. In addition, the worker may also be serving a valuable social-work function by assisting the client in sorting out fac from fantasy—for example, that the Social Security worker was following regulations in this matter rather than simply giving the client a hard time.

Thus a gerontological social worker has a three-step process: (1) identifying the relevant area of law and, if possible, its specific provisions; (2) gathering the facts of the situation as relevant to the specific law; (3) deciding whether to assis the client directly in coping with the problem or to seek legal assistance.

In many areas related to the elderly, there is no definite line separating the role of a social-work advocate from that of a lawyer. As discussed in the next section social-work representation at an administrative hearing may well be the bes advocacy route. When *is* a lawyer needed, then? The following are rough guidelines for seeking a lawyer:

1. When a catastrophic result is imminent without court intervention (e.g. eviction or surgery the client opposes)
2. When the client has been served with legal papers
3. When other administrative remedies have failed and been exhausted (e.g., denial of a Social Security claim up to the Appeals Council level
4. When the client wants to achieve a goal that must comply with certain legal requirements in order to be valid or enforceable (e.g., divorce, will general power of attorney)
5. When the client needs information about legal options in order to decide what course of action to take (e.g., eligibility for Medicaid if money is transferred to a child or an action for age discrimination).

If the decision is made that the client's situation requires a lawyer, private and public resources should be pursued with all the networking skills social workers employ in other situations. If the decision is made that the situation does not so require, there are various modes of proceeding without a lawyer.

Proceeding Without a Lawyer

There are three routes for acting without a lawyer: the client acts on his/he own; the client acts with the assistance of a nonlawyer (often a relative or a socia worker); and the client or worker uses nonlegal dispute-resolution mechanisms

First, some proceedings are set up with the *intention* that cases will be handled by the aggrieved person himself/herself. Small-claims courts, fo example, are set up by many civil-court systems to handle the small-dollar-value grievances of one person against another or against a business (the person whose dry cleaner has lost laundry, or whose landlord has not returned a security deposit). Self-help books found in many bookstores and those listed in the Bibliography contain resources for handling these procedures alone, although it is wise to check what is useful in each particular state or locality.

Other proceedings *permit* a person to act on his or her own, to be represented by a lawyer, or to be assisted by a nonlawyer. Usually, when the government has an obligation to provide certain benefits generally or to specific population groups—often through state and federal income, health, housing, tax, employment, and antidiscrimination agencies—due process requires a hearing to contest a decision *not* to grant such benefits. In these hearings an individual may choose whether and how to be represented. In an administrative hearing (i.e., the meeting that is the final step of an agency's review of objections to decisions it has made), nonlawyers are often as skilled as lawyers. Thus this is a crucial arena for social workers to exercise advocacy skills. This is particularly true if the nonlawyers are well versed in the relevant law, or if the problem is not so much one of disagreement about the law as confusion about the facts, as often is true in agency proceedings. Then the hearing may be viewed as an opportunity to present an organized, clear view of the facts—and supporting documents or spoken testimony—to someone (called a judge but really a hearing officer) who comes to the situation without the bias of having dealt with the particular case previously. Various organizations have manuals about lay hearing representation in general or in specific substantive areas; some of these manuals are listed in the Bibliography (e.g., Arnason, 1983).

In addition, there is a general legal principle that even in a court that permits representation by *another* person only if that other person is a lawyer, an individual can still represent himself/herself entirely alone (*pro se*). How this general legal principle is carried out varies according to specific state and federal laws. However, claimants who carry out all prior Social Security, Medicare, or SSI appeals steps and still receive unfavorable decisions, or individuals who believe their civil rights have been violated, may go on their own to the *pro se* clerk of the nearest federal district courthouse. An individual who goes to state or federal court on his/her own and who also files a "poor person's" (*in forma pauperis*) petition indicating that he or she cannot pay court fees, will often—although not necessarily—have a free (*pro bono*) lawyer appointed by the court. A poor client who is charged with a crime will also usually have a free lawyer appointed by the judge.

Finally, over the last decade or so there has been an increasing interest in nonlegal dispute resolution—either mediation (in which an impartial person simply helps the antagonists resolve the dispute) or arbitration (in which the antagonists agree ahead of time that the impartial person will make a decision to which they will adhere) (Denenberg and Denenberg, 1981). Such conflict resolution may be particularly useful when individuals might otherwise attempt to sue to settle something that's not really a legal matter, or where legal expenses and procedures are out of proportion to the dollar value of the actual issue—for example, disputes between relatives or neighbors, or between a client and a small business.

Government-Funded Legal Services

If referral to an attorney is needed, many gerontological agency social workers will first contact local legal services (often called legal aid) funded by the Legal Services Corporation (LSC) and/or the Administration on Aging (AoA) of the U.S. Department of Health and Human Services. The LSC, established by Congress in 1974 as a private nonprofit corporation and successor to the legal-services programs under the 1964 Economic Opportunity Act (the Kennedy-Johnson "War on Poverty"), provides free civil legal assistance to all poor persons, not just the elderly. LSC-funded legal assistance is for those who have incomes below 125 percent of the federal Office of Management and Budget poverty line. In 1982, these limits were $4,738 yearly income for one person and $6,263 for a couple. The Older Americans Act, not providing specifically for legal services until the 1975 amendments to Title III (and thus often referred to simply as Title III Legal Services), provides free aid for those 60 and over. These services are not targeted specifically for the poor, although in 1980 over half the clients served were low-income. Rather, the OAA requires preference for older persons with the greatest economic or social need without imposing a means test. This preference is most often manifested by targeting issues most relevant to the elderly (income, health care, housing, protective services) or geographic areas where the elderly are concentrated. The effect is an informal but not a rigid means test.

Both LSC and AoA legal services are forbidden to take fee-generating cases (i.e., ones where the individual is suing for money) and have many other limitations. On the whole they specialize in civil, not criminal, cases having to do with income maintenance, health benefits, consumer complaints, and family, and housing law. Some specialize even further—particularly in these days of cost containment—in order to use their services most effectively for their target population.

An urban legal-services program, whether funded by AoA or LSC, might have three or four lawyers, possibly assisted by paralegals and law students. It might have a social worker, but probably would not. Each attorney might well have a caseload of over one hundred, typically involving landlord-tenant disputes, protective services and homecare issues, and questions of eligibility for government income and medical-care programs. Frequently, more than one legal issue would be involved. For example, a client might be referred because he or she had received an eviction notice for nonpayment of rent. Upon investigation, the attorney might discover the client's nonpayment of rent to be related to a problem with SSI or Social Security or to an inability to manage his or her funds.

Elderly clients would first come in contact with this office by telephone or by referral of family, social agencies, or other lawyers. Home visits might occasionally be made. At the initial contact, some brief information about the client and his or her problem would be taken. If the client seemed appropriate for government-funded services in terms of broad characteristics such as age, financial status, and type of problem, the client would be given an appointment for a more thorough intake interview. In an emergency, a client would be scheduled for an initial interview as soon as possible.

After the initial interview, the supervising attorney would determine whether the office would handle the problem. If another referral were more appropriate, it would be made. At all stages of this process and subsequent legal representation, a social worker or family member might well be involved if the client so desired; the lawyer would probably wish to see the client alone at least once to ascertain the client's wishes. Such assistance would be particularly crucial if the client had some diminished ability to understand the legal proceedings or to carry out necessary actions.

Legal-services offices for the elderly take other forms around the country. As AoA funding must be given to the best possible provider, in 1981 one-third of the AoA funds went to other than LSC grantees; for example, the New York City Office on the Aging each year since 1978 has awarded funds to one law-school clinic, one social-service agency, and two different LSC grantees. In small communities and rural areas, AoA legal services are often provided by contract with local private lawyers.

Currently, both AoA and LSC legal services are under federal and state political and economic attack. Title III legal services are additionally vulnerable to local political pressure since, unlike LSC funding decisions (made federally and with the obligation that all allotted funds go to legal services or administration), the decisions on allocating AoA funds to legal services are made by the local Area Agency on Aging (AAA). An AAA is required only to spend "some funds," no amount specified, on legal services—and indeed since 1982 it is required *not* to spend any funds if it finds the legal needs of the elderly in the community are already being met. Since the AAA is usually a branch or a neighbor of the state human-services/welfare agency, many AAAs are reluctant to fund legal services that may represent clients against these agencies, especially when the block grant must also fund homecare and access services. Thus many AAAs resolve this political dilemma by allocating negligible resources, primarily for information and referral, not direct representation to legal services. In 1982 proportionately fewer dollars were spent on legal services by AAAs than the previous year: an average of less than $20,000 per AAA, ranging from 1.5 percent to only 22.6 percent of the total state Title III grant.

Occasionally an LSC grantee or another organization receives funding from other government sources. In particular, Title XX Social Security Act funds are to be used by states for services to prevent or reduce economic dependency and inappropriate institutional care. As an example, a Connecticut LSC grantee has received major Title XX funding since 1977 through the State Department of Income Maintenance (DIM). The project, called Legal Assistance for Medicare Patients (LAMP), carries out both major lawsuits and highly replicable administrative appeals of denials of Medicare reimbursement for skilled-nursing care in hospitals and nursing homes. LAMP has generated interest in social service departments of other states. Since early 1982, LAMP has had an additional contract with DIM, using Title XIX (Medicaid) funds to appeal the Medicare denials of patients also Medicaid-eligible. Because of the nature of Title XX block grants, which do not mandate funds specifically for *legal* assistance, such programs are politically vulnerable. Similarly, VISTA and CETA were formerly major sources of labor in legal-services programs but proved politically vulnerable.

To maximize the chances of getting needed legal assistance for a client in these days of restricted public funding, workers should keep several factors in mind. First, as already discussed, the worker should have a clear statement of the legal problem in order to facilitate communication with a probably overworked lawyer. Second, the possibility that a private attorney would be more appropriate, or necessary, should have been examined, as discussed in the next section of this article. Third, as the presence of income and population restrictions just discussed implies, both programs are themselves entitlement systems, like the government bureaucracies against which they often act for their clients; this means that only some individuals, who meet certain criteria, are entitled to free legal services. Further, neither system has a due-process mechanism for a person who has been denied representation to appeal that decision. Thus, knowing what kinds of case and client categories are served by a particular office is crucial to client advocacy. Information is available from the federal Legal Services Corporation on all grantees nationwide; each state's office on aging has information on Title III services statewide, as does the federal Administration on Aging. A question to the local Area Agency on Aging or to the state office on aging should reveal whether a particular LSC grantee is also receiving Older Americans Act funds; such recipients are precluded from using a rigid means test, although services may be targeted for those with the greatest economic need (Landrum, 1982; U.S. Administration on Aging, 1982).

Private Lawyers and Bar Associations

Many workers with the elderly avoid the use of private attorneys on the assumption that a private lawyer is likely to be too costly and not attuned to the psychosocial needs of older clients. However, at times private attorneys could and should be used. First, some elderly clients, despite low fixed incomes, do have savings and other assets; these resources will make them ineligible for LSC-funded legal assistance and most AoA-funded assistance. In turn, the clients' possession of economic resources may necessitate taking legal precautions to ensure that these resources will be transferred or managed well in case of death, institutionalization, or decreased mental ability; it is exactly these areas of law that are often best known by private attorneys.

Second, in some areas of law there are provisions for lawyer reimbursement if the client wins. In such cases, a prepayment of fees (retainer) is usually not required. For example, up to 25 percent of a retroactive Social Security benefit won in a hearing by an attorney may be paid directly to the attorney. (Note that this is *not* applicable to SSI.) It may well be worth that payment for an elderly client to receive denied past benefits as well as future ones (Sweeney and Lyko, 1980). As another example, a client's case might result in a money settlement (out of court) or judgment (in court)—for example, when a physically injured client wishes to sue the person who caused the injury for money damages (a fee-generating case LSC and AoA grantees cannot take). An attorney may be willing to take on such cases on a "contingency fee" basis, meaning that the lawyer will get a preestablished proportion (usually one-third) of whatever is won. Obviously, a lawyer is usually willing to take on a case without a retainer only when the probability of winning is high.

It should be noted that if a client—or a relative—is contemplating such a suit or other legal action, it is worth a consultation with a private lawyer on the probable outcome of such a case, potential contingency fee, and willingness to take the case. In fact, such a consultation is necessary in order to decide whether to proceed. It is standard in legal practice to ask when setting up the appointment what the consultation fee (if any) for a specified length of time is. During the consultation, discussion should include both the fee for the lawyer's services *and* the fee for court and other costs. A consultation does not imply a commitment to use that lawyer.

How to find a private attorney? Networking is critical. With an elderly person, it might be wise to check first whether there is a family friend or relative who would be willing to handle the particular problem, if put in touch with relevant legal manuals or a specialist in this kind of law. Other workers or clients might know private attorneys who are skilled in the particular substantive law. The local LSC- or AoA-funded legal-services office might refer a client to a private attorney; because of the recent decrease in federal legal-assistance funding, as well as because the legal problems of the elderly cut across all economic classes, some legal-services attorneys have recently moved into private practice with a partial specialization in legal problems of the elderly.

Another source is a bar association, which may be organized by municipality, county, state, or, in urban areas, by particular groups of attorneys (women, blacks, etc.). Since the mid-1970s a number of bar associations have developed special programs for the elderly that may either provide or refer for the services needed. These elderly-specializing private-bar services tend to be of three basic types: (1) *pro bono* (volunteer), usually in a few legal areas, like wills; (2) reduced-fee referrals for the elderly with fixed incomes; (3) prepaid "judicare" programs (ABA and American Bar Foundation, 1982; Lardent and Coven, 1981; Schmidt 1980). In addition, many bar associations have a general telephone-referral service in which attorneys are listed by areas of law they practice in return for agreeing to see referred clients for an initial consultation at a flat fee that is somewhat below the market rate. Every referral lawyer must be a member in good standing of the local bar, but the amount of screening and attorney monitoring varies considerably among bar referral services. A consultation should provide necessary data to decide on the costs, necessity, and feasibility of pursuing a particular legal course, as well as the skills of the particular lawyer. Again the worker's or client's network may be needed to confirm that impression.

Advertised "legal clinics" have developed since the mid-1970s, particularly in urban areas. For highly repetitive legal problems (for example, a simple will or an uncontested divorce that does not involve property, alimony, or child support), a clinic may have low fees because the case-handling can be replicated on a volume basis, often by paralegals. A clinic should not be used if there are any complications in a problem, and its reputation should be checked through the client's or social worker's network.

A final possibility is to look around for lawyers or law-related groups that have a particular interest in the *issues* your client is concerned with (employment discrimination, mental illness), the *population* your client is a member of (retirees of a particular union, Masons), or the *kind* of case (Social Security appeal, immigration problem). A local law school may well have a practice component geared to one of the above, in which students handle the cases of clients unable to pay under the supervision of a faculty member/attorney. Most schools select only a few categories of cases that have been determined to be both educationally useful and where students can offer significant services to clients (Harbaugh, 1976; Nathanson, 1982).

Lastly, if ever a lawyer's service—whether public or private—to a client is unsatisfactory, it is possible to complain about that lawyer, usually through a local, county, or state bar association (ABA, 1982). An investigation and response to a written complaint will usually be made. If a court has appointed a lawyer to represent a client or a guardian *ad litem* (obligated to represent the client's best interests, not his or her choice), a complaint may also be made to that court. Finally, it is possible—although more difficult—to consult another attorney about a legal malpractice suit if there has been harm to a client as a result of the first attorney's failure to act by the standards of the legal profession.

DEVELOPING LEGAL SERVICES FOR THE ELDERLY

Direct Provision of Legal Services to Agency Client

In most cases, direct provision of legal assistance by a gerontological-services agency is not financially possible. However, putting aside the question of money, there is the difficulty in many social-service agencies of persuading top executives and board members, whether social workers or lawyers, of the need for legal services for the elderly. Although those with direct client contact know the importance of law-related areas to the daily lives of the elderly, those not in direct practice often do not realize that the problems of the elderly cannot be managed simply by information, referral, and counseling but require intensive and costly advocacy. Social-worker board members may not recognize that the legal issues of clients cannot ethically be handled by the same lawyers who handle questions, like those of incorporation, of the agency itself. Lawyer board members unfamiliar with entitlement law are probably not aware of the adversarial nature of entitlement systems.

If this threshold obstacle is surmounted, two primary organizational problems must be dealt with. First, the overhead costs for legal services are higher than those for social services and will probably not be covered even by a sliding-scale fee structure. Costs include both the higher salary of even the lowest-paid starting attorney, as well as that of a secretary able to type legal documents. Legal supplies will be needed, funds for court fees and transcripts, malpractice insurance, and expensive books and subscription reporter services in crucial areas of the law. Donations of or access to some legal materials can perhaps be arranged, but without basic materials immediately at hand the lawyer will be unable to work efficiently and effectively.

Second, the gerontological-services agency must consider how to handle conflicts between the lawyer's and the social worker's goals in working with a shared client (Malick and Ashley, 1980). Preparation for such conflicts includes mutual education about the differences between the professional stances so that they can be recognized as just that — different rather than right or wrong in any absolute sense. Equally important is establishing guidelines for what cases will be handled and structure for decision-making when consensus breaks down on those cases that are handled.

Of course lawyers and gerontological social workers are often in harmony on their work with clients. However, at times there will be conflict between the ways that each profession regards as essential to assist a client, consistent with its professional theory, ethics, and practice. For example, social workers in a gerontological agency might decide, as a matter of professional judgment, that an elderly person is unable to manage Social Security benefits and therefore needs a representative payee to receive and spend those checks on behalf of the actual beneficiary. The in-house lawyer might be called in to obtain the representative payee but perceives his/her professional obligation as representing the client's expressed desire to continue to receive benefit checks and spend them, however inappropriately. Social workers and lawyers might also find themselves in conflict when the professional confidentiality obligation of one precludes sharing certain information with the other (Bernstein, 1977).

The Lawyer's Code of Professional Responsiblity, available from most state bar associations, requires the lawyer to make legal decisions in conjunction with the individual client, not allowing agency or other interests to control that judgment. Even a lawyer board of directors can set only broad policy parameters, for example on the kinds of cases that may be taken, not specific directions on what course of action may be taken in a specific case. Of course, many gerontological services agencies would be reluctant to pay for an in-house lawyer who would have ultimate say in such conflicts. Consequently, it is critical to establish, as part of the development of a legal-assistance program, what kinds of cases will be handled (e.g., administrative hearings only or, further, more costly court appeals). These guidelines can be made clear to an attorney being hired as well as to clients. Because of the practical and ethical problems of one profession supervising another (Barton and Byrne, 1975; Ehrlich and Ehrlich, 1979) it is probably best to have the legal-services unit of a social-service agency operate within those guidelines but somewhat separately from the usual agency lines of authority.

An alternative would be for a gerontological-services agency to use available funds to pay an outside lawyer, lawyers, or firm to handle clients' cases, which would avoid in-house professional conflict on how to assist an elderly client. Further, if the arrangement were with just one or a few attorneys, it might be possible to select one who has knowledge of legal and interpersonal issues relevant to the elderly, which would be less possible if the referrals were to a large firm where the case might be assigned to one of a number of lawyers.

It would again be important to discuss service issues fully, in an atmosphere of mutual education, before the agreement is reduced to a written document. These issues would include fee, unit of service, case preferences or limitations, referral mechanisms, and reciprocal confidentiality concerns. Defining the unit of service and payment for it is particularly important because of the different professional assumptions on what is appropriate service. Finally, it would be advisable to have an ongoing review of the terms of the agreement, as both social workers and lawyers develop a fuller sense of what the working arrangement actually entails.

Expansion of Legal Services Available to Elderly Clients in the Community

A gerontological services agency might choose to expand legal services in the community through a small- or large-scale mobilization of the community bar association. A connection with the private bar should tend toward institutionalizing legal services in the locality rather than having them depend on one agency's fiscal choices. The skills required for such mobilization are those social workers use in other community-organization tasks, with due attention to particular strategy issues raised by the formal and informal authority structure of local bar groups as well as the status difference between social workers and lawyers. Such an effort would capitalize on recent interest in the private bar's involvement in provision of legal services to the elderly. This movement, born in the mid-1970s, has come partly from within the organized bar itself. Since 1976 the American Bar Association (ABA) Young Lawyers Division has been active in encouraging state and local bar associations to supply legal information and services to the elderly; since 1978 the ABA has had a special interdisciplinary Commission on Legal Problems of the Elderly (ABA Commission, 1981b) with the delivery of legal services to the elderly as one of its four priorities. The movement can be traced to a recognition that many of the elderly who are too poor to pay private attorneys still have middle-class legal needs, including the need for wills, trusts, and other arrangements that care adequately for the older generation, in the community and in institutions, as well as their offspring. The result is that when some attorneys decide to fulfill their ethical obligation to do legal work *pro bono publico* (volunteer; literally "for the public good"), the elderly are an appealing section of the public to assist (ABA, 1977). Pressure to mobilize the private bar has also come from the government-funded legal-services sector. Since 1978, AoA grantees have been required to foster involvement of the local private bar to provide reduced-fee and *pro bono* services to those over 60, while since 1982 LSC grantees have been mandated to expend 10 percent of funding on involvement of private attorneys in provision of legal services to the poor.

The potential for such service must not be overestimated, since in the current straitened economy there is much competition for scarce *pro bono* lawyer resources. However, since even slight assistance from local lawyers may be of major assistance to elderly clients, it is an approach worthy of consideration. The most modest approach — and the most common nationwide — would be for the bar association to provide a number of limited (in time and scope) services of the kind the member attorneys are already likely to be expert in — for example, executing a number of wills or providing brief consultations on consumer or other issues, perhaps at a senior citizens' center. An example is an individual attorney who recently took a leave from his firm and in five weeks wrote a large number of "wills on wheels" for homebound clients of the local LSC office. The essence of less glamorous versions of this approach is that the volunteer attorney incur no obligations outside of the specific amount of time for the basic task. If the client's social worker can ensure that the client will get to the appointment with relevant documents and facts, this will help the success of such a project.

There are, of course, other examples of private-bar legal assistance to the elderly of varying degrees of complexity. Many of these examples are described in state bar association publications (Schmidt, 1980). A project in rural Colorado sponsored by the state bar association and run by a nonlawyer director uses 120 *pro bono* attorneys to serve clients spread out over eleven countries (Paine, 1982). Volunteer lawyers through the Cleveland Bar Association aid that city's Hospice Council. The large-scale Volunteer Lawyers Project in Boston uses lawyers and paralegals with background in special areas of law to provide technical assistance and close working relationships with volunteer attorneys who handle a variety of cases for low-income clients (Lardent, 1980). The same project (listed in Appendix 15-2) recently announced that it had received a grant to assist legal-service programs in developing private-attorney-involvement projects keyed to local needs and circumstances.

Several issues should be kept in mind as more complex models are considered. First, because much law related to the elderly—particularly government-benefit law—is esoteric, private attorneys will need training and on-going technical assistance in order to do high-quality work and feel comfortable in the process. Similar requirements emerge as the representation becomes larger scale, more complex, or of longer duration. Related is the problem of monitoring the quality of representation either when a project becomes large scale or when the referral system means that the lawyer may perceive ongoing communication with the referral source as a breach of confidentiality or of decision control. Those who have developed successful large-scale *pro bono* projects indicate that the best way to maintain volunteer attorney investment and quality performance is to key the work to the volunteer's particular interests, with substantial ongoing technical assistance for areas of law in which private lawyers are not expert (ABA Commission, 1981b; Lardent, 1980; Lardent and Coven, 1981; Paine, 1982).

Obviously, these additional needs would require a director to coordinate, train, and monitor volunteers, as well as to raise funds. Another important function would be close coordination between this service and other available legal resources, including LSC- and AoA-funded projects, and perhaps attempts to utilize funds from these sources. To enter the competition engendered by scarce funds is, of course, possible as the local AAA is mandated to locate the best possible provider. Better, however, might be to develop a community consortium of gerontological service agencies, the private bar, and government-funded legal services. In such a way might the legal and social-service resources of a community pull together to use their energy to improve the status of the country's legally underserved elderly.

REFERENCES AND BIBLIOGRAPHY

American Bar Association. (1977). *Implementing the lawyer's public interest practice obligation.* Chicago: American Bar Association.
American Bar Association. (1982). *Grievance referral list of lawyers disciplinary agencies.* Chicago: American Bar Association.

American Bar Association Commission on Legal Problems of the Elderly. (1981a). *Involving the private bar in the aging community.* Washington: American Bar Association.

American Bar Association Commission on Legal Problems of the Elderly. (1981b). *Legal services for the elderly: Where the nation stands.* Washington: American Bar Association.

American Bar Association Commission on Legal Problems of the Elderly. (1981c). *Reduced fee lawyer referral service for the elderly.* Washington: American Bar Association.

American Bar Association Commission on Legal Problems of the Elderly and the Committee on Delivery of Legal Services to the Elderly. (1981d). *The law and aging resource guide.* Washington: American Bar Association.

American Bar Association and American Bar Foundation, Legal Services Section (1982). *The ABA catalog.* Chicago: American Bar Association.

Arnason, S. (1983). *Administrative appeals manual.* New York: Institute on Law and Rights of Older Adults, Brookdale Center on Aging, Hunter College.

Barton, P. N., and Byrne, B. (1975). Social work services in a legal aid setting. *Social Casework, 60*, 226-234.

Bernstein, B. (1977). Privileged communications to the social worker. *Social Work, 22*, 264-268.

Bernstein, B. (1980). Lawyer and social worker as an interdisciplinary team. *Social Casework, 65*, 416-422.

Binder, D., and Price, S. (1977). *Legal interviewing and counseling: A client-centered approach.* St. Paul: West Publishing.

Blumberg, R. E., and Grew, R. (1978). *The rights of tenants: ACLU handbook.* New York: Avon Books.

Brieland, D., and Lemmon, J. (1977). *Social work and the law.* St. Paul: West Publishing.

Brown, R. N. (1979). *The rights of older persons: ACLU handbook.* New York: Avon Books.

Clearinghouse Review (National Clearinghouse for Legal Services, Chicago, Ill.), monthly.

Denenberg, T. S., and Denenberg, R. V. (1981). *Dispute resolution: Settling conflicts without legal action.* New York: Public Affairs Pamphlets.

Dickson, D. (1976). Law in social work: Impact of due process. *Social Work, 21*, 274-278.

Drew, E. (1982, Feb. 27). A reporter at large: Legal services. *New Yorker.*

Edelman, C. D., and Siegler, I. C. (1978). *Federal age discrimination in employment law: Slowing down the golden watch.* Charlottesville, Va.: The Michie Company.

Ennis, B. J., and Emery, R. D. (1978). *The rights of mental patients: ACLU handbook.* New York: Avon Books.

Ehrlich, I., and Ehrlich, P. (1979). Social work and legal education: Can they unite to serve the elderly? *Journal of Education for Social Work, 15*(2), 87-93.

Foster, M. G., Pearman, W. A. (1978). Social work, patient rights, and patient representatives. *Social Casework, 59*(2), 89-100.

Handler, J. (1979). *Protecting the social services client.* New York: Academic Press.

Harbaugh, J. D. (1976). Clinical training and legal services for older people: The role of the law school. *Gerontologist, 16*(5), 447-450.

Health Advocate (National Health Law Program, Los Angeles, Calif.), monthly.

Hemphill, C. F. Jr. (1981). *Consumer protection handbook: A legal guide.* Englewood Cliffs, N.J.: Prentice-Hall.

Jankovic, J., and Green, R. D. (1981). Teaching legal principles to social workers. *Journal of Education for Social Work, 17*(3), 28-35.

Krauskopf, J. M. (1983). *Advocacy for the aging.* St. Paul: West Publishing.

Landrum, R. (1982). *Report of the legal services corporation conference on legal services and the elderly.* Washington: Legal Services Corporation.

Landsman, S., McWherter, D., and Pfeffer, A. (1977). *What to do until the lawyer comes.* Garden City, N.Y.: Doubleday Anchor.

Lardent, E. F. (1980). Pro bono that works. *NLADA Briefcase, 37*, 54-71.

Lardent, E. F., and Coven, I. M. (1981). *Quality control in private bar programs for the elderly.* Washington: American Bar Association.

Malick, M. D., and Ashley, A. A. (1980). Politics of interprofessional collaboration: Challenge to advocacy. *Social Casework*, **62**(3), 131-137.

McCormick, H. L. (1983). *Social Security claims and procedures*. St. Paul: West Publishing.

Miller, J. (1980). Teaching law and legal skills to social workers. *Journal of Education for Social Work*, **16**(3), 87-95.

Nathanson, P. (1982). An innovative approach to elders' unmet legal needs. *Generations*. **6**(3), 37.

NCSLC Washington Weekly (National Senior Citizens Law Center, Washington), weekly.

1981 Medicare explained. (1981). Chicago: Commerce Clearing House.

1982 Social Security explained. (1982). Chicago: Commerce Clearing House.

Paine, K. (1982). Stretching resources for legal services: Nontraditional approaches in two settings. *Clearinghouse Review*, **16**(6), 559-565.

Schmidt, L. (1980). *Bibliography of selected materials: Private bar involvement in legal services delivery*. Washington: Legal Services Corporation.

Schuster, M. R. (1981). *Social Security and Supplemental Security Income disability programs: Practice manual*. Washington: Legal Counsel for the Elderly.

Shaffer, T. L. (1976). *Legal interviewing and counseling*. St. Paul: West Publishing.

Slonim, S. (1982). *Landlords and tenants: Your guide to the law*. Chicago: ABA.

Social Security Forum (National Organization of Social Security Claimants' Representatives, Pearl River, N.Y.), monthly.

Spring, J. C. (1981). Medicare: An advocacy perspective for social workers. *Social Work in Health Care*, **6**(4), 77-89.

Stone, L. M. (1978). Due process: A boundary for intervention. *Social Work*, **23**(5), 402-405.

Striker, J. M., and Shapiro, A. O. (1977). *Super threats: How to sound like a lawyer and get your rights on your own*. New York: Rawson Associates.

Striker, J. M., and Shapiro, A. O. (1981). *How you can sue without hiring a lawyer: A guide to winning in small claims court*. New York: Simon & Schuster.

Sweeney, D. M., and Lyko, J. J. (1980). *Practice manual for Social Security claims*. New York: Practicing Law Institute.

U.S. Administration on Aging. (1982). *Legal services programs under Title III of the Older Americans Act*. Washington Office of Field Services, Legal Services Corporation.

Warner, R. (1980). *Everybody's guide to small claims court*. Berkeley, Calif.: Addison-Wesley.

Weiss, J. (1976). *Law of the elderly*. New York: Practicing Law Institute.

Appendix 15-1: Basic Legal Issues for the Elderly, Sources, and Agencies

Subject Matter	Statute	Regulations	Agency Responsible for Administration
1. Income maintenance			
(a) Old age, survivors, and disability insurance (Social Security)			
(i) Social security retirement	42 U.S.C.A. § 401 *et seq.*	20 C.F.R. § 404 *et seq.*	Social Security Administration (SSA), U.S. Dept. of Health and Human Services
(ii) Social security disability	" "	" "	
(b) Supplemental security income (SSI)	42 U.S.C.A. § 1381 *et seq.*	20 C.F.R. § 416 *et seq.*	Social Security Administration, U.S. Dept. of Health and Human Services
(c) General assistance (home relief, welfare)	State public assistance statutes	State public assistance regulations	State public assistance agencies (e.g., State Dept. of Social Services)
(d) Food stamps	7 U.S.C.A. § 2011 *et seq.*	20 C.F.R. § 27 *et seq.*; regulations of state	State public assistance agencies under the direction of the U.S. Dept. of Agriculture
(e) Railroad retirement benefits	45 U.S.C.A. § 231 *et seq.*	20 C.F.R. § 200 *et seq.*	Railroad Retirement Board (federal)
(f) Veterans benefits	38 U.S.C.A. § 301 *et seq.*	38 C.F.R. § 3 *et seq.*	Veterans Administration (federal)
(g) Private pensions	Employee Retirement Income Security Act of 1974 (ERISA), 29 U.S.C.A. § 1001 *et seq.*; Internal Revenue Code of 1954, as amended, 26 U.S.C.A. § 401 *et seq.*	29 C.F.R. § 2560 *et seq.*	Labor Management Service Administration, Pension Benefit Guaranty Corp.; Internal Revenue Service

(continued)

Appendix 15-1: (Continued)

Subject Matter	Statute	Regulations	Agency Responsible for Administration
(h) Age discrimination in employment	Age Discrimination in Employment Act of 1967 (ADEA), 29 U.S.C.A. § 621 et seq.; state fair employment practice laws; state human rights laws	29 C.F.R. § 5 et seq. State regulations	Equal Employment Opportunity Commission (Federal) State agencies (e.g., State Division of Human Rights)
2. Health Care (a) Medicare	42 U.S.C.A. § 1395 et seq.	42 C.F.R. § 405 et seq.; 20 C.F.R. § 405 et seq.	Health Care Financing Administration (HCFA) and Social Security Administration (SSA), U.S. Dept. of Health & Human Services (HHS)
(b) Medical assistance program (Medicaid)	42 U.S.C.A. § 1396 et seq.; state medical assistance statutes	42 C.F.R. § 430 et seq.; state regulations	State public assistance agencies under the direction of HCFA and SSA of U.S. Dept. of Health & Human Services
(c) Veterans benefits	38 U.S.C.A. § 601 et seq.	38 C.F.R. § 17.30 et seq.	Veterans Administration (Federal)
(d) Nursing homes (licensing, patients' bill of rights, abuse reporting)	42 U.S.C.A. § 1395; § 1395 X(j)(SNF); 42 U.S.C.A. § 1396 d(c)(ICF); state public health laws	42 C.F.R. § 405.1120 et seq. (SNF); § 442.250 et seq. (ICF); state public health regulations	U.S. Dept. of Health & Human Services; state depts. of health
3. Social Services	Social Services Block Grant Act (Title XX of the Social Security Act) 42 U.S.C.A. § 1397 et seq.	45 C.F.R. §1397 et seq.	State agencies under the direction of the U.S. Dept. of Health & Human Services

4. Housing

	Statute	Regulation	Agency
(a) Public housing	42 U.S.C.A. § 5301 et seq.	24 C.F.R. § 860.1 et seq.	U.S. Dept. of Housing & Urban Development (HUD) with local public housing authorities
(b) Housing subsidy	Section 8 of the U.S. Housing Act of 1937. 42 U.S.C.A. § 1437c	24 C.F.R. § 882 et seq.	U.S. Dept. of Housing & Urban Development with local public housing authorities
(c) Housing loans (rural housing loans and grants to the elderly to improve/repair homes)	§ 504 of the Housing Act of 1949. 42 U.S.C.A. § 147 et seq.	7 C.F.R. § 1904; 1904.301 et seq.	Farmer's Home Administration (Federal)
(d) Adult homes	See SSI # 1(b)	See SSI # 1(b)	See SSI # 1(b)
(e) Rent control, exemption from increased rent, protection from eviction in a condo/co-op conversion	State housing statutes; local housing statutes	State housing and local regulations	State agencies; local housing boards

5. Consumer Affairs

	Statute	Regulation	Agency
(a) Consumer fraud	Federal Trade Commission Act, 15 U.S.C.A. § 2301 et seq.; Magnuson-Moss Warranty FTC Improvement Act, 15 U.S.C.A. § 2301 et seq.; state unfair trade practices and consumer protection acts	16 C.F.R. § 700 et seq.; state consumer protection regulations	Federal Trade Commission; state consumer affairs agencies

6. Legal Services

	Statute	Regulation	Agency
(a) Legal services	Legal Services Corporation Act, 42 U.S.C.A. 2996 et seq.	45 C.F.R. § 1600 et seq.	Legal Services Corporation; local grantee corps.

(continued)

361

Appendix 15-1: *(Continued)*

Subject Matter	Statute	Regulations	Agency Responsible for Administration
(b) Older Americans Act	Title III of the Older Americans Act. as amended. 42 U.S.C.A. § 3021 et seq.	45 C.F.R. § 1321 et seq.	Federal Administration on Aging; state aging agencies; areas agencies on aging
7. Protective Services			
(a) Conservatorship (of property)	State mental hygiene/mental-health statutes	State mental health/mental-hygiene regulations	State mental health/mental-hygiene agencies; state courts
(b) Committee/guardian (of the person)	State mental hygiene/mental-health statutes	State mental health/mental-hygiene regulations	State mental-hygiene agencies; state courts
(c) Commitment (involuntary)	U.S. Constitution; state mental health/mental-hygiene statutes	State mental health/mental-hygiene regulations	State mental health/mental-hygiene agencies; state courts
(d) Power of attorney (durable)	State statutes (e.g. N.Y. General Obligations Law)	Not applicable	Not applicable
(e) Surrogate payees	Social Security Act	20 C.F.R. §§ 404 and 416	Social Security Administration (Federal)
8. Property Transfers			
(a) Wills, trusts, lifetime gifts	State statutes (e.g., N.Y. Estates. Powers & Trusts Law)	Not applicable	Not applicable
(b) Probate: living wills	State probate statutes (e.g., Uniform Probate Code)	Rules of the state court	Surrogate's court/probate court (state)
9. Tax Relief			
(a) Income tax	Internal Revenue Code of 1954 as amended. 26 U.S.C.A. § 151	26 C.F.R. § 1.151-1(c)	Internal Revenue Service (Federal)
(b) Property tax/utility rates	State/local statutes	State/local regulations	State/local tax commissions

**APPENDIX 15-2: NATIONAL ORGANIZATIONS DEALING
WITH LEGAL ISSUES
RELEVANT TO THE ELDERLY**

American Arbitration Association
140 West 51st St.
New York, N.Y. 10020

American Bar Association
1155 East 60th St.
Chicago, Ill. 60637

ABA Commission on Legal Problems of the Elderly
1800 M St., N.W.
Washington, D.C. 20036

Center on Social Welfare Policy & Law
95 Madison Ave., Room 701
New York, N.Y. 10016

House Select Committee on Aging
712 House Office Bldg. Annex No. 1
Washington, D.C. 20515

Institute on Law and Rights of Older Adults
Brookdale Center on Aging/Hunter College
425 East 25th St.
New York, N.Y. 10010

Legal Assistance to Medicare Patients (LAMP)
P.O. Box 258, 902 Main St.
Willimantic, Conn. 06226

Legal Counsel for the Elderly
American Association of Retired Persons/National Retired Teachers Association
1909 K St., N.W.
Washington, D.C. 20049

Legal Services Corporation/Office of Field Services
733 15th Ave., N.W.
Washington, D.C. 20005

Legal Services for the Elderly
132 West 43rd St.
New York, N.Y. 10036

National Clearinghouse for Legal Services
407 S. Dearborn, Suite 400
Chicago, Ill. 60605

National Consumer Law Center
11 Beacon St., Room 925
Boston, Mass. 02108

National Health Law Program
2639 South La Cienaga Boulevard
Los Angeles, Calif. 90034

National Housing Law Project
2150 Shattuck Ave., Suite 300
Berkeley, Calif. 94704

National Institute for Dispute Resolution
1901 L St., N.W.
Washington, D.C. 20036

National Organization of Social Security Claimant Representatives
P.O. Box 794
Pearl River, N.Y. 10965

National Senior Citizens Law Center
1424 16th St., N.W., Suite 300
Washington, D.C. 20036

Pension Rights Center
1346 Connecticut Ave., N.W.
Washington, D.C.

Practicing Law Institute
810 Seventh Ave.
New York, N.Y. 10019

Senate Special Committee on Aging
Room G—225 Dirksen Senate Office Bldg.
Washington, D.C. 20510

Volunteer Lawyers Project
73 Tremont St., Suite 1001
Boston, Mass. 02108

16

Assistance to Crime and Abuse Victims

Jordan I. Kosberg, Ph.D.

University of South Florida, Tampa

Those working in the helping professions are in vantage points to detect, prevent, and treat elderly who are victimized by the criminal or abusive behavior of others. Whether in hospital emergency rooms, in family-service agencies, in mental-health centers, or other such settings, professional care providers should be sensitized to detect cases of elder abuse and victimization, trained to help the victimized elderly person, and committed to needed social-policy changes to better protect the elderly, especially the most dependent and vulnerable.

This chapter deals with the victimization of the elderly on the street and in the home by strangers and with the abuse of the elderly by informal care providers — family members, friends, and neighbors. Explanations of the problems are followed by suggestions for prevention of victimization and abuse and for treatment of the elderly victims. Because of the author's background of study in the area of elder abuse and the "invisibility" of this problem, the chapter emphasizes the problem of abusive behavior against the elderly.

GENERAL VULNERABILITY

The following examples of elder abuse, elicited in hearings before the Subcommittee on Retirement Income and Employment of the House Select Committee on Aging (U.S. Congress, 1981), reflect the variety and severity of the abuse to which the dependent elderly are peculiarly vulnerable:

The North Carolina County Department of Social Services reported finding a 91-year-old widow lying on her bed. She had multiple severe bruises on her face, hands, arms and chest. She was incoherent and very confused. She was assessed to have been beaten approximately a week before. The daughter of the elderly woman had been beaten by her own son, also, and that was why she had not reported her own mother's condition. The elderly woman was transported to an emergency room where she eventually died. Her grandson is being held on charges of murder (p. 171).

Caseworkers in West Virginia were alerted that an 80-year-old couple might be having problems. Upon investigation they found the husband ill to the point of being comatose. The man was described as "unable to respond, barely breathing with eyes glazed." The wife was exhausted and distraught from trying to care for her husband to the point where her mental condition was unstable. The wife would not allow authorities to remove the man to a hospital for treatment. She charged them with engaging in a plot to take her husband away from her. Caseworkers contacted the couple's daughter to assist them in persuading the wife that the man needed attention. They were unsuccessful and the husband died two days thereafter (p. 174).

California officials report that an 87-year-old widow in frail health and generally confined to a wheelchair, unable to care for her day-to-day needs, was allegedly the victim of physical and financial abuse from 1974 through 1980. A nurse companion who was also her conservator and three children depleted her financial resources by more than $300,000 while depriving the woman of proper medical attention, food and clothing. Caseworkers helped the woman to institute legal proceedings (p. 175).

In California, an 87-year-old woman in ill-health, confined to a wheelchair, and unable to care for her daily needs, was repeatedly and systematically abused by her family and nurse companion. The mental and physical torture lasted six years. During this time, the woman was threatened, held prisoner, deprived of all contact with the outside world, not permitted to see friends and family, and battered (p. 176).

In Washington, an 84-year-old woman terminally ill with cancer was refused proper medical attention by her grandson who did not want the woman's property and income dissipated by doctor and hospital payments. The woman was found in tremendous pain living in truly wretched conditions. The victim was transferred to a nursing home where she died a few weeks later (p. 177).

There are many reasons why the elderly are especially vulnerable to criminal or abusive behavior (Kosberg, 1983). Some pertain to social values and attitudes toward the elderly, and others pertain to their physical and economic needs. Still other reasons for the vulnerability of the aged are related to their social and psychological losses.

The elderly are likely to live alone, which is especially true for elderly women. This fact combined with residence in a high-crime-rate area increases the vulnerability of the elderly and the probability of isolation (through fear of leaving one's dwelling) or the actual commission of crime against the elderly.

Because of their diminished physical strength and stamina, older people are less able to defend themselves or to escape from threatening situations (Goldsmith and Tomas, 1974). Related to this is the fact that they are likely to suffer from physical disabilities and have impairments affecting hearing, sight, touch, and mobility. The result is a lessened ability to resist crimes of a physical nature, whether the aggressor is a stranger or a relative.

There is a likelihood that the elderly will be additionally vulnerable to crime because of residence in high-crime-rate neighborhoods where they are in close proximity to groups likely to victimize them—the unemployed and teenage dropouts (Goldsmith and Tomas, 1974). There are at least two reasons why the elderly often live in high-crime areas. First, low incomes may necessitate moving to low-rental areas. Second, there is a reluctance to leave the neighborhood (and home) where one has lived for many years, even when the neighborhood has greatly changed. The economic, social, and psychological meaning of one's dwelling may be more important than the extent of crime or incongruity of population in one's neighborhood.

Many elderly persons rely on walking or on public transportation to get around in the community. Accordingly, they are visible and vulnerable. Walking to and from public transportation, waiting at stops, getting on or off a bus or subway, and being in crowded situations all have ramifications for the possiblity of accidents as well as for victimization.

Given low fixed incomes, the elderly are especially vulnerable to fraudulent promises and quick-wealth schemes (Butler, 1975; Pepper, 1983). Poor health conditions, with little if any hope for improvement, can make an elderly person vulnerable to health-care quackery or schemes to evoke anxiety about health or economic security. Expensive or excessive health insurance, funeral arrangements, cemetery plots, and health devices are but a few of the many gambits to part the elderly from their financial resources. In addition, the loneliness of elderly persons makes them vulnerable to overly friendly and solicitous clerks, salespersons, or strangers. Many elderly have had their savings "stolen" by a variety of confidence games and unscrupulous salespersons.

The dates when monthly pension and benefit checks are received in the mail are widely known. Such knowledge results in mail boxes being broken into and checks stolen, robberies, and purse snatchings. These crimes are especially frequent around banks, shopping malls, and grocery stores.

Beside these reasons for the vulnerability of the elderly to criminal activity, there are also reasons why the elderly are especially vulnerable to abusive behavior by members of their informal care system.

Elder abuse by family members occurs within the home, outside of public scrutiny. If a problem is detected by outsiders, it is considered a "family affair." Even professionals are reluctant to intervene. Finally, the informal care system has been used as a panacea by those in the legal, social-service, and health-care systems; yet such individuals turned to for care of ill and dependent elderly may be ill-suited, ill-prepared, and unmotivated to provide necessary care or may be motivated for all the wrong reasons (e.g., exploitation). "In the eagerness to find an easy and inexpensive solution to care for an elderly person, those making referrals . . . may turn too quickly to family members without assessing the appropriateness of the family or pressures on the family to be caused by having to care for an elderly relative" (Kosberg, 1983, p. 267).

In addition to these factors associated with vulnerability of the elderly to criminal or abusive behavior is the social perception of the elderly in society as worthless. Such a negative view of the elderly can result, it is believed, in aimless and senseless crimes against them. Too often one reads about muggings, beatings, psychological abuse, killings, etc. with no apparent motives. The only conclusion is that the criminal or abusive behavior was based upon thrills, taking out aggression on a defenseless scapegoat, or seeking out a (perceived) value-less individual. It is further believed that if an elderly person is also perceived as a deviant (e.g., alcoholic, drifter, handicapped, mentally ill, etc.), the greater the likelihood of his/her becoming a victim. In American society, being dependent is also an undesirable status. Katz (1979-80) has suggested that ageism and bias against the handicapped can result in the creation of abusive situations.

DIMENSIONS OF THE PROBLEM

According to the Senate Special Committee on Aging, of 1,000 persons aged 65 and over studied, 22 had been victims of theft (19 of personal larceny without contact). Eight had been victims of violent crimes, including five instances of robbery and three of assault (U.S. Congress, 1978).

Research findings on the most prevalent forms of elder abuse are inconclusive and reflect variations in the definitions of elder abuse as well as the methods by which abuse is measured and reported. The House Select Committee on Aging found that physical trauma was the most prevalent type of abuse in a Massachusetts study, psychological abuse in a Maryland study, passive neglect in a Michigan study, and lack of personal care in an Ohio study (U.S. Congress, 1981).

It is difficult to know the exact extent of criminal victimization of the elderly and abusive behavior against the aged. First, the elderly may fail to report their victimization. Second, the problem of criminal or abusive behavior may not be detected or correctly identified.

Criminal activity by strangers against the elderly has been rather widely studied (Malinchak and Wright, 1978). While elderly individuals are victims of personal larceny (e.g., purse snatching) more so than younger persons, the elderly have much lower rates of homicide, robbery, rape, assault, burglary, larceny from the household, and motor-vehicle theft than younger persons (Hindelang and Richardson, 1978). Tomas (1974) concluded that, for several cities, the rates of victimization for robbery with injury, personal larceny, and fraud of the elderly were equal to or higher than that of younger age groups. Certain groups of elderly were found to be more likely to be victimized. For example, Liang and Sengstock (1983) found the risk of criminal victimization among the elderly higher for urban dwellers, the young-old, those who are not married, nonwhite persons, and men.

Often the fact that the aged do have lower levels of crime committed against them is interpreted to mean that the problem is not a significant one. Such a conclusion glosses over important considerations. First, the consequence of crime may be an injury from which convalescence is slow or may result in institutionalization; the loss of possessions or financial resources may greatly affect the quality of life; and damages to property cannot be repaired or replaced. Second, the older person is more likely to be victimized repeatedly—often by the same offender (Goldsmith and Tomas, 1974). Third, low crime rates reported for the elderly may result, in part, from the failure of the elderly to report the commission of a crime (such as theft or fraud) because of embarrassment, fear or intimidation, or because they believe the reporting of a crime to be futile. Liang and Sengstock (1983) found that 45 percent of aged victims failed to report the commission of the crime.

The fourth, and final, consideration glossed over by crime statistics is fear. As insidious as being the victim of a crime is the anticipation of becoming a victim. Fear of crime has been found to be a more prevailing emotion for the elderly than for younger persons (Clemente and Kleiman, 1976). Whether the fear is based upon real or imagined danger of crime, the results limit the comings and goings of elderly persons and adversely affect the quality of their lives by being—in many cases—an all-consuming preoccupation. Finley (1983, p. 22), however, notes that fear of crime is not all bad, for it has "an important role in reducing actual victimization [of the elderly], as it does for all age groups."

Less empirical work has been done on elder abuse. Given the invisibility and underreporting of the problem, coupled with methodological difficulties and differing definitions (Kosberg, 1979), the limited number of studies on elder abuse preclude definite conclusions about the scope of the problem. This author has concluded that a comprehensive definition of elder abuse should include the following:

1. *Passive Neglect.* Characterized by a situation in which the elderly person is left alone, isolated, or forgotten. The abuser is often unaware of the neglect or the consequences of the neglect, due to the abuser's lack of intelligence or lack of experience as a care provider (Hickey and Douglass, 1981).
2. *Active Neglect.* Characterized as the intentional withholding of items necessary for daily living, such as food, medicine, companionship, and bathroom assistance (Hickey and Douglass, 1981).
3. *Verbal, Emotional, or Psychological Abuse.* Characterized by situations in which the older person is called names, insulted, infantilized, frightened, intimidated, humiliated, or threatened.
4. *Physical Abuse.* Characterized by the older person being hit, slapped, bruised, sexually molested, cut, burned, or physically restrained.
5. *Material or Financial Misappropriation.* Characterized by actions including monetary or material theft or misuse (when not being used for the benefit, or with the approval, of the elderly person).
6. *Violation of Rights.* Characterized by efforts to force an elderly person

from his or her dwelling or to force him or her into another setting (most often a nursing home) without any forewarning, explanation, opportunity for input, or against the older person's wishes.

Self-abuse is a special type of problem and, since it is mainly done without assistance, is not included for discussion. When, however, informal care providers are cognizant of the self-abuse and either do not intervene or, indeed, knowingly assist in the self-abuse (e.g., by buying alcohol or medication, not seeking professional assistance), then the problem can be considered an example of neglectful behavior.

Several studies on elder abuse were undertaken during the late 1970s. Rathbone-McCuan (1980) presented information on the existence of inter-generational family violence and neglect affecting elderly relatives. Steinmetz (1978) was also one of the first to identify and discuss the maltreatment of the elderly by their families. The University of Maryland's Center on Aging undertook a study of battered elderly persons (Block and Sinnot, 1979) and found that 4.1 percent of the elderly respondents in their study reported abuse. If projected to a national population of elderly, the researchers concluded that there would be nearly 1 million cases of elder abuse each year. Other estimates of elder abuse range from 500,000 to 2.5 million cases per year (Rathbone-McCuan and Hashimi, 1982).

In an exploratory study of professional and paraprofessional encounters with abuse in Massachusetts (Legal Research, 1979), it was found that 55 percent of the respondents knew of at least one incident of abuse in an eighteen-month period. A study in Michigan (Hickey and Douglass, 1981) was based upon recollections of care providers (i.e., police, social workers, physicians) in five study areas. While they found little or no direct physical abuse, 50 percent reported contact with passive neglect. Finally, in a study of abuse of elderly clients at the Chronic Illness Center in Cleveland, Ohio (Lau and Kosberg, 1979), it was found that 10 percent of all clients had been abused. Informal care providers, mainly relatives, were the abusers.

The flurry of empirical research findings of abusive behavior by family and friends of elderly persons produced hearings by the U.S. House of Representatives Select Committee on Aging in June, 1979, and in 1980 a Senate-House joint hearing took place. In 1981 a National Conference on Abuse of Older Persons was held and experts' testimonies were presented to the House of Representatives Select Committee on Aging. The Committee (U.S. Congress, 1980, pp. xiv-xv) concluded that ". . . some four percent of the nation's elderly may be victims of some sort of abuse from moderate to severe. In other words, one out of every twenty-five older Americans, or roughly one million elder Americans may be victims of such abuse each year." The report went on to indicate that abuse was most likely to be a recurring event rather than a single incident, and that elderly victims were likely to be the very old, women, and those dependent on others for care and protection. Generally, the abused older person lives with the abuser, who is most often a relative. Finally, the research studies concluded that no aged person is immune to the possibility of abuse, for it is not associated with social class, educational level, race or nationality, or geographic location.

EXPLANATIONS

Crime against the elderly is, of course, a reflection of the pervasive nature of crime in general. The elderly are victimized for the same reasons that younger persons are victimized. And the motivations of those who victimize the elderly are the same for those who victimize younger persons. Yet the characteristics of the elderly do make them especially visible, vulnerable, and defenseless.

The causes of abuse and maltreatment of the elderly by informal care providers are complex and varied. Those in the helping professions should be aware of differing explanations for the abuse of elderly persons (mainly by family members), so that appropriate intervention and treatment can be provided. The following is a summary of the major theoretical explanations for elder abuse (or those explanations extrapolated from research on child or spouse abuse).

Psychopathology Model

Elderly individuals may be maltreated by individuals who exhibit abnormal or deviant behavior, including drug addiction, alcoholism, mental illness, and senile dementia, among others. Steele and Pollock (1968) found child abusers to be impulsive, immature, and depressed; abusive behavior displaced aggressive and sadistic inclinations. Parents may have cared for schizophrenic, retarded, or alcoholic children who became adults. "As aged parents weaken and need care, their adult children become abusing and neglectful care givers because of an inability to make appropriate judgments and perceptions" (Lau and Kosberg, 1979, p.13).

Sociological Approach

Gelles (1973) discussed sociological interpretations of child abuse that have, it is believed, application to elder abuse. Vulnerability of children to abuse was explained as due to their lack of physical ability to withstand physical force, and the fact that they are not capable of much meaningful social interaction, resulting in parent frustration. Further, the infant (or elderly person) may create stress by imposing economic hardships or interfering with professional, occupational, or educational plans.

Intrafamily violence may be caused by stress-producing conditions. An overrepresentation of abusing fathers have been found to be unemployed (O'Brien, 1971). Another contextual factor is that child abuse is often associated with an unwanted pregnancy; often the parents had to get married, were ill-prepared to become parents, or the unwanted child caused stress in the family. "The child may be a financial burden, an emotional burden, or a psychological burden . . ." (Gelles, 1973, p. 618). So, too, might the elderly parent be an unwanted or unexpected responsibility.

Social Exchange Theory

Edwards and Brauburger (1973) studied the exchange system between parents and their adolescent children. They found that when exchange between them breaks down, conflict develops. This exchange incorporates a system of rewards, power, the costs of compliance, and reciprocity. Conflict was found related to coercive control techniques used to resolve problems. While, for adolescents, increased independence from parents can produce tension and conflict, it may well be that increased dependence of elderly parents upon grown children can result in conflict. The conflict, in turn, may result in maltreatment or abuse.

Adding to the understanding of exchange phenomena, Richer (1968, p. 464) suggested that the greater the availability of resources and alternative sources of rewards available to children ". . . the less likely parental dictates are to be followed and the more conflict-ridden the relationship with parents will be." It is interesting to speculate whether the relationship problems of earlier times are reproduced in the old age of the parents, or whether a role reversal occurs whereby the elderly parent is expected to comply with the directions of the adult children. In this latter case, the earlier social-exchange relationship is altered, if not reversed.

Life Crisis Model

Justice and Duncan (1976) discussed stress resulting in child abuse. They focused upon life-changing events that require readjustment in the life-style of a person or family. When an excessive number or magnitude of such life-change events occur, a "state of life crisis" may be said to exist. The researchers found such "states" associated with abusing parents. They utilized the forty-three events requiring some readjustment by the person or family to whom the event occurred (Holmes and Rahe, 1967). These events include physical illness, occurrence of an accident or injury, and personal, social, economic, or interpersonal changes. Such a multicausal model of abuse focuses upon life crises, caused by excessive changes, as predisposing factors. The life crises, a series of change events rather than situational day-to-day problems that are often unpredictable, result in abuse. "... [T]he end state of the life crisis is a stage of exhaustion, of decreased ability to adjust, and increased risk of losing control" (Justice and Duncan, 1976, p. 112).

Social-Structural Theory of Family Violence

This view of conflict focuses, in part, upon the socialization of aggression. "The theory states that parents who punish more severely produce children who are more aggressive" (Lystad, 1975, p.330). This socialization of violence is seen for certain groups with lower educational achievements and lower socioeconomic status as well as among broken families.

The power structure of the family is also considered in relationship to family violence. Each family has a hierarchy of interpersonal relationships with superordinate and subordinate roles. Each family has different structures, values, and beliefs regarding power relationships. Moreover, the power structure of the larger society affects violence in the family. Societal abuse of children (through hunger, poverty, poor education)—or any dependent population (including the aged)—can be seen to be more serious than individual abuse (Gil, 1971). Cultural values support the view that the aged are unimportant, and cultural norms toward dependent populations (use of physical force) may sanction abusive behavior.

Finally, the social-structural variables of race and ethnic subcultures have been discussed as "cultures of violence." It is suggested by some that such systems of values justify and support violent behavior (Lystad, 1975), although Cazenave (1983) believes that the "culture of violence" is more an impression than an empirical fact.

Intergenerational Conflict

Less empirically based are efforts that focus specifically upon the intergenerational problems between the elderly and their grown children. Tensions between older mothers and adult daughters have been discussed in terms of personality conflicts that are worsened by the passing of years (Farrar, 1955). Failure to redefine family roles with the passing of years has been seen to result in either hostility (Blenkner, 1965) or overt violence (Glasser and Glasser, 1962). It has been suggested that conflict betwen family members and aged relatives is more likely in situations where the family—as individuals or a unit—has difficulty coping with an elderly parent suffering from a chronic disease (Maddox, 1975). Miller (1981) has written about the stress to adult children, facing their own aging process and the needs of their own children, of having to care for elderly parents. Conflict between generations has also been viewed as reflecting a lack of normative definition with regard to the rights and responsibilities of middle-aged children vis-à-vis their aged parents (Cavan, 1969).

ASSESSMENT

As Rathbone-McCuan (1980, p. 296) states: "Identification of and intervention in cases of physical abuse and purposeful neglect of the elderly within the context of the family are rare; because professionals in the field seem unaware that the phenomenon exists, they fail to recognize cues of willful abuse and neglect." Indeed, to discuss assessment and—especially—intervention without first alluding to the need to address sensitivity to the possible existence of criminal or abusive behavior against an elderly person is rather meaningless.

Those working with and for elderly persons should not expect elderly persons to necessarily verbalize their adversities. As has been discussed, elderly victims are often reluctant to report the criminal action against them because of embarrassment, fear, or belief that it would be futile. Research on elder abuse has found that abused elderly, too, do not report their adversities. In their study of elder abuse, Lau and Kosberg (1979) found that denial was the most prevalent reaction of elderly persons, followed by resignation. Failure to report abusive behavior or denial of its existence by an elderly person may arise from the following reasons (Kosberg, 1983): fear of reprisals by the abuser, embarrassment about the behavior of a family member who is the abuser, anticipation that the solution to the problem will be worse than the problem (e.g., removal from one's home, institutionalization), fear that legal and criminal action might be taken against the abusing family member, belief that the problem is a family affair that should remain within the confines of the family, or feelings of guilt in being dependent and causing tensions and pressures on informal care providers.

If there is a reluctance to report criminal and abusive behavior by the elderly, then those in the helping professions have a special responsibility for detecting and assessing such problems. The consequences of certain types of adverse action are obvious, if proper assessment is undertaken: injuries, bruises, burns, etc. Other consequences are more subtle to discern and can be best identified through assessment of a person's affect and demeanor. Depression, fear, confusion, anger, withdrawal, etc. may result from a variety of causes. Criminal or abusive behavior can be one such cause and should not be overlooked. Physical assessments to determine elder abuse (Falcioni, 1982) or criminal activity against the elderly seem further developed than more subtle social or psychological assessments for such problems.

Ideally, those in the helping professions who are in contact with elderly persons who might be victims should be able to establish a relationship with an elderly person in a quiet and private location. The interviewer's role should be clarified, and the appropriate use of information should be mentioned. Emphasis should be placed on assistance and support, not on criminal charges against an individual. Especially in cases of suspected abuse, there should not be anyone else present (such as a family member who brought the older person to the hospital emergency room, social-service agency, etc.). The relative should be interviewed separately, and the explanations for what happened to the older person should be compared to the report by the older person. When there is incongruence in stories, or suspected collaboration in a fabricated story, there is reason to further pursue the actual events leading up to a problem situation (whether of a long-term or episodic nature). The skills and personality of the professional or paraprofessional will determine the success in securing factual information about the older person and the occurrence of criminal or abusive behavior.

In assessing the problem of criminal or abusive behavior, there is a danger in viewing problems too simplistically. Assessment should include information on the type of criminal or abusive behavior, the frequency and duration of such behavior, and the sequence of events leading to the adversity. In addition, the elderly person (or witnesses to events) should be questioned about events surrounding the adversity in terms of the time and place of occurrence and number of offenders and characteristics. For abusive behavior, information should be obtained as to the conditions under which the abuse occurred and the motivation of the abuser. (While the results of the action on an older person may be similar, intervention with one who abuses out of ignorance is different than with one who abuses out of hostility.) Also, it is important to learn whether there was more than one abuser and whether the abuse took place with the knowledge or in the presence of others.

Finally, the interpretation by the elderly person to the adverse actions of another, or others, is important. Some elderly persons may see the criminal or abusive behavior to be a result of their own actions, limitations, or needs: "I was too interested in getting something for nothing" or "I was desperate for a cure" in cases of fraud; "I was a burden to my daughter" or "I beat my son when he was a child" in cases of abuse. In other situations, the older person does not see the problem in the same way as the professional: "There was no maltreatment. My family has always been very physical and emotional with one another." And, in cases of elder abuse, the assessment of the abuser's explanation of the problem is vital to the type of recommended treatment plan. Some abusers remain hostile and deny any wrongdoing in their treatment of an older person; some are confused and do not understand what they have done; and some are embarrassed and saddened by events and situations that erupted in their abuse of an elderly relative.

INTERVENTIONS

Activities to assist the elderly include both prevention before and treatment after abuse or criminal victimization has occurred. There are prodigious roles for those concerned with the vulnerability of the elderly to criminal and abusive behavior. A variety of direct, programmatic, and policy interventions follow.

With Crime Victims

As has been discussed, research findings have helped identify high-risk elderly and situations related to the commission of crime. "When older persons can learn to identify criminal opportunities in their environment and assess their risk, they can then take simple precautions to divert the criminal's behavior" (Jaycox and Center, 1983, p. 319). Community care providers can assist the elderly in preventive activities. Jaycox and Center (1983) have identified individual and collective crime-prevention activities. The former include home inspections by trained individuals to determine the security status of the home and particular risks, property-marking programs for the identification of possessions, improved precautionary activities (e.g., using locks, leaving lights or radios on), and increased precaution on the street (e.g., sensitivity to one's appearance and the environment). Collective activities include block clubs, neighborhood watch, building patrols, escort service, and telephone assurance programs, among others.

Curtis and Kohn (1983) have discussed preventive activities in age-segregated settings for the elderly and emphasized the importance of environmental design as a detriment to criminal activity against the elderly. Such preventive strategies can include access controls that create barriers for visitors, formal surveillance, programs to increase prevention awareness, and fostering protective behaviors.

Those working with aged who have been victimized (whether by personal attacks, theft of possessions, fraud, or exploitation) or immobilized by fear need a special sensitivity and skills to deal with the trauma of the criminal act and its aftermath on the older person. While the clinical skills of those working with the elderly are covered in other chapters, public policy is needed to create victim-assistance programs for the elderly. "Programs which are primarily concerned with helping people recover from their crime-induced stress usually offer counseling and social services, and may lobby for sensitive handling of victims by social agencies and criminal justice professions" (Jaycox and Center, 1983, p. 323). Examples of victim-assistance efforts are rape-crisis centers and battered-women shelters.

Jaycox and Center (1983) have identified three main objectives of victim-assistance programs for older crime victims. First, there is the need to assist the elderly to recover from the psychological and emotional impact of being a victim. This necessitates clinical skills as well as providing support and empathy. Second, assistance should be provided to get whatever benefits are available as compensations for losses. For example, some states have victim-compensation programs. Third, assistance is needed to provide either directly or indirectly (through referrals) services needed by the older person to recover from the criminal act (e.g., medical care, transportation, homemaker services, etc.) and to participate in the criminal-justice process (e.g., assistance and support in dealing with the law enforcement and judicial bureaucracies). The setting for such victim-assistance activities can be located within police departments, social-service and health-care resources, or the court system.

With Abuse Victims

Hopefully, those working with older persons, in whatever the setting, will be sensitive to the possibility of abusive behavior. Research and practice experience has identified high-risk elderly persons: the old old, the impaired and dependent, and women. Findings from research studies and conclusions from social-science theory in the areas of child and spouse abuse extrapolated to an elderly population have identified individual or situational conditions that are associated with abusive behavior.

From a preventive perspective, there are several mechanisms that can be used to preclude placing an elderly person in a situation that could well lead to abuse. Social workers and other professionals in social- and health-service systems should make a careful assessment of the appropriateness of an informal care provider. "Designating a relative a guardian, placing an elderly client with a child, or discharging an elderly patient to the family without adequate assessment may be viewed as a panacea by service providers but may result in great problems for the elderly person" (Kosberg, 1983, p. 271). Those who care for dependent elderly persons should be mentally, socially, physically, and economically able to provide the needed care and attention. Further, the informal care system should be assessed. This refers to the number, location, and health of family members and friends who can either share in the care of an elderly person or who can be available to relieve the major care provider from ongoing responsibilities.

Inasmuch as there are often economic pressures on those caring for elderly persons, those in the helping professions should advocate social policies that seek to relieve some of the economic burdens of such care. Among various proposals are those for tax incentives, direct subsidies, or direct cash payments through a family-allowance program. Such proposals may encourage family members to share in the care of an elderly person and can reduce the economic burden of such care. The enactment of policies need, however, some mechanism to ensure that the motivation for care is not an economic one.

Supporting community services for those caring for elderly persons is important for preventive reasons. Especially for those caring for elderly relatives who do not have extensive informal support systems, formal supporting services are vital to relieve family members from the constant and demanding care of a dependent elderly relative. Such needed community services include adult day care, day hospitals, friendly visitors, respite care, homemaker and home health aides, and chore services, among others. The existence of these supporting services can assist in precluding the institutionalization of an elderly relative by a family that can no longer cope with the constant demands for care and can relieve some of the pressures and tensions upon the family that could result in abusive behavior.

The areas of prevention and treatment of elder abuse are not mutually exclusive, and each has elements of the other. Protective services have elements of both prevention and treatment. In 1980, twenty-five states had some type of protective services legislation (Salend, Satz, and Pynoos, 1981), and it is likely that other states have enacted such legislation since 1980. All states should have protective-service legislation that would permit social workers and other professionals entry into private homes (to investigate cases of suspected abuse), provision of services, legal intervention, and authority for the removal of an elderly person (being abused) without the consent of family members. Of course, removal of an elderly person from the home should be the last resort and would follow (1) efforts to work with family members to resolve problems and (2) the mobilization of supporting community services or informal resources in the effort to assist the family in the care of their elderly relative.

Counseling or casework with the elderly person and family is another area that embraces elements of both prevention and treatment. As for prevention: "Counseling should be available during the time a family is making decisions regarding care for [an] elderly person. Families endure enormous social pressure to care for their own, and the professional's role should be to aid the family to make an intelligent decision, not on social values or guilt, but on what they want or are able to do" (Steuer, 1983, p. 245).

Steuer (1983) suggests that once abusive behavior has been identified, intervention with the abuser and the entire family is necessary to work out feelings of conflict and guilt. Rathbone-McCuan and Hashimi (1982) have indicated that clinical intervention in cases of elder abuse was both "ill-defined" and in need of evaluation. Rathbone-McCuan, Travis, and Voyles (1983) have attempted to fill this practice gap in their discussion of a task-centered model for family intervention in cases of elder abuse. If social or psychological interventions do not resolve the problem and elder abuse continues, legal action should be taken. Removal of the elderly person from the customary dwelling should always be the last resort, after all else fails. It is hoped that, as a result of the publicity given to the existence and causes of elder abuse, those caring for the dependent elderly persons will voluntarily seek out professional guidance to deal with their feelings or the consequences of excessive demands upon them prior to an eruption of abusive behavior. But in cases of identified elder abuse, those who mistreat elderly persons should be required to seek professional intervention, at the very least.

Professionals need to consider legal protection against irate relatives who are either elder abusers or are under suspicion of being elder abusers. Given the difficulty of securing conclusive evidence of abusive behavior by a family member, accusations or confrontations may result in actions against the professional. Certainly, personal professional liability insurance is needed; often an agency's policy covers individual professional staff. Professionals need to be protected as well from false accusations of abusive or unprofessional behavior by the elderly client, who may be suffering from delusional or distorted perceptions. In this regard, it is necessary for those working with elderly persons to judge very carefully the accuracy and validity of any charges of abusive behavior. Such accusations need to be substantiated by a very careful assessment of the elderly person's cognizance of reality, at the least, and by the statements of others whose testimony corresponds to that of the older person.

Foster Care as a Preventive Measure

Foster care for the elderly has come to be considered a viable alternative to independent living, on one hand, and to institutional living, on the other. However, foster care has been subject to the criticism that elderly persons can be quite vulnerable to abusive behavior at the hands of foster-care providers. Brody (1977), for example, questions the motivations of foster care:

Discussions of foster home care constantly refer to the family, to the family setting and to participation in normal family activities as essential ingredients. . . . If six people or 10 people . . . are in such a home, is it really a "family residence"? Or, is it a congregate facility of some type such as the many "Mom and Pop" boarding homes that almost invariably are without a "Pop"? Or, is it an unlicensed nursing home? Are these really "families" as we know them, with a variety of motivations for providing foster care . . . ? Or, are they small business concerns?

A report of the Senate Special Committee on Aging (U.S. Congress, 1976b) concluded that foster homes are less capable of meeting the needs of discharged mental patients:

Most often, they are converted residences but they may also be new high rise buildings or converted hotels, in some cases they may be converted mobile homes or renovated chicken coops. What they have in common is that they offer board and room but no nursing care and that most States do not license such facilities.

Lack of licensure pertains both to the characteristics of the foster home and the characteristics (training, motivation, and suitability) of the foster-care providers.

Further, there has seldom been any mandated professional surveillance or follow-up to a foster-care placement of an elderly person. The possibility of abuse of a vulnerable elderly person in a foster home is thus great and may continue undetected. As Dr. Robert N. Butler testified to a joint hearing of the House Subcommittees on Long-term Care and on Health of the Elderly, "From the perspective of civil liberties, as well as health care, of the two sides of the right-of-treatment concept, such facilities as foster care homes have even less protection than do mental hospitals" (U.S. Congress, 1976a).

Upgrading foster-care homes for the elderly can be achieved by educational or training requirements for care providers as well as by assessment of their backgrounds, commitments, and motivations. The homes themselves should be subject to licensing standards pertaining to issues of safety, sanitation, and privacy, as well as limitations on the number of foster-care recipients within each home. How many individuals can be cared for in a foster home before it is no more a "family" but an institution or "small business concern"? Sherman and Newman (1977) point to a perplexing paradox: regulations will drive out small foster homes. "The advantage of these homes is their small size, but if the regulations are made too stringent, there will not be sufficient incentive for the small homes and they simply may become unfeasible."

CONCLUSIONS

Crime and abusive behavior against the elderly are, ultimately, affected by social values and attitudes toward dependency and the importance of older persons. Accordingly, professionals have a role to play not only in assessment and intervention but also in influencing changes in public education, the mass media, and efforts by the aged themselves to challenge popular myths, stereotypes, and negative perceptions of the old, the ill, and the dependent. In addition to safeguards for the elderly, which will minimize their chances for being victims of crime and abuse, these more elementary and pervasive changes of attitudes and values are needed. Such changes are the first steps in true and lasting prevention of adverse behavior against the aged.

REFERENCES

Blenkner, M. (1965). Social work and family relationships in later life with some thoughts on filial maturity. In E. Shanas and G. F. Streib (Eds.), *Social structure and the family: Generational relations*. Englewood Cliffs, N.J.: Prentice-Hall.

Block, M., and Sinnot, J. (Eds.). (1979). *The battered elderly syndrome: An exploratory study*, College Park: Center on Aging, University of Maryland.

Brody, E. M. (1977). Comments on Sherman/Newman paper. *Gerontologist*, **17**(6), 520-522.

Butler, R. M. (1975). *Why survive? Being old in America*. New York: Harper & Row.

Cavan, R. (1969). *The American family* (4th ed.). New York: Crowell.

Cazenave, N. A. (1983). Elder abuse and black Americans: Incidence, correlates, treatment, and prevention. In J. I. Kosberg (Ed.). *Abuse and maltreatment of the elderly: Causes and interventions.* Boston: Wright-PSG.

Clemente, F., and Kleiman, M. B. (1976). Fear of crime among the aged. *Gerontologist,* **16**(3), 207-210.

Curtis, L. A., and Kohn, I. R. (1983). Policy responses to problems faced by elderly in public housing. In J. I. Kosberg (Ed.), *Abuse and maltreatment of the elderly: Causes and interventions.* Boston: Wright-PSG.

Edwards, J. N., and Brauburger, M. B. (1973). Exchange and parent-youth conflict. *Journal of Marriage and the Family,* **35**(1), 101-107.

Falcioni, D. (1982). Assessing the abused elderly. *Journal of Gerontological Nursing,* **8**(1), 208-212.

Farrar, M. S. (1955). Mother-daughter conflicts extended into later life. *Social Casework,* **36**(5), 202-207.

Finley, G. E. (1983). Fear of crime in the elderly. In J. I. Kosberg (Ed.), *Abuse and maltreatment of the elderly: Causes and interventions.* Boston: Wright-PSG.

Gelles, R. J. (1973). Child abuse as psychopathology: A sociological critique and reformulation. *American Journal of Orthopsychiatry.* **43**(4), 611-621.

Gil, D. G. (1971). Violence against children. *Journal of Marriage and the Family,* **33**(4), 637-648.

Glasser, P. H., and Glasser, L. N. (1962). Role reversal and conflict between aged parents and their children. *Journal of Marriage and the Family,* **24**(1), 46-51.

Goldsmith, J., and Tomas, N. E. (1974). Crimes against the elderly: A continuing national crisis. *Aging,* nos. 236-237, pp. 10-13.

Hickey, T., and Douglass, R. L. (1981). Neglect and abuse of older family members: Professionals' perspectives and care experiences. *Gerontologist,* **21**(2), 171-176.

Hindelang, M. J., and Richardson, E. H. (1978). Criminal victimization of the elderly. In U.S. Congress. House. Select Committee on Aging. *Research into crimes against the elderly,* part 1. Washington: Government Printing Office.

Holmes, T. H., and Rahe, R. H. (1967). The social readjustment rating scale. *Journal of Psychosomatic Research,* **11**(2), 213-218.

Jaycox, V. H., and Center, L. J. (1983). A comprehensive response to violent crimes against older persons. In J. I. Kosberg (Ed.), *Abuse and maltreatment of the elderly: Causes and interventions.* Boston: Wright-PSG.

Justice, B., and Duncan, D. F. (1976). Life crisis and precursor to child abuse. *Public Health Reports,* **91**(2), 110-115.

Katz, K. D. (1979-80). Elder abuse. *Journal of Family Law,* **18**(4), 695-722.

Kosberg, J. I. (1979). *Family conflict and abuse of the elderly: Theoretical and methodological issues.* Paper presented at the 32nd Annual Scientific Meeting of the Gerontological Society of America, Washington.

Kosberg, J. I. (1983). The special vulnerability of elderly parents. In J. I. Kosberg (Ed.), *Abuse and maltreatment of the elderly: Causes and interventions.* Boston: Wright-PSG.

Lau, E. E., and Kosberg, J. I. (1979). Abuse of the elderly by informal care providers. *Aging,* nos. 299-300, pp. 10-15.

Legal Research and Services for the Elderly. (1979). *Elder abuse in Massachusetts: A survey of professionals and paraprofessionals.* Boston: Legal Research and Services for the Elderly.

Liang, J., and Sengstock, M. C. (1983). Personal crimes against the elderly. In J. I. Kosberg (Ed.), *Abuse and maltreatment of the elderly: Causes and interventions.* Boston: Wright-PSG.

Lystad, M. H. (1975). Violence at home: A review of the literature. *American Journal of Orthopsychiatry,* **45**(3), 328-345.

Maddox, G. (1975). Families as context and resource in chronic illness. In S. Sherwood (Ed.), *Long-term care: A handbook for researchers, planners, and providers.* New York: Spectrum.

Malinchak, A. A., and Wright, D. (1978). The scope of elderly victimization. *Aging,* nos. 281-282, pp. 10-16.

Miller, D. A. (1981). The "sandwich" generation: Adult children of the aging. *Social Work*, **26**(5), 419-423.

O'Brien, J. E. (1971). Violence in divorce prone families. *Journal of Marriage and the Family*, **33**(4), 692-698.

Pepper, C. D. (1983). Frauds against the elderly. In J. I. Kosberg (Ed.), *Abuse and maltreatment of the elderly: Causes and interventions*. Boston: Wright-PSG.

Rathbone-McCuan, E. (1980). Elderly victims of family violence and neglect. *Social Casework*, **61**(5), 296-304.

Rathbone-McCuan, E., and Hashimi, J. (1982). *Isolated elders: Health and social intervention*. Rockville, Md.: Aspen.

Rathbone-McCuan, E., Travis, A., and Voyles, B. (1983). Family intervention: Applying the task-centered approach. In J. I. Kosberg (Ed.), *Abuse and maltreatment of the elderly: Causes and interventions*. Boston: Wright-PSG.

Richer, S. (1968). The economics of child rearing. *Journal of Marriage and the Family*. **30**(3), 462-466.

Salend, E., Satz, M., and Pynoos, J. (1981). *Mandatory reporting legislation for adult abuse*. Los Angeles: UCLA/USC Long-Term Care Gerontology Center.

Sherman, S. R., and Newman, E. S. (1977). Foster-family care for the elderly in New York state. *Gerontologist*, **17**(6), 513-520.

Steele, B., and Pollock, C. (1968). A psychiatric study of parents who abuse infants and small children. In R. E. Helfer and C. H. Kempe (Eds.), *The battered child*. Chicago: University of Chicago Press.

Steinmetz, S. K. (1978). Battered parents. *Society*, **15**(5), 54-55.

Steuer, J. L. (1983). Abuse of the physically disabled elderly. In J. I. Kosberg (Ed.), *Abuse and maltreatment of the elderly: Causes and interventions*. Boston: Wright-PSG.

Tomas, N. E. (Ed.). (1974). *Reducing crimes against aged persons*. Report of the Mid-Atlantic Federal Regional Council Task Force Workshop, U.S. Department of Health, Education, and Welfare.

U.S. Congress. House. Select Committee on Aging. (1976a). *Mental health problems of the elderly*. Washington: Government Printing Office.

U.S. Congress. Senate. Special Committee on Aging. (1976b). *Nursing home care in the United States: Failure in public policy*. Washington: Government Printing Office.

U.S. Congress. Senate. Special Committee on Aging. (1978). *Developments in aging, 1977, part 2*. Washington: Government Printing Office.

U.S. Congress. House. Select Committee on Aging. (1980). *Elder abuse: The hidden problem*. Washington: Government Printing Office.

U.S. Congress. House. Select Committee on Aging. (1981). *Physical and financial abuse of the elderly*. Washington: Government Printing Office.

PART V

HOME-BASED SERVICES

17

Housing

Susan R. Sherman, Ph.D.

State University of New York at Albany

This chapter focuses on housing services to individual clients and their families. Much of the material may also be used by social workers involved in policy development and program planning for the elderly.

Although this chapter is concerned with housing, housing cannot be considered in isolation. Thus there are many linkages between topics covered here and topics covered elsewhere in this handbook. Housing for the elderly, whether age-segregated or age-integrated, must be considered as part of the elderly's wider environment (Gelwicks and Newcomer, 1974; Hochschild, 1973; Schooler, 1970; Sherman, 1979). This environment includes, for example, transportation, medical and social services, shopping, recreation and activity centers, potential social networks, vulnerability to crime—all components whose impacts extend beyond the individual dwelling unit. Housing for the elderly must be considered in the context of service provision, both hard services and social networks.

The major premise of this chapter is that the client must be given a choice of housing, that is, available alternatives and the information necessary to make a wise decision. While this should not need to be stated in a handbook for social workers, it is far from realization in the case of housing for the elderly. In this chapter, many types of housing alternatives are described. Unfortunately, a complete continuum of housing is unavailable to a large number of elderly, sometimes because of financial restrictions and at other times because of local gaps in service. The distribution of special housing for the elderly bears little relationship to the numbers of elderly in the states or in localities (Kamerman and Kahn, 1976).

Not only at the macro policy level of making a broader choice of housing available, but at the micro level, choice is the issue. The client must be involved in the decision about his/her housing (including preoccupancy visits and possibly temporary stays). No one type of housing is best for all. The important issue is to make choices available and, once an individual has made a choice, to provide what is desired.

NEED

In order to analyze the issue of housing need, we must first subdivide the population of elderly persons. Among persons aged 65 and over, about 5 percent live in institutions. That group is discussed elsewhere in this handbook and will not be considered in this chapter. Lawton (1980) estimates that only about 4 percent of the elderly population live in specialized planned housing. This leaves about 90 percent living in the community. The present chapter discusses both the 4 percent in special planned housing and the 90 percent in ordinary housing dispersed in the community. (A study recently completed by Marans, Feldt, and Pastalan estimates that 2.5 million older Americans now live in age-segregated residential environments [Institute of Gerontology, 1982].) It is likely that social workers will have contact with both groups.

Housing need may be described in terms of household composition to understand the need for social support; in terms of housing tenure to assess the security and flexibility of the current situation; and in terms of housing quality to understand the need for relocation to different housing arrangements.

Household Composition

Approximately 80 percent of men 65 and over live in families (76 percent as head of family). About 56 percent of women live in families (44 percent as head of family or wife of head). About 15 percent of men but 37 percent of women live alone (U.S. Bureau of the Census, 1976). Although Shanas (1979) has dispelled the myth that families abandon their older members, the overwhelming number of older persons prefer not to live with their children. For example, 96 percent of Sherman's (1972) sample of older persons agreed that it is better not to live with their children. If there is need for support and supervision, and if no alternatives are available, some older persons may have to live with their children. But despite sentimental revisions of history, three-generation family households have never been the norm.

Housing Tenure

Seventy-one percent of all household heads 65 and over own their homes and 84 percent of these homes are mortgage free (Allan and Brotman, 1981; Brotman, 1981). Although for many this represents an element of security, both psychological and financial, for other elderly this may be more of a "trap." The unit may be too large, there may be unnegotiable stairs, the house may be located in a high-crime neighborhood, and taxes and fuel costs may be consuming too large a share of the person's monthly income. Additionally, the owner may not be able to afford maintenance of the house. Real-property-tax exemptions have been applied unevenly, and reverse equity has not been widely accepted (N.Y. Legislature, 1982). However, the sale of the house may be difficult and may not bring enough money to ensure a secure future in rental housing. Furthermore, the older person may be reluctant to leave a familiar setting and friends.

Sometimes housing tenure, rental or owned, is threatened by forced relocation due to urban renewal, conversion to condominiums, or "gentrification." The lack of affordable rentals affects the medium-income elderly as well as the poor elderly (N.Y. Legislature, 1982). Renters aged 65 and over spend nearly one-third of their incomes on housing costs.

Housing Quality

Manney (1975) estimates that 30 percent of all older Americans and 40 percent of poor elderly live in substandard housing. According to a survey by the U.S. Department of Housing and Urban Development, 9 percent of units with household heads 65 and older had physical deficiencies or flaws; the rate for the population as a whole was 9.7 percent (Allan and Brotman, 1981). Struyk and Soldo (1980) estimate that 15 percent of elderly renters and 6 percent of elderly homeowners live in units with deficiencies in one or more of the following areas: plumbing, kitchen (incomplete or shared use), sewage, heating, and maintenance. Lawton (1980), in analyzing the Annual Housing Survey 1976 public-use tape, also found that housing deficiencies are more frequent in rented dwellings than in owner-occupied dwellings, though about one-quarter of each group had a room lacking heat, about 10 percent of each group had coal, wood, or no heating fuel, and rodents were present in about 10 percent of homes in each group.

Despite these deficiencies, Carp (1976) cited several studies reporting favorable assessment, by residents, of housing that investigators rated as poor. She suggested that if persons have no choice, a positive assessment may be a defensive reaction. When residents were given a choice, Carp found that housing evaluation become more negative.

Groups who are most deprived with respect to housing include inner-city elderly, farm dwellers, Hispanic-Americans, Asian-Americans, blacks, and Jewish slum dwellers (Carp, 1976; Lawton, 1980).

ASSESSMENT

Because the array of housing types is so diverse, it would be difficult to have an all-purpose instrument to match a specific client with a specific housing alternative. (However, a particular agency or housing counseling program may devise its own tool. See, for example, Pastalan's assessment schedule in Lawton [1975]. This survey, derived from Pastalan [1972], asks respondents about what type of housing they would prefer, where they would prefer the housing to be [in terms of rural/urban continuum, access to services and to friends], what services they wish provided within the building, important neighborhood and dwelling-unit features, plans to move, causes for move, current housing arrangements and cost, transportation, need for in-home services in current home, health problems and perceived need for housing and other services in the community.) A good conceptual tool for assessment is the Lawton/Nahemow adaptation model described more fully in the "Theory" section of this chapter. In essence, this model indicates that, for a given environment, a person of a specified level of competence will be optimally adjusted. Likewise, for a given level of competence, an environment of a given level of demand will be optimal. This necessitates a very careful understanding of the client's capabilities and of the environment's requirements. When various options are described below, they will be arrayed roughly in terms of decreasing environmental demand. Although clients will be described who are particularly appropriate for each modality, such guidelines should be used with great caution. There is much overlap between optimal types for each housing alternative, depending on client's wishes and coping style and the availability of other formal and informal supports.

Clearly, one type of housing assessment is that of determining what interventions are necessary in current housing. Are repairs necessary? Are there services that need to be brought in? Another kind of assessment is required for relocation (perhaps involuntary) to an institution. For this a medical assessment is required. This chapter, however, emphasizes moves that are relatively voluntary and that are to other types of relatively independent housing.

As in all good social-work assessment, the client should be asked his/her preferences in housing. Some of the major dimensions that need to be decided are:

Age-segregated or age-integrated housing
Need and desire for services—for example, meals, housekeeping, and
   activities

Maximum distance willing to move—that is, increasing (or decreasing) distance from relatives, friends, and familiar places
Type of location

When persons in the community are asked whether they would prefer age-segregated or age-integrated housing, the large majority prefer age-integrated. For example, Sherman (1971) found that only about 15 percent of a (non-random) sample of older persons in the community indicated that they would like to move to retirement housing. Sherman et al. (1985) found that 22 percent of a sample of persons 60 and over would prefer to live in housing limited to people their own age. On the other hand, when persons already living in age-segregated housing are queried, a large majority report being satisfied (Lawton and Nahemow, 1975). Eighty percent of Sherman's (1972) sample of persons in retirement housing said that it is better for retired people to live in special housing.

Social workers need to be concerned with being sure that older persons considering a move relocate so as to be near needed resources and that transportation for older persons to services is available. But a further question is what services—for example, medical, meals—should be available at the housing facility itself. This issue is somewhat controversial. On the one hand, a major advantage of special housing for the elderly is the efficiency of providing centralized services within the housing setting, since a population with relatively high need is concentrated there. On the other hand, there are those (both consumers and providers) who fear that the provision within housing of too many services will generate an institutional atmosphere. Perhaps even more crucially, this argument proceeds, if too much is provided too early, over-dependency might be encouraged, leading to further loss of function and negative change in self-concept (Carp, 1976). Lawton (1980) cites some findings that indicate the possibility of some reduction in engagement with the external environment, but suggests that considerably more research is needed to settle the question definitively.

The provision of recreational activities may be beneficial for those to whom this is an important part of their life-style. However, for some this would represent an intrusion. Carp (1968) found that among those who were not previously involved, and who highly valued their privacy, a move to new housing with activities was not evaluated favorably. This pertained, however, only to a minority of the residents.

A related question is how much modification is needed or desired in the housing unit itself. For example, some special housing facilities offer emergency call buttons, easy to reach electric outlets and cupboards, elevators or single-level facilities, walk-in/sit-down showers, and grab bars. Although, ideally, these features would be useful for a person of any age, one must determine how essential they are to the client contemplating a move.

A further question to be considered when deciding whether one would be satisfied in retirement housing is how much dislocation would be required. There was some alienation found at the one site studied by Sherman (1972) where a substantial proportion (30 percent) had recently moved from out of state. Relocation does not necessarily mean an increase in distance from children. For example, at a retirement hotel and an apartment building studied by Sherman (1975b), residents had actually decreased the distance from their children by making the move. These findings are not unlike those of Bultena and Wood (1969), who established that only one-fourth of the migrants (from Wisconsin to Arizona) they studied had had a child located in their home community. Furthermore, a disproportionate number of old persons who seek special housing are childless (Bultena and Wood, 1969; Carp, 1966; Sherman, 1975b).

Finally, probing must be conducted as to the type of location desired: urban, suburban, rural, and in what part of the country. Even the types of facilities commonly associated with the Sunbelt—for example, retirement villages—are available in other parts of the country as well. Clients must be clear in their minds as to the priorities given climate and social networks.

The most essential step in assessment is to arrange for the client to visit the prospective housing. This means not only an inspection of the facility but a more extended stay—a meal, an activity, perhaps even an overnight stay. If the client is moving to a different climate or community, a longer visit is necessary—perhaps two or three visits at different times of the year. In some smaller programs such as shared housing, visits are important not only to determine if the client likes the site but to determine if he or she is compatible with the other residents. Before buying into a retirement community, some clients may be offered an opportunity to rent a unit temporarily.

Before leaving the topic of assessment, some mention should be made of the issue of relocation stress. Most of the research on relocation stress has been on the move within institutions or from community to institution, and that will be covered in another chapter of this handbook. With respect to relocation in the community, Lawton (1980), in summarizing several studies, notes a risk of deterioration in physical health with relocation (but not in social and psychological functioning or in mortality), but this is dependent on preparation, the quality of the new environment, and perceived choice in the situation. In Schulz and Brenner's (1977) review of within-community relocation, both choice and the quality of the new environment appeared to be important determinants of positive outcome. Finally, it should be recognized that, for some people, change or novelty is enhancing, such as is predicted by the Lawton/Nahemow model described below.

INTERVENTION

Unlike some programs in other chapters of this handbook, housing is not a specific "program." Rather, it is a disparate collection of environments, some of which have arisen out of specific governmental policies, others of which have emerged "in the marketplace." Because housing is not one specific program, there is not a well-defined path nor a typical sequence for social-work intervention. The role of the social worker will be defined below as each modality is described. A very useful role for social workers, rarely realized at the present time, is as part of a housing counseling service.

Range of Services

The first division that needs to be made when discussing the range of housing services is between independent, unplanned housing in the community and special, planned housing. As was explained previously, about 90 percent of all persons age 65 and over live in housing dispersed in the community, and about 70 percent of all household heads 65 and over own their homes. The housing may be too large, old and run-down, in high-crime areas, and subject to rising property taxes and fuel costs, leaving little money for maintenance and repairs. If the person desires to move, he or she may not be able to make enough from the sale of the house to be able to afford future rents. Furthermore, many people are reluctant to leave a familiar community with well-established social networks.

Unplanned, dispersed community housing, whether owned or rented, is particularly appropriate for independent, healthy elderly with available social networks or for more dependent elderly who have strong family support, usually a spouse (Lawton, 1981).

Social workers will be involved with persons who live in unplanned housing as needs for additional services arise, either those specifically related to housing, such as home repairs, or those concerning in-home social and medical services, described elsewhere in this handbook. The social worker may also be involved in helping to make a decision to relocate and sell a house, and must consider accessibility to shopping and medical services. In protective-services cases, the older person may have to move when he or she can no longer live alone safely or maintain the dwelling. This suggests a further role for the social worker when the elderly person is reluctant to leave and needs to be assisted in handling this crisis. (Schooler, 1976, and Fried, 1963 discuss grief engendered by involuntary moves.) While not considered in detail in this chapter, it is important for the social worker involved in helping to plan a relocation to understand the importance to the client of bringing cherished objects from home, even if it is only some favorite pieces of jewelry, photographs, etc. (Sherman and Newman, 1977-78).

The other general category of housing for the elderly is that of special planned housing. The impetus for special planned housing has come primarily from nonprofit organizations, private enterprise, and the federal government. A few types could be described more accurately as having evolved into senior housing rather than having been planned as such. Sherman (1971) found that reasons given for moving to retirement housing included easy maintenance, health and personal needs cared for, change in physical strength, wish to be with own age group, quality of the dwelling, proximity to facilities and services, proximity to children, relatives, or friends, and provision of meals. In summarizing a number of studies, Lawton (1980) concluded that low-intensity medical services are most highly valued, while meal services are lower in priority.

We shall array planned housing according to the amount of *independence* required by the *typical* occupant. This is a very rough ordering, not only because the names of the types vary from locality to locality but because each category itself includes a range of housing, and a particular facility may house a range of occupants. Some staff in comparable sites offer more assistance than others. Thus, in terms of independence, there is much overlap between categories; the requirements may not be visible on the outside; much depends on what goes on inside the facility. Three other dimensions upon which to order planned housing are financial arrangement, type of dwelling unit, and government program. Financial arrangements include purchase, rental, cooperative, condominium, and life-care. Type of units include detached houses, apartments — either high-rise or garden-type — mobile homes, single rooms. Government programs are described in the section entitled "Policy." There is a certain degree of correlation among these four dimensions, and financial and dwelling arrangements will be described when they typify one of the categories below.

Lawton (1980) describes two developmental models of planned housing:

Constant: The housing maintains the same level of capability among the residents. The residents must leave as soon as they cannot maintain themselves at that level of demand.

Accommodating: The housing is able to maintain a resident as his or her capability changes, up to twenty-four-hour nursing. The facility changes its programs, physical space, and requirements for new tenants.

Whether a facility is constant or accommodating is very important for the social worker to consider when he or she is counseling a client who is making a move. Sherman (1972) described a type of planned housing in which a variety of units are available, so that the client may stay in one facility but, within the facility, move from a detached house to an apartment, then to a single room, and eventually to an infirmary. Although rated favorably by residents, such opportunities are rare and, when available, are generally very expensive.

Retirement Villages

Although retirement villages have received the most publicity in sunbelt areas, they appear in many parts of the country. They frequently offer hundreds of units, either apartments or detached houses or both. Some have congregate housing and institutional care on the premises, in which case they could serve throughout the independence continuum applied here (Lawton, 1981). They are usually for purchase (including cooperatives and condominiums) (Walkley et al., 1966a, 1966b). The advantages of retirement villages are:

1. They may have a complete package of on-site services, such as shopping, medical clinics, activity programs, social clubs, golf course, swimming pools, and arts and crafts rooms.
2. They may offer on-site maintenance of the dwelling, both inside and outside. Frequently a great deal of care is given to maintenance of very attractive grounds.
3. They may have special security arrangements, such as a gate, guard, etc.
4. There is the potential for an extensive network, offering both instrumental and expressive support.

The disadvantages of retirement villages are:

1. Usually the resident is dependent on an automobile, either within the site or off-site. Some retirement villages have their own transportation systems, but they are not usually extensive enough to make the person completely self-sufficient. Transportation may only be within the village, but shopping, entertainment, hospital, etc. may be off-site at some distance. When the person is no longer able to drive, this might necessitate a move.
2. Many villages are oriented to married couples. When a person becomes widowed, he or she may be left out of social networks.
3. Most villages are expensive.
4. Some villages are isolated from an urban area, from services, and from previous social networks. There may be reduced contact with families (although significant possibilities for new friendships).
5. Many retirement villages are constant rather than accommodating environments, as in Lawton's designation, and the resident may have to move again if, for example, his or her health declines.

Retirement villages are particularly appropriate for financially well-off, independent, healthy elderly, who can drive an automobile, and who are interested in an extensive opportunity for activities. It is unlikely that the social worker would be involved in this type of housing beyond helping a client with a decision to move.

Mobile Homes

While most mobile-home parks are not exclusively for the elderly, some have a policy of adults only, and some specifically have programs for the elderly. In 1976, 4.9 percent of all older persons lived in mobile homes, and they represented

17 percent of the total population in mobile homes (Lawton, 1980). Most parks have the spaces for rent while the mobile homes are owned by the individuals. Mobile-home subdivisions are those with a mobile home placced on a permanent foundation; the owner of the mobile home owns the space as well.

The advantages of mobile-home living are:

1. Low cost
2. Informality
3. Active social life and sense of community (Johnson, 1971) in some mobile-home communities

The disadvantages of mobile-home living are:

1. Possible lack of privacy
2. Lack of space
3. Lack of accessibility to the community and services
4. Nonaccommodating
5. Necessity to drive an automobile

Mobile-home parks are particularly appropriate for healthy elderly who like the opportunity to combine independence with the availability of informal support in time of need. Again, it is unlikely that a social worker would be involved with this type of housing other than in assisting the client to make a decision to move in, or helping to decide when the client needs a greater degree of support.

Retirement Hotels and Single Room Occupancies (SROs)

Retirement hotels can range from expensive to inexpensive. Some older hotels in central cities, in order to maintain reasonable occupancy, have specialized as senior-citizen hotels. This ordinarily involved little adjustment, since by that time the hotel had already become occupied primarily by senior citizens. In some cases, meals are provided. There may be a few activity rooms and a few organized activities such as cards and bingo. Goode, Hoover, and Lawton (1979) estimated that slightly more than 80,000 units in hotels were occupied by persons 65 and over in 1975, half permanent and half transient. Of the transients, 25 percent were female, while of the permanent, 50 percent were female.

A type of housing that has been receiving increasing attention is the SRO (Ehrlich, 1976). The number of elderly who choose SROs appear to be increasing (Siegal, 1978). SRO housing is found in large commercial hotels, specialty retirement hotels, rooming houses, and converted apartment buildings. These facilities contain furnished rooms, usually without kitchens and frequently without bathrooms. The facilities may be old and deteriorated, and they are usually in or near transitional or commercial inner-city locations, thus accessible to services (Blackie et al., 1983; Eckert, 1979). They may be used by welfare clients and discharged mental patients as well as by the elderly. "Contrary to commonly held assumptions, the majority of SRO residents are not vagrants or social deviants . . . [they] have simply chosen this type . . . because of its affordability" (Blackie et al., 1983, p. 37).

Thus, while there is overlap between the categories of retirement hotels and SROs, there are some more luxurious hotels with meal plans that would not share many of the characteristics of SROs, and some SROs that are not in hotels. Many of the advantages, however, are the same.

The advantages are:

1. For a relatively reasonable cost, provision of services — for example housekeeping and/or meals.
2. Accessibility to the services of the city, including restaurants, and to transportation.
3. Privacy and the ability to continue a life-style of independence (what others might call isolation) and autonomy (Erickson and Eckert, 1977; Plutchik, McCarthy, and Hall, 1975; Stephens, 1975).
4. Sociability and some limited support provided by the other residents, when desired.
5. Sense of security provided by twenty-four-hour staff.

The disadvantages are:

1. The hotels are frequently located in high-crime areas.
2. The units may be unattractive.

Hotels are particularly appropriate for self-reliant elderly who wish to continue a life-style of independence. They are appropriate for those who wish to be near the amenities of a city and who need public transportation, or for those who simply prefer the urban life-style. For the more affluent elderly who prefer to have meals prepared, specialized retirement hotels would be appropriate. But more generally, this type would be for people who do not desire housekeeping responsibilities.

A caseworker in a local social-services department might very well be involved in placing an elderly client in a hotel. The worker would need to know the availability of such residences, whether meals are offered, and the availabilty of localized services. It is also more likely that a social worker would be involved in housing placement for hotel clients, as they tend to represent a disproportionate share of the childless (Wilner et al., 1968).

Independent Apartments

Apartment complexes that provide meals and other more intensive services will be discussed under congregate housing; in this section we refer to a relatively common type of housing in which meals are not provided, requiring an intermediate degree of independence on the part of residents. (Some may require more independence than do some retirement hotels, discussed previously.) There may be some common rooms for social activities. Some facilities may offer some meals through a nutrition program operating in the building. Project sizes vary widely. Much of this housing has been built under some form of government program, such as public housing, Section 202, or Section 236, described later in this chapter. This category presently houses a wide range of income groups.

The advantages are:

1. Quality and cost of the dwelling unit. Frequently this is of a quality much higher than the residents had ever hoped to have (Sherman, 1971).
2. Central location. While this is not intrinsic to the housing type, much of such housing is in urban areas, if not in central cities.
3. The opportunity to form social networks (Hochschild, 1973).
4. The availability of on-site activity programs.

Independent apartments are particularly appropriate for persons who want the privacy of their own apartment, who want to and are capable of preparing their own meals, and who seek the opportunity to have new friends available when needed for either instrumental or expressive support. It may be an economical way to achieve an attractive living environment. These arrangements are quite popular, and many facilities have long waiting lists.

The social worker could be involved in helping the client find such housing, and perhaps in negotiating the system of eligibility requirements, waiting lists, etc. In some larger complexes and in nonprofit lower-middle-income housing, there may be a staff member with social-service training (Lawton, 1980).

Congregate Housing

While buildings in this category may look like those in the previous category, congregate housing has a special meaning; it designates housing with a central kitchen and common dining (although residents may also have their own kitchens). It may provide space for other services. There may be activity programs, resident councils, etc. "In . . . 1978 legislation authorized the Department of Housing and Urban Development to award grants to public housing authorities and section 202 sponsors to provide meals and supportive services . . . [to keep people] out of . . . institutions. Over 2200 elderly are now being served by the congregate housing services program. The demand for this and similarly designed programs that coordinate housing and supportive health-care and housekeeping services can be expected to grow" (U.S. Congress, 1982, p. 212). The more supportive these other services become, the more the distinction between congregate housing and homes for aged/adult homes becomes blurred. Following the distinction suggested by Lawton (1975, 1981), congregate housing will be used to refer to the provision of on-site services for the more independent — for example, activity program, outpatient clinic, transportation, and possibly congregate meals. Homes for the aged/adult homes, described below, can offer personal services (assistance with ADL skills) in addition, and are more institutional, though again there is a great deal of overlap between categories.

The advantages of congregate housing are:

1. The provision of nutritious meals
2. The sociability of eating together
3. The opportunity to form social networks

Unfortunately, "the supply of congregate and subsidized housing is shrinking . . . throughout the country. Some housing and loan grants . . . have been phased out" (N.Y. Legislature, 1982. p. 10).

Congregate housing is particularly appropriate for older persons who need some support in order to remain on their own in the community. This housing offers a range of services that may be used when needed. It would be particularly appropriate for those who desire social contact. Unfortunately, there frequently are long waiting lists for this type of housing.

Social workers could be part of the staff in congregate housing to help in times of crisis — for example, bereavement counseling, obtaining medical services, working with the families of residents, etc. More generally, they would be involved in helping a client determine if this is the level of support needed and then locating a facility.

Shared Housing

This option recently has received increasing attention (Blackie et al., 1983; N.Y. Legislature, 1982; N.Y. Office for the Aging, n.d.; Streib, 1978). "Shared housing refers to a household of two or more unrelated persons residing in one dwelling unit. The members of the household share in the financial responsibilities as well as in household duties such as cooking and cleaning" (Blackie et al., 1983, p. 1), although in the managerial model staff take care of such tasks as cooking, cleaning, shopping, laundry, and transportation. "The kitchen, bathroom, and other public areas of the unit are shared, while each person maintains a private area, such as a bedroom" (Blackie et al., 1983, p. 1).

At a November 1981 Congressional hearing on shared housing, three models were identified as shared-living environments: residences of individuals who open their homes to others, groups of unrelated individuals who live in a single housekeeping unit, and single-occupancy apartments with common dining areas. (A related form is intermediate housing in which residents share only a living room, but have some support from the sponsoring long-term-care institution [Lawton, 1981].) The formation and operational structure of shared homes fall into three categories: naturally occurring shared homes, generally accommo-dating three to five persons; agency-assisted; and agency-sponsored, generally serving two to twenty persons (Blackie et al., 1983; N.Y. Legislature, 1982). The first and sometimes the second type are not sheltered or supported housing and would belong earlier in the independence continuum. The "enriched housing" program in New York state, for example, serves unrelated elderly living in a single housekeeping unit. Such services as homemaker, social worker, and transportation are provided. Public assistance for shared housing has come from such programs as Section 8, Community Development Block Grants, Title XX, Older Americans Act monies, and state, city, and county governments.

The advantages of shared housing are:

1. Companionship and social support
2. Maintenance of ties with the community
3. Income for the homeowners
4. Sustained involvement in the household
5. Safety and protection from crime
6. In some cases supervision with activities of daily living (one such program is referred to as "enriched housing")
7. Financially efficient

The disadvantages are:

1. Difficulty for strangers to share living quarters, kitchens, etc., problems with territoriality
2. Loss of privacy

Shared housing is particularly appropriate for someone who needs support in order to prevent institutionalization, for someone who wishes to have the opportunity to form social networks, and for homeowners who want someone to share expenses or maintenance. Good interpersonal skills are important. This model may not be appropriate for persons who are used to living alone.

The social worker will be involved in screening and matching clients and in case management. Matching is absolutely critical to the success of this program.

Additionally, such housing requires ongoing follow-up to be sure residents receive necessary services and to provide counseling when conflicts arise among residents.

Licensed Boarding Homes

This is an old form of assisted housing for the elderly. These homes are generally licensed by state or local social-welfare departments or the Veterans Administration to provide personal care and services (Walkley et al., 1966a, 1966b). This category may overlap with the following category. (Some elderly, of course live in boarding homes that are not licensed and that might be placed higher on the independence continuum.) Meals are provided. A subcategory of boarding homes is foster-family-care homes (Sherman and Newman, 1977), generally housing no more than six residents and usually fewer. Frequently a part of the mental-health system, these homes provide some supervision for the residents. This is an option that has not been sufficiently explored for the frail elderly who are not in need of institutionalization but who need some supervision.
The advantages are:

1. Permits a person needing a protective setting to live in the community, perhaps delaying institutionalization
2. Offers the possibility of a family atmosphere, although research has indicated that the clients themselves may be what constitutes a family, rather than being introduced into some model family form (Newman and Sherman, 1979).

The disadvantages are:

1. May be of poor quality because of lack of regulation (Carp, 1976)
2. May lack stimulation
3. May increase dependency

Licensed boarding homes or foster-family-care homes are particularly appropriate for persons in need of a protective environment but not requiring institutionalization. They are appropriate for persons who have lost contact with their own families and who have limited social networks.
Caseworkers in local social-services departments are responsible for the recruitment, initial evaluation, visitation, and continued supervision and evaluation of small foster-family homes. In the Veterans Administration, social-work staff screen and approve the homes and make ongoing supervisory visits (Sherman and Newman, 1977). Caseworkers could also be involved in helping clients find such homes, in matching clients and homes (Sherman and Newman, 1979), and in providiing training for caretakers.

Homes for the Aged/Adult Homes/Domiciliary-Care Facilities/Personal-Care Residences

These homes, both nonprofit and proprietary, provide supportive services on a twenty-four-hour basis for aged, frail, or disabled adults (Snider, Pascarelli and Howard, 1979). Services include room and board, housekeeping, personal care, supervision, and other nonmedical services. The National Center for Health Statistics defines a domiciliary-care residence as offering one or two of eight personal-care services, while a personal-care residence is one that offers three or more such services (Lawton, 1981). As part of the long-term-care continuum offering a lower level of care than health-related or skilled-nursing facilities, these homes are described in more detail in other chapters of this handbook. Facilities are diverse, ranging in size from under a dozen beds to a few hundred. In some institutions life-care arrangements are available. These facilities tend to be more luxurious and offer a greater diversity of services. In other homes, recreation facilities may be no more than a TV room. This is such a diverse category that it is difficult to specify general advantages and disadvantages. Homes for the aged are particularly appropriate for persons requiring support services but not a formal medical component.

Caseworkers would be involved in determining that this is the proper level of care, in locating a facility, and in making the referral. In some large homes, there could be a social worker on staff, involved with admission, activities, etc.

Other alternatives, which deserve further examination but which will not be discussed in great detail here, include:

• "An accessory apartment, also referred to as a single-family conversion, is a small, self-contained unit within a larger building, most often a single family home. Approximately 2.5 million accessory apartments were built into existing buildings between 1970 and 1980, many in homes owned by an elderly person. After the conversion, the elderly homeowner may reside either in the accessory apartment or in the remaining part of the home ... Benefits [are] extra income ... [and] increased security . . ." (Blackie et al., 1983, p. 2).

• "Elder cottage housing opportunity (ECHO) [also called 'Granny Flats'] refers to the concept of a small, mobile, self-contained housing unit which is placed in the yard of an existing host house. The elderly person resides in this unit in close proximity yet independent of his/her child or relative" (Blackie et al., 1983).

Client Contact with Services

This would depend greatly on the type of housing. For example, retirement villages advertise privately. Mobile-home parks are listed in various directories, as are shared-housing programs. Retirement hotels are listed in telephone directories. Social-service departments have lists of licensed boarding homes. Some aging-related agencies also have lists of available housing.

Effectiveness of Current Forms of Intervention

Most research on the effectiveness of special planned housing has been either on housing for the economically advantaged elderly or on public housing. Neither group is particularly representative of most older persons, and the results may not be generalizable. Some of the studies cannot be conclusive because of design problems, such as self-selection. Furthermore, when we discuss special planned retirement housing, we include a number of characteristics besides age segregation, such as new construction, service access, etc. The literature has tended to equate the study of age segregation with the evaluation of planned housing (Carp, 1976). However, the issues need to be distinct; Sherman (1971) found that for many persons moving to retirement housing, a wish for easy maintenance and having health and personal needs cared for were more salient than a wish to be with their own age group. A few of the studies of planned housing programs may be summarized here, keeping in mind that they are not studies of age segregation per se but of a special type of environment with many diverse features, only one of which is age segregation.

Carp (1966) found that movers, as compared to nonmoving controls, who had applied for special housing, rated higher on housing satisfaction, neighborhood satisfaction, service access, increased morale, increased health, and increased social interaction and amount of participation in activities.

Sherman, Newman, and Nelson (1976) found that among elderly in public housing, there was less fear of crime and less crime experienced in age-segregated buildings than in age-integrated buildings.

Lawton and Cohen (1974), in comparing movers to controls who had not applied for such housing, found that movers rated higher on housing satisfaction, involvement in external activities, and satisfaction with the status quo. However, there was no change due to new housing in morale or breadth of activities, and there was a decline in functional health.

Sherwood, Greer, and Morris (1979) found greater housing satisfaction, participation in formal social activities, and likelihood of being admitted to an acute-care hospital and less likelihood of becoming institutionalized, less time spent in a long-term-care facility as well as a lower death rate among movers to a medically oriented public-housing project as compared to matched controls.

Sherman (1975c) found that, with respect to caring for health needs, desire for counseling services, and expected support in crises, a good match between personal need and environmental provisions was reported at five of the six retirement-housing sites studied. During a two-year period (both interviews after the move to retirement housing) there was an increase in leisure-activity scores for retirement-housing residents and a decrease for community residents (Sherman, 1974). Sherman (1975b) also found that retirement housing residents interacted less than did their controls in ordinary housing with their children, grandchildren, and other relatives, and fewer had friends younger than 40.

However, they had more new friends and visited more with neighbors and with age-peer friends. There was little test-control difference in sufficiency of contact or in assistance patterns (Sherman, 1975a). Bultena and Wood (1969) also found that retirement-housing residents interacted less with family, but had more friends available. They had higher morale and self-rated health.

THEORY

A few theories or models that are particularly relevant to housing selection will be summarized here.

Lawton and Nahemow's (1973) adaptation model is perhaps most useful for the social worker. This model characterizes two dimensions: environmental press, referring to the demands of the setting, and individual competence, including such dimensions as biological health, sensorimotor functioning, cognitive skill, and ego strength. The social worker can attempt to maximize adaptive behavior and positive affect either by improving the individual's competence level or by adjusting the demands of the environment. In practice, this frequently means assessing the competence of the client and helping to determine that he/she needs a less demanding environment — for example, one with no stairs, one that offers meal service, etc.

Lawton and Simon's (1968) environmental docility hypothesis asserts that the less competent the individual, the greater the impact of environmental factors on that individual, which would suggest that the choice of housing is particularly important for the vulnerable client who is most likely to come to the attention of the social worker. It also means that it is the vulnerable client who is most likely to be affected by even a small change in environment, either positively or negatively. Contrastingly, elderly who are healthy and economically secure would be least likely to have aspects of their behavior dependent on external conditions of the housing environment. Sherman (1974) found that moving to retirement housing did not increase the leisure-activity level for persons of high economic and health status relative to community residents. Persons in the community group had the economic means and health to maintain an activity level as high as that of their counterparts who chose to move into special housing.

In Kahana's theory of person/environment congruence (Kahana, Liang, and Felton, 1980), a person may be characterized by the types and relative strengths of his or her needs; the environment may be characterized by the extent to which it is capable of satisfying these needs. It is the role of the social worker to enhance morale by matching a person's needs with the environment in question. An aid to this match may be found above, in the discussion of assessment, and in the descriptions of clients who can benefit the most from each housing type.

Dowd's (1975) exchange theory has relevance for issues of housing for the elderly. Since the bargaining position of older persons is weakened because of devalued status, an age-segrated environment may be strategic to minimize the costs inherent in ordinary social exchange. In such an environment, exchange networks will be formed within age categories rather than between categories, and the older person will not be at such a disadvantage.

Newman's (1972, 1976) theory of defensible space is important in both selecting housing and in building new housing. Defensible space refers to a physical environment constructed so that residents are encouraged to monitor their own setting. These characteristics engage the sense of territoriality and community among the residents. "This is accomplished by designing housing developments in which dwelling units are grouped together to facilitate associations of mutual benefit; by delineating areas for particular functions; by clearly defining paths of movement; by defining outdoor areas of activity for particular users through their juxtaposition with interior living areas; and by providing inhabitants with natural opportunities for the continued visual surveillance of their public areas, in buildings and outside them" (Newman, 1976, pp. 4-5). In this way, residents are in control and intruders are observed and challenged. When Newman's design principles are applied, greater security and quality of life are afforded to older residents.

In Kuypers and Bengtson's (1973) social reconstruction model, housing is viewed as an intervention that can help to reverse a cycle of social breakdown. By improving housing conditions, dependence will be reduced and self-reliance will be increased. This will lead to self-labeling by the client as able, and to an internalization of an effective self-image. The social worker can be a critical catalyst for such a reversal.

In analyzing the effect of planned retirement-housing facilities, Sherman (1979) employed the concept of site permeability. Retirement housing facilities can vary from a relatively closed community (i.e., low site permeability) to one that allows for frequent penetration and movement in and out of its boundaries (i.e., high permeability). In Sherman's model, perceived community support in crises is a joint function of site permeability and service availability: given a situation of good service availability, the lower the site permeability, the greater the perceived community support; given a situation of poor service availability, the lower the site permeability, the less the perceived community support. The social worker thus needs to look beyond the dimension of service availability to the dimension of site permeability. Those elderly who prefer and select a site with low permeability may be in greater need of service augmentation and supportive assistance at times of crisis—for example, of illness or bereavement —than those elderly who select a site with high permeability. At those sites where services are present, the less permeable the boundaries, the less is the need for additional support during crises. Once a threshold of services is available, the very sense of enclosure provides security.

POLICY

The major federally assisted housing programs are described in a report of the Senate Special Committee on Aging (U.S. Congress, 1982):

The section 8 program is currently the largest of the Federal programs providing subsidized housing to households with incomes too low to obtain decent housing in the private market. Under the program, HUD enters into assistance contracts with owners of *existing* housing or developers of *new* or *substantially* rehabilitated housing for a specified number of units to be leased by households meeting Federal eligibility standards. Payments made to owners and developers under assistance contracts are used to make up the difference between what the rental household can afford to pay for rent and what HUD has determined to be the "fair market rent" for the dwelling. At the end of June 1981, it was estimated by HUD that approximately 597,000 or 37 percent of the more than 1.5 million total section 8 units were occupied by older persons. Over 283,000 or 54 percent of the newly constructed units were occupied by the elderly (p.214).

The section 202 program is the primary Federal financing vehicle for constructing housing for older persons that will enable them to remain self-sufficient and independent in our society. Under the program, the Federal Government makes a direct loan to private, non-profit project sponsors to use in developing section 8 housing that is specifically designed to the needs of the low-income elderly and handicapped. Since the program's authorization in 1974, over 79,000 units for the elderly have been constructed (p.216).

The 202 program, first authorized in the 1959 Housing Act and discontinued in 1969, provided direct construction loans at 3 percent interest to nonprofit sponsors to serve moderate income renters. The old 202 program produced 45,275 units (Lawton, 1980).

The low-rent public housing program is the oldest of those Federal programs providing housing for the elderly. It was established by the United States Housing Act of 1937. Over 45 percent of the Nation's more than 1.2 million public housing units are occupied by older Americans. It is a federally financed program which is operated by locally established, nonprofit public housing agencies (PHAs). . . . In many communities there is a long waiting list for admission to these projects serving the elderly and such lists can be expected to increase as the demand for elderly rental housing continues in many parts of the nation (p.218).

Other Federal programs include rural-housing loans, rural rental housing, mortgage insurance, Indian housing, community-development block grants, urban-development block grants, rehabilitation-loan programs, energy-assistance programs, and monies obtained from Title III of the Older Americans Act or from Title XX of the Social Security Act.

There are many gaps in our public policies regarding housing for the elderly. First, there is insufficient housing offered in an intermediate range between independent housing and an institutional setting, which makes the job of the social worker working with a frail but not seriously impaired client far more difficult.

Second, federal housing policy has been primarily that of construction of rental housing (N.Y. Office for the Aging, n.d.). Since 70 percent of all elderly heads of housholds own their homes, it is clear that this cannot possibly be sufficient to address fully the housing needs of older persons. It is only with drastic federal cutbacks that increased attention is being paid to more innovative programs, primarily at the local level.

According to Lawton, "The overriding policy issue in the area of housing for the aged concerns the relative lack of federal programs designed to aid the more than 90% of all older people who live in ordinary, unplanned communities" (1980, p. 72). It is generally agreed that federal policy has paid insufficient attention to programs for maintenance/rehabilitation and weatherization of existing housing, much less to offering housing counseling services. Other programs that also have been used only sparsely are local property-tax rebates. According to an analysis by the N.Y. State Senate Committee on Aging, "HUD's 1983 budget emphasis on preservation and protection of existing housing stock is indicative of a policy shift from new construction to rehabilitation . . ." (N.Y. Legislature, 1982, p. 11).

Some of the public- and private-sector policy options under discussion by the federal government and others include voucher programs (housing allowance), housing-assistance block grants, home-equity conversion plans (U.S. Congress, 1982).

All of the programs described above together do not approach meeting the housing needs of older Americans. The theory is that new programs can serve a wider population. Whether they do, remains to be seen. Social workers can be involved in helping to organize some of these innovative programs.

REFERENCES

Allan, C., and Brotman, H. (Comps.). (1981). *Chart book on aging in America.* Washington: White House Conference on Aging.

Blackie, N., Edelstein, J., Matthews, P. S., and Timmons, R. (1983). *Alternative housing and living arrangements for independent living.* Ann Arbor: National Policy Center on Housing and Living Arrangements for Older Americans, University of Michigan.

Brotman, H. B. (1981). *Every ninth American.* Draft prepared for "Developments in Aging, 1980" for the Senate Special Committee on Aging.

Bultena, G. L., and Wood, V. (1969). The American retirement community: Bane or blessing? *Journal of Gerontology,* **24**(2), 209-217.

Carp, F. M. (1966). *A future for the aged: Victoria Plaza and its residents.* Austin: University of Texas Press.

Carp, F. M. (1968). Person-situation congruence in engagement. *Gerontologist,* **8**(3), 184-188.

Carp, F. M. (1976). Housing and living environments of older people. In R. H. Binstock & E. Shanas (Eds.), *Handbook of aging and the social sciences.* New York: Van Nostrand Reinhold.

Dowd, J. J. (1975). Aging as exchange: A preface to theory. *Journal of Gerontology,* **30**(5), 584-594.

Eckert, J. K. (1979). The unseen community: Understanding the older hotel dweller. *Aging,* nos. 291-292, pp. 28-35.

Ehrlich, P. (1976). A study: Characteristics and needs of the St. Louis downtown SRO elderly. In *The invisible elderly.* Washington: National Council on the Aging.

Erickson, R., and Eckert, K. (1977). The elderly poor in downtown San Diego hotels. *Gerontologist,* **17**(5), 440-446.

Fried, M. (1963). Grieving for a lost home: Psychological costs of relocation. In L. J. Duhl (Ed.), *The urban condition.* New York: Basic Books.

Gelwicks, L. E., and Newcomer, R. J. (1974). *Planning housing environments for the elderly.* Washington: National Council on the Aging.

Goode, C., Hoover, S. L., and Lawton, M. P. (1979). *Elderly hotel and rooming-house dwellers.* Philadelphia: Philadelphia Geriatric Center.

Hochschild, A. R. (1973). *The unexpected community.* Englewood Cliffs, N. J.: Prentice-Hall.

Institute of Gerontology, University of Michigan. (1982, October). Retirement communities continue to change. *Gerontology at Michigan.*

Johnson, S. K. (1971). *Idle haven: Community building among the working-class retired.* Berkeley: University of California Press.

Kahana, E., Liang, J., and Felton, B. J. (1980). Alternative models of person-environment fit: predictions of morale in three homes for the aged. *Journal of Gerontology,* **35**(4), 584-595.

Kamerman, S. B., and Kahn, A. J. (1976). *Social services in the United States.* Philadelphia: Temple University Press.

Kuypers, J. A., and Bengtson, V. L. (1973). Social breakdown and competence: A model of normal aging. *Human Development,* **16**, 181-201.

Lawton, M. P. (1975). *Planning and managing housing for the elderly.* New York: Wiley.

Lawton, M. P. (1980). *Environment and aging.* Monterey, Calif.: Brooks/Cole.

Lawton, M. P. (1981). Alternative housing. *Journal of Gerontological Social Work,* **3**(3), 61-80.

Lawton, M. P., and Cohen, J. (1974). The generality of housing impact on the well-being of older people. *Journal of Gerontology,* **29**(2), 194-204.

Lawton, M. P., and Nahemow, L. (1973). Ecology and the aging process. In C. Eisdorfer and M. P. Lawton (Eds.), *Psychology of adult development and aging.* Washington: American Psychological Association.

Lawton, M. P., and Nahemow, L. (1975). *Cost, structure, and social aspects of housing for the aged.* Philadelphia: Philadelphia Geriatric Center.

Lawton, M. P., and Simon, B. (1968). The ecology of social relationships in housing for the elderly. *Gerontologist,* **8**(2), 108-115.

Manney, J. D. Jr. (1975). *Aging in American society.* Ann Arbor: Institute of Gerontology, University of Michigan.

Newman, E. S., and Sherman, S. R. (1979-80). Foster-family care for the elderly: Surrogate family or mini-institution? *International Journal of Aging and Human Development,* **10**(2), 165-176.

Newman, O. (1972). *Defensible space.* New York: Macmillan.

Newman, O. (1976). *Design guidelines for creating defensible space.* Washington: National Institute of Law Enforcement and Criminal Justice, Law Enforcement Assistance Administration, U.S. Department of Justice.

New York (State). Legislature. Senate. Standing Committee on Aging. (1982). *Shared housing for the elderly.* Albany.

New York (State). Office for the Aging. (n.d.). *Innovative housing programs for the elderly in New York state.* Albany: New York State Office for the Aging.

Pastalan, L. (1972). *Retirement housing study.* Madison: Methodist Hospital of Madison, Wisconsin.

Plutchik, R., McCarthy, M., and Hall, B. H. (1975). Changes in elderly welfare hotel residents during a one-year period. *Journal of the American Geriatrics Society,* **23**(6), 265-270.

Schooler, K. K. (1970). Effect of environment on morale. *Gerontologist,* **10**(3), 194-197.

Schooler, K. K. (1976). Environmental change and the elderly. In I. Altman and J. Wohlwill (Eds.), *Human behavior and environment: Advances in theory and research,* vol. 1. New York: Plenum.

Schulz, R., and Brenner, G. (1977). Relocation of the aged: A review and theoretical analysis. *Journal of Gerontology,* **32**(3), 323-333.

Shanas, E., (1979). The family as a social support system in old age. *Gerontologist*, **19**(2), 169-174.

Sherman, E. A., and Newman, E. S. (1977-78). The meaning of cherished personal possessions for the elderly. *International Journal of Aging and Human Development*, **8**(2), 181-192.

Sherman, E. A., Newman, E. S., and Nelson, A. D. (1976). Patterns of age integration in public housing and the incidence of fears of crime among elderly tenants. In J. Goldsmith and S. S. Goldsmith (Eds.), *Crime and the elderly: Challenge and response*. Lexington, Mass.: Lexington Books.

Sherman, S. R. (1971). The choice of retirement housing among the well-elderly. *International Journal of Aging and Human Development*, **2**(2), 118-138.

Sherman, S. R. (1972). Satisfaction with retirement housing: Attitudes, recommendations, and moves. *International Journal of Aging and Human Development*, **3**(4), 339-366.

Sherman, S. R. (1974). Leisure activities in retirement housing. (1974). *Journal of Gerontology*, **29**(3), 325-335.

Sherman, S. R. (1975a). Mutual assistance and support in retirement housing. *Journal of Gerontology*, **30**(4), 479-483.

Sherman, S. R. (1975b). Patterns of contacts for residents of age-segregated and age-integrated housing. *Journal of Gerontology*, **30**(1), 103-107.

Sherman, S. R. (1975c). Provision of on-site services in retirement housing. *International Journal of Aging and Human Development*, **6**(3), 229-247.

Sherman, S. R. (1979). The retirement housing setting: Site permeability, service availability, and perceived community support in crises. *Journal of Social Service Research*, **3**, 139-157.

Sherman, S. R., and Newman, E. S. (1977). Foster-family care for the elderly in New York state. *Gerontologist*, **17**(6), 513-520.

Sherman, S. R., and Newman, E. S. (1979). Role of the caseworker in adult foster care. *Social Work*, **24**(4), 324-328.

Sherman, S. R., Ward, R. A., LaGory, M. Socialization and aging group consciousness: The effect of neighborhood age concentrations. *Journal of Gerontology* (in press).

Sherwood, S., Greer, D. S., and Morris, J. N. (1979). A study of the Highland Heights apartments for the physically impaired and elderly in Fall River. In T. O. Byerts, S. C. Howell, and L. A. Pastalan (Eds.), *The environmental context of aging: Life-styles, environmental quality, and living arrangements*, New York: Garland STPM Press.

Siegal, H. A. (1978). *Outposts of the forgotten*. New Brunswick, N.J.: Transaction Books.

Snider, D. A., Pascarelli, D., and Howard, M. (1979). *Survey of the needs and problems of adult home residents in New York state: Final report*. Albany: Welfare Research, Inc.

Stephens, J. (1975). Society of the alone: Freedom, privacy, and utilitarianism as dominant norms in the SRO. *Journal of Gerontology*, **30**(2), 230-235.

Streib, G. F. (1978). An alternative family form for older persons: Need and social context. *Family Coordinator*, **27**(4), 413-420.

Struyk, R. J., and Soldo, B. J. (1980). *Improving the elderly's housing*. Cambridge: Ballinger.

U.S. Bureau of the Census. (1976). Demographic aspects of aging and the older population in the United States. *Current Population Reports*, Series P-23, No. 59. Washington: Government Printing Office.

U.S. Congress. Senate. Special Committee on Aging. (1982). *Developments in aging, 1981*, vol. 1. Washington: Government Printing Office.

Walkley, R. P., Mangum, W. P. Jr., Sherman, S. R., Dodds, S., and Wilner, D. M. (1966a). The California survey of retirement housing. *Gerontologist*, **6**(1), 28-34.

Walkley, R. P., Mangum, W. P. Jr., Sherman, S. R., Dodds, S., and Wilner, D. M. (1966b). *Retirement housing in California*. Berkeley: Diablo Press.

Wilner, D. M., Sherman, S. R., Walkley, R. P., Dodds, S., and Mangum, W. P. Jr. (1968). Demographic characterisitcs of residents of planned retirement housing sites. *Gerontologist*, **8**(3), 164-169.

18

Homecare

Lenard W. Kaye, D.S.W.

Columbia University

The evolution of a coherent system of homecare services for older people has been painfully slow. For many years institutional solutions (nursing homes, homes for the aged, state hospitals) were promoted in response to problems of dependency, illness, and disability among the aged. Only in the last fifteen or twenty years have public policy and societal values begun to reflect a more balanced view of the place of homecare among the range of social and health services provided for the aged. Legislation, such as Title XX of the Social Security Act and the various titles of the Older Americans Act, as well as a gradual easing of restrictions in Medicare and Medicaid home-health-care regulations, are evidence of this partial change in philosophy. Even so, a genuine, widespread commitment to in-home services for the aged remains substantially unrealized.

Pressures growing out of an increasingly large and more sophisticated elderly population, coupled with the skyrocketing costs of institutional care, first forced the community-care issue into open debate. In the 1970s the media and public commissions documented scores of cases of nursing-home abuses. At state and national hearings, social and health researchers, program planners, and policy analysts stressed the economic, physical, and psychological advantages of home health care. Accompanying this renewed interest in what is in fact a service approach dating back to the nineteenth century has been a growing body of literature addressing a variety of topics in gerontological homecare. In many cases the available data reflect the underdevelopment and disagreements to be expected of a stunted service modality. Even so, we have sufficient data to describe the current status of in-home services for older people and to foresee their probable future development.

NEED

The rapid growth of the aged population, the increased incidence of chronic and disabling conditions, and the imperfect association between those conditions and service dependency make it difficult to measure the homecare needs of the elderly. A complicating factor is the difficulty of determining the number of institutionalized elderly who might be better served in their homes.

The usual approach to estimating homecare needs is in terms of the extent of functional incapacity—that is, the inability to perform one or more of the basic activities of daily living. While this method overstates the actual demand for services, it is useful in providing an upper estimate of the need for formal and informal support systems.

In 1978, almost 46 percent of the noninstitutionalized population 65 and over—approximately 10.5 million persons—reported some activity limitation due to chronic conditions. Activity limitation increased dramatically with age. It was reported by 41 percent of persons 65 to 74, by 51 percent of persons 75 to 84, and by 60 percent of persons 85 and over (U.S. National Center for Health Statistics, 1979). The number of persons with activity limitation due to chronic conditions is expected to increase by 13 to 23 percent by 1990, chiefly among older persons (U.S. Department of Health and Human Services, 1981).

The proportion of aged persons living in the community and in immediate need of homecare services has been variously estimated at 14 to 18 percent, or 3.2 to 3.9 million persons. These numbers include persons who are bedfast, homebound, or unable to carry out their major activities of daily living (Kovar, 1977; Lavor, 1979; Morris, 1974; Nagi, 1976; Shanas, 1971).

When the institutionalized aged population is considered, an additional group of candidates for homecare can be identified. Estimates of the institutionalized elderly who might be better served at home range from 10 to 50 percent (Barney, 1977; Bell, 1973; Lawton, 1978; Morris, 1974; Mossey and Tisdale, 1979; U.S. Department of Health, Education, and Welfare, 1976; Weiler, 1974). One study of 348 elderly referrals to two mental hospitals concluded that the needs of 77 percent could have been met at home (Markson et al., 1973). The U.S. Congressional Budget Office (1977b) found that intermediate-care patients were more likely to be wrongly placed (20 to 40 percent) than those in long-term facilities (10 to 20 percent). More recently, however, the U.S. Health Care Financing Administration (HCFA) (1981) concluded that estimates of inappropriate placements may have been overstated because of an emphasis on medical criteria in making such judgments. The inclusion of social and psychological criteria, according to the HCFA, would have led to significantly reduced estimates of the percentage of patients not in need of nursing-home care.

A different perspective on the need for homecare services is provided by the ratio of home helpers to the population at risk. Home helpers, or homemakers/ home health aides as they are called in the United States, are considered the core service providers in most homecare delivery systems. The National Council for Homemaker/Home Health Aide Services (recently renamed the National Homecaring Council) has placed the overall need for such personnel at over 300,000, or approximately one homemaker for every 1,000 persons under 65 and one for every 100 persons 65 and over. In 1978, approximately 82,000 homemakers were employed in the United States by 3,700 home health agencies—a ratio of one homemaker for every 2,700 persons (Somers and Moore, 1976; Winston, 1977, 1978).

Using data compiled by the International Council on Home Help, Little (1982) reports that the United States in 1976 had approximately 60,000 home helpers, or a ratio of 28.7 per 100,000 population. By contrast, Sweden, Norway, and the Netherlands had ratios of 923.0, 840.0, and 599.0 per 100,000 population.

Home health care is currently provided by about 5,000 certified and uncertified agencies, such as Visiting Nurse Associations, hospital-based programs, state and local health departments, voluntary nonprofit organizations, and proprietary (profit-making) groups. Uncertified, profit-making groups constitute 40 percent of the total (Mayer and Engler, 1982). In January 1981, 3,014 home health agencies were Medicare-certified, of which 2,908 were also certified through Medicaid (Lloyd and Greenspan, 1983; Palmer, 1983).

In measuring the extent of need, it is important to note that the elderly themselves have repeatedly made clear their desire for community and home-based solutions to long-term-care needs rather than for service plans requiring relocation to unfamiliar settings (Barron, 1974; Bell, 1973; Griffith, 1971; Oktay and Sheppard, 1978; Riley and Foner, 1968; Shanas, 1962).

ASSESSMENT

Just as the method used to determine the overall homecare-service needs of a community's elderly population vary widely, so too do the methods used to determine eligibility for participation in local homecare programs.

Little (1982) identifies three methods of assessing community homecare needs: rational, empirical, and relative. The rational method entails a professional determination of the extent to which the elderly deviate from a state of ideal well-being. The empirical method bases its estimate on the level of demand for service at a particular time; in this case, utilization levels are presumed to reflect the full extent of need. The relative method, as Little writes, "is based on a process of consensus-building in the community, and is considered politically realistic, although possibly overinfluenced by providers at the expense of consumers."

At the program level, variability in methods of determining client need and eligibility prevails. No standardized assessment procedure has yet been adopted nationally by homecare providers to determine the physical and mental status of the elderly or an appropriate level of service. Little (1982) notes that "there is an unfortunate tendency for each new project to reinvent the wheel and make up its own interview form; the resulting information is then not comparable with that gathered elsewhere by other methods." Assessments made by service providers tend to be based on medical evaluations. The social and emotional status of the client is less often considered. Furthermore, assessments by specialized homecare programs tend to be provider-oriented rather than client-oriented—that is, they are heavily influenced by the resources available at a particular agency, the interests of the dominant profession, and financial eligibility criteria rather than by the actual needs of the older person.

The absence of a uniform system of assessment employing universally accepted definitions can probably be traced to the lack of a national mandate for the development of common measures of service assessment, provision, and utilization. Nevertheless, the growth of the number of homecare programs and demonstration projects has increased the likelihood that sound multidisciplinary patient assessment and classification procedures will emerge.

The Chicago Five Hospital Homebound Elderly Program's criteria for acceptance includes consideration of medical, psychiatric, and architectural conditions that cause homeboundedness (Schreiber and Hughes, 1982). The assessment visit is always made by a social worker/nurse team who observe the client's home environment and physical condition. They also consider the strength of the existing formal and informal support network. Standardized assessment tools include medical histories, physical examinations, social histories, discussions with significant others, and application of the Older Americans Resources and Services Program (OARS) Multidimensional Functional Assessment Questionnaire. This instrument takes into account five areas of functioning: social, economic, mental, physical, and activities of daily living.

The ACCESS Program of the Monroe County Long Term Care Program in New York State considers the client's health and psychological, financial, and environmental needs and resources (Eggert et al., 1980). A unified "Pre-Admission Assessment Form" allows for a comprehensive evaluation of such needs. The assessment consultation also includes a review of home architectural barriers. The Wisconsin Community Care Organization reports use of the Geriatric Functional Rating Scale (GFRS)—a measure of the client's risk of institutionalization—in combination with a determination of Medicaid eligibility and satisfaction of residency requirements (Applebaum et al., 1980). Most comprehensive assessment instruments can serve as both eligibility screening devices and research and evaluation tools.

The Coordinated Care Management Corporation of Buffalo, New York, a nonprofit, voluntary organization established to coordinate and integrate community services for the frail elderly, has developed a comprehensive assessment device that elicits objective responses, is computer compatible, and can be administered by both professionals and paraprofessionals (Anderson, 1982). The tool comprises questions divided into sixteen sections:

1. *Identifying Data*—sex, date of birth, race, marital status, income and resources, next of kin, most recent hospitalization
2. *Administrative Data*—referral source, services requested, living arrangements, household composition
3. *Social and Health Supports*—family members, neighbors, or volunteers who provide care in the home, agencies that recently provided services
4. *Home Assessment*—quality and characteristics of the home
5. *Social/Emotional Status*—client's affect or current mood, ability to relate to others, short-term changes in mental status, mental impairment
6. *Personal Care/Activities of Daily Living and Identification of Needs*—assistance needed and source in the areas of bathing/showering, walking, wheelchair, transfer, eating, dressing, appearance, hygiene, use of toilet
7. *Personal Business and Household Chores*—extent of community-living skills such as capacity to do shopping, housework, meal preparation, laundry
8. *Services/Treatment*—need for skilled nursing, physical therapy, occupational therapy, speech therapy, nutrition, medical social work, mental health
9. *Medications*—capacity to self-administer medications and name, type, and frequency of administration
10. *Sensory Impairment*—extent of impairment of speech, sight, hearing, and skin as well as allergies and sensitivities and required aids (dentures, glasses, hearing aids)
11. *Elimination Problems*—status of bladder and bowel
12. *Diet*—nutritional restrictions and appetite problems
13. *Medical Information*—diagnosis, prognosis, nature of surgery, medical equipment required, client awareness of diagnosis
14. *Care Plan*—services recommended (scope and duration), services ordered (provider, unit cost, when ordered, when delivered), date of next assessment
15. *Problems*—social and health problems, interventions and outcomes
16. *Community and Residential Services*—services in the areas of home support, community support, health support, and residential services

This instrument aims to translate a client's functional status into service needs and to coordinate the delivery of a variety of services beyond those traditionally defined as homecare.

INTERVENTION

A system of care for the homebound elderly may encompass any or all of the following service components:

1. Homemaker, home health aide, home attendant
2. Friendly visiting, escort, telephone reassurance
3. Professional nursing; social work; nutritional, medical, dental, psychiatric, and legal services; physical, occupational, and recreational therapy; speech and language therapy

Homemaker/home-health-aide services, the core services in homecare, comprise social care, health care, personal ("hands on") care, household maintenance, and home management. Specific tasks may include: marketing; meal preparation; house cleaning; companionship; assistance with bathing, eating, dressing, and toileting; paying bills; writing letters.

Few programs provide all the homecare services outlined above. The type of funding source and organizational auspice often determines the mix of components available in a program's service package. An exception to the rule was the Triage project in Connecticut, which was able to offer a wide spectrum of home-delivered services through special Medicare reimbursement arrangements and additional reimbursements from other statutory sources (Hodgson and Quinn, 1980). Another exception was the Georgia Alternative Health Services Project, a large-scale demonstration project supported by the Health Care Financing Administration. This program, through contracts with eighteen separate agencies and with Medicaid reimbursement, provided a comprehensive package of home health and support services (Skellie and Coan, 1980).

More common are small-scale programs composed of two or three social workers or nurses and six to twelve part-time homemakers, chore workers, and home health aides. Waiting lists are usual, as are frustrated program administrators forced to perform multiple functions while juggling high demand for services and shoestring budgets. Requests for such common services as twenty-four-hour home attendants, heavy housekeeping, home repairs, transportation, and extended periods of social support or companionship often go unheeded in these programs.

The Homecare Client Pathway

The sequence of stages along the client pathway to homecare services generally includes:

1. Intake/Screening
2. Needs assessment
3. Case planning
4. Service delivery
5. Monitoring/Evaluation

Stage 1: Intake/Screening

The older person may reach the entry point to service through self-referral or referral by a relative, friend, neighbor, physician, hospital social-service department, or another social-service agency. Outreach by program staff can lead to the discovery of homebound elderly cut off from the service network. In this stage the appropriateness of the referral and an initial determination of whether the older person satisfies the program's eligibility requirements are made. Ineligible persons are referred elsewhere, while eligible persons move to the next stage along the pathway.

Stage 2: Needs Assessment

Needs assessment is most frequently performed by a social worker or nurse who visits the client in his or her home. When resources allow and program philosophy dictates, a multidisciplinary team approach is utilized so that medical, nursing, and psychosocial problems are evaluated by the appropriate disciplines. The kinds of services that may be needed and the capacity of the client's informal support system to share in homecare are considered. A decision whether or not to provide homecare marks the completion of the needs assessment stage.

Stage 3: Case Planning

This stage, which sometimes overlaps the preceding one, includes a review of case information and the development of a specific service plan that responds to the needs and preferences of the client. Failure of program staff to match specific services to client needs and expectations can have serious consequences. For example, the absence of mutual contracting among client, family, and program staff may lead to grossly inaccurate perceptions of service (Friedman and Kaye, 1979):

1. Clients may expect homecare workers to perform tasks different from those in their job descriptions.

2. Clients may expect workers to provide companionship after normal work hours.
3. Clients may harbor unrealistic standards with regard to the performance of the homecare worker.
4. Clients may expect homecare workers to be similar to themselves in race, religion, and age.
5. Families of clients may be confused about their roles in the homecare plan.

Stage 4: Service Delivery

The actual provision of homecare services begins in this stage. In addition to the skills unique to the various disciplines involved in homecare, there are certain basic skills needed by professionals and paraprofessionals alike for which specific training is desirable. These include:

1. Knowledge of the aging process and sensitivity to the impact of disability, dependency, and loss of privacy on the homecare patient
2. Appreciation of the merits of the team approach to homecare in addressing the multiple needs of the homebound
3. Observational and diagnostic capacity for identifying change in client symptomatology and needs
4. Appreciation for maintaining the integrity and viability of the client's natural helping network by means of supplementation rather than substitution
5. Ability to withstand strain and to respond flexibly to client demands
6. Skill at navigating the bureaucratic tangle of health and social entitlements and services available to the elderly in the community

Stage 5: Monitoring/Evaluation

This final stage in the service-provision process is perhaps the least articulated and respected. Necessarily embedded in the service-delivery stage, it includes periodic reviews and reassessments of the homecare service plan with a view to determining whether the plan should be continued, modified, or terminated.

Failure to monitor service can aggravate worker-client relationships already tense and angry, allow for client exploitation or for blackmail and abuse of workers, and increase the likelihood of delivery of services no longer needed by clients (Friedman et al., 1977). Professional supervision, effective case management, and in-service training of homecare personnel are necessary to maintain service quality and accountability (Cassert, 1970; Houghton and Martin, 1976;

Moore, 1977; National Council for Homemaker/Home Health Aide Services, 1974; Shinn and Robinson, 1974; Trager, 1973).

Social Work and Homecare

Historically, family social-service agencies and other social-welfare organizations had a large part in the development of homecare services. The connection between social casework and housekeeper/homemaker services was recognized by the voluntary sector as far back as the 1920s, and this relationship was made an integral part of subsequent federal policy (Kepecs, 1929; Long, 1957). Indeed, services delivered in the client's home have been a cornerstone of social work practice in America. While public health, medicine, and nursing may all rightly claim roles in the administration and delivery of certain components of home health care, the nonmedical, socially oriented character of many home-care tasks (e.g., personal care, household maintenance, home management, emotional support, social advocacy) suggests a powerful connection between this interventive system and the social services.

Some commentators advocate placement of in-home support services within the social-service sector. They believe that the personal social services constitute an emerging sixth system of public-sector services that, by definition, includes in-home support services (Kahn and Kamerman, 1980; Kamerman and Kahn, 1976). In this system they see the social-work profession as offering substantive field expertise as well as research, planning, and management capabilities. Such a conceptualization is closely akin to that currently in place in European countries—for example, the British system of home helps.

Since social or personal care has been identified as a core element of the social services, social work has been urged to solidify its identification with the caretaking of the functionally disabled (Axelrod, 1978; Morris, 1974; Morris and Anderson, 1975). Dinerman (1979) stresses the role of social workers in maintaining fragile persons in the community. The scope of social caretaking is potentially considerable when we consider that, although the aged may be the most numerous users of home health services (Abdellah, 1978), the need for this type of assistance is shared by people of all ages—children, the handicapped, the mentally ill, the terminally ill.

The practice of social casework has been most characteristic of the social-work role in homecare. The skills of individual and family assessment and appreciation of the multiple influences on behavior are especially transferable to care in the older person's home. Techniques of therapeutic support, counseling, crisis intervention, problem identification, and problem resolution, so basic to traditional social-work practice, are essential ingredients of many homecare programs. Important too is the social worker's broad theoretical perspective and respect for the collaborative team process (Oktay and Sheppard, 1978). Kirschner and Rosengarten (1982) emphasize the importance of professional expertise in the psychology of somatic illness, psychogeriatrics, ego psychology, theories of personality, and family dynamics as well as knowledge of community resources and government entitlements.

A recently established role of social workers in homecare is that of case manager or service coordinator. The effective case manager, in addition to supervisory functions, needs to assume the following responsibilities (Friedman et al., 1977):

1. Developing a mutually agreeable work plan by matching elderly clients to homecare workers when possible, and preparing clients, along with their families and the homecare worker, for the homecare plan
2. Incorporating the clients' social network into the homecare plans at a level that is both sound and acceptable to all involved
3. Providing casework services to families, as needed, which would afford them the opportunity to explore their feelings, to contribute constructively to the homecare relationship, and to remain connected with their elderly family members
4. Identifying and screening clients with special counseling or protective-service needs prior to the initiation of service, so that a greater measure of case management can be provided in response to need
5. Assessing clients' expectations and resolving conflicts in the homecare relationship
6. Linking clients to the larger social systems
7. Assisting clients and their families in making the transition between care modalities, if and when a different level of care becomes necessary

There are several reasons why social workers so infrequently administer homecare programs and rarely engage in education, program design, and evaluation.

First, homecare services are considered ancillary services of low priority. Workers (both professional and nonprofessional) occupy positions of relatively low status within the human-services field (Kaye, 1982a, 1982b). In part because some authorities consider in-home services to consist of a supportive-maintenance component only, without therapeutic, preventive, and remedial elements, there are limited career opportunities and little chance to develop positive occupational identities (Callahan et al., 1980; Caro, 1973, 1974; Friedsam, 1974; Harris and Axelrod, 1972).

Second, reimbursement formulas are primarily tied to medical and health-related homecare services. The absence of legislation ensuring that social work services in the home will be reimbursed by third parties further inhibits participation by social workers.

The Effectiveness of Homecare

The application of even elementary evaluative-research measures to service programs for the homebound elderly is of recent origin. There have been few rigorous studies of the effectiveness and efficiency of these programs (Callender and LaVor, 1975; Dunlop, 1980; Kane and Kane, 1980). Because of variable targeting techniques, comparability across programs has not been possible (Rosenfeld, 1982; Rosenthal and Holmes, 1981; Seidl et al., 1978).

Studies have generally addressed the commonly accepted homecare goals of reducing rates of institutionalization and improving the quality of life of service recipients. Other outcome variables include postprogram institutionalization rates, morbidity and mortality rates, collateral stress, levels of functional attainment, change in morale and life satisfaction, and degree of contentment (Bloom, 1975; Caro, 1981).

Blenkner et al. (1971), reporting on the now-classic findings from a controlled protective service demonstration project, cited mixed results for certain of the just cited outcome variables. Findings on preservice, ongoing, and five-year-follow-up measurements of participant functioning showed significant relief of alternate caregiver stress following provision of casework and environmental supports and improvements in the service recipients' physical surroundings. But there was no significant impact on physical or mental competence and level of contentment. The likelihood of institutionalization actually increased among the service group, which also had a higher death rate than the control group.

Breslau and Haug (1972) also reported higher institutionalization rates among service recipients compared to controls but lower mortality rates and improvement in levels of well-being and contentment.

A protective-service research and demonstration project under public-welfare auspices that relied heavily on personal care, household management, and other concrete services reported more positive findings (U.S. Community Services Administration, 1971). Operating in both rural and urban settings, the National Protective Services Project for Older Adults realized a higher percentage improvement among clients given services compared to those not receiving services. Categories of greatest improvement for both rural and urban samples were (1) suitability of living arrangements, (2) physical functioning, and (3) mental and emotional adjustment. Institutionalization and guardianship rates were low.

Nielsen et al. (1972), in examining the effects of an organized program of home-aide service on elderly patients discharged from a geriatric rehabilitation hospital, considered survival, contentment, and institutionalization as their major dependent variables. The independent variable, home-aide service, consisted of personal care, housekeeping, shopping, and escort services. Findings indicated no significant difference in survival rates between the experimental and the control groups, but favorable differences in levels of contentment, morbidity, and institutionalization.

More recent research has reported generally positive findings on the potential effectiveness of homecare services, suggesting that interventive strategies have achieved higher levels of sophistication. Homecare services are increasingly seen as effective in reducing institutionalization (Barney, 1977; Brickner et al., 1976; Noelker and Harel, 1978; U.S. General Accounting Office, 1979) and compare well with such alternative services as care in nursing homes and intermediate-care facilities (Mitchell, 1977; Smyer, 1977; Smyer et al., 1978). Consumer satisfaction with homecare services also appears adequate (Fashimpar and Grinnell, 1978; Jette et al., 1981; Weissert et al., 1979), although the capacity of beneficiaries to make objective judgments is questionable (Kaye, 1982a, 1982b).

Findings from a time-limited project addressing the impact of functionally impaired older persons on other family members as well as the effects of supplementary services on older persons and their natural supports demonstrate that formal and informal supports can together maintain the elderly in the community (Gross-Andrew and Zimmer, 1978). Short-term effects included the reduction of emotional, physical, social, and financial stress felt by family members actively involved in caring for older relatives (U.S. Health Care Financing Administration, 1981). More research is needed in this area, especially research that considers the consequences of caregiver stress felt by homecare agency staff as well as family members (Kaye, 1983).

Weissert et al. (1979) reported the results of a randomized experiment assessing the effects and costs of day-care and homemaker services on a Medicare-eligible, chronically ill population. Services included home management, personal care, supportive activities, and health-care management. Compared to the control group, the experimental group had significantly more favorable outcomes on measures of contentment, mental functioning, social activity, and mortality. However, it also displayed somewhat greater use of hospital care.

A number of authors caution against premature conclusions concerning the savings potential of homecare services due to lack of rigor, comparability, and comprehensiveness of available research (Doherty et al., 1978; Kane and Kane, 1980; Seidl et al., 1977). Seidl et al. (1977) present a framework for determining comparative costs based on five essential considerations: (1) how the target population for the service is defined; (2) how homecare clients are identified; (3) the structure of case management; (4) the relative efficiency and quality of available services; and (5) the determination of who is to bear the costs. They concluded that increased savings would be realized if less severely disabled clients are serviced; if social service rather than medical professionals provide the initial assessments and the ongoing reassessments of need; if "preventive" interventions are not stressed; if centralized case management is employed; and if fewer hours of training are provided to service personnel. Clearly, such cost-saving measures would result in diminished quality and accessibility of services.

Doherty et al. (1978) and Caro and Frankfather (1981) point out that average costs alone are not satisfactory bases for efficiency comparisons. Internal program costs that reflect the efficiency of different aspects of administrative and service activity are essential as well. Secondary (additional health-related costs) and tertiary (nonhealth-related living expenditures) costs need to be accurately assessed in addition to institutional and homecare costs. A person's level of disability or impairment is believed to be the determining per diem cost factor (Greenberg, 1974; Pollack, 1974).

The recent rise in the popularity of homecare is due in part to the belief that it is cheaper than nursing-home care. At low levels of client impairment, homecare is apparently a more efficient and less costly delivery design. Beyond a certain point, however, higher levels of impairment can be more efficiently if not more effectively addressed in institutions. Total population costs might well increase were homecare services to be significantly expanded, since a new population would be served (U.S. Health Care Financing Administration, 1981; Weissert et al., 1979).

THEORY

Homecare programs have emerged through trial and error without the benefit of preconceived conceptual frameworks. As a result, current delivery models incorporate a "mixed bag" of philosophies, values, technologies, and skills. No two programs seem to render the same set of services in the same way. Future homecare systems may benefit from greater recognition of the inter-dependence of homecare and other gerontological services as well as appreciation of the complex relationship between formal and informal networks.

The interactive association in homecare among the service provider, the elderly client, and his or her primary support network may be usefully viewed in the light of exchange theory, according to which interactions among individuals or aggregates is characterized by desire to maximize rewards and minimize costs (Emerson, 1972; Knipe, 1971).

In the homecare relationship, the reward for the elderly client is the receipt of a particular set of services. These services are most likely to be instrumental, since they are delivered by a formal organization (Litwak and Figueira, 1968; Litwak and Meyer, 1966). However, the client also demands affective services, especially if he or she lacks an informal support network of friends, relatives, and neighbors. Service packages must include components that respond to both instrumental and affective needs. For the service provider, the reward may be more affective (e.g., personal satisfaction, client friendship) than instrumental (e.g., salary, fringe benefits, promotion opportunities) since the economic rewards in the homecare field are so limited. Simply put, the homecare worker may enter the field for personal/expressive reasons more often than for remuneration.

For the elderly recipient of homecare services, the cost is sometimes economic but more often is measured in sociopsychological terms. Free homecare service may cause the elderly client to feel pressed to (1) accept whatever service package is offered, (2) accept the particular worker assigned to deliver the service regardless of match, and (3) acquiesce in the loss of privacy at times convenient to the provider rather than the recipient. But the homecare worker also experiences costs. However inadequate salaries and benefits may be, these "rewards" are still needed. As a result, the worker may not be able to afford to give up the job and consequently may have to suffer the costs of poor working conditions in the client's home, abusive or critical clients, and the stigma of low status assigned by other human-services professionals. High turnover rates among homecare workers and their supervisors suggest that these costs will be borne only so long.

The exchange theorist maintains that individuals will remain in an exchange relation only so long as rewards outweigh costs. When one participant is more dependent on the relationship than the other, that dependence is manifested by compliance to the greater power of the other. In the current service environment, where there is a scarcity of homecare programs, the homebound aged person is more often the dependent party. This dependency, in fact, characterizes all exchanges between older people and societal institutions (Dowd, 1975, 1980). Their decreasing power is due both to their loss of instrumentally valued skills and goods and to the devaluation of those resources that they retain.

Designers of homecare programs, trainers, and workers could benefit from viewing the service from this social-exchange perspective. It would better attune them to the socioemotional and economic complexities of the homecare relationship. It would also serve to explicate those contributions that natural supports can make better than formal agency programs to the overall plan of care. Finally, it would serve to better prepare the homecare worker for the expansion of role behaviors required when serving those older people who are without viable support networks. A proper balancing of instrumental and affective functions would enhance the likelihood that the delicate "host-guest" relationship in homecare is respected. In turn, the client's capacity to cope with his or her entire life space—both the internal microenvironment and the external macro-environment—would be encouraged as homecare takes on an environment-restorative function (Monk, 1978).

POLICY

Public homecare policy in the United States lacks comprehensiveness, coherency, and consistency. (An undetermined amount of homecare is financed through private and commercial insurance companies and charitable organizations or paid for directly by clients.) Funding at all levels of government is uncoordinated and restrictive or else underutilized. In general, national health policy has emphasized long-term institutional care and short-term hospital and community care despite the fact that the in-home needs of the functionally impaired elderly population are increasingly viewed in the context of long-term chronic disability (Brody, 1979; Jivoff, 1977; Morris, 1977; State Communities Aid Association, 1977; U.S. National Clearinghouse on Aging, 1977; Weiler, 1974).

Morris (1977) maintains that the current complex structure is the result of professional practices and cultural values. Since the medical model has served as the basis for most national policy, legislation has been biased toward health-intensive services (institutional care, acute hospital care, and time-limited, medically related community care). Similarly the social-work profession, when it has succeeded in impacting on policy formulation, has tended to stress the primacy of the income or interpersonal needs of the elderly as opposed to basic home-maintenance requirements. Thus both health and, to a lesser degree, social-service professionals have understated the need to develop comprehensive in-home service policy.

There are at least five major federal programs with mandates for financing gerontological homecare services. Medically oriented homecare is funded through Titles XVIII and XIX of the Social Security Act. Social and personal care service grant programs are more directly promoted under Title XX of the Social Security Act and Title III of the Older Americans Act. The Veterans Administration program incorporates both medical and social emphases. These reimbursement sources vary considerably in types and coverage, funding, service duration, service eligibility, target group, and utilization provisions.

Title XVIII of the Social Security Act (Medicare)

Coverage of home health care is authorized by sections 1812, 1832, and 1835 of Title XVIII of the Social Security Act. Eligibility criteria stress the need for intermittent skilled-nursing or therapy services rather than nonhealth-related care. Until 1 July 1981, Medicare home-health visits were limited to 100 in a benefit period, and eligibility under Part A (Hospital Insurance) required three days of prior hospitalization. The Omnibus Reconciliation Act of 1980 (P.L. 96-499) removed these limitations and added occupational therapy to skilled-nursing care and physical or speech therapy as qualifying for benefits. The act also, however, eliminated the application of the Supplementary Medical Insurance (Part B) deductible to home-health-aide services under this section of the program and retained physician certification and the need to be confined to one's home. Coverage is not available to individuals who are in need solely of medical social services, custodial care, or assistance in carrying out the activities of daily living. Reimbursement of in-home support services is limited to personal care provided by a home health aide. Homemaker services are not covered. A health-intensive acute-care orientation appears to have been largely retained even in the face of the recent liberalization of provisions. In 1977, 96 percent of those served received nursing care, 32.5 percent received home-health-aide services, and 20 percent received physical therapy (Palley and Oktay, 1981).

Funding for Medicare home health services is open-ended but highly underutilized. In 1979, payments amounted to slightly more than 1.8 percent of total Medicare payments. Approximately 92 percent was expended for persons 65 and over (U.S. Health Care Financing Administration, 1980). Reimbursable homecare personnel must be employed by federally certified home health agencies. The primary intent in establishing coverage seems to have been to help eligible persons meet the costs of health-care services rather than to optimize consumer independence or to avoid unnecessary institutionalization.

At the local level, Medicare reimburses certified agencies delivering home health services in the same way as hospitals. Insurance companies and other fiscal intermediaries assist in administering the Medicare program, judging the appropriateness of claims, and reimbursing all reasonable costs. Disagreement is common between fiscal intermediaries and certified agencies in the interpretation of Medicare regulations and instructions.

Title XIX of the Social Security Act (Medicaid)

Title XIX of the Social Security Act authorizes reimbursement for nursing, home-health-aide, and personal-care services in the home. Like Medicare, such personnel must be employed by a certified home health agency and adhere to federally approved standards. Services are part-time and intermittent. Eligibility criteria include low income, nursing supervision, and physician's authorization for service. However, a person does not require prior hospitalization nor are the number of covered visits limited by federal law (although states may and do impose their own limitations). In 1980 only nine state Medicaid plans provided reimbursement for in-home personal care (Callahan et al., 1980).

Title XIX homecare regulations do not demand that recipients be in need of professional nursing or therapy to qualify for personal care, although many states continue to impose this limitation to coverage. Furthermore, existing regulations, while allowing for assistance with household maintenance and activities of daily living, are seldom tapped by the individual states. An acute-care, medical orientation prevails in practice if not in statutory design.

Medicaid homecare expenditures are not subject to a dollar ceiling yet remain severely restricted, especially for the elderly population. In fiscal year 1979, total reimbursements for home-health-agency services amounted to about 1.3 percent of the total reimbursed for all services; only 0.08 percent benefited persons 65 and over (U.S. Health Care Financing Administration, 1980).

424 L. W. Kaye

Medicaid reimbursement procedures for local services vary considerably by state. In general, they are based on schedules of maximum allowances established at the state level. As a rule, Title XIX provides for 50-50 federal/state matching, though this too may change depending on regional differences in per capita income. Homecare providers have been highly critical of Medicaid allowances as poorly matched to actual costs of service delivery.

Title XX of the Social Security Act

Title XX, the social services amendment to the Social Security Act, authorizes a wide array of home-based services. At least one of the following services must be provided by each state, although the actual configuration and scope are left to the state's discretion: homemakers, chore, home health aide, home management, personal care, consumer education, and counseling. Some home-based services provided by states under this Title seek to provide all categories of individuals with opportunities to remain in their homes and avoid inappropriate institutionalization. Others choose to limit eligibility to income-maintenance recipients. Training guidelines and provider standards are determined by individual states, and reimbursable in-home personnel may include agency providers, relatives, neighbors, and friends.

Title XX stresses homemaker service and thus tends not to be overly medically oriented. Services address chronic as well as acute needs. There is a ceiling on the funds available, and federal funding levels are determined by a state's proportion of the nation's population rather than the prevalence or severity of functional incapacity. State utilization of the homecare provisions in Title XX is considerably higher than for Medicare and Medicaid legislation, but expenditure levels can vary considerably from state to state. Approximately 15 percent of allocated funds is used to provide home-based services (Callahan et al., 1980).

Title XX mandates a 75-25 federal/state matching formula. Local reimbursement methods are quite variable. As Trager (1980) reports, these methods include purchasing on a contract basis, including competitive bidding models (California), purchasing through negotiated rates, and even contracting with individuals for services. A single community may utilize several reimbursement methods at one time.

Title III of the Older Americans Act

Since 1965, Title III of the Older Americans Act has been extended, revised, and expanded through a series of amendments. It currently authorizes closed-ended formula grants to individual states and designated areas therein. Comprehensive and coordinated services seek to enable persons 60 and over to remain in their homes as long as possible. Priority is placed on the needs of the low-income, isolated, and minority aged.

The Comprehensive Older Americans Act Amendments of 1978 (P.L. 95-478) mandated that priority be placed on the provision of in-home, legal, and access services, for which area agencies are required to spend 50 percent of their Title III allocations. In-home services include homemaker, home health aide, chore, friendly visiting, and telephone reassurance. On the other hand, access services include transportation, outreach, and information and referral. Home-delivered meals are included in a separate section of the title. While the Older Americans Act program operates under extremely limited funding, homecare expenditures are considerable and growing. Local contractors are awarded start-up grants through their Area Agency on Aging on an annual basis with no guarantees of renewed funding. Services tend to be oriented toward those provided by Title XX homemakers and are similar to tasks normally performed by primary-group members. Coverage is time-limited, the nature of standards and training is determined locally, and service programs tend to be locally situated as well as substantially underfinanced. The Administration on Aging, the federal agency with administrative authority for the Older Americans Act, provides up to 75 percent of local program costs.

The Veterans Administration

The Veterans Administration (VA) is one of the few sources of funding that directly supports the involvement of the older person's natural supports (e.g., kin) in providing homecare. "Aid and attendance" cash allowances are earmarked for family members able to provide relatively nonspecialized in-home services for their aged family members. The VA also operates a hospital-based home-health-care program whose services become available following discharge from an acute-care hospital. The professional delivery team is composed of a physician, nurse, rehabilitation therapist, dietician, and social worker. Eligibility criteria stress the medical model, including the requirements of prior hospitalization, physician certification, and the availability of an informal caregiver (Mitchell, 1978; Scanlon et al., 1979).

Expenditures are limited for both segments of the VA homecare program. In 1975, 98 percent of total expenditures was allocated for the Aid-and-Attendance Program (U.S. Congressional Budget Office, 1977a).

Future Directions

Recent analyses of the adequacy and equity of the various national programs of homecare for the elderly indicate that in-home services remain highly inadequate (Palley and Oktay, 1981.) At the service level, workers, too, voice frustration with the limited range of services they have been authorized to provide (Kaye, 1982a, 1982b). In particular, service workers have found that client needs and expectations almost always exceed agency capacity.

Proposed legislative, financial, and organizational solutions include: front-end investments; capitation prepayments; modification or merger of current funding mechanisms; family-care incentives; and homecare tax subsidies, premiums, or voucher advances (Callahan et al., 1980; Caro, 1972; Moore, 1977; Morris, 1974; Morris and Pendleton, 1976; Packwood, 1981; Shinn and Robinson, 1974.)

Innovative programs include the New York State Long Term Home Health Care Program, commonly referred to as Nursing Home Without Walls, established in 1978. It mandates the provision of comprehensive home health care to those patients who have been determined to need either skilled nursing or health-related facility placement. Total expenditures for patient care in the home may not, however, exceed 75 percent of the average reimbursement for maintaining that same person at a corresponding level of care in an institution. Fourteen Nursing Homes Without Walls programs were operating in 1982 with an additional seven approved (New York State Council on Home Care Services, 1982).

Another recent approach to improving the balance in utilization between community-based and institutional care in New York State is that of Community Alternative Systems Agencies (CASA). This statewide system of coordinating agencies seeks specifically to assist the frail elderly and the physically disabled to avoid inappropriate institutionalization and to make better use of community alternatives. These objectives are to be realized through the establishment of a system of service coordination, gatekeeping, and community systems-development activities.

The National Long Term Care Channeling Demonstration Program, with administrative authority residing in state units of the Administration on Aging, is currently testing the financial and programmatic effectiveness of centralized assessment procedures and individualized case management for persons requiring a variety of long-term-care services, including in-home care.

These initiatives look to resolve one or more problems inherent in the current system by promoting comprehensive systems of care and streamlining mechanisms of payment. The problems have been summarized by Trager (1980):

Home health services have been reimbursed or funded from multiple sources with complex and differing requirements that impede coordination.

Intent with respect to target populations is confusing and contradictory.

Definitions of the services vary widely and are frequently illogical and inappropriate.

Minimal attention has been directed to capacity building with the result that the services are inadequate, inaccessible, or absent.

Regulations differ with respect to the range of services, the duration of services, eligibility of the target populations, and the circumstances, both financial and physical, that govern and control access.

Federal/state/local matching requirements differ, as do reimbursement methods and service procedures.

Standards that regulate quality assurance and accountability are inconsistent across public programs and are generally inadequate.

Unfortunately, the adoption of solutions comes far more gradually than clear statements of the problem. A series of uncertainties face the future of homecare for the elderly and disabled.

First, there continue to be no valid guidelines as to the potential need for and utilization of homecare at present or in the future. Homecare utilization data are either totally unavailable or incomparable across funding sources. Furthermore, the impact that new homecare alternatives would have on aggregate demand is unclear, although current data certainly reflect a strong mismatch between supply and demand.

Second, projections of homecare costs for both statutory sources and the user population should be accepted with the greatest caution. We do not have a clear understanding of the comparative costs and potential savings of different forms of home versus institutional care.

Finally, feasibility of new initiatives is likely to be strongly influenced by factors such as the vested interests of professional organizations and other groups as well as traditionally uncoordinated federal funding streams. The permanence of an austere budgetary climate in Washington may well be the determining factor that will ultimately shape future homecare policy for the aged and disabled.

In the final analysis, policymakers should not be misled by the movement afoot suggesting that traditional family supports have the capacity and desire to fulfill the full range of needs of the functionally impaired aged living in the community. Without minimizing the critical contributions of informal supports in community care for the aged, the limits of their beneficence must be recognized. This is particularly true when service demands take on a quality of permanence due to chronic or prolonged impairments of the older person. Moreover, family supports are simply nonexistent for a large segment of the aged population. Cost savings and the severity of functional need alone should not serve as ultimate justifications for expanding organized homecare for the aged. Rather, responding to the personal preferences of older people and arriving at a more equitable sharing of community homecare responsibilities between government and family is essential.

REFERENCES

Abdellah, F. G. (1978). Long-term care policy issues: Alternatives to institutional care. *Annals of the American Academy of Political and Social Science,* **438**, 28-39.

Anderson, E. 1982, November. *Standardization of the Assessment Process in a Decentralized Service Delivery System.* Paper presented at the 35th Annual Scientific Meeting of the Gerontological Society of America, Boston, Mass.

Applebaum, R., Seidl, F. W., and Austin, C. D. (1980). The Wisconsin community care organization: Preliminary findings from the Milwaukee experiment. *Gerontologist*, **20**(3), 350-355.

Axelrod, T. B. (1978). Innovative roles for social workers in home-care programs. *Health and Social Work*, **3**(3), 48-66.

Barney, J. L. (1977). The prerogative of choice in long-term care. *Gerontologist*, **17**(4), 309-314.

Barron, J. (1974). Home is the place—Health care for the aged. In *Community health services in the health care delivery system*. New York: Department of Home Health Agencies and Community Health Services, National League for Nursing.

Bell, W. G. (1973). Community care for the elderly: An alternative to institutionalization. *Gerontologist*, **13**(3), 349-354.

Blenkner, M., Bloom, M., and Nielsen, M. (1971). A research and demonstration project of protective services. *Social Casework*, **52**(8), 483-499.

Bloom, M. (1975). Evaluation instruments: Tests and measurements in long term care. In S. Sherwood (Ed.), *Long-term care: A handbook for researchers, planners, and providers*. New York: Spectrum Publications.

Breslau, N., and Haug, M. R. (1972). The elderly aid the elderly: The senior friends program. *Social Security Bulletin*, **35**(11), 9-15.

Brickner, P. W., Janeski, J. F., Rich, G., Duque, T., Starita, L., LaRocco, R., Flannery, T., and Werlin, S. (1976). Home maintenance for the home-bound aged: A pilot program in New York City. *Gerontologist*, **16**(1), 25-29.

Brody, E. M. (1979). Long-term care of the aged: Promises and prospects. *Health and Social Work*, **4**(1), 29-59.

Callahan, J. J., Jr., Diamond, L. D., Giele, J. Z., and Morris, R., (1980). Responsibility of families for their severely disabled elders. *Health Care Financing Review*, **1**(3), 29-48.

Callender, M., and LaVor, J. (1975). *Home health care: Development problems and potential*. Washington, D.C.: U.S. Department of Health, Education, and Welfare, Office of Social Services and Human Development, (mimeographed).

Caro, F. G. (1972). *Organizing and financing personal care services: An alternative to institutionalization for the disabled*. Waltham, Mass.: Levinson Gerontological Policy Institute, Brandeis University.

Caro, F. G. (1973). *The personal care organization: An approach to the maintenance of the disabled in the community*. Waltham, Mass.: Levinson Gerontological Policy Institute, Brandeis University.

Caro, F. G. (1974). Professional roles in the maintenance of the disabled elderly in the community: A forecast. *Gerontologist*, **14**(4), 286-289.

Caro, F. G. (1981). Objectives, standards, and evaluation in long-term care. *Home Health Care Services Quarterly*, **2**(1), 5-26.

Caro, F. G., and Frankfather, D. (1981), November. *Aggregate costs of home care: Regulating demand and costs of production*. Paper presented at the 34th Annual Scientific Meeting of the Gerontological Society of America and the 10th Annual Scientific and Educational Meeting of the Canadian Association on Gerontology/Association canadienne de gerontologie, Toronto.

Cassert, H. P. (1970). Homemaker service as a component of casework. *Social Casework*, **51**(9), 533-543.

Dineman, M. (1979). In sickness and in health: Future social work roles. *Health and Social Work*, **4**(2), 5-23.

Doherty, N., Segal, J., and Hicks, B., (1978). Alternatives to institutionalization for the aged: Viability and cost effectiveness. *Aged Care Services Review*, **1**(1), 1-16.

Dowd, J. J. (1975). Aging as exchange: A preface to theory. *Journal of Gerontology*, **30**(5), 584-594.

Dowd, J. J. (1980). Exchange rates and old people. *Journal of Gerontology*, **35**(4), 596-602.

Dunlop, B. D. (1980). Expanded home-based care for the impaired elderly: Solution or pipe dream? *American Journal of Public Health*, **70**(5), 514-519.

Eggert, G. M., Bowlyow, J. E., and Nichols, C. W. (1980). Gaining control of the long term care system: First returns from the ACCESS experiment. *Gerontologist*, **20**(3), 356-363.

Emerson, R. M. (1972). Exchange theory, parts 1 and 2. In J. Berger, M. Zelditch, Jr., and B. Anderson (Eds.), *Sociological theories in progress,* vol. 2. Boston: Houghton Mifflin.

Fashimpar, G. A., and Grinnell, R. M., Jr., (1978).The effectiveness of homemaker-home health aides. *Health and Social Work,* **3**(1), 147-165.

Friedman, S. R., and Kaye, L. W. (1979). Homecare for the frail elderly: Implications for an interactional relationship. *Journal of Gerontological Social Work,* **2**(2), 109-123.

Friedman, S. R., Kaye, L. W., and Farago, S. (1972, November). *Maximizing the quality of home care services for the elderly.* Paper presented at the 30th Annual Scientific Meeting of the Gerontological Society of America, San Francisco.

Friedsam, H. J. (1974). Some issues in manpower for parallel services. *Gerontologist,* **14**(1), 19-26.

Greenberg, J. (1974). The costs of in-home services, part II. In N. Anderson and the Governor's Citizens Council on Aging, *A planning study of services to non-institutionalized older persons in Minnesota.* Minneapolis: School of Public Affairs, University of Minnesota.

Griffith, E. (1971). Home health agencies today. In *Home health agency concerns.* New York: Department of Home Health Agencies and Community Health Services, National League for Nursing.

Gross-Andrew, S., and Zimmer, A. H. (1978). Incentives to families caring for disabled elderly: Research and demonstration project to strengthen the natural supports system. *Journal of Gerontological Social Work,* **1**(2), 119-133.

Harris, S., and Axelrod, S. (1972). Allied health personnel: Some problems. *Gerontologist,* **12**(3), 289-293.

Hodgson, J. H., Jr., and Quinn, J. L. (1980). The impact of the triage health care delivery system upon client morale, independent living and the cost of care. *Gerontologist,* **20**(3), 364-371.

Houghton, L., and Martin, A. E. (1976). Home vs. hospital: A hospital-based home care program. *Health and Social Work,* **1**(4), 89-103.

Jette, A. M., Branch, L. G., Wentzel, R. A., Carney, W. R., Dennis, D. L., and Heist, M. M. (1981). Home care service diversification: A pilot investigation. *Gerontologist,* **21**(6), 572-579.

Jivoff, L. 1977, December. *The long term care system in New York: An appraisal.* Paper prepared for the Institute on Continuity of Long-Term Care, Arden House, Harriman, N.Y.

Kahn, A. J., and Kamerman, S. B., (1980). *Social services in international perspective: The emergence of the sixth system,* New Brunswick, N.J.: Transaction Books.

Kamerman, S. B., and Kahn, A. J. (1976). *Social services in the United States: Policies and programs.* Philadelphia: Temple University Press.

Kane, R. L., and Kane, R. A., (1980). Alternatives to institutional care of the elderly: Beyond the dichotomy, *Gerontologist,* **20**(3), 249-259.

Kaye, L. W. (1982a, November). *The adequacy of the Older Americans Act home care mandate: Provider experience.* Paper presented at the 35th Annual Scientific Meeting of the Gerontological Society of America, Boston, Mass.

Kaye, L. W. (1982b, May). *Home care services for older people: An organizational analysis of provider experience.* Final report on AOA Grant No. (OHDS) 90-AT-0044/01.

Kaye, L. W. (1983, May). *The influence of family and friends on agency-delivered homecare services for the aged: A fragile partnership.* Paper presented at the 3rd Annual Meeting of the Northeastern Gerontological Society, Newport, R.I.

Kepecs, J. (1929). More about housekeeping services. *Child Welfare League of America Bulletin,* **8**, 115.

Kirschner, C., and Rosengarten, L. (1982). The skilled social work role in home care. *Social Work,* **27**(6), 527-530.

Knipe, E. E. (1971). *Attraction and exchange: Some temporal considerations.* Paper presented at the Annual Meeting of the Southern Sociological Society, Atlanta.

Kovar, M. G. (1977). Health of the elderly and use of health services. *Public Health Reports,* **92**(1), 9-19.

LaVor, J. (1979). Long term care and home health care: A challenge to service systems. *Home Health Care Services Quarterly,* **1**(1), 19-74.

Lawton, M. P. (1978). Institutions and alternatives for older people. *Health and Social Work,* **3**(2), 108-134.

Little, V. C. (1982). *Open care for the aging: Comparative international approaches.* New York: Springer Publishing.

Litwak, E., and Figueira, J., (1968). Technical innovation and theoretical functions of primary groups and bureaucratic structures. *American Journal of Sociology,* **73**(4), 468-481.

Litwak, E., and Meyer, H. J., (1966). A balance theory of coordination between bureaucratic organizations and community primary groups. *Administrative Science Quarterly,* **11**(1), 31-58.

Lloyd, S., and Greenspan, N.T. (1983). Nursing homes, home health services, and adult day care. In R. J. Vogel and M. C. Palmer (Eds.), *Long-term care: perspectives from research and demonstrations.* Washington, D.C.: Government Printing Office.

Long, E. (1957). *Homemaker Service in Public Assistance.* Washington, D.C.: Government Printing Office.

Markson, E. W., Levitz, G. S., and Gognalons-Caillard, M., (1973). The elderly and the community: Reidentifying unmet needs. *Journal of Gerontology,* **28**(4), 503-509.

Mayer, M. J., and Engler, M., Demographic change and the elderly population: Its implications for long term care, *Pride Institute Journal of Long Term Home Health Care,* **1**(1), 21-28.

Mitchell, J. B. (1977). *Alternatives in extended medical care: A comparative study of post-acute treatment programs in the Veterans Administration.* Unpublished doctoral dissertation, The Florence Heller School for Advanced Studies in Social Welfare, Brandeis University.

Mitchell, J. B. (1978). Patient outcomes in alternative long-term care settings. *Medical Care,* **16**(6), 439-452.

Monk, A. (1978). Home support services and the ecology of aging. *Journal of Sociology and Social Welfare,* **5**(6), 765-772.

Moore, F. M. (1977). New issues for in-home services. *Public Welfare,* **35**(2), 26-37.

Morris, R. (1974). The development of parallel services for the elderly and disabled: Some financial dimensions. *Gerontologist,* **14**(1), 14-19.

Morris, R. (1977). *Approaches to long-term chronic illness: Dilemmas and opportunities.* Paper prepared for the Institute on Continuity of Long-Term Care, Arden House, Harriman, N.Y., December.

Morris, R., and Anderson, D., (1975). Personal care services: An identity for social work. *Social Service Review,* **49**(2), 157-174.

Morris, R., and Pendleton, S. (1975). *A Local approach to public home care insurance.* Waltham, Mass.: Levinson Gerontological Policy Institute, Brandeis University.

Mossey, J., and Tisdale, W. (1979, November). *Measurement and development of functional health indicators among the institutionalized aged.* Paper presented at the 32nd Annual Scientific Meeting of the Gerontological Society of America, Washington.

Nagi, S. Z. (1976). An epidemiology of disability among adults in the United States. *Millbank Memorial Fund Quarterly,* **54**(4), 439-467.

National Council for Homemaker/Home Health Aide Services. (1974). *Widening Horizons: The teaching aspect of homemaker services.* New York: National Council for Homemaker/Home Health Aide Services.

New York State Council on Home Care Services. (1982). *Annual Report to the governor and legislature, April 1981-April 1982.* New York: New York State Council on Home Care Services.

Nielsen, M., Blenkner, M., Bloom, M., Downs, T., and Beggs, H. (1972). Older persons after hospitalization: A controlled study of home aide service. *American Journal of Public Health,* **62**(8), 1094-1101.

Noelker, L., and Harel, Z. (1978). Aged excluded from home health care: An interorganizational solution. *Gerontologist,* **18**(1), 37-41.

Oktay, J. S., and Sheppard, F. (1978). Home health care for the elderly. *Health and Social Work,* **3**(3), 35-47.

Packwood, B. (1981). Long-term care: Public and private sector policy options. *Journal of the Institute for Socioeconomic Studies,* **6**(3), 13-26.

Palley, H. A., and Oktay, J. S. (1981, November). *In-home health and social programs: Adequacy and equity of U.S. policy.* Paper presented at the 34th Annual Scientific Meeting of the Gerontological Society of America and the 10th Annual Scientific and Educational Meeting of the Canadian Association on Gerontology/Association canadienne de gerontologie, Toronto.

Palmer, M. C. (1983). Home care. In R. J. Vogel and M. C. Palmer (Eds.), *Long-term care: Perspectives from research and demonstrations.* Washington. D.C.: Government Printing Office.

Pollack, W. (1974). *Modeling the costs of federal long term care programs.* Washington. D.C.: The Urban Institute.

Riley, M. W., and Foner, A. (1968). *Aging and Society,* vol. 1. *An inventory of research findings.* New York: Russell Sage Foundation.

Rosenfeld, A. S. (1982, April). *Home health services and long term care: A two state comparison.* Paper presented at the University Health Policy Consortium, Brandeis University, Waltham, Mass.

Rosenthal, M., and Holmes, M. (1981, November). *A synthesis of findings based on AoA model projects serving the homebound elderly.* Paper presented at the 34th Annual Scientific Meeting of the Gerontological Society of America and the 10th Annual Scientific and Educational Meeting of the Canadian Association on Gerontology/Association canadienne de gerontologie, Toronto.

Scanlon, W., Difederico, E., and Stassen, M. (1979). *Long term care: Current experience and a framework for analysis.* Washington, D.C.: The Urban Institute.

Schreiber, M. S., and Hughes, S. (1982). The Chicago five hospital homebound elderly program: A long term home care model. *Pride Institute Journal of Long Term Home Health Care,* **1**(1), 12-20.

Seidl, F. W., Austin, C. D., and Greene, D. R. (1977). Is home health care less expensive? *Health and Social Work,* **2**(2), 5-19.

Seidl, F. W., Mahoney, K. D., and Austin, C. D. (1978, November). *Providing and evaluating home care: Issues of targeting.* Paper presented at the 31st Annual Scientific Meeting of the Gerontological Society of America, Dallas.

Shanas, E. (1962). *The health of older people: A social survey.* Cambridge: Harvard University Press.

Shanas, E. (1971). Measuring the home health needs of the aged in five countries. *Journal of Gerontology,* **26**(1), 37-40.

Shinn, E., and Robinson, N. D. (1974). Trends: In homemaker-home health aide services, *Abstracts for Social Workers,* **10**(3), 3-8.

Skellie, F. A., and Coan, R. E. (1980). Community-based long-term care and mortality: Preliminary findings of Georgia's alternative health services project. *Gerontologist,* **20**(3), 372-379.

Smyer, M. A. (1977, November). *Differential effects of services for impaired elderly.* Paper presented at the 30th Annual Scientific Meeting of the Gerontological Society of America, San Francisco.

Smyer, M. A., Sorell, G., and Gimmel, M. (1978, November). *Improvement and decline among impaired elderly.* Paper presented at the 31st Annual Scientific Meeting of the Gerontological Society of America, Dallas.

Somers, A. R., and Moore, F. M. (1976). Homemaker services—Essential option for the elderly. *Public Health Reports,* **91**(4), 354-359.

State Communities Aid Association, New York. (1977, December). *Report of Arden House Institute on Continuity of Long-Term Care.* Harriman, N.Y.

Trager, B. (1973). *Homemaker/home health aide services in the United States.* Washington, D.C.: Government Printing Office.

Trager, B. (1980). Home health care and national health policy. *Home Health Care Services Quarterly,* **1**(2), 1-103.

U.S. Community Services Administration. *Report of the national protective services project for older adults.* Washington, D.C.: Government Printing Office.

U.S. Congressional Budget Office. (1977a). *Long term care: actuarial cost estimates.* Washington, D.C.: Government Printing Office.

U.S. Congressional Budget Office. (1977b). *Long term care for the elderly and disabled.* Washington, D.C.: Government Printing Office.

U.S. Department of Health, Education, and Welfare. (1976). *Home health care: Report of the regional public hearings.* Washington, D.C.: Government Printing Office.

U.S. Department of Health and Human Services, Office of Planning and Evaluation/Health. (1981). *Working papers on long term care.* Washington, D.C.: Government Printing Office.

U.S. General Accounting Office. (1979). *Entering a nursing home: Costly implications for medicaid and the elderly.* Washington, D.C.: Government Printing Office.

U.S. Health Care Financing Administration. (1980). *Medicare: Use of home health services, 1979.* Washington, D.C.: Government Printing Office.

U.S. Health Care Financing Administration. (1981). *Long term care: Background and future directions.* Washington, D.C.: Government Printing Office.

U.S. National Center for Health Statistics. (1979). *Current estimates from the health interview survey, United States, 1978.* Washington, D.C.: Government Printing Office.

U.S. National Clearinghouse on Aging. (1977). *Homemaker-home health aide services.* Washington, D.C.: Government Printing Office.

Weiler, P. G. (1974). Cost-effective analysis: A quandary for geriatric health care systems. *Gerontologist,* **14**(5), 414-417.

Weissert, W. G., Wan, T. T. H., Livieratos, B. B. (1979). *Effects and costs of day care and homemaker services for the chronically ill: A randomized experiment.* Hyattsville, Md.: National Center for Health Services Research.

Winston, E. (1977). Rx for independent living. *Perspectives on Aging,* **6**(1), 12-14.

Winston, E. (1978, April 17). *Shaping in-home care for the eighties.* Paper presented at the Annual Meeting of the National Council on the Aging, St. Louis, Mo.

PART VI

LONG-TERM CARE AND INSTITUTION-BASED SERVICES

19

Long-Term-Care Institutions

Ann Burack-Weiss, M.S.S.W.

Columbia University

Long-term care for the aged has historically referred to the site of service delivery for the chronically impaired who require ongoing medical, rehabilitative, and maintenance care: the institution — sometimes identified as the nursing home, old-age home, or extended-care facility — was this site. Today, long-term care refers to the range of services themselves, which may be provided in the community as well as in the institution. The contemporary definition recognizes the continuum of need and care experienced by the frail elderly, the similarities of population across practice sites, and the necessity for a comprehensive, coordinated approach to service delivery; yet within the continuum there are differentials of social-work practice dictated by the settings themselves. This chapter discusses those differentials of the long-term-care institution.

Excluded are those forms of congregate living arrangements for elders that are not funded or administered as health services. These forms include boarding homes, foster placements, group apartments, enriched housing, and senior-citizen residences and hotels that serve both the well and the frail elderly. Such arrangements, quite different from one another, are run under a variety of auspices, many subject to minimal public regulation. Disparate as they are, however, they share a characteristic that separates them from the nursing home: they are not total institutions.

The total institution has been defined as "a place of residence and work where a large number of like-situated individuals, cut off from the wider society for an appreciable period of time, together lead an enclosed, formally administered round of life" (Goffman, 1961). It is this "formally administered round of life" that differentiates the nursing-home setting from those settings with more permeable boundaries and that dictates the social-work role within it.

For elders who live there twenty-four hours a day, often for many months or years, the long-term-care institution is a home-in-name within which they seek the home-in-spirit that they have lost. For staff, the institution is the workplace in which social, professional, and economic expectations endemic to any employment situation are played out. For administration, the long-term-care institution is an organization to be managed in a humane and cost-effective manner, which in proprietary homes includes showing a profit. Because the social-work intervention can and should take place at all points of the organizational cycle, and will have reverberating effects throughout the system, the practice role is a multifaceted one.

This chapter thus places the social-work role within the long-term-care institution in a systems perspective, addressing work with each major constituency and the worker's mediating function between them. The typical sequence of the service-rendering process, in this case the career of the elder in institutional care, provides the framework for this discussion. It is preceded by an examination of the service need, the policy considerations that underlie its delivery, and the theoretical and value base on which all rests.

THE NEED

The need for nursing homes for the aged and the feasibility of community alternatives to lessen this need has dominated professional and public concern for over a decade. Concern was simultaneously stimulated by recognition of a growing population of impaired elders in need of care, the rapid increase in the number of institutions fostered by the Medicare and Medicaid legislation of 1965-1966, and the ensuing disenchantment with these institutions because of low quality and high cost of care. This concern was fueled by a growing societal sense that there is something inherently unnatural in the removal and segregation of the old from the mainstream of life. The absolute and relative numbers of the aged placed in institutions and their reasons for being there however are often obscured in the controversy. Some facts about the elderly population who require long-term-care services place these arguments in perspective.

Although only 5 to 6 percent of the elderly may reside in a long-term-care facility on any given day, it is estimated that 20 to 25 percent will spend time there at some point in their lives (Kastenbaum and Candy, 1973). Currently, over 1 million elderly are in nursing homes.

Those over age 75, known as the "old old," are repeatedly cited as a target population for services because of the correlation of increasing age and functiona[l] impairment. By the year 2000, 45 percent of the old will be within this group, with one out of eleven living beyond the eighty-fifth birthday (U.S. Federal Council on the Aging, 1979).

For these elders, primarily female, chronic health problems such as arthritis, cardiovascular conditions, and sensory and cognitive losses are common. Acute illnesses occur more often and last longer. Disabling conditions such as stroke and hip fracture occur with greater frequency. These impairments of later life rarely exist singly but are multiple and cumulative, interacting with one another to produce a population who have been defined as "frail," "vulnerable," and "at risk." Ongoing medical supervision and reliance on others for help in carrying out activities of daily living are frequently dictated by these conditions. Moreover, in old age, internal assaults to independent functioning are often worsened by external circumstances such as lessened social supports, reduced finances, and unsafe or inadequate living arrangements.

Community resources that provide services to chronically impaired elders in their own homes include visiting-nurse, day-care, home health and housekeeping services. In addition, rent and utility allowances, escort, transportation, and home-repair services may contribute to environmental improvements. Respite and counseling services give a boost to families maintaining elders in the community. Social workers, or others designated as case managers, often coordinate care plans, buying time for the frail elder in the community, postponing and sometimes avoiding institutionalization. The availability and quality of these services varies in different locales; however, they share the characteristic of frequently being inaccessible or inadequate to meet the needs of all impaired elders in the area.

Contrary to the prevailing myth, families do not abandon their aged, but rather provide the bulk of care to them in the community for as long as they are able to do so. Placement is sought only at such time as the family has exhausted themselves and their resources or the elder needs an amount or type of care that cannot be provided elsewhere. Thus the elders in long-term-care institutions are predominantly those who have no family or those who have a concerned but overwhelmed family rather than those who have been dumped there by uncaring relatives.

The health-care community is currently directing attention to the shortage of nursing-home beds to which to discharge elders in acute-care hospitals who no longer require such a costly or intensive level of care but need more attention than they can receive in their own homes. Pressure is being brought to bear for the provision of additional nursing-home beds at the same time that an increase in community resources is being urged for less impaired elders. As of now, the supply of both alternatives is not sufficient to meet the demand, a consequence of technological advances that allow those who would previously have died to live on for years, albeit with incapacitating conditions. It is clear that there will be many more elders in the twenty-first century, but projections of need are difficult as their health status and preferences for care are, as yet, unknown. For the present, however, the need for institutional as well as community services for the frail elderly outstrips the supply.

POLICY

The public policy mandating long-term-care institutions is grounded in the Medicare and Medicaid acts of 1965-1966 and the amendments that have grown out of this legislation; the "med" in each title highlights the medical as contrasted with the social intention of the policy.

Medicare, a nearly universal entitlement for those over 65, is funded and administered federally through the Social Security Administration. It accounts for only 7 percent of the funding for nursing-home beds. Regulations are stringent, necessitating that the elder enter directly from an acute-care hospital and require skilled nursing, psychiatric, or rehabilitative care for a time-limited period. Excluded are those elders who enter long-term-care institutions from the community, those who require maintenance rather than rehabilitative care, and those whose needs are for an indefinite length of time. They, of course, account for the majority of the long-term-care population and illustrate the limitation of Medicare as a funding resource for the institutionalized aged.

Medicaid, a public-assistance program for those of all ages who are medically indigent, is jointly administered and funded by federal and state governments. It accounts for 60 percent of the funding for nursing homes. Although exact amounts and regulations vary by state, the eligibility procedure is essentially similar. For Medicaid reimbursement in a nursing home, the recipient must "spend down" savings, if any, for care until the minimum allowable level is reached. Once the elder is deemed eligible, monthly income sources (typically Social Security and private-pension checks) must be signed over to the institution, which in turn collects from Medicaid the difference between the income and the rate for the level of care received as set by the state. The resident then receives a small monthly allowance, often divided and distributed bimonthly, for sundry expenses.

Administrative regulations pursuant to the Medicaid legislation on spouse and filial financial responsibility for an institutionalized elder are interpreted differently by states. Legislation deems the community spouse responsible, but precedent has been set by fair hearing decisions that reversed this requirement when an undue hardship would result (Monk, 1979). On the other hand, although adult children are not deemed financially responsible, there has been a resurgence in some states of the concept of filial responsibility, which harkens back to the Elizabethan Poor Law principle that the public will help only after family resources are tapped. The primary justifications offered for this are cost containment and moral obligation. Aging advocates challenge both points, citing that administrative costs to implement such programs would outweigh the benefits and that detrimental effects on the aging and their families would be far reaching: elders abased at becoming burdens and adult children unable to also provide for their families and save for their own old ages. "Filial maturity" or the emotional and social imperative acted out by families to their elders has been empirically and conceptually documented (Blenkner, 1965; Shanas, 1979). It is argued that the addition of financial responsibility would weaken rather than strengthen this existing bond.

Levels of care covered by Medicaid again vary, according to name and definition, by state. Differentiation is usually made between the highest, most expensive level of care for the significantly impaired, often called "skilled nursing," and the lower, less costly level of care for the higher-functioning elder, often called "health related" or "intermediary care."

Objective measurement forms, signed by a physician, are thus a requisite for admission and continuing recertification of residents in long-term-care institutions. For example, in New York State the DMS 1 form assigns a numerical score to each functional requirement for care. A minimum of 60 points is required for the lower level of Medicaid reimbursable care and 180 for the higher. This form was composed to ensure appropriate placement level.

The fact that almost 40 percent of Medicaid expenditures are for nursing-home care while less than 1 percent goes to home health care is disturbing to social workers when it is obvious that so many more elders reside in the community, or would like to do so if services could be provided there. It is more disturbing when it is evident that this expenditure is based on a definition that does not address the elder as a whole person of interlocking biological, psychological, emotional, and social needs but rather as an array of ailments suffered and treatments administered. It is within this context that the problems involved in standard setting and staffing patterns for the social-work profession in long-term-care institutions are most clearly understood.

There are over 24,000 nursing homes in the United States today; 8 percent are under the aegis of government, 17 percent are not-for-profit, and 75 percent are profit-making enterprises (Lowy, 1980). Standards for social work in these institutions refer to the presence, qualifications, and ratio of social workers to residents as defined by federal, state, and professional mandates. Federal guidelines are based on amendments to the original legislation of 1972 that removed the requirement that social workers hold at least a master's degree in social work. Some states have retained the more rigorous earlier standards while others followed the federal example. The National Association of Social Workers (NASW) also has a set of standards that focuses on the need for "qualified" social-work participation in intake and discharge planning, services to clients and their families, and staff consultation. The Joint Commission on Accreditation of Hospitals (JCCA) is less emphatic, but also stresses the need for a "qualified" social worker in such tasks as admission, discharge planning, advocacy, and interdisciplinary case planning. Only NASW defines "qualified" as the master's level of training. No standards address staffing ratios (Silverstone, 1981).

In any setting, the prevailing staffing, though minimally set by regulations, may be above these levels. Government and not-for-profit institutions, which also tend to be larger, voluntarily employ master's level professionals. Ongoing opportunities for training and supervision are also usually available. In contrast, many smaller proprietary homes are staffed by untrained social workers who do double duty as clerical employees and have mandated, though limited, access to an MSW consultant. Consultants typically function in a supervisory capacity to staff designated as social workers by the employing facility. It has been suggested that this practice does not, and should, move beyond consideration of the worker's performance in specific situations to a broader emphasis on the administrative and managerial aspects of the social-service role throughout the institution (Mercer and Garner, 1981).

Although institutional settings differ, the social worker's role as mediator among the needs of elders (and their families), staff, and administration is essentially the same. In the state-of-the-art institution, identification with a department will serve as a buffer and a source of power; but the problems too will be more complex. In the less-endowed setting, the social worker has fewer resources, but with this may come independence and greater possibility for innovation.

The theoretical framework and typical sequence of the service-rendering process that follow are thus presented with the expectation that they will be generally applicable, but require modification as indicated by the specific setting of practice.

THEORY

Three bases of theory underlie the following discussion: those that arise from the profession, from the population, and from the practice setting. They are clearly not exhaustive, but reflective of current professional thinking on work with the aged in institutions.

The objectives of social-work practice, and the values underlying them, were most currently set forth by NASW in 1981. Monk (1981) upholds them as valid with the aging population but notes the need for a "specific gerontological perspective that can be used as a kind of corrective lens" for translating them into practice. He reviews the objectives (that appear here in italics), in each instance suggesting guidelines appropriate for the aged. The ideas, in summary, follow.

Help people enlarge their competence and increase their problem-solving and coping abilities. This objective requires a positive attitude toward old age based on an understanding of its place in the developmental life cycle, an appreciation of each individual's uniqueness as represented by lifelong coping capacities, and an assessment of remaining strengths with a commitment to maximize them no matter how great the impairment, which includes realistically adapting treatment plans with recognition of achievement in even small gains and the enhancement of elder self-esteem necessary in the face of dependence on others.

Help people obtain resources. This objective requires worker sensitivity to the personal, physical, social, and bureaucratic barriers to the aged in receiving services and a commitment to overcome these barriers through interventions that build elder trust and enhance access as well as through interventions with service providers through case management and coordination and, in both cases, avoiding worker overprotectiveness by helping the informal support network to perform these functions.

Make organizations responsive to people.

Influence interactions between organizations and institutions. These objectives require awareness of the care requirements of the aged population and a commitment to define service priorities in a way that is responsive to them, including enlarging the options for care as well as providing improved access to the system. In all cases, preferences of the elderly as to the care plan of choice is to be respected.

Facilitate interaction between individuals and others in their environment. This objective requires recognition of the losses of significant others through death that have been experienced by the elderly, and the compensatory human relationships necessary to take their place, including promoting mutual helping efforts and resocialization of elders and sensitivity to the special needs of their adult children.

Influence social and environmental policy. This requires knowledge of the legislation that both mandates and constrains practice, including eligibility requirements, restrictions, and service priorities. Commitment to increase needed services may involve participation in formulation of new policies or advocacy on behalf of them.

The overall objectives of long-term care, whether in the community or in the institution, have been stated as: maximizing functional independence, including rehabilitation and maintenance; humane care, including placement in the least restrictive environment and death with dignity; prolonging longevity; and prevention of avoidable medical and social problems (Callahan and Wallack, 1981). These objectives are echoed by social-work goals within the nursing home, which have been defined as: participation in the provision of a comprehensive, integrated, and continuous program of care; planning and treatment; and enabling residents and families to use their personal resources as well as institutional and community resources to maximize their functioning (Brody, 1977; Brody et al. 1974). The role is thus defined as simultaneously addressed to work with the organization and with the client group. Of late, social-work goals have been expanded to include reducing excess disability and meeting residual dependency to promote independence and well-being (Brody, 1979). This is in recognition of the unwarranted degree of "learned helplessness" often witnessed in settings where opportunities for client mastery and control of the environment are not afforded (Hooker, 1979; Van Hook, 1979).

Studies of total institutions speak to their all-encompassing nature, the leveling or stripping of the individual's personal characteristics necessary to blend with the group, and the myriad factors that act against maintenance of self-image and a sense of personal efficacy in surroundings where all is public and under the control of others (Goffman, 1961; Tobin and Lieberman, 1976). Opportunities and gratifications for as much autonomy as possible provided through enhancement of remaining strengths is clearly of primary importance.

It has been noted that the future goal for the nursing home is "a mix of a medical and social environment that has not yet been achieved . . . the real frontier of institutional care" (Brody, 1979). It is the facilitating of this mix, or the humanizing aspect of the delivery of care to elders in institutions, that sets the parameters of the social-work role.

SEQUENCE OF SERVICE DELIVERY

The career of the elder in the long-term-care institution follows several distinct, though overlapping stages: it commences at the time the nursing home is first considered as a possible option for care and ends at the time of discharge or death. Staff and administration are involved throughout this sequence, with the potential at each stage for easing or impeding the process. The following section addresses the social-work role with these constituencies at each stage of the service-delivery sequence. The conceptual framework on which it is based is a practice model specifically developed for work with the frail elderly, the auxiliary-function model (Silverstone and Burack-Weiss, 1982, 1983).

The auxiliary-function model is based on the salient characteristics of frailty and the responses required by the environment to counteract its force. Although closely associated with advanced age, illness, and loss, frailty is not the sum of these; it is rather the functional consequence. Reliance on someone else to fulfill tasks once handled independently is necessitated by depletions in crucial areas of life.

Primary depletions are intrinsic to the aging process; secondary depletions are extrinsic to the individual but accompany biological aging in our society. Both characterize the aged in institutions. The consequences of depletion require a strategic approach with elder, staff, and administration to counteract their force and promote adaptation at the optimum level possible.

Sometimes that which was lost is recovered through healing, spontaneous remission, or external replenishment. Restitution may occur, as in the case of restored eyesight after cataract surgery or increased mobility after physical therapy for a hip fracture. Sometimes that which was lost cannot be totally recovered, but through the use of prosthetic devices or substitutions, compensation to a limited degree or in regard to specific functions may occur. Hearing aids and eyeglasses may compensate for primary depletion of the senses. New relationships and activities may compensate for the loss of spouse or peers. Sometimes, however, that which was lost is not and cannot be restored. Accommodation to diminished functioning and an altered physical or mental state becomes necessary.

Understanding the processes of depletion and adaptation leads away from any propensity to globalize "frailty" in the elderly. The task becomes an individualized one, to identify the adaptive processes that are already in motion when and where the elder is met, to question if these processes are the best that can be achieved given the individual circumstances, and to lend a boost to those adaptations that need strengthening. Whether the optimum will be achieved in the specific situation depends largely on the coping capacities of the elder, including the unimpaired areas of functioning and the particular style of meeting adversity developed over a lifetime; the resources available in the environment, including both informal supports (family and friends), formal supports (service providers and professionals), and prosthetic arrangements; the transactions between the elder and the environment; or the way that resources are tailored to meet elder need.

The name of the auxiliary-function model is based on metaphor—the image of an auxiliary lighting system triggered to action by failure of a permanent one, then fading when power is restored. An auxiliary adds to, fills in for, bolsters that which is depleted. The model is bounded by the study, assessment, and plan for the individual elder, and the environmental interventions needed for optimal functioning, which are linked to the elder through the auxiliary role.

The auxiliary role, or the relationship of significant others to the elder, contains instrumental and affective components that together serve to unite the frail elder and needed services while maximizing self-esteem and mastery. The affective component fills the emotional needs of the frail elder for affirmation and human connection. The instrumental component fills the concrete needs of the frail elder for environmental resources to supplement failing powers. The auxiliary role is commonly filled by family in the community, who should be encouraged to continue to the extent possible within the institution. However, placement may itself be indicative of their declining capacity to meet at least the instrumental component of elder need.

In summary, the application of the auxiliary-function model to practice within the long-term-care institution dictates simultaneous consideration of elder dependency, environmental resources, and the social-work task of maximizing adaptation by uniting these factors through orchestration of the auxiliary role. With the elder, the affective component must be continued to the extent possible with family and friends, the social worker acting as a bridge to extend these affective components to new relationships after placement; the instrumental component will involve utilization of services. These components are primarily enabling functions. With family, staff, and administration, the instrumental component is primary, helping with the provision and utilization of necessary resources. This is primarily an interpretive and mediating function.

The systems perspective that underlies this discussion indicates that a change in any area may affect all others. Thus there is no inherently better way to work, no either-or, with client, family, staff, or administration. All are interrelated, and the point of intervention will vary depending on an assessment of the issue at hand.

Entering the Institution: Application, Intake, Admission

Application, intake, and admission are separate phases of elder beginnings with institutions; however, for the purpose of this discussion, and because functions of each often overlap in practice, they are consolidated here.

The waiting period and that immediately following entry have been found to be the most stressful for the aged, with the greatest likelihood for deterioration and death specifically among those who are most passive and dependent (Tobin and Lieberman, 1976). It has also been empirically demonstrated that, although the event of relocation is undeniably difficult for elders, negative effects can be mitigated by careful preparation, voluntary participation, and perceived control over the new environment (Pablo, 1977). The social worker in the long-term-care institution is the staff person most appropriate for facilitating this task.

The elder or family who approach the nursing home for admission generally come to this step with reluctance and fear. Often a crisis situation has precipitated the application, which originates from an acute-care hospital currently holding the older person who is awaiting transfer because the aftereffects of illness, surgery, or accident preclude a return home. Or, as is often the case when mental impairment is the primary difficulty, family or other community-service providers have come to the end of their resources and see no other alternative.

Whatever the case, the elder's need is to mourn the loss of the past while being prepared for the massive changes in his/her life that will soon take place. The family and other significant people in the elder's personal world must also face the ending of one era and the beginning of another. The process through which the social worker helps with these tasks is geared to the capacities of the client to assimilate the experience.

The auxiliary role with the elder is instrumental in helping with the provision of information that will aid in preparedness and initial control, and affective in according empathy and support over the difficult transition: with the family, who have assumed an auxiliary role in the community, it is finding a way to continue their support to the extent possible within the institution. Individualization takes place through the study, assessment, and plan. This may begin with a medical or functional form used for reimbursement and placement determination (like the DMS 1 cited earlier) but must reach beyond it if the worker is to differentiate between elders sharing common diagnoses to affirm and address the uniqueness of each.

Knowledge and understanding of psychosocial information, specifically of family background and past life experiences as they affect the present, is uniquely the social-work province within the institution. Exploration at the point of application is the basis of this information. Such individualization is useful not only for easing the admission process but for making referrals to community agencies if and when placement is found not to be indicated. It is often argued that there is no time for social workers to conduct such an exploration, yet the task of completing the many forms required for financial or medical eligibility in nursing homes affords a natural entry point for the skilled practitioner. Collection of demographic data can be accompanied by reflection on current and past living arrangements. Financial data lead easily into a discussion of past employment and the changes entailed by retirement. Listing of persons to be contacted in an emergency similarly yields insight into relationship patterns. Information that is not needed administratively will nevertheless be of use for the psychosocial assessment and beginning plan.

Care must be taken that irrevocable decisions are not made at a time of crisis. Helping elder and family keep options open at the time of admission will be a difficult task. It is often financially difficult to maintain a community residence even when rehabilitative efforts have a good chance of rendering the elder capable of discharge. This places a particular responsibility on the worker to explore less final alternatives to care than placement and to make all choices known to the applicant.

First impressions that elders and families receive of the institution will be long lasting and will provide a model for future interactions with the facility. Although situations vary, common principles hold true for all and suggest a range of individual, family, and group strategies.

Decision-making for placement should include all responsible or concerned others, not just the person or agency who initiated the admission procedure, which may involve the worker's reaching out to all family members individually or in a family conference. Of particular importance to note is the precipitating event of application, how the decision was made, and coping styles until the present crisis. This information yields indicators of strengths, past and present adaptive patterns, and life-styles and interests; all are important as related to potential adaptation to the demands and constraints of institutional life. Whatever is expected, hoped for, or feared in the placement situation must also be explored for the purpose of responding to perceptions and clarifying misconceptions with corrective information.

The elder should be included, to the fullest extent possible, in the planning process. Anticipation of a negative response is no reason to abrogate this step, but indeed underscores the reason for it. Anger, depression, and anxiety are the usual responses to the fact of placement. If not amenable to resolution prior to admission, these feelings at least must be recognized and addressed.

Mourning the loss of one's home and independence, even if presented as temporary as when rehabilitation is anticipated, will usually precede or accompany acceptance of institutionalization. The elder may lose many prior roles—householder, church member, spouse—in exchange for one other, that of nursing-home resident. The new role necessitates a more regimented, compliant pattern of life; meals, medication, and personal hygiene, once private affairs, become public, which will act against the maintenance of a positive self-image and diminish feelings of competence. Bridges from the past to the present, with as many opportunities for individualization as possible, and an empathic recognition of what cannot be replaced are an important auxiliary function of the worker. This is accomplished through help with deciding what to bring and the decoration of private space with personal objects, plants, and pictures from the home that was left. Preparation is fostered through tours of the facility in advance, opportunities to visit or share in a meal or activity, and groups specifically planned for new applicants and new residents. Printed brochures on services or a cadre of old-time residents in a welcoming committee are also helpful.

For the family, relief from daily caregiving concerns may be quickly superseded by feelings of loss and anticipatory grief heralding the total loss of the parent. Disappointment in themselves for a perceived failure to live up to their own or others' expectations of filial caring, or conflicting feelings about the parent, if not recognized and handled, may be displaced onto the facility and manifested by complaints about service and care. The family will need a new role vis-à-vis the elder, one that is in partnership with the institution (Dobrof and Litwak, 1977). Informational brochures, explanation of organization procedures, and new family orientation groups will help answer their questions and provide relief in sharing their concerns with others experiencing similar problems.

Elders and families who have had some time to prepare for admission and have notable strengths within themselves may need no more than a beginning individual interview with the worker before being linked up with group sources of support within the institution. But for those who enter at a time of crisis with little preparation, and for those who are particularly troubled or have still unresolved issues, a longer period of individual contact in the initial phase will be necessary. It is useful to tag these "high risk" cases and alert staff to the need for individualized intensive attention to begin at admission. (This is especially the case if the elder or family are withdrawn or nonassertive: passivity may be misinterpreted by staff as indicative of good adjustment when actually it often masks depression.)

The social worker is often the first personal contact that the new admission has with the nursing home. The affective component of the auxiliary role is introduced to the elder through affirmation that his/her uniqueness and dignity will be respected in the new setting. The instrumental component of the auxiliary role is introduced to the elder through the beginning connections made between him/her and the many other helping systems within the institution.

Some staff of the long-term-care facility such as nurses and dietary aides will have maximum contact with the residents in a very personal way; others, such as physicians or special therapists, will respond only to one aspect of the elder's condition. Whatever the degree or type of involvement, however, the primary need of staff is for information about the elder that will aid in delivery of the service they provide and for a quick integration of the newcomer into their work routines.

To help staff with their beginnings with residents, the instrumental role of the worker is an interpretive one, selectively sharing information about the entering elder and family. This serves two purposes: it helps the staff immediately begin to individualize the new resident and suggests fruitful ways to offer services and develop a working relationship with the family. The social worker might share elements of the elder's past that may be reawakened in positive or negative ways in the placement, the language or style the elder communicates in, and the approach he/she is most responsive to. Interests, activities, and hobbies of the recent past that can be continued in the nursing home are of particular note.

The methods the worker uses to impart this information may include pre-admission or immediately postadmission team meetings and staffing conferences and individual briefings of key institutional caregivers. In a large facility, psychosocial profiles may be transmitted to department heads for circulation to those of their staff who will be relating to the new individual. These one-paragraph summaries are introductions of the entering individual and serve as a complement to the team meeting.

The administrative need that parallels the admission processes of elder and staff is the necessity for maintaining the census of the institution at full capacity—in other words, keeping the beds filled in order to receive maximum financial reimbursement. This policy sometimes results in the institutional definition of admission as a business rather than as a social-work task, particularly in a proprietary or for-profit home. Recognition of the crucial role of the beginning stages in the well-being of the elder throughout his/her institutionalization and the importance of reaching out to families in distress before they lump accumulated grievances into an attack against the nursing home will inform the social worker's advocacy stance with administration in the interests of access to the clients as early in the process as possible. This is a cost-effective as well as a professionally responsible approach.

The Middle Phase: Settling In

There will be a continuing need for social-work services to elder and family after the admission phase is over, the amount and modality depending on the individual situation.

All residents experience strangeness adjusting to roommates and new care arrangements. Energies, however limited, that were used to cope with surviving on the outside may now lie fallow, atrophying from disuse. New outlets and experiences will be needed to encourage their expression. New opportunities for mastery and control, for socialization and life enhancement, must be provided. Although the auxiliary role of the worker will continue on an individual basis with elders around idiosyncratic matters, the commonality of the resident situation, the time limitations of the worker, and the unique properties of the institutional setting dictate that groups are primary in the delivery of social services.

Groups for the aged foster communication, mutual aid, and self-affirmation for members. At the same time, they offer opportunity for goal-directed activity on common concerns (Miller and Solomon, 1980). Resident councils, and floor groups whose contributions flow into them, are excellent mechanisms for fostering elder mastery over the environment (Getzel, 1982; Silverstone, 1974).

The range of possible special-interest groups is limited only by the worker's creativity and skill. In larger institutions, recreation or activities departments may share in or administer such groups, which include poetry groups, oral-history groups, current-event discussions, adult education, and a variety of crafts. Groups for subpopulations with special needs are useful in providing education and support. In larger institutions, nursing, speech, or physical therapy departments may share in or administer such groups, which include diabetic groups, stroke clubs, and reality orientation or resocialization groups for the mentally impaired. Social-work texts on group work with the aged are most useful in generating ideas and the specific skills needed to implement them (Burnside, 1978; Hartford, 1980).

The group experience will be an unfamiliar one to many elders, and much outreach, invitation, and explanation may be necessary to get the groups underway, not to mention transport difficulty and the necessity for coordinating resident-care schedules, arranging space, etc. The worker should not be deterred, however, as initial time invested in planning and instituting group services will be more than repaid when these groups become an integral part of the social-service program. At the same time, it must be remembered that groups will be contraindicated for some residents due to the nature of their impairments or, simply, their preferences. Those who cannot or wish not to participate must be reached in other ways.

The total nature of the institutional experience and the feeling of being closed off from the rest of the world that it generates can be alleviated by interventions that open doors to the community. Foster-grandparent programs that bring elders into the schools or children into the nursing home are enriching to both populations. RSVP programs can be instituted within the nursing home. Volunteers of all ages can be utilized as friendly visitors, which is especially useful for the lonely elder who has no pressing problems but welcomes the chance for conversational interchange with someone outside of his/her daily orbit. High-school and college students exploring careers in gerontology may be enlisted to help in social and recreational activities; some may be used for aid in feeding and transport. More able residents may benefit from sheltered-workshop activities in which they can earn extra spending money as well as regain a lost role. Screening, training, and ongoing supervision play major parts in the success of these endeavors, and the social worker is the staff person best equipped by education and skill to either perform the tasks or to provide consultation to the department charged with it.

Families will enter into a partnership with the institution in the care of their elders and benefit from ongoing help with their sharing of the auxiliary role. Friends and relatives groups serve both an educative and supportive function. Through participation, families may learn about the aging process, particular disease entities, or common treatment strategies as well as the workings of the institution. A forum is provided for registering their concerns. The example of others can thus serve as a corrective role model for those less able to cope with the deterioration or demands of a parent in the home (Silverman, Kahn, and Anderson, 1977). The social worker may need to invest considerable energies in beginning family groups, but in time indigenous leadership inevitably emerges and the professional task may then be limited to staffing and consultation.

The need for more individual interventions with residents and families than time permits will be strikingly apparent and a source of concern to the conscientious social worker. Priorities must be set. As a general rule, the more recent the origin of the difficulty, the more amenable to intervention; a timely if necessarily short-term response will often suffice. Problems in access to and utilization of the nursing home's services, the pain around the loss of a close relationship, upset over a declining health situation are all responsive to the instrumental and affective aid of the worker. Similarly, interpersonal difficulties that have arisen with family or other residents around a specific occurrence can often be handled with the basic counseling skills that are the social worker's stock-in-trade. In contrast, dysfunctional conditions of long standing such as chaotic family relations and pathological behavioral manifestations may intrigue but will ultimately envelop the worker, syphoning off time more profitably spent elsewhere. In such situations, it is necessary to extricate and direct a strictly problem-solving approach to the current reality concerns.

Eighty-three-year-old Mrs. Baskin and her 60-year-old unmarried son had always lived together until her admission to the nursing home following a hip fracture. Each sought to engage the worker's support in a lifelong, ambivalent struggle for separation: the mother, suggesting that he stay home and rest, then hurt because he did not visit enough, the son entreating the worker to advocate on his behalf. The worker helped the son instead by referral to a community counseling agency for his personal problems and inclusion in a monthly family group to handle more general concerns he had about the placement and foster socialization. Work with the mother involved hastening assimilation to institutional life through introductions to residents with similar ethnic backgrounds and engagement in a history class in which she had expressed interest.

Residents who were lifelong loners may be expected to continue this pattern in the nursing home; their manner of coping should be respected and socialization not forced. On the other hand, residents who were isolated before admission because of health or environmental factors may now be ready to resume peer relationships that were once satisfying, but their social skills may have become rusty. A brief period of individual/worker involvement that may center on reminiscence as well as on enhancement of conversational skills may precede group involvement or friendships with peers (Kaminsky, 1978; Liton and Olstein, 1969).

Mental impairment of the resident, except of the most extreme degree, should not rule out any of the interventions just discussed. The confused, forgetful, or disoriented elder is nevertheless a feeling human being, acutely responsive to the attitudes of others. For those in whom fear, anxiety, and anger are generated by this condition, a structured, predictable round of institutional life, designed to offer the optimum amount of stimulation without overwhelming, provides a needed sense of security. At the same time, the need for human connection remains. Often family and staff need help in communicating with the cognitively impaired in a calming, accepting manner; the worker can role model effective methods for them.

Work with staff, sometimes as teamwork or interdisciplinary collaboration, begun at admission continues through the settling-in period. The social worker's relationship to other staff will be *the* decisive factor in his or her ability to be helpful to residents in the long-term-care facility. As one of the team, participation in formal and informal encounters must be approached with an appreciation of the perspective of and the demands upon other members that may differ from the worker's own.

A common institutional problem is the complaint of elder or family that necessary care has not been provided or that it was rendered in an unsatisfactory manner. The staff member responsible will cite the organizational constraints of his/her department or place the blame on the resident for misrepresenting the facts or not participating in the treatment plan as indicated. Social-work advocacy on behalf of the client, while often successful with service providers in a community setting, is not useful in the institution where cooperative efforts with the same people over time are essential. Here the instrumental component of the worker's auxiliary role with staff is seen in the mediating function performed. Involvement of the elder helps to role model the way in which intrainstitutional conflict can be resolved.

Mrs. Roman, an 87-year-old woman suffering from congestive heart failure, and her daughter who visited daily, deluged the worker with complaints about the "callous" and "inhuman" care at the home. Exploration with them revealed that specific complaints were delay in getting evening medications and lack of answers to their medical questions.

The worker had only to mention the resident's name to the charge nurse to release a torrent of frustration. She was constantly stopped by them and so detained from doing her work which was already overwhelming because of staff shortages. Everyone got their evening medications an hour later because of this. And, finally, questions should have been answered by the doctor and were not her responsibility. A meeting with the doctor revealed that he was not aware of any of the above. With respect for the views of all concerned, the worker scheduled and led a meeting of doctor, nurse, elder and daughter, facilitating the communication among them. The medical condition was explained; it was decided that evening medications could be administered by the daughter before she left; and a procedure for registering future problems was arranged. However, the worker, realizing that ongoing reinforcement and support of resident and daughter would be necessary to curb their dysfunctional patterns of reaching out, stayed involved to monitor the plan. This was perceived as caring by the clients and as a great help to staff as well.

In another typical instance, the instrumental component of the worker's auxiliary role is seen in the interpretive function performed: staff is helped to understand and so more appropriately respond to the resident's needs.

The occupational therapist complained that Miss Montgomery refused to participate in the rug-making project prescribed to widen the range of upper torso movement. She saw the resident as unmotivated and was prepared to terminate the service. The worker, who over time had gained the trust of this quiet and retiring client, learned that she had been a fine craftswoman in her earlier years and that the childish efforts which were now all that she could produce were humiliating for her, especially in the presence of others. This information was interpreted to the therapist who was then able to select another activity that would serve the same purpose but that the resident could perform in the privacy of her room.

Social workers have much to learn from other members of the helping team, including hands-on providers as well as professionals, and much to contribute. The sharing of expertise in a consultative fashion, as well as the personal peer relationships that grow with familiarity over time with those engaged in the same effort, is an achievable goal; this improves the work environment for all as well as service delivery to elders. Understanding and facilitating team dynamics is of use to the worker in exploiting their full potential (Brill, 1976; Kane, 1975). The determination and coordination of a care plan for each resident is a mandated task around which such collaboration can begin.

Administrative sanction is necessary for the aforementioned social-work activities, and will be easier to achieve in some areas than others. Group activity is often wrongly perceived as generating and giving voice to feelings of discontent with the institution. The contrary is more often the case, with organized elders and families ready to defend their institution against outside threats to cut services. An active, satisfied client population is a good reflection on an institution, and efforts on the residents' behalf that may not otherwise be approved can often be advanced on these grounds.

Social-work services that troubleshoot incipient problems before they escalate into crises, as well as needs that remain unmet because of inadequate staffing, should be documented to administration.

The administrative need for paperwork, a requirement of funding and regulating sources, is reflected in three-month or six-month notes required on each resident in institutional care. These notes typically include an assessment and plan defined in operational terms, accompanied by goals, short- and long-term objectives, and a time frame in which this is to be achieved. The social worker's prompt and skillful performance of this unpopular task not only meets organizational needs but validates in writing the helpfulness of the intervention provided.

Quality-of-life issues such as enhancement of the physical environment, providing a measure of privacy for each resident, and relations with the surrounding community are not the exclusive province of the social worker but one in which he/she is uniquely able to stimulate interest on the part of all involved systems and to assist in the framing of solutions.

While working within even the most advanced institution, the social worker will identify gaps in service delivery and posit ideas for organizational change. Such efforts can be successful but must be informed by knowledge about the particular properties of human-service organizations and with a careful consideration of the implications of each action for all constituencies (Brager and Holloway, 1978).

Leaving the Institution: Discharge, Transfer, Death

Leaving the institution, or even one's floor on it, for any reason can be as traumatic to the elder as entering. Now-familiar routines and relationships must be ended; the future is unknown. If rehabilitation efforts have resulted in improvement, discharge to the community or tranfer to another facility or area of the nursing home that offers a lower level of care will arouse fears of functioning in a less secure environment. If the move is to a higher level of care necessitated by increased impairment, the scenario of the admission phase may be reenacted with even greater intensity for the elder. Family doubts or guilt about the original placement will be reawakened. The institution may be blamed for not making the elder better. The worker's auxiliary role with elder and family will closely parallel that of the beginning phase, simultaneously working on giving up the past and preparation for next steps.

For the client who will be expected to function more independently, preparation must anticipate and minimize all that can go wrong. Community services and firm commitments from informal supports as to who will do what should be in place before discharge. A home visit by the interdisciplinary team will provide necessary information for the planning of aftercare. A trial visit home, while keeping the institutional bed, will help elder and family to make the adjustment. Day-care programs, where available, are excellent intermediary steps between the institution and the community.

For the client who is moving to a higher level of care, the move is more often precipitous, based on a sudden decline. The resident and/or family must deal not only with the reality of deterioration but its occurrence in an unfamiliar situation with strange caregivers. At this point it is often helpful to review, and take guidance from, the admission experience.

Mr. Olson's oldest son had been out of town at the time of his entry to the home, and had caused great difficulty to staff at the time of his return, maintaining that he had not been informed or consulted on planning for his father. When hospital transfer was necessary a year later, special attention was directed to involving this son at the outset.

Resident and family may lack understanding of the reasons for transfer or misinterpret information given, adding to the distress experienced. Global explanations such as that the resident is growing weaker or needs more care are unsatisfactory. Clients are entitled to specific diagnoses, prognoses, and explanations of these transfers, a task that the social worker will share with medical or nursing staff, in so doing exercising both affective and instrumental components of the auxiliary role.

The specter of death surrounds the long-term-care institution, especially in the most intensive level of care where many residents are in the dying process and death is a relatively common event. Although death is more "natural" in extreme old age and more welcome in the face of severe depletions than it might have been earlier in life, the worker must be aware of the salient characteristics of death in the nursing home. Often the greatest fear is of abandonment. Additional concerns such as fear of becoming a burden, undergoing extreme pain, and not receiving needed care will vary with the individual and must be explored and addressed with factual explanations, instrumental interventions, and affective support. The mentally impaired resident may not be able to identify concerns but become more agitated and demanding, responding to a structured and calming approach.

The well-known stages of the dying process are by now familiar to many (Kübler-Ross, 1969). Helpful in identifying common elements, these stages sometimes obscure individual variations and are not universally applicable to the elderly (Kastenbaum, 1978). Concrete help with burial and financial plans will be appreciated by some. Many will experience a resurgence of reminiscence or life review in a last attempt to put their lives into perspective. The worker's participation in this, and helping the family or significant others to do so, is very helpful.

The family of the transferred or dying resident will need individual attention at the point of crisis. Self-blame, mourning, and a guilty sense of relief will often coexist. Helping members of the family review steps they went through from when frailty began until the present will often yield insight and reassurance that they did all they could.

Mrs. Callahan lamented that she should never have placed her husband in the home; if she had only kept him with her he would be much better off today. The worker asked what it was like when he was home. Mrs. Callahan remembered the sleepless nights, her own deteriorating health and the complaints of neighbors about his behavior and concluded for herself that it could not have gone on that way.

Terminating with the family after the death of a resident should not be overlooked. Completion of this phase of their lives, which may include both handling of concrete details and review of the resident experience in the home, helps worker and family.

Resident responses to the death of peers will vary according to the individual and to the relationship to the deceased. A readiness to begin "where the client is" rather than rushing in with an assumption of grief is appropriate. Denial of death's importance is a common defense mechanism of elders surrounded by it and may serve an adaptive function; yet those who wish to express their feelings should be provided an opportunity to do so.

Staff as well as family are often grieved and guilty about the deterioration of residents in their care, and also angry at the additional demands this places upon them. They, along with the social worker, have defenses against these feelings, some helpful in performance of the caregiving function, others resulting in distancing and poor care. The worker's use of self as a catalyst for discussing this issue with team members and sharing ways of dealing with it will improve service and job satisfaction at the same time.

The administrative need of residents leaving the institution, for whatever reason, is for replacement. Full bed utilization, necessary for maximum financial reimbursement, may thus precipitate hasty moves that bypass resident and family process and participation in their acceptance. The worker's appreciation of the administrative perspective will lead to creative ways of bridging facilities the resident may be transferred to or from.

The worker knew that Mr. Roberts would be transferred from the health related to the skilled nursing facility of the home when the next bed became available, but that the period of time from notification to move would be less than a day. She began preparation in advance, taking the elder for visits to a typical floor, discussing differences in staffing and care, etc. When the day arrived, Mr. Roberts and the niece who came to help him were physically and emotionally ready to go within the afternoon.

Often news of death in an institution is hushed on grounds that it will distress other residents; this adds to mystery and confusion. Posted or announced mention of those who have died, funeral plans, and next of kin will allow those who wish to pay their last respects to do so. Mention of the recently deceased and reminiscence, individually and in groups, assures that memory and life go on.

SUMMARY

The social-work role within the long-term-care institution is grounded in a systems perspective; work with elders, families, staff, and administration is of equal importance. The modalities of intervention are reflective of the individual circumstances of the situation at hand, but always with the goal of maximizing functioning and enhancing quality of life for the resident.

Each stage of the typical sequence of service delivery—from the moment when decision for placement is made to the time of discharge and death—poses particular challenges. The social worker in a nursing home, whether buttressed by a department or on his/her own, will have a multifaceted, demanding, and often overwhelming job. Priority setting and parsimony in interventions will be necessary, the knowledge of work undone being eased by the understanding of the reverberating effect of each small intervention throughout the system.

Tobin and Lieberman (1976) note: ". . . the institution is too much a world of sickness and death, of schedule and staff, to be that comfortable, warm and relatively free and unstructured place properly called 'home'."

The extent to which these definitions can be brought together is the social worker's challenge; the small steps taken in this direction each day are the sources of his or her gratification in work in long-term-care institutions.

REFERENCES

Blenkner, M. (1965). Some thoughts on filial maturity. In E. Shanas and G. F. Streib (Eds.), *Social structure and the family: Generational relations*. Englewood Cliffs, N.J.: Prentice-Hall.

Brager, G., and Holloway, S. (1978). *Changing human service organizations: Politics and practice*. New York: Free Press.

Brill, N. I. (1976). *Teamwork: Working together in the human services*. Philadelphia: Lippincott.

Brody, E. M. (1977). *Long-term care of older people: A practical guide*. New York: Human Sciences Press.

Brody, E. M. (1979). Long-term care of the aged: Promises and prospects. *Health and Social Work*, **4**(1), 29-59.

Brody, E. M., et al. (1974). *A social work guide for long-term care facilities*. Rockville, Md.: National Institute of Mental Health.

Burnside, I. M. (1978). History and overview of group work with the elderly. In I. M. Burnside (Ed.), *Working with the elderly: Group process and techniques*. North Scituate, Mass.: Duxbury Press.

Callahan, J. J. Jr., and Wallack, S. E. (Eds.). (1981). *Reforming the long-term-care system: Financial and organizational options*. Lexington, Mass.: Lexington Books.

Dobrof, R., and Litwak, E. (1977). *Maintenance of family ties of long-term care patients: Theory and guide to practice*. Rockville, Md.: National Institute of Mental Health.

Getzel, J. (1982). Resident councils and social action. *Journal of Gerontological Social Work*, **5**(1/2), 179-185.

Goffman, E. (1961). *Asylums: Essays on the social situation of mental patients and other inmates*. Garden City, N.Y.: Anchor Books.

Hartford, M. (1980). The use of group methods for work with the aged. In J. E. Birren and R. B. Sloane (Eds.), *Handbook of mental health and aging*. Englewood Cliffs, N.J.: Prentice-Hall.

Hooker, C. E. (1979). Learned helplessness. *Social Work*, **21**(3), 194-198.

Kaminsky, M. (1978). Pictures from the past: The use of reminiscence in casework with the elderly. *Journal of Gerontological Social Work*, **1**(1), 19-32.

Kane, R. A. (1975). *Interprofessional teamwork*. Syracuse, N.Y.: Syracuse University School of Social Work.

Kastenbaum, R. (1978). Death, dying and bereavement in old age: New developments and their possible implications for psychological care. *Aged Care and Services Review,* **1**(1), 1-9.

Kastenbaum, R., and Candy, S. E. (1973). The 4% fallacy: A methodological and empirical critique of extended care facility population statistics. *International Journal of Aging and Human Development,* **4**(1), 15-21.

Kübler-Ross, E. (1969). *On death and dying.* New York: Macmillan.

Liton, J., and Olstein, S. C. (1969). Therapeutic aspects of reminiscence. *Social Casework,* **50**(5), 263-268.

Lowy, L. (1980). *Social policies and programs on aging.* Lexington, Mass.: Lexington Books.

Mercer, S. O., and Garner, J. D. (1981). Social work consultation in long-term care facilities. *Health and Social Work,* **6**(2), 5-13.

Miller, I., and Solomon, R. (1980). The development of group services for the elderly. *Journal of Gerontological Social Work,* **2**(3), 241-257.

Monk, A. (1979). Family supports in old age. *Social Work,* **24**(6), 533-538.

Monk, A. (1981). Social work with the aged: Principles of practice. *Social Work,* **26**(1), 61-68.

Pablo, R. Y. (1977). Intra-institutional relocation: Its impact on long-term care patients. *Gerontologist,* **17**(5), 426-435.

Shanas, E. (1979). Social myth as hypothesis: The case of the family relations of old people. *Gerontologist,* **19**(1), 3-9.

Silverman, A. G., Kahn, B. H., and Anderson, G. (1977). A model for working with multigenerational families. *Social Casework,* **58**(3), 131-135.

Silverstone, B. (1974). *Establishing resident councils.* New York: Federation of Protestant Welfare Agencies.

Silverstone, B. Long-term care. (1981). *Health and Social Work,* **6**(4), 28S-34S.

Silverstone, B., and Burack-Weiss, A. (1982). The social work function in nursing homes and home care. *Journal of Gerontological Social Work,* **5**(1/2), 7-33.

Silverstone, B., and Burack-Weiss, A. (1983). *Social work practice with the frail elderly and their families; The auxiliary function model.* Springfield, Ill.: Thomas.

Tobin, S. S., and Lieberman, M. A. (1976). *Last home for the aged: Critical implications of institutionalization.* San Francisco: Jossey-Bass.

U.S. Federal Council on the Aging. (1979). *Public policy and the frail elderly.* Washington: The Council.

Van Hook, M. (1979). Female clients, female counselors: Combating learned helplessness. *Social Work,* **24**(1), 63-65.

20

Respite and Adult Day-Care Services

Eloise Rathbone-McCuan, Ph.D.

University of Vermont

Raymond T. Coward, Ph.D.

University of Vermont

The purpose of this chapter is to offer practical information about the means by which social-service practitioners can facilitate the effective use of two distinct, but equally important, services by older persons and their families. The first service, respite care, is temporary and supportive, whereas the second, adult day care, provides longer-term health and social services to older community residents. On both conceptual and practical dimensions, these two service concepts are promoted as components of community-service systems. Unfortunately, seldom is either service available or accessible at the community level in proportion to need.

Each service is valuable for elderly persons who are unable to perform essential activities of daily living safely or adequately or to experience meaningful social interactions without assistance. Elderly persons who utilize one service are often able to benefit from the functions provided through the other service. An elderly day-care-center participant, for example, might receive respite care either through the auspices of the center or another provider source. The utilization of respite services may in no way change, either increase or decrease, the need for day-care-center participation. Each of these services can have a beneficial outcome for both the elder and those individuals who comprise the informal-care network.

Sections of this chapter will address the need for respite and day-care service, the composition and structure of both, and the development and delivery of such programs. Social-service practitioners assume numerous and diverse roles in the delivery of these services, such as functional assessment, direct service referral, care-plan management, service-eligibility determination, and service monitoring. Additionally, practitioners may accept responsibility for developing or expanding the availability of services or improving the quality of existing resources. Social-service expertise is central to the success of respite services and day-care-center programming.

Increasingly, social-service practitioners desire to provide services to the elderly in a manner that supports the care-giving efforts of families. The outreach of formal-care sources to the informal-care network is a pattern relevant in many social-service systems to reduce discontinuities in care (Froland, 1980). Families and the informal helping network bear the brunt of providing in-home services for elders. This help far exceeds the amount of services available for elders through arrangements such as nursing homes, congregate housing, or day-care centers (Atchley et al., 1981). Therefore, we have adopted a family perspective throughout this chapter as a means of directing practitioners to focus on the relevancy of family systems to the provision of respite and adult-day-care services.

RESPITE CARE AS A SERVICE ALTERNATIVE

In the context of this chapter, the individuals who are unable to perform self-care tasks are elderly persons who are at-risk because they cannot be fully independent in the performance of important tasks. Estimates of the need for assistance among the elderly were gathered in the 1978 National Health Interview Survey. Limitations of task performance are associated with chronic conditions that increase as people age. Data from that survey indicated that the percentage of elderly individuals unable to carry on a major activity jumped from 14 percent among those age 65 to 74 to 31 percent for those age 85 and older. Between 21 and 24 percent of the population age 65 and older experience limitations in the amount and kind of major activities they can perform. Of those age 85 and older, 18 percent needed assistance to dress, 11 percent needed help to bathe, 7 percent needed aid to toilet, and 4 percent needed facilitation to eat (U.S. National Center for Health Statistics, 1978).

Branch and Jette (1983) noted that there continues to be a data gap on the role of the informal-support network to provide long-term-care assistance to the elderly. Much of the data available have been collected on hypothetical situations that do not indicate or measure actual support. In these studies, elderly people are asked where they would seek assistance if it was needed. Informal-network members are questioned about potential circumstances they have not encountered in the caregiving process. Clinical information is available from studies of operational networks performing tasks under specific conditions. An analysis of the need for respite is clearly understood in situations where family members are caring for Alzheimer's disease victims (Mace and Rabin, 1981; Silverstone and Kandel, 1982; Thorton and Fraser, 1982) and the mentally confused (Eisdorfer and Cohen, 1981).

Studies of actual caregiving in situations of major dependency contribute evidence for the need to structure and provide respite functions in a manner that meets the expectations of both the person who is needy and the helping-network members for whom temporary assistance is sought (Silverstone, 1982). Federal policy defines respite care as temporary services for an individual who is unable to care for himself on a full-time basis because of the absence of the person who typically cares for the individual (U.S. Congress, 1980). That limited definition should be expanded to include preventive concerns for the stresses of the caregiver. Respite care is not a single mode of care but an array of different patterns that will be explored in the following section.

Models of Respite Care

Gerontological practitioners often define the sources of respite care very narrowly or very loosely. The concept gets joined with very specific categories of special care arrangements now popular in England. For example, night care, weekend care, vacation care, and floating beds are approaches that are built into the approved use of institutional and quasi-institutional settings. They represent "bed-space strategies" that rely on out-of-home resources for respite care. Only limited use has been made of these strategies in the United States. The American planners' perceptions of what strategies to employ to provide relief for families from caregiving responsibilities are directly related to the scope or the sponsors of the services that fit into restrictive third-party cost regulations. We believe, however, that social-service providers should view respite as broadly defined and diversely provided for the aged. The most useful specification of respite-service alternatives that we identified emerged from the field of developmental disabilities in conjunction with family advocacy efforts. Kinney (1979) noted five models of respite care as potentially valuable to the parents of handicapped children. These models, with their various strengths and limitations, are all potentially applicable to some segment of the aged population requiring respite care:

1. *In-Home Respite Care.* Specifically trained respite providers (preferably persons who already know the family) go to the home while the primary caregiver(s) are away.
2. *Out-of-the-Home Respite Care.* The impaired person moves into the home of the respite provider, which serves as a temporary foster home.
3. *Respite Group Home.* The impaired person moves into a setting specif-

ically planned to be a respite facility for multiple persons who need respite care and is planned to approximate the permanent residential environment.

4. *Group-Home Respite.* The impaired person moves into a permanent residence group home that is equipped with the capacity to accommodate a short-term-stay person living in another permanent residence.

5. *Institutional Respite.* The impaired person moves into space designated for short-term respite use within a twenty-four-hour-care facility that is primarily devoted to ongoing institutional service to patients.

Table 20-1 presents the beginning of a typology that illustrates the variety of ways in which respite care can be organized and delivered for the elderly. Although the listing is not exhaustive, it should serve to increase awareness that repite care for elders is not an undimensional program, nor are all respite services the same. At present, none of these adaptations have been extensively implemented for the elderly. Nevertheless, communities and agencies have demonstrated definite interest in exploring their potentials.

In-Home Respite

Although there are similarities, the in-home respite arrangement should not be confused with an elder-companion service. Respite typically involves care for a length of time that exceeds the brief five-hour period that is available from companion services. Given the current limits of resources in most communities, the practitioner attempting to create respite alternatives may begin by contacting an agency that coordinates companion personnel or at least maintains a register of independent individuals available to provide such services. Examples of agencies where companions might be identified include home-health agencies, visiting-nurse services, and senior-citizen employment referrals. Through programs funded through ACTION, such as RSVP or Senior Companions, it is sometimes possible to identify older persons who will come to the home and provide care for another elder for up to a weekend period. Listings from home-health and in-home nursing-care agencies vary widely on such factors as (1) the extent to which the listing is current, (2) the types of situations acceptable to the person who comes into the home, (3) the references or other indicators of competency for the provider, (4) the geographcial area within which the provider is willing to travel, and (5) the liability or insurance arrangements. The positive features of in-home respite arrangements include a lower cost than other forms of respite, less disruption to the older person because he/she remains in his/her own surroundings, and more quickly arrangable than some other respite forms that require that space be available at the needed time. A negative feature of in-home respite is the discomfort that can be felt by both the aged person and

Table 20-1. Critical Characteristics of Respite Care for Elders: The Beginning of a Typology

Respite care characteristics	Alternative program approaches
Location	Respite care can be delivered either in the home of the elder or by transporting the elder to a location where respite care is available. *In-Home Respite Care* is when specially trained respite providers travel to the home of the elder to provide care. *Out-of-Home Respite Care* is characterized by three primary approaches: (1) a *Respite Home* is where the elder temporarily moves into the home of the respite care provider; (2) a *Respite Group Home* is a facility that can accommodate more than one elder at a time for respite care; and (3) *Institutional Respite* is where public and private institutions (e.g., hospitals or nursing homes) maintain a few beds that are used for respite care on a rotating basis.
Timing	The need for respite care is sometimes a consequence of an *emergency*. The primary caregiver may be suddenly hospitalized, incapacitated, or overwhelmed by a personal crisis and unable to meet the needs of the elder. At other times, the timing of the respite care may be *planned*. Plans for a necessary business trip, vacation, or visit to kin may be made well in advance and respite care arranged for the dependent elder.
Arranging for respite care	In many instances, the *family or primary caregiver* makes all of the necessary arrangements for respite care — identifying providers, checking references, arranging for transportation, and negotiating fees. In other cases, these details are handled by a formal *social-service agency*.
Service orientation	Most respite-care services are focused exclusively on providing for the physical, safety, and social needs of the elderly *individual*. Recently, however, there have been a growing number of services that use respite care as a vehicle for attending to the distinct needs of the entire *family*.

his or her family if the provider is a stranger. Also, unanticipated behavioral problems can arise because of a lack of familiarity between the individuals or with the caregiving procedures.

Little data is available regarding how families, independent of any agency assistance, find and utilize in-home respite providers. Some rely on the friendship network to identify help or turn to the church or similar organizations to find a reliable person (Rathbone-McCuan and Hashimi, 1982). Other families will utilize word-of-mouth or advertisements to generate a list of potential helpers. Still others will fulfill this need through their contacts with "caregiver support groups"—that is, self-help support groups formed by individuals who are the primary source of care for an elder. Many families, however, would not consider contacting a professional service to find a suitable individual or, if they did feel comfortable seeking professional help, would not know which agency within the community to contact to find assistance.

Out-of-Home Respite

The concept of a respite home may reflect many similarities to foster-home care for the elderly. It is a concept that has evolved in the care of handicapped children as part of the strong and widespread pattern of self-support among family groups, service-advocacy organizations, and citizen-participation mechanisms. It is considered to be a relatively inexpensive approach that can be modified during emergency periods of crisis or illness (Kinney, 1979). The highly organized parent and family networks that give support to this model of low-cost respite, however, do not necessarily characterize the informal support systems of the elderly. Thus the adaptation of this form of respite as a model for the elderly will require strong family-advocacy networks to sustain the volunteer respite resources. While such a self-helping cadre would be a desirable aspect of the informal community-resource network, the closest equivalent for elder respite would seem to be the foster-home approach.

Practitioners regularly mention the possibility of foster-home care as an alternative for homeless isolated older people or those being discharged from mental institutions. However, frequently there is less understanding of the potential of foster-home care as a type of respite. Often it is difficult to identify foster-home settings. Also, the methods used to select homes varies greatly among states. The invisibility of these resources to both families and practitioners is related to such factors as a confusion about how these facilities are classified, the extent to which they are uncoordinated with larger community-care information systems, and the regulations and standards that control them (Steinhauer, 1982). The respite home is a variation of the foster home because respite is not intended to be more than a brief-stay arrangement. Many foster-home care providers, in contrast, prefer that the residence and care arrangement be relatively stable. Therefore, these providers may not desire to use their homes as respite resources because payment/reimbursement would be less predictable.

If communities lack foster homes that are also willing to serve as respite placements, practitioners could initiate a development effort intended specifically to generate a list of foster-home selections exclusively for respite care. There are several values in developing such a list. First, communities could expand their resources for elders without competing for limited space in foster-home placements intended for longer stays. Second, more coordination of these facilities could be introduced as part of a respite-care resource pool instead of an alternative institutional-care directory. Lastly, it might be possible to coordinate some special training for those who provide only respite foster-home care as compared to longer placements.

Group-Home Respite

Some of the features of foster-home respite are similar to group-home respite. The group-home alternative has lagged behind other approaches in the evolution of noninstitutional alternatives for the aged. Realistically, there is too limited a supply of placement opportunities in geriatric group homes. There are few respite group homes that are designed to serve multiple elderly people living with family who need periods of respite support. The typical geriatric group home has no resources for taking a short-term-stay person. This is because of lack of space and/or skill to help a respite-stay elder integrate into the routine of other permanent residents in the setting. The options that are available tend to service the elderly who do not have a family-based support system. The expansion of the group-home model would seem to require more than the mere designation of a few existing group-home placements as reserved for respite. Also, the cost of a vacant space (i.e., a bed reserved for respite care but not in use—a circumstance that is not uncommon in respite systems) may be prohibitive to the overall operation of the facility. The program could be developed exclusively as a respite group home, but the logistics of financing and staffing such a facility would be difficult. In addition, unforeseen family needs to extend the respite period or the rapid decline of the health status of the elder beyond the ability of the prerespite situation to provide proper care could create major operational dilemmas.

Institutional Respite

Institution-based respite, utilizing existing long-term or acute-care hospital beds, has received considerable attention among professionals. Less effort has been expended in exploring the viability of adapting these types of inpatient facilities for respite functions that can be reimbursed through third-party sources. Most practitioners are acquainted with the undiscussed practice of admitting elderly people to acute-care hospitals for what is essentially a need of the family for respite. Often, family members and health professionals do not believe that this is the optimal means of offering respite, though it may be perceived as the only alternative available. Respite needs of this type frequently result from the failing health of the primary caregiver. The same situation may also produce an effort to provide short-term nursing-home placement. But in communities where there is a serious shortage of Medicaid nursing-home beds this alternative is often unavailable.

While there is a definite need to explore the feasibility of institution-based respite for the most impaired elderly, social-service practitioners must proceed with a full understanding of the disadvantages of this option. For many elders and their families, a short-stay institutional admission is unacceptable because it is perceived as contrary to their goal of preventing institutionalization. Furthermore, if there is no third-party reimbursement the cost of even a short stay can be a substantial burden on resources. However, the most important drawback to use of institutional respite is the potential negative effect on the aged person, who must endure a series of disruptions associated with entry and discharge. The personal and emotional difficulties of hospital or nursing-home admission are sufficiently great for the individual and family even when institutionalization is necessary. To promote this approach as an acceptable service manifestation of respite would be to move backward in the significant effort to minimize inappropriate institutionalization. At most, institutional respite is an option with limited potential.

Counseling as a Component of the Respite Process

Practitioners would benefit from envisioning respite as a multidimensional process that involves significant social-exchange efforts within the caregiving network and the management of diverse needs within the family system. The respite-service models briefly described above reflect only one dimension of the full respite process. Having a means for providing short-term relief from care duties is a necessary resource for families, but alone it is insufficient to accommodate the full range of ongoing support required by many families as they struggle with the long-term care of their elders. A respite-care service as outlined above is not intended to resolve interactional or resource problems within the family.

Additional services have been recommended as valuable to at-risk families caring for the elderly. For example, Archbold (1982) has suggested that stress-related health screening be available to the caregiver, that coping skills be fostered as part of the caregiving process, that accurate and comprehensive information on referrals be readily available, and that social and emotional support be extended. The National Supports Program, developed by the Community Service Society of New York, experimented with delivering minimal respite for elders for a few hours every month to allow caregivers time for themselves. That service, combined with education, information skills training, and some counseling, was useful to caregivers (Zimmer and Mellor, 1982).

Family therapy, either individual or groups of families, might also be added to the array of professional services that blend into those needs associated with respite. Problems such as coping with parental limitations, working with parental resistance, establishing expectations around caregiving and communication among the aged and younger family members are all situations that might be resolved through family therapy (Zarit, 1980). The Adult Counseling Center of the Andrus Gerontology Center has demonstrated the clinical value of developing groups for relatives of dependent older people. Participation in a time-limited, closed-membership group was offered to individuals who wanted assistance in dealing with older relatives. This method provided a means for resolving concerns about relocations, appropriate family caregiving roles, emotional reactions to caregiving, improving communication and conflict management skills, and mental and physical age changes (Hartford and Parsons, 1982).

Families always have the option of defining their own respite needs and locating appropriate resources to meet those needs without the involvement of a formal social-service agency. When families approach an agency for help in locating a source for respite, no other social services may be requested or required. When additional services are needed and sought by the family, short-term counseling to facilitate service selection and utilization may be appropriate. Research on the caregiving process repeatedly indicates that the kind and amount of support needed varies from case to case depending upon the degree of frailty of the elder, his or her level of independent functioning, and the number of people who comprise the caregiving network (Zimmer and Mellor, 1982). Practitioners need to be aware that counseling efforts can be directed toward assisting families to map their own service priorities as a function of their assessment of the support needed to continue to offer caregiving without undue and dangerous stress to the family. Even practitioners whose primary function is to provide therapeutic counseling should have a working and updated knowledge of community resources.

Respite Care in the Community-Service Context

A number of communities in the United States have been awarded federal funds to implement and evaluate community-care systems. Despite variations in the populations served, the affiliations of programs, the strategy for coordinating the services, and the funding base, there is a common philosophy to these programs that includes (1) promoting community and in-home care for as long as possible for those elders with disabilities, (2) coordinating health and social services, (3) some variation of a holistic approach, (4) overall systems planning, (5) stable and common funding, and (6) the availability of quality services within reasonable costs (Sklar and Zawadski, 1981). None of these projects was directly concerned with respite care per se, but each project experimented with the larger community-service structure. The National Long Term Care Channeling Demonstration Projects (U.S. Department of Health and Human Services, 1981), San Francisco's On Lok Senior Health Center (Zawadski, 1979), Connecticut's Triage Project (Hodgson and Quinn, 1980), New York's Monroe County Project Access (Eggert, Bowlyow and Nichols, 1980), Wisconsin's Community Care Organization (Applebaum, Seidl, and Austin, 1980), and Georgia's Alternative Health Service Project (Skellie, Mobley and Coan, 1982; Skellie and Coan, 1980) have each advanced our knowledge of the structure of coordinated community care. Unfortunately, many communities continue to lack highly developed noninstitutional long-term-care programs, case-management systems, or strategies for client assessment.

If these community-level, coordinating features are not present, the respite-care resources, if they exist, may function as yet another separate resource operating without integration into the larger service context. Any of the various respite models could be developed and managed as a single service; however, the overall impact of such an approach is considerably less than those respite services that are linked to at least some other services.

In-home respite-care services are less formal and smaller in scale than those requiring a specialized facility or some linkage with an acute-care hospital or a long-term-care facility. Nonprofessionals, indeed families, can assume a prominent role in the development and continuation of the less formal respite service. In contrast, professionals with more knowledge about geriatric-service planning are needed to join with the consumer sector to work toward the establishment of more bureaucratically connected respite services. The ultimate challenge for communities is to find a complementary role for practitioners to work with families to increase the availability of respite services and, when appropriate, to link such services to the emerging community-care systems that encompass and try to coordinate the resources necessary to maintain the elderly in community and home settings.

ADULT DAY CARE

The continuous evolution of geriatric day-care services, like home-health services, is being influenced by the current restrictive policy environment. The cost-benefit logic of long-term care may well be ignored in the survival efforts of the most established agencies to protect their existing services (Morris, 1980). A serious implication of these circumstances is that limited fiscal resources will be spent on continuously inflationary institutional chronic-care costs rather than being balanced with other community options. Adult day care is one of the many program alternatives that hold the potential for reducing the predicted rise in nursing-home expenditures from $16 billion in 1976 to a projected $76 billion in 1990 (U.S. Federal Council on Aging, 1981). Furthermore, adult day care is a service-delivery concept that can distribute the support needed by the elderly between the formal services in the community and the informal supports in the home.

The growth of adult day-care services has been slow but consistent over the past ten years. It has developed unevenly among the states, yet each year the place of adult day care in the long-term-care continuum has become more fixed. Programs that developed throughout the 1970s were largely the result of local initiatives. In spite of the silence of federal policies on adult day care, programs were launched and many have experienced significant expansions in their service capabilities because financial reimbursement was made available at the state level. Estimates of the magnitude of adult day care range from more than 600 programs serving approximately 13,500 elders (Robins, 1981) to more than 800 programs serving approximately 20,000 persons (National Institute on Adult Daycare, 1982).

The purpose of this section is to describe the concept of adult-day-care services, to discuss its programmatic characteristics and availability in America, to analyze successful approaches to incorporating such programs into the care plans of individual elders, and to establish adult day care as a viable option in the community. Since the beginning of the adult-day-care movement, social-work practitioners and nurses have played a very instrumental role in the planning and operation of these programs. New challenges will face all of the major professionals who in the coming years will act as providers of and advocates for adult day care.

Overview of Adult-Day-Care-Service Development

One of the persistent dilemmas faced by those who develop adult-day-care services is to formulate a definition of the service that can be useful in planning a program, developing policy, devising a reimbursement strategy, proposing regulations, and educating the community to the goals of the program. The difficulty in defining adult day care is a function of the extent to which the concept is flexible and, therefore, subject to programmatic variations. The lack of definitional uniformity has been a point of frustration to policymakers with responsibility for creating orderly rules and regulations and a point of stimulation for practitioners who have undertaken to design specific programs at the local level.

The most recent federal definition of adult day care was written by the U.S. Congress in 1980. U.S. Senate Bill 2809 defined adult day care as:

Services provided on a regular basis, but less than 24 hours per day, to an individual in a multi-purpose senior center, intermediate care facility, or agency for the handicapped or other facility licensed by the state, which are provided because such individual is unable to be left alone during the day time hours but does not require institutionalization. Such services may include (but not limited to) provision of meals, personal care, recreational and educational activities, physical and vocational rehabilitation, and health care services (U.S. Congress, 1980).

This particular definition attempts to specify the range of organizational settings where day-care services can be provided. (Organizational sponsorship is one aspect of adult day care that has major variation among programs.) Also, this definition makes the assumption that the person needing day care cannot be left alone, whereas other definitions merely suggest that the person would benefit from not being left alone in a residence.

An alternative definition, which seems to be more acceptable to many practitioners, was developed by the National Institute of Adult Daycare under the sponsorship of the National Council on the Aging. This umbrella definition emphasizes the service consistency that exists among programs. (These programs have very different labels but typically include certain general features.) The definition used by the National Council on the Aging is:

An adult day care program provides a gamut of services in a congregate setting, enhancing the daily lives of its participants and supporting their continued involvement in the community. Adult day care is a generic term that applies to a variety of programs offering services that range from active rehabilitation to social and health related care. Various terminology is applied: day care, day treatment, day health care, psychiatric day treatment, partial hospitalization, day hospital care, etc. Adult day care is coordinated with, and relates to, other agencies such as senior centers, in-home services, and institutional and hospital care. It is an innovative way to organize and blend traditional health and social services for disabled older persons (National Institute on Adult Daycare, 1982).

Both of the above definitions exclude a reference to adult-day-care services as an alternative to institutional care. The first definition indicates clearly that the services are provided to those who do not require institutionalization, whereas the second definition makes no mention of it. In addition, neither definition refers to the inclusion of family or caregivers as part of the clientele. The notable lack of reference to the service benefits of adult day care to the family suggests that traditionally these services are perceived as having major benefits for the individual. A definition of adult day care that specifically identifies the family as part of the client system is rare but has been suggested as an appropriate adjunct (Rathbone-McCuan, 1976; Weiler and Rathbone-McCuan, 1978).

There has been a tendency to categorize specific adult day-care programs according to the models that they most closely parallel on such factors as target population, sponsorship, and pattern of funding (Rathbone-McCuan and Elliott,

1976-77; Robins, 1981). A recent survey of existing or proposed adult-day-care standards reviewed data from thirty states. Two general types of programs were evident: (1) programs funded under Medicaid had a tendency to emphasize the delivery of medical and health services; and (2) programs funded under Title XX of the Social Security Act or Title III of the Older Americans Act tended to place greater emphasis on social services with complementary health-related services (Issacs, 1981). The 1980 Adult Day Care Directory classified programs into three broad clusters:

1. *Restoration Programs.* Those offering intensive health-supportive services prescribed in individual-care plans for each participant. Where prescribed, therapeutic services are provided on a one-to-one basis by certified specialists with constant health monitoring and provision of a therapeutic activities program.
2. *Maintenance Programs.* Those with the capability (in terms of health professionals on the staff and appropriate equipment) to carry out a care plan for each participant based on recommendations from the personal physician (or clinic) and developed by the multidisciplinary program team. Services provided include health monitoring, supervised therapeutic individual and group activities, and psychosocial services.
3. *Social Programs.* These show wide variations in nature and scope. Some social programs place great stress on health maintenance, with nursing services an integral part of the total program; other social programs create formal linkages with local clinics or health departments and transport participants to needed services; still others are concerned solely with socialization and lunches (Robins, 1981).

Day care first evolved as an alternative to mental hospitalization in Russia in the 1920s. Eventually the concept spread to this country and was used in programs for both the psychiatrically ill and the mentally retarded. The use of the concept in programs for the elderly took much longer to develop. Lionel Z. Cousin introduced the idea at the Oxford Hospitals in 1950, and a separate facility with its own staff was established in 1958 (Padula, 1981). The concept of day care for the elderly grew successfully in England as part of their effort to develop a comprehensive system of geriatric care (Farndale, 1961). It minimized institutionalization and coordinated and integrated hospital and community resources for the elderly (Brockelhurst, 1973). Two major themes dominated the early American debate about geriatric day care. First, whether or not adult day care was an alternative to institutional care (specifically nursing homes). This theme reflected the increasing recognition that the alarmingly escalating costs of nursing-home care in the late 1960s was going to continue unabated unless an alternative programming strategy established a different trend. Second, the assimilation process focused on whether adult day care was a cost-beneficial service. This theme was the result of trends in program-evaluation research to measure programmatic success on dollar-and-client-outcome ratio data. These two themes were closely tied to an overall question of whether third-party reimbursement coverage, especially Medicare, could be expanded to include repayment for adult-day-care services.

Federal policymakers were successful in creating research and demonstration projects focused on the effectiveness of adult day care. These demonstrations were authorized in the 1972 amendments to the Social Security Act (mainly through P.L. 92-603, Sec. 222), which granted permission for special waivers of standard Medicare coverage and, thus, afforded a means of covering the cost of services provided in select adult-day-care centers. The selected sites were included as part of the sample for federally sponsored randomized experiments to measure the effects and costs of day care and home-health services for the elderly (Weissert, 1976, 1977, 1978; Weissert, Wan, and Livieratos, 1980). The results of these studies were unfavorable and inhibited movement by the federal government toward routing Medicare coverage for adult day care. The results described adult-day-care services as an add-on cost and asserted that such services did not contribute significantly to patient functional abilities, patient contentment, or social-activity level. Numerous qualified researchers and practitioners have challenged the results of this study, have publicly demanded a reevaluation of the original data, and have produced detailed critiques of the methodological limitations of the study (Baker, 1980; Clauser, 1980; Klapfish, 1980; Shinn, 1980; Tufts and Hall, 1980; Weiler, 1980; Zawadski, 1980).

The battle that has been waged over the results of the day-care evaluation studies has slowed down the progress of obtaining third-party reimbursement coverage for adult-day-care services—except for the occasional program that has been able to obtain a "222 waiver" (referring to Section 222 of P.L. 92-603, which granted the original special waivers for coverage). However, this significant financial battle has not eliminated the expansion of day-care programs.

At the center of the debate generated by federal research and demonstration projects on day care are hard questions that preclude a simple approach to policy and reimbursement regulations. First, research on day care has promoted the "levels of care" mentality that divides medical care from all other forms of service. Information on day-care services consistently shows that health and social services are intermingled more consistently than in other long-term-care situations. Second, the pattern of day-care service utilization is an ongoing service support. Some individuals attend day-care programs for long periods of time. These clients show slow and small rehabilitative gains, but such types of progress are hard to measure in the context of short-term evaluations. A third feature of many successful day-care programs is the nontraditional setting and sponsorship, often lacking connection to a medical facility. These qualities or characteristics of day care deviate from other patterns of long-term care that are more medical or institutional in design. It is simpler to establish bed levels in a nursing home, where special units can have more or less nursing-service concentration, than in day-care programs, where more-impaired persons are integrated with those who have a higher functional ability. One of the particular advantages of a day-care program is that mixture of disabilities without visible labels attached to participants. The evolution of day-care staffing and administration/management has not consistently produced medical leadership. In many situations, physicians have a consultative role. The development of day-care programs outside of health-care settings is an important variation from other types of ambulatory services.

Designs of cost analysis for day care are fraught with problems about what to include for true costs and comparative costs. These research-method issues cut across much of the health-finance research (U.S. Health Care Financing Administration, 1982). A nursing-home cost is a per-diem unit that is fixed and easily measured, but day-care charges are not appropriate for the same approaches to cost calculation. Living in the community alone or with other people and using day-care services as one of possibly several supportive services entails actual costs for community living of a day-care client. Participation in day care does not remove community-living costs—elderly people do not live at centers but attend centers and live elsewhere. The Weissert final cost rate for day care was $52 per day, which was an average of four programs ranging from $18.54 to $88.17 per day; however, services in the four varied greatly. Klapfish (1980) challenged the Weissert cost data for failure to obtain additional cost information from other comparable programs. At that time, Massachusetts had forty-eight-day-health programs operating at an average all-inclusive cost of $22 to $25 per day, and similar cost figures were available from New Jersey, Washington, and California.

A more localized and within-state effort emerged both prior to and after the completion of the federally funded experiments. This alternative strategy for developing new service programs and policies reflected a national trend that emphasized noninstitutional, small-scale, and informal methods for meeting the needs of elders. Thus the developmental history of many of the adult-day-care programs now operating throughout the country represents planning within the community where the programs operate. These local initiatives have prompted state governments to support the delivery of day-care services through funding and the development of regulations, licensure, and policies.

The most up-to-date, readily available data on the status of adult day care was generated by Isaacs (1981) under the sponsorship of the National Institute on Adult Daycare. Table 20-2 provides a summary of funding information. Results of the Isaacs survey indicated that thirty-four of the fifty states (plus the District of Columbia and Puerto Rico) had established state-level standards for adult day care. Of the thirty-four with these standards, thirteen had standards for both funding and licensure certification, twelve had standards for funding only, eight had standards for licensure/certification, and one had standards for approval.

Table 20-2. Funding Sources for Adult Day Care among the Various States

Title XX Only	*Title III Only*
Alabama	Kentucky
Arkansas	Nevada
Hawaii	South Dakota
Idaho	
Louisiana	*Titles XIX, XX, and III*
Mississippi	Florida
North Carolina	Kansas
Oklahoma	Maryland
Rhode Island	Minnesota
South Carolina	Nebraska
Utah	New York
Puerto Rico	
Titles XIX, XX, III and XVIII	*Titles III and XVIII*
California	Missouri
Georgia	
State Only	*Private Funding Only*
Alaska	Montana
	Oregon
Title XIX Only	*Titles XX and III*
Colorado	Arizona
North Dakota	Delaware
	Illinois
Titles XIX and XX	Indiana
New Jersey	Iowa
Texas	Maine
Washington	Michigan
	New Hampshire
Titles XIX and III	New Mexico
District of Columbia	Ohio
Massachusetts	Pennsylvania
	Vermont
Titles XX and XVIII	Virginia
Connecticut	West Virginia
Tennessee	Wisconsin

Source: B. Issacs, *A description and analysis of adult day care standards in the U.S.* Unpublished monograph, National Council on the Aging, Washington, D.C., 1981.

The study found a great diversity in the standards that existed. Some states emphasized rehabilitative programs while others gave greater priority to maintenance or supportive services. The funding of programs was equally diverse. Funding from Titles XIX and XX of the Social Security Act and Title III of the Older Americans Act were and continue to be the major sources for programs. An array of other funding sources have been used to create or to continue adult-day-care centers combining a mix of local, public, private, and philanthropic resources. In addition, generous community support has contributed to the survival of some programs and the expansion of others. Volunteer efforts are another important contribution that is encompassed within the realm of local economic contributions.

Summary of Day-Care Services

Given considerable programmatic variations in the design and delivery of adult day care, it is difficult to articulate a core of services that should be included in such programs. Padula (1972) was the first practitioner in the United States to propose general program guidelines that went beyond the scope of a description of services provided in a single day-care center. Recently a new version of these guides was produced that reflects a decade of program development (Padula, 1983). Weiler and Rathbone-McCuan (1978) have provided detailed suggestions for the content of programs attached to public-health services and long-term-care institutions.

Presented below is a detailed checklist of services included in a very comprehensive adult-day-care program. This listing might serve as a useful tool for practitioners to assist elderly persons or concerned family members to choose a day-care service or to select from among several programs. The indicators are organized into eighteen program dimensions.

1. *Counseling*
   a. Is there counseling available to individuals and families?
   b. Are mental-health referrals and linkages readily available?
   c. Do program participants receive encouragement to discuss personal issues in a relaxed and informal context?
2. *Education*
   a. Have program staff received appropriate training to provide care to the mentally or physically impaired elderly?
   b. Are education programs made available to program participants in a stimulating and appropriate format?
   c. Does the day-care center serve as an educational training site for student or have a linkage with an educational program?
3. *Exercise*
   a. Is there adequate space for program participants to safely exercise?
   b. Is exercise a part of the daily program?

   c. Are appropriate devices and instructions available to program participants with special exercise needs or limitations?

4. *Group and Individual Activities*
   a. Are there a combination of both group and individual activities available for each program participant every day?
   b. Are group and individual activities recorded and monitored as part of an individual care plan?
   c. Are the special needs of each program participant recognized within the scope of group activities?

5. *Health Care*
   a. Is health-care provision a major goal of the program?
   b. What is the health-care expertise of the program staff or consultants?
   c. How are the health needs of individual program participants assessed?

6. *Health Screening*
   a. Is health screening required before an individual is accepted into the program?
   b. Is general health screening done at the program?
   c. Is there a policy for follow-up if health-screening results indicate the existence of a problem?

7. *Information and Referral*
   a. Is the program known to local information and referral services in the community?
   b. Are information and referral functions performed by the day-care-service staff for individual program participants?
   c. Are information and referral functions performed by the day-care-service staff for family member or other caregivers connected to individual program participants?

8. *Meals*
   a. Are there resources to provide for special diets?
   b. Do program participants enjoy the food served at meal times?
   c. Are meals and eating treated as a dignified personal and meaningful social activity?

9. *Medical and Social Evaluation*
   a. Is medical and social information required and/or gathered at the time of admission?
   b. Is evaluation information used for initial and ongoing individual-care planning?
   c. If requested, will important information be available to other agencies serving program participants?

10. *Occupational Therapy*
   a. Is occupational therapy available in the program?
   b. Is occupational therapy included in the assessment of the needs of the program participant at the times of admission and discharge?
   c. When appropriate, is occupational therapy introduced as part of the individual-care plan?

11. *Physical Therapy*
   a. Are there resources to provide physical therapy to program participants?
   b. Are the physical-therapy services integrated into a larger rehabilitation care plan?
   c. Are program staff skilled at dealing with the potential problems of program participant resistance?
12. *Reality Orientation*
   a. Is there a range of reality-orientation techniques that are used according to the individual needs of program participants?
   b. Are program staff trained to employ other complementary behavior-modification approaches as needed?
   c. Are program participants who do not need reality orientation given the option not to participate?
13. *Recreation*
   a. Is recreation conceived and offered as a special part of the daily program?
   b. Is recreation programming planned with the ongoing input of program participants?
   c. Are opportunities for recreational events available outside the day-care setting?
14. *Remotivation Therapy*
   a. Is motivation therapy offered in the program based on individual assessments of need?
   b. Does an atmosphere of general program-participant motivation dominate throughout the program?
   c. Are efforts made to have continuity of remotivation efforts supported in the program participant's residential environment?
15. *Speech Therapy*
   a. Is speech therapy available at the center from an appropriately trained person?
   b. Can speech-therapy consultation be used for program participants with special communication problems?
   c. Are program staff prepared to assist and provide consistent support of speech-improvement goals?
16. *Socialization*
   a. Are the socialization needs of a program participant objectively assessed at admission?
   b. Are the goals of socialization clearly distinct from recreation?
   c. Are the opportunities for socialization matched to individual backgrounds and preferences?
17. *Supervision*
   a. Is supervision available for program participants throughout the daily regime of the program?
   b. Does the program provide for an individualized plan of supervision

that varies according to the functional disability and specific daily program schedule of program participants?

c. Are all day-care staff and volunteers provided with some overall training and supervision related to their service?

18. Transportation

a. Is transportation a stable and dependable component of the day-care program?

b. Is there a means of accommodation for participants with special transport problems?

c. Are there consistent policies regarding a transportation emergency or breakdown?

As more day-care programs have reached a point where there are some special state regulations that control or at least guide the staffing pattern, it is possible to identify a typical staffing with qualifications. Table 20-3 is adapted from the Isaacs (1981) study overviewing day care.

It is also advisable for a practitioner to know whether a particular day-care center conforms to the standards or regulations that may be established within the individual state. It should be a matter of public record whether or not a program is in violation of a standard. Practitioners should also acquire information regarding the cost of programs and their methods of payment, medical and emergency hospital backup, and policies on participant absenteeism due to illness or hospitalization. How much information practitioners must have about individual day-care programs depends largely on their roles and responsibilities. At one extreme, the practitioner may be a source of information and referral to older persons and their families, while at the other extreme the practitioner may administer a day-care program or be in charge of its social-services component. The greater the administrative or direct-service responsibility, in either a planning or management capacity, the more important it is to have first-hand knowledge about the day-care-service concept and the programs that are in operation.

The administrative responsibilities for day-care-program operation vary according to the structure of the individual program, organizational sponsorship, community resources, state licensure requirements, and participant and staff composition. Numerous differences in the administrative roles and functions are present at different stages of program development. At the onset of a program, the person may have few tasks and responsibilities that are not traditional administration because program development means community development. The amount of community-development work required depends on whether or not other day-care programs operate in the area. Briefly, resource development is the key factor in the early stages, and resource maintenance is certainly central once a program is operating. Prevailing conditions such as the numerous changes and cuts in third-party reimbursement, competition for private contributions, reduction of grant money, and economic hardships among

Table 20-3. Day-Care Staff Qualifications

Staff	Qualifications	Functions
Activity/recreational specialist	Training in therapeutic recreation and one or more years in an adult social or recreational program.	Plans leisure events, works with residents in planning and preparing for events, conducts socialization groups, and designs individual plans for participants with special needs.
Social worker	Training at master's level and one or more years of work experience, preferably with programs for disabled and elderly.	Does in-home assessments; participates in the admission and treatment planning; may do individual, group, or family counseling as well as case management and possible program administration.
Program nurse	A registered nurse with current state licensing and at least one year of experience in a health-care setting.	Evaluates intake health data, plans health-care component of individual's plan, does treatments and medication supervision, may do health education, and connects with physicians as well as program administration.
Medical consultant	Licensed to practice medicine by the state.	Reviews adequacy of medical data at intake and may consult participant's physician; reviews policy and procedures in the program; may do staff consultation and provide emergency medical backup as required.
Rehabilitative therapist	A bachelor's degree from an accredited program and licensed, registered, or certified in accordance with state standards.	Does individual assessment and treatment planning and implements the therapy; does preventive work in group programs and may work with families to handle special in-home needs.
Dietary aide	Training in food handling and one year experience in meal preparation and serving.	Does meal planning, reviews special diets, involves participants in nutrition interests, and may prepare and or coordinate food service.

Source: B. Issacs, *A description and analysis of adult day care standards in the U.S.* Unpublished monograph, National Council on the Aging, Washington, D.C., 1981.

participants and families demand that administrators keep a program economically stable. In some instances, administrators are having to work double time to keep their programs operational.

A decade ago, developing a day-care program was little short of an adventure into the outer limits of community long-term care. The first centers that were planned and operated in the United States were stimulated, as well as burdened, by their reputation as innovative programs. Those who worked in the field of day care then, as now, must believe in the process of experimentation, critical evaluation, modification, and reevaluation. The presence of high-quality clinical and administrative evaluation and the commitment to share results through publications and professional meetings characterized the efforts of people associated with the Burke Rehabilitation Center in White Plains, New York, On Lok Senior Health Center in San Francisco, California, the Lexington Adult Day Health Program in Lexington, Kentucky, and the Levindale Day Treatment Center in Baltimore, Maryland. The staffs of these programs demonstrated willingness to speak and write in professional arenas about the possibilities of day care as an innovative concept; their activity helped to initiate the day-care movement.

The tradition of information sharing continues to operate in the 1980s. Many states now have adult-day-care associations that provide meeting grounds for professionals, advocates, and concerned citizens. These associations have been a critical force in stimulating state legislation and regulation. They have also served to establish a better linkage within communities and regions between adult-day-care programs and other services in the long-term-care network. As state associations developed, their leadership felt the need to formulate a national vehicle for information exchange and adult-day-care-center advocacy. The National Council on the Aging emerged as the organization capable and willing to become the focal point for integrating national efforts and facilitating communication among state associations and individual programs. As an organization, it has sponsored the preparation and distribution of the most recent handbook on day-care programming.

In the opinion of these authors, any group wanting to plan a program should make a complete study of the existing knowledge base about day care. A variety of data about the experiences of other groups is useful in the planning of an adult-day-care center. Information is readily available through state associations and the National Institute on Adult Daycare. In addition, the annual meeting of the National Council on Aging (Washington, D.C.) provides a major program commitment to issues relevant to adult day care. Furthermore, it is the role and responsibility of the National Institute on Adult Daycare to be the captial-based legislative advocacy group for this particular long-term-care service.

FUTURE DIRECTIONS OF RESPITE AND DAY-CARE SERVICES

The concept of adult-day-care services captured the attention of the aging-service network and the long-term-care provider system in the 1970s. While the definition of the concept deemphasizes the respite component, that component should not be overlooked. Nevertheless, day-care services are therapeutic, supportive, and rehabilitative for the aged person. Focus on the elderly participant should remain the major thrust of programs. Future directions to expand and strength both services should include a reexamination of the potential of planned complementarity between day-care and respite services.

Research on the role of informal networks in the provision of services to the elderly indicates that numerous sociological, economic, psychological, and residential variables influence elder support (Coward, 1982). These variables must be examined with an eye toward developing a dynamic equilibrium between direct services to the elderly person and support to the family.

Coward (1982) strongly cautioned practitioners and policymakers to avoid overlooking some of the negative and detrimental forces of informal networks in the lives of the elderly. Families can be the information brokers for the elderly and distribute misinformation with an array of negative outcomes, reinforcing unhealthy practices and encouraging destructive behaviors even though they are involved with the best intentions. The presence of a supportive network may delay access to formal or professional services because the network is trusted, judged adequate, and available. Coward's (1982) analysis to the illusion of coping within the network is an issue of major importance in day-care and respite-service delivery. Families vary in their ability to tolerate stress, judge the existence of pressure and tensions in the network, and find solutions to problems. Both respite services and day-care facilities can be of immediate value to adult children who are overburdened in caregiving, aged spouses who also need assistance, and nonfamily members who want to be involved but share responsibilities with formal organizations. A frequently forgotten component of respite and day-care programming is the appropriate interface between the formal and informal sources of support.

It would seem that the staffs of adult-day-care centers are in an excellent position to maintain a continuous communication with family members because of their frequent contact with them. Center staff may be better able to detect the family's need for respite care than the family members themselves. The primary informal caregivers of the estimated 20,000 aged who participate in day-care programs are among a very fortunate minority. Those families at least have the possibility of forming close linkages with professional service providers who daily share their concerns about the well-being of aged persons. This generalization may also be extended to the families of elderly people who receive home-health care.

Professionals in the field of aging are now campaigning for an end to the neglect of the needs of family members who provide care for elders. It is rather clear that any program for the frail elderly that offers services to assure continued home-based living cannot ignore the prominent role of families. The existence of family does not preclude the possibility of isolation among the aged (Rathbone-McCuan and Hashimi, 1982); indeed, the family can be a deterrent to effective coping (Coward, 1982). However, a recognition of the role of families does offer the possibility of applying a systems definition to the boundaries of the "life-in-community" of the older client. From the perspective of family systems, it is possible to both assess and intervene within the family context when warranted (Rathbone-McCuan, 1985).

How the future needs for respite among the informal caregivers of the elderly will be influenced by the continual increase of adult-day-care services remains an unanswered question. Unless the number of adult-day-care centers in the United States is expanded to the point where they number in the thousands rather than hundreds, it is assistance to a very small proportion of those who are in need of respite. The concern for family respite, however, is probably a necessary but insufficient reason to make an all-out commitment to develop a national policy and reimbursement mechanism for adult day care. The motivation to rectify the neglect of adult day-care-service expansion in this country must emerge because of a greater appreciation of the needs of elders. But as adult day care becomes more prevalent so does the possibility of its capacity to help fill the gap created by undeveloped family respite options.

REFERENCES

Applebaum, R., Seidl, F. W., and Austin, C. D. (1980). The Wisconsin community care organization: Preliminary findings form the Milwaukee experiment. *Gerontologist,* **20**(3), 350-355.

Archbold, P. G. (1982). All-consuming activity: The family as caregiver. *Generations,* **6**(2), 12-13.

Atchley, R. B., Sklar, B. W., Weismehl, R., and Kerschner, P. A. (1981). A symposium: The family and long term care. *Generations,* **5**(3), 10-13.

Baker, J. A. (1980). Critique of the Weissert study. *Home Health Care Services Quarterly,* **1**(3), 114-121.

Branch, L. G., and Jette, A. M. (1983). Elders' use of informal long-term care assistance. *Gerontologist,* **23**(1), 51-56.

Brockelhurst, J. C. (1973). Geriatric services and the day hospital. In J. C. Brockelhurst (Ed.), *Textbook of geriatric medicine and gerontology.* Edinburgh: Churchill Livingstone.

Clauser, S. B. (1980). Comments on the 222 adult day care and homemaker service experiments. *Home Health Care Services Quarterly,* **1**(3), 103-106.

Coward, R. T. (1982). Cautions about the role of natural helping networks in programs of the rural elderly. In N. Stinnett et al. (Eds.), *Family strengths 4: Positive support systems.* Lincoln: University of Nebraska Press.

Eggert, G. M., Bowlyow, J. E., and Nichols, C. W. (1980). Gaining control of the long term care system: First returns from the Access experiments. *Gerontologist,* **20**(3), 356-363.

Eisdorfer, C., and Cohen, D. (1981). Management of the patient and family coping with dementing illness. *Journal of Family Practice,* **12**(5), 831-837.

Farndale, J. (1961). *The day hospital movement in Great Britain.* New York: Pergamon.

Froland, C. (1980). Formal and informal care: Discontinuities in a continuum. *Social Service Review,* **54**(4), 572-587.

Hartford, M. E., and Parsons, R. (1982). Groups with relatives of dependent older adults. *Gerontologist,* **22**(4), 394-398.

Hodgson, J. H., and Quinn, J. L. (1980). The impact of the Triage health care delivery system on client morale, independent living and the cost of care. *Gerontologist,* **20**(3), 364-371.

Issacs, B. (1981). *A description and analysis of adult day care standards in the United States.* Unpublished research report for the National Council on the Aging, Washington.

Kinney, M. (1979). *A handbook for home-based services*. New York: Educational Resources Information Center.

Klapfish, A. (1980). Problems with the Weissert report's conclusions about adult day health services. *Home Health Care Services Quarterly*, **1**(3), 112-114.

Mace, N. L., and Rabin, P. V. (1981). *The 36-hour day: A family guide to caring for persons with Alzheimer's disease, related dementing illnesses, and memory loss in later life*. Baltimore: John Hopkins University Press.

Morris, R. (1980). Designing care for the long-term patient: How much change is necessary in the pattern of health provision? *American Journal of Public Health*, **70**(5), 471-472.

National Institute of Adult Daycare. (1982). *Why adult day care?* Washington: National Council on the Aging.

Padula, H. (1972). *Developing day care for older people*. Washington: National Council on the Aging.

Padula, H. (1981, March). Toward a useful definition of adult day care. *Hospital Progress*, pp. 42-45.

Padula, H. (1983). *Developing adult day care: An approach to maintaining independence for impaired older persons*. Washington: National Council on the Aging.

Rathbone-McCuan, E. (1976). Geriatric day care: A family perspective. *Gerontologist*, **16**(6), 517-521.

Rathbone-McCuan, E. (1985). Task-centered approach with older families. In A. E. Fortune (Ed.), *Task-centered practice with groups and families*. New York: Springer.

Rathbone-McCuan, E., and Elliott, M. W. (1976-77). Geriatric day care in theory and practice. *Social Work in Health Care*, **2**(2), 153-170.

Rathbone-McCuan, E., and Hashimi, J. (1982). *Isolated elders: Health and social intervention*. Rockville, Md.: Aspen Systems.

Robins, E. G. (1981). Adult day care: Growing fast but still for lucky few. *Generations*, **5**(3), 22-23.

Shinn, E. (1980). Critique of the Section 222 day care and homemaker experimental study. *Home Health Care Services Quarterly*, **1**(3), 99-103.

Silverstone, B. (1982, Summer) The effects on families of caring for impaired elderly in residence. *Benjamin Rose Institute Bulletin*, pp. 1-2.

Silverstone, B., and Kandel, H. (1982). *You and your aging parents* (2nd ed.). New York: Pantheon.

Skellie, F. A., and Coan, R. E. (1980). Community-based long-term care and mortality: Preliminary findings of Georgia's alternative health services project. *Gerontologist*, **20**(3), 372-379.

Skellie, F. A., Mobley, G. M., and Coan, R. E. (1982). Cost-effectiveness of community-based long-term care: Current findings of Georgia's alternative health services project. *American Journal of Public Health*, **72**(4), 353-358.

Sklar, B. W., and Zawadski, R. T. (1981). Comprehensive coordinated: Community-based care. *Generations*, **5**(3), 14-16.

Steinhauer, M. B. (1982). Geriatric foster care: A prototype design and implementation issues. *Gerontologist*, **22**(3), 293-300.

Thorton, S. M., and Fraser, V. (1982). *Understanding senility: A lay person's guide*. Buffalo: Potentials Development for Health and Aging Services.

Tufts, J., and Hall, H. D. (1980). Reactions to the Weissert report. *Home Health Care Services Quarterly*, **1**(3), 106-108.

U.S. Congress. Senate (1980). *Comprehensive community-based non-institutional long-term care services for the elderly and disabled* (Senate bill 2809). Washington: Government Printing Office.

U.S. Department of Health and Human Services. Office for Planning and Evaluation. (1981). National long term care channeling demonstration program. *Generations*, **5**(3), 30.

U.S. Federal Council on Aging. (1981). *The need for long term care: Information and issues*. Washington: U.S. Department of Health and Human Services.

U.S. Health Care Financing Administration. (1982). *Research and demonstrations in health care financing 1980-1981*. Baltimore: U.S. Health Care Financing Administration.

U.S. National Center for Health Statistics. (1978). *1978 national health interview survey*. Unpublished data, Washington.

Weiler, P. G. (1980). Response to the study, "Effects and costs of day care and homemaker services for the chronically ill: A randomized experiment." *Home Health Care Services Quarterly,* **1**(3), 97-99.

Weiler, P. G., and Rathbone-McCuan, E. (1978). *Adult day care: Community work with the elderly.* New York: Springer.

Weissert, W. G. (1976). Two models of geriatric day care: Findings from a comparative study. *Gerontologist,* **16**(5), 420-427.

Weissert, W. G. (1977). Adult day care programs in the United States: Current research projects and a survey of 10 centers. *Public Health Reports,* **92**(1), 49-56.

Weissert, W. G. (1978). Costs of adult day care: A comparison to nursing homes. *Inquiry,* **15**(1), 10-19.

Weissert, W. G., Wan, T. T. H., and Livieratos, B. B. (1980). *Effects and costs of day care and homemaker services for the chronically ill: A randomized experiment.* Hyattsville, Md.: U.S. Department of Health, Education and Welfare.

Zarit, S. H. (1980). *Aging and mental disorders: Psychological approaches to assessment and treatment.* New York: Free Press.

Zawadski, R. T. (1979). *On Lok senior health services: Toward a continuum of care.* San Francisco: On Lok Senior Health Services.

Zawadski, R. T. (1980). Methodological constraints of the Medicare 222 day care/homemaker demonstration project. *Home Health Care Services Quarterly,* **1**(3), 109-112.

Zimmer, A. H., and Mellor, M. J. (1982). The role of the family in long term home health care. *Pride Institute Journal of Long Term Home Health Care,* **1**(2), 20-25.

21

Protective Services

Elias S. Cohen, J.D., M.P.A.

Community Services Institute, Narberth, Pa.

Improvements in mortality rates have brought about an unprecedented blessing of very old age on large numbers of people. The blessing is not unmixed. The increase has brought with it an ever-increasing number of very old people who are unable to protect themselves, unable to give effect to their choices and their preferences, and—for reasons of physical impairment, mental impairment, severe social and environmental obstacles, or poverty—who are at risk or potential risk of serious harm. Although we can trace the historical antecendents of adult protective services all the way back to the fourteenth century,[1] it is largely within the last twenty years that adult protective services, and particularly protective services for the elderly, have received specific attention. Since 1963, scholars and practitioners have wrestled with definitions of protective services that attempted to define them in terms of the characteristics of the recipients of the services, in terms of the nature of the service, or in terms of the objectives the services were intended to achieve. Those definitions are not always helpful because they encompass too much and confuse *protective services* with the broad array of social services in general. Nonetheless, those early definitions are useful because they explicate the intent, the techniques, the populations, and the kinds of services that are frequently called into play.

In addition to these early definitions, more recent attempts have been made in such volumes as *Protective Services for Adults*, a 1982 publication of the U.S. Department of Health and Human Services, and in various state statutes that have established protective services by law. The following definitions are drawn from materials presented in *Protective Services for Adults:*

1. The federal definition set forth in 45 CFR 222.73 pursuant to Title XX of the Social Security Act:

Protective services means a system of services (including medical and legal services which are incidental to the service plan) which are utilized to assist seriously impaired eligible individuals who, because of mental or physical dysfunction, are unable to manage their resources, carry out the activities of daily living, or protect themselves from neglect or hazardous situations without assistance from others and have no one available who is willing and able to assist them responsibly.

2. The Administration on Aging, in a "Guide on Protective Services for Older Persons," set forth in an appendix to *Protective Services for Adults* defines protective services as follows:

Protective service is a social service with medical and legal aspects provided to an older person, who, as a result of physical or mental dysfunction (or both), abuse, neglect or extreme social or economic need is at risk of harm to self or to others. The purpose of protective services is to protect that older person from such harm, by stabilizing his (or her) situation in order to maintain him in the least restrictive setting, or by providing institutional care where it is needed. Community protective service involves case work services and occasionally medical and legal intervention. Medical interventions are needed to identify the type and severity of functional disability and abuse and neglect (physical, emotional, mental). Legal interventions to protect the individual's money or his person may be required when the older individual appears unable or incompetent to use judgement or unable to make decisions for himself. These legal procedures may include conservatorship, guardianship, admission to a chronic care institution or commitment to a mental institution in the case of a seriously mentally impaired individual. Such legal procedures are necessary to authorize Protective Service intervention when an older person is unable or incompetent to authorize or consent to protective service intervention himself.

3. New York State offers the following definition:

Protective services for adults is a system of care which includes the availability of a constellation of services bearing individually or in concert upon a problem situation of an adult requiring a planned approach of intervention. As a preventive, supportive and surrogate service, it is aimed at maintaining individuals in the community as long as feasible rather than institutionalizing them, though, in some cases, the latter may be necessary. More specifically it can be stated that a protective service system aims at the prevention, reduction or elimination of neglect, exploitation or crisis breakdown through the provision of services appropriate to the individual's needs which will strengthen his capacity to function and maximize his ability at self direction.

Most such definitions, however, are either so broad as to include virtually all medical and social services or so narrow as to include only services brought into being through the use of formal judicial interventions. In fact, most social, medical, psychiatric, and legal services may be regarded as "protective services" since an individual may require them in order to avoid extraordinary vulnerability. On the other hand, to suggest that protective services are those that come into being in conjunction with, or immediately following, judicial intervention is to avoid an important middle ground that both law and practice envision.

It is the premise of this chapter that protective services are those that are invoked or that accompany as a natural result the alteration in legal relationships undertaken to protect and preserve the best interests of the adult individual, including the interests associated with self-determination.

This definition admits to the array of services under the rubric of *protective services* any and all of the traditional social services provided to adults, *provided that these services emerge following recognition and action on the recognition that an individual's decision-making power has been altered through legal means by the individual himself or by judicial intervention.* Similarly, it excludes from the definition all those services that may in some way "protect" or "serve" the best interest of the client" without any deliberate effort or action to alter legal relationships. Furthermore, the definition encompasses a wide array of legal devices ranging from those that are "preventive" in nature and entirely under the control of the adult individual to those that are involuntary, massively intrusive, and involve entirely the judgments of others that an individual is incompetent and unable to make decisions for himself/herself. Thus protective services may include assisting an individual to understand and execute a power of attorney (including a "durable power"), establishing a trust for oneself, assisting the attorney-in-fact with providing certain services or amenities, doing the same for a trustee, on up to petitioning for guardianship, conducting the investigation, responding to requests for assistance in dealing with an alleged incompetent, assisting a guardian, assisting an alleged incompetent to secure representation, and many other activities. The common thread in all these services is the alteration of legal relationships that, in some way, permits — on a temporary and revocable basis or on a more "permanent" court basis — the transfer of the client's decision-making power to another person or persons.

Critical to the definition is the notion that the interests to be served are first and foremost those of the client, subject only to the limitations customarily invoked in the exercise of the police power to protect individuals from their own actions. These limitations do not usually justify intervention to protect individuals from their own willful, rationally arrived at, though foolish decisions. The right to folly is reasonably well preserved in both law and, hopefully, the philosophy of protective services.[2] It is too often honored in the breach — a breach more difficult to close than usual because it derives, in general, from beneficent motives.

LEGAL STATUS AND THE RIGHT TO BE PROTECTED

Given a definition that has at its heart the alteration, voluntarily or otherwise, of legal relationships, the question of *legal status* is an important consideration.

The legal status of elderly people is determined by a great many things. First and foremost, however, is the status conferred by having reached adulthood, however defined and for whatever purposes.[3] In addition to status achieved through adulthood, older individuals also receive special status as taxpayers; Supplemental Security Income beneficiaries; social-services beneficiaries: users of public transportation, social services, educational and recreational programs; renters or home owners; and workers. Furthermore, "old age" may grant special protection, and hence special status, relative to mandatory retirement or other discrimination in employment based on age.These special statuses all give rise to interests to be protected. In addition to these interests that grow out of age, there are the usual interests that grow out of adulthood, namely, the interests arising from our status as parties to contracts, as renters, home owners, taxpayers, citizens, residents of particular jurisdictions, and so on.

On the other hand, there are some "negative" statuses that may be conferred by law (however wrongheaded they may be) and that are of significance here because they frequently concern the basis for invading the rights of older people. There continue to be, in too many states, definitions contained in statutes setting forth standards for determination of incompetency that incorporate negative stereotypes of old age. Just a few of these might be cited here (emphases added):

Incapacitated person means any person who is impaired by reason of *advanced age* . . . to the extent that he lacks sufficient understanding or capacity to make or communicate responsible decisions concerning his person (Arizona Rev. Stat. 14-5101).

An "incompetent" . . . is a person who is incapable by reason of . . . *senility* . . . *old age*, or other incapacity, of either managing his property or caring for himself or both (Indiana Stat. Ann. 29-1-13-1(c)(2)).

"Person of unsound mind" means . . . one whose mind, because of . . . *old age* has become imbecile or unsound as to render him incompetent to manage his estate (Kentucky Rev. Stat. Ann. 387.010).

A guardian may be appointed for . . . any person who, by reason of extreme *old age* . . . is mentally incompetent to have the charge and management of his property (Nebraska Rev. Stat. 38-201).

The Supreme Court and the County Courts outside the City of New York have jurisdiction over the custody of a person or his property, if he is incompetent to manage himself or his affairs by reason of *age* . . . (New York Standard Civil Practice Service—Mental Hygiene 78.01).

WHAT ARE THE INTERESTS TO BE PROTECTED?

Virtually all the interests to be protected can be grouped under the overarching interests of the older individual, indeed of all adults, in maintaining and

maximizing autonomy—the exercise of self-determination, of making preferences and choices operational, of controlling one's destiny and fate in both
short- and long-range time frames. This translates into choosing where and how
one lives, where and how one eats, imbibes, dresses, recreates, associates, votes,
contracts, maintains personal hygiene, withholds or gives consent for medical
procedures, and otherwise engages with (or without) the rest of society.

Related to the interests of autonomy are the interests associated with property,
currently or potentially available, that may give meaning to those interests
associated with autonomy and the exercise of free choice. Thus an interest in a
potential money benefit is an interest to be protected since it may give rise to the
exercise of more choice if secured than if not.

One interest deserves special mention because of the frequency with which it
appears to arise, its apparent relationship to the rights of privacy arising from the
Fourth Amendment, and the very recent emergence of "recognition" of this
interest—namely, the interest or right to be left alone. This interest will be
discussed in greater detail below in the so called "right to die" cases or similar
situations like *Northern v. State.*[4]

Interest analysis is crucial in any approach to protective services, whether
theoretical or clinical. Key questions to be raised *always* are:

What interests are involved?
Whose interests are involved?
What limitations are being considered for which party?
Whose autonomy is being limited?
Who will bear the burden if particular remedies are imposed?
Who will bear the burdens if the remedies are not imposed?

It is out of this kind of interest analysis that the paradox and dilemma of
protective services arises, particularly for social workers. The paradox in which
the social worker finds himself/herself is: How can limitations on free choice in
decision making increase the range of autonomy for the objective of the
protective service? Viewed obversely, the question becomes: If no benefits
accrue to the increased autonomy of the individual, what justification exists for
limiting freedom and autonomy?

TYPICAL LIFE SITUATIONS APPEARING TO CALL FOR PROTECTIVE SERVICES

There is an array of older people—whose numbers are increasing at a
furious pace—for whom protective services appear to be required:

The old man with a severely impaired memory who can't recall what he did
with his funds, where his money comes from, what amount he gets, or

what he has spent it for. He manages somehow to have a little bit of food in the cupboard. He sometimes forgets to cash checks or spend money, and at other times spends it foolishly and comes down to the end of the month without enough to provide himself with food. Somehow neighbors and a few friends step in, although he lives on the verge of starving, suffers leg ulcers and may be filthy and bewildered.

The old man or lady constantly moving from place to place, unable to stay rooted very long, frequently without funds.

The wanderers, street people, "vent men," bag ladies, and others who have no permanent living quarters but who use bus stations and other public places in which to live.

The dischargee from the mental hospital, disoriented as to time and place, living in a boarding home, foraging for scraps in garbage cans, wandering in the street, shouting obscenities, dressing bizarrely, and appearing to neglect himself/herself.

The bedridden, crippled, or arthritic individual dwelling in a building he/she owns that is full of rubbish and infested with vermin, refusing hospitalization for treatment of infection, seclusive and fearful.

The recluse living in an apartment using a portable kerosene heater and a hot plate for cooking, living in filth and regarded as something of a danger because he or she set a fire accidentally nine months before while cooking a meal.

The mildly forgetful, physically well busybody who is intrusive, garrulous, mildly paranoid, an unabashed beggar, often demanding food or money, living in his or her own home that is packed with the "treasures" accumulated over the years including both valuable paper ephemera as well as collections of old milk bottles (now grown valuable) and pure unmitigated junk that represents a horrendous fire hazard.

The 55-year-old mentally retarded individual never adjudged incompetent and, in fact, never institutionalized. Such individuals may have lived with parents all their lives and may find that they are alone following the death of parents and in possession of very considerable amounts of property.

The neatly dressed old man in good shape physically but forgetful and confused who continues to operate a small neighborhood store with his business affairs hopelessly tangled. He may be heavily in debt, but his entire life is wrapped up in his business. He is without known relatives or friends to whom he can turn.

The proud and independent old lady in imminent danger of sustaining serious personal injury by reason of her infirmity who refuses to consider leaving her home and who will not accept any help in the home.[5]

These are the people into whose lives social workers may be called upon to intervene. They may be well-to-do or they may be poor. They may be alone or they may have family. They may be wise or they may be foolish. And they may or may not meet the tests the law prescribes for incompetency.

HISTORICAL LEGAL ANTECEDENTS OF PROTECTIVE SERVICES

The legal antecedents of protective services are to be found in the laws and decisions concerning the mentally ill. The historical evolution has moved from the seizure of the individual who was "furiously mad" in order to protect the public to protection of the individual himself and subsequently his estate. In more recent years, courts have modified the powers of the state to intervene and have imposed (or relaxed) strictures concerning the need for and meaning of informed consent, while legislatures have been busy tinkering with the uniform probate code, with durable-power-of attorney statutes, and with natural-death or right-to-die acts. Protective services have their roots both in the police power (narrowly construed) and in the state's power as *parens patriae*.

Under the police power, the state has authority to confine dangerous individuals so that the health and safety of others may be protected. The most familiar exercise of this power is under the criminal law. However, in some instances, as in the exercise of mental-health commitment laws, the police power may be exercised to commit to mental institutions individuals who are dangerous to others and who are, by reason of mental illness, unable to control their activities.

However, where the harm that the individual might visit is not upon others but rather upon himself or herself, the power the state exercises is that of *parens patriae*. It grows out of the notion that the sovereign, as the political father and guardian of the kingdom, has a special obligation to care for those who, because of their lack of mental capacity, are unable to take care of themselves.[6]

An 1845 Massachusetts Supreme Judicial Court decision in *Re Josiah Oakes*[7] blended the police and *parens patriae* powers. Josiah Oakes, it was alleged, was mentally deranged, the evidence of which was that he had become engaged to a young woman of questionable character shortly after the death of his wife. There was no indication in the report of the case that he was violent and it wasn't clear whether his involuntary confinement was for his benefit or for the safety of the community. Nonetheless, it represents the earliest case in which involuntary confinement was used to justify therapeutic benefit for the patient as well as a measure to protect the safety of the community.[8]

There is now little question that states have the power to confine mentally ill or mentally retarded persons for therapeutic purposes, although that power has been moderated somewhat to require that, if individuals aren't confined to protect the public or to protect themselves, then they must be confined for therapeutic purposes (*O'Connor v. Donaldson*[9]). The ruling in this case is a far cry from a right to treatment. The court held only that a nondangerous patient was entitled to release if he received no treatment.

Courts have not been imaginative in dealing with the issues presented by protective services. It is only recently that some states have begun to develop specific statutory bases for intervening in cases of vulnerable, potentially incompetent individuals in ways that will not necessarily and inevitably lead to the violent act of imposing a guardianship—violent because it strips an individual of his personhood in virtually every relevant facet of his life.

Protective services, as we are beginning to know them, are a recent phenomenon for a variety of reasons. It is less than half a century since the Social Security Act radically altered the way in which vulnerable people in society were provided for. Prior to 1935, "indoor relief" was a common mode of care. The idiot, the insane, the derelict, the alcoholic, the ne'er-do-well, the unemployed, and the inadequate were housed together in the county home or almshouse. The Social Security Act made clear that the preferred method of "treatment" was to provide economic relief in the community. Federal relief was not available for those in institutions. This beginning was following some thirty years later by the so-called Services Amendments added to the Social Security Act in the 1960s that made further provision for the delivery of a wide variety of social services to past, present, and potential dependents. At that point, the federal government reimbursed the state for 75 percent of expenditures for services in behalf of such persons. The appropriation was open-ended. In the late 1960s the Community Mental Health Act reinforced that declaration with the development of community mental-health centers. It was no accident that the National Council on Aging, the American Public Welfare Association, and other organizations began to look at the issue of protective services in a serious way.[10]

The issue, however, was not informed by very much research in the area. Alexander and Lewin's landmark study, *The Aged and the Need for Surrogate Management*,[11] pointed out that, in examining over 400 cases in which guardians were appointed for certain mental-hospital patients, not a single case could be found in which any benefit accrued to the incompetent person.

The U.S. Senate Special Committee on Aging commissioned a paper on protective services for the elderly by John J. Regan and Georgia Springer (1977). Once again, the issues were well explicated and an attempt was made to present a model guardianship, conservatorship, and power-of-attorney legislation.

That relatively little progress has been made is attested by the persistence of statutes and probate-court practices that make guardianship easy to obtain, make no provision for intermediate remedies, and provide minimal due-process protections for those who need help and assistance in altering legal relationships.

BASIC LEGAL CONCEPTS IN PROTECTIVE SERVICES

Underpinning any development of protective services are two fundamental concepts: First is the presumption of competence on the part of the impaired individual. To be sure, the presumption is a rebuttable one, but all efforts must be made to support the basic presumption. One must raise this presumption even for those who are uncommunicative and who appear not to understand or to be unresponsive. One must inquire whether they need an interlocutor because they are not conversant in English, may be hard of hearing, may suffer aphasia, or may not understand the questions being put. A presumption of competence requires an inquiry into a determination of precisely what areas of behavior are impaired and what areas are unimpaired. It requires a determination of those areas in which the individual can express or articulate preferences, choices, and wishes and whether the impairment is limited to the ability to give effect to those wishes. The bedridden patient who cannot visit a benefit office, who may not have a phone, who certainly can't go shopping, and who is utterly dependent on others is not necessarily incompetent. Incompetence is not synonymous with dependence. Quadriplegia renders one almost totally dependent but does not deprive one of competence.

The second legal concept crucial to protective services is the Doctrine of the Least Restrictive Alternative. The doctrine was perhaps best articulated in *Shelton v. Tucker*[12] as follows: "Even though the governmental purpose be legitimate and substantial, that purpose cannot be pursued by means that stifle fundamental personal liberties when the end can be more narrowly achieved. The breadth of legislative abridgement must be viewed in the light of less drastic means for achieving the same basic purpose." What this means in protective-services terms is that guardianship must not be imposed if conservatorship will do as well; a total guardianship must not be imposed if a limited guardianship will achieve the result; involuntary processes must not be used if such voluntary processes as the use of agency or power of attorney or a joint bank account or trusteeship will serve as well.[13]

The least-restrictive alternative has been most directly applied to the elderly in Judge David Bazelon's opinion in *Lake v. Cameron.*[14] While this was a commitment proceeding, the least-restrictive-alternative principles are well laid out. In this particular situation, Ms. Lake was detained as she was leaving a government building where she had gone to inquire about a tax matter. She appeared to be confused. She was taken into custody and subsequently committed to St. Elizabeth's Hospital. Judge Bazelon held that the presence of "mental illness" without more was insufficient to deny basic freedom rights to an individual. He pointed out that it was the way in which an individual functioned and the alternatives that would least impinge upon civil rights that mattered most. Thus, confronted with a petition for commitment to an institution, the court held that there must be an inquiry as to the possibility of employing less restrictive measures to compensate for the functional problems that were present.

As a matter of law, the Lake case has no real precedential value. It was grounded primarily in District of Columbia law and, while it has been cited as support for similar issues (deservedly so), it cannot really govern. There is little evidence that the kind of inquiry suggested by Judge Bazelon is routinely made.

And there is little to suggest that options for less-restrictive alternatives are presented to the court or that services in the community are ordered for the mentally impaired elderly.

In the Lake case, Judge Bazelon ordered the District of Columbia Department of Public Welfare to explore and secure less-restrictive alternative services (i.e., alternatives to commitment to St. Elizabeth's Hospital) in order to avoid institutionalization. The issue here was to find services that would help Ms. Lake with her shopping and activities of daily living in her home. While the decision and the decree were admirable, the results were less so. Ms. Lake ended her days in St. Elizabeth's Hospital because the District of Columbia could not fashion a program of less-restrictive alternatives for her. Among other things, the lesson here may be that the judicial forum, despite its power to issue orders and decrees, is very frequently at the mercy of the executive branch of government for implementation.

Of course, in addition to these less-restrictive-alternative considerations, it goes without any further explication that due-process protections normally available in criminal and involuntary commitment cases are no less important in involuntary protective-services proceedings.

Less fundamental, but no less important to the development of a gamut of protective legal devices ranging from voluntary and revocable transactions to involuntary transactions is an understanding of the law of agency. The law of agency does *not* govern what social agencies or organizations can or can't do, nor does it deal with such agencies' behavior. The law of agency concerns the duties, obligations and privileges that arise when one person, an *agent*, undertakes to carry out the orders of another, the *principal*. In such an arrangement, the agent, having agreed to the undertaking, agrees to carry it out and to exercise no more discretion and to do no more or less than the undertaking calls for (if possible). The principal will be liable for the acts of his/her agent carried out within the scope of the duty. A principal may change his/her mind at any point. The authority given to an agent is always revocable (except in a durable power of attorney as described below). The law of agency is the basis of all powers of attorney. It is a venerable doctrine of high utility in protective services that has not been utilized appropriately.

While there are some other legal concepts that come into play in the course of protective services (such as those embodied in the law of trusts), it is not necessary to review those here. Suffice to say that a starting point of presumptive competence, the knowledge and application of the doctrine of least-restrictive alternative, and some understanding of the law of agency will provide a basis for assisting in the resolution of the paradox of liberating through intrusion and may assist social workers as they attempt to understand the role they play in relationship to their clients and the duties they owe to the agencies for which they work.

LEGAL DEVICES FOR PROTECTIVE SERVICES

Voluntary Devices

Legal devices for protective services for adults are at an early stage of conceptual development, although the devices discussed here have, as noted, ancient origins. The adoption or rejection of any of them is predicated upon the employment of sensitive assessment mechanisms that take into account not only the psychological and physical capabilities of an individual but also his or her social situation and how he or she has been able to adapt to it. The question of which legal device to employ is not and cannot be a matter of precise formula or scoring system that produces a computerlike response. The legal devices noted below are nothing more than available patterns that social workers, together with lawyers, can utilize to tailor-make a solution for any given individual and any given set of problems.

Agency

Agency, as noted above, is the shorthand description for a relationship between a principal and an agent. Agents are utilized in those situations where the client is sufficiently well-oriented to be able to make choices, express preferences, and enjoy the benefits of a degree of autonomy. Agents can be advantageously utilized even where clients suffer a degree of impairment such that they may not be completely oriented to time, may suffer some short-term memory loss, and may even have some difficulty in managing money. Nonetheless, such a person might sincerely enjoy the utility of an agent if one were provided. An agent might help the client pay his bills, deposit his funds in the bank, and assist in many ways in giving effect to the client's preferences and wishes. One analogy might be that of a beneficent son or daughter, son-in-law or daughter-in-law, brother or sister who has undertaken to assist a relative whose powers are somewhat diminished but who, nonetheless, has preferences, expresses them, and needs help in bringing those preferences to fruition.

An agent is something more than an informal helper and something different from a friend who drops in occasionally and gives the client a ride to the senior citizens center. An agent is one who owes a fiduciary duty to the client. He is bound to carry out his or her principal's instructions and exercises judgment only to the extent that the principal has delegated such power to the agent. This authority is spelled out in some detail in writing. The written instrument is called a power of attorney. Control of the scope and duration of the relationship is squarely in the hands of the principal. It is not unusual for some impaired persons to terminate agency relationships with some degree of frequency, especially if the impairment is accompanied by even a mild paranoia. That a principal may change his or her mind with what may be maddening frequency is not necessarily an indication that the principal is too demented to utilize an agent. It may be an indication of fickleness, frustration over the loss of capabilities, or one of the last gestures of authority that a diminished older person can exercise. Agents are, after all, agents. They are not "friends," they are not "relations," and they are not "angels of mercy." Their function is to proceed at the direction of their principal and to give effect to his/her preferences and decisions.

"Agents" have not yet found their way into the array of social services. There are a few very limited experiments and demonstrations utilizing agents in the way described here. Some Senior Companion Services and RSVP programs have made some attempt at this, and there is at least one demonstration program funded by the Administration on Aging through a grant to the South Orange, New Jersey, section of the National Council of Jewish Women. Beyond that, however, social agencies, Area Agencies on Aging, and other organizations that serve older people must fashion and train (not to mention provide legal, medical, psychiatric, and social-work back-up to) their own cadres of agents.

Power of Attorney

A power of attorney is a legal instrument through which a principal grants power to an agent to act for him or her. Powers of attorney may be very broad and general and provide for the agent to buy and sell property, make investments, enter into contracts, receive and disburse funds, sue, receive service in suit, defend the principal, and expend funds in either suit or defense thereof, and otherwise act for the principal. On the other hand, the power of attorney may be extraordinarily narrow, authorizing the agent only to expend funds from the principal's bank account for the sole purpose of paying the principal's rent, which shall not exceed for example $227.50 per month. Powers of attorney are what we give to stockbrokers who execute orders on our behalf, real-estate agents who undertake to sell our homes, and attorneys-at-law who undertake to represent us. Many people execute a power of attorney when they are going into a hospital or when they take a vacation out of the country where they may not be reached easily in the event that their business or personal affairs require some immediate action.

A power of attorney is revocable at will by the principal. As long as it is not revoked, it is said to be renewed at each and every moment that the principal has the capacity to renew it. This represents a serious limitation on the use of the ordinary power of attorney. If, for example, a principal is ill and slips into a coma, the power of attorney he executed would automatically expire and would be invalid while he was in that coma. Similarly, if a power of attorney were executed and the principal became incompetent, or so demented that he could not properly extend the power to his attorney-in-fact (the term used for an agent named in a power-of-attorney instrument), the power of attorney would automatically expire. There has now developed in a majority of the states a device intended to overcome this problem. It is commonly known as a "durable power of attorney." A durable power of attorney is a special instrument, authorized by state statute, that permits a power of attorney to endure beyond the incapacity of the maker or grantor of the power. Depending upon the particular state law, a durable power of attorney must declare the intent of the maker of the power for it to endure beyond his incapacity, may require special witnessing or notarization of signatures, may require that the attorney-in-fact be a relative of the maker of the power, and may have other special requirements. In many ways, the durable power of attorney is a major breakthrough in what we might call "preventative protective services." In a manner of speaking, it permits an individual while still competent to select someone to manage his affairs at some future time when he (the principal) is no longer able to do so. In some ways, it is almost like selecting one's own guardian. If the durable power of attorney is sufficiently broad, it can cover virtually all eventualities.

Joint Bank Accounts

Another method of determining in advance who will have control over liquid financial assets is through joint bank and stock accounts or other jointly held property in which either party is permitted to deposit, withdraw, expend, invest, or liquidate accounts, funds, securities, and real or personal property jointly held. This, like the power of attorney, permits an individual to make plans in advance of incapacity so that funds can be managed. It provides, however, only for management of property and, unlike the power of attorney, does not permit application for public or private benefits that might accrue, as for example through public or private pension plans, disability plans, and similar matters.

Trusts

A trust is a legal device whereby an individual (technically known as the settlor) transfers title of property to another, known as the trustee, for the explicit purpose or purposes of being used for the benefit of a beneficiary. The beneficiary may be the settlor himself and the trust may be limited to particular purposes. The beneficiary may be one or more persons and the settlor may designate residual beneficiaries who will acquire an active interest in the trust upon the death of the named primary beneficiary(ies). Beneficiaries can be named to enjoy benefits during their lifetimes or for a term of years (or months). Trusts can be created that are either revocable or irrevocable. The trustee is bound to carry out the terms of the trust, and the trust can be enforced through state courts. Trustees can be surcharged for mismanagement, and they are bound to a high-level duty to manage the property in the way that the settlor intended. Here again is a device that can be used by an individual or individuals to provide for the management of property in advance of incapacity. Trusts can be established that will become effective upon the occurrence of a certain event, such as a determination of incapacity. Trusts may be formed during an individual's lifetime or may be established upon death as a part of the devolution of one's estate. That is to say, one may leave a portion of one's estate to a trust to be administered by a trustee for the benefit of one or more beneficiaries.

Involuntary Devices

The preceding devices are those that one would term "voluntary." All require action and volitional expression by a competent adult. With the exception of the irrevocable trust, the individual maintains absolute control and can withdraw any powers or participation that he or she may have authorized or entered into. The two following devices, conservatorship and guardianship, are, for the most part, involuntary. In some states that provide for conservatorships, there may be provision for application for a conservator by an individual himself. This, however, is rare, and accordingly conservatorship and guardianship are treated here as involuntary devices.

Conservatorship

Conservatorship is generally a procedure that is involuntary, involving a petition to a court, an investigation, a hearing, and a court finding. Conservators are appointed by the court, typically (but not always) to manage the estate (i.e., the property) of the conservatee. Conservatorships do not typically require a finding of incompetency. That is generally said to be the value of a conservatorship. Being a device that manages only the property, it leaves the conservatee's control of his or her person in tact. Conservatorships, however, have left unanswered in too many instances questions of who determines where the conservatee lives, what control a conservatee may have over any allowance he or she may receive, what control a conservatee may have over wages or salary earned, and similar matters.

Recognizing the importance of being able to tailor-make protective arrangements, the California legislature modified the California probate code to provide for conservatorships that do, in fact, take account of the variations that may arise between and among people with different disabilities. In California, conservators may be appointed for both the person or for the estate. The state's probate code provides for appointment of a conservator of the person for one "who is unable properly to provide for his or her personal needs for physical health, food, clothing, or shelter" (Sec. 1801). A conservator of the estate may be appointed for a person who is substantially unable to manage his or her own financial resources or resist fraud or undue influence. The statute also provides that substantial inability may not be proved by isolated incidents of negligence or improvidence (Sec. 1802).

Most important, however, for our purposes are the explicit provisions that address the rights that a conservatee may retain. The new probate code provides that the court may limit the powers of the conservator and reserve those powers to the conservatee. The court may do so in accordance with the capacity and abilities of the conservatee (Sec. 2351). The court may grant the conservatee certain explicit rights (Sec. 1873). And the statute explicitly grants the conservatee the right to control an allowance or any wages or salary, the right to make a will, and the right to enter into transactions to provide necessaries. It is possible, under the California statute, for the conservatee to retain powers to grant or withhold informed consent for medical treatment if the court so finds (Sec. 1880). The appointment of a conservator does not affect the right to marry *ipso facto*. The right to marry is determined independently of whether a conservator was appointed or not; the law that would apply would be that which is applied to the validity of all marriages. And finally, a conservatee may retain the right to vote if the court does not determine that he or she is unable to complete the necessary affidavit for voting.

Conservatorship in the California context attempts to provide surrogate authority that comports with the doctrine of least-restrictive alternative. It provides safeguards through court investigation, court follow-up, and court review. The statute, however, is nothing more than the legal framework on which social services must be placed in order to achieve the hoped-for results for the individual, namely, assistance with the management of one's property and personal affairs in a way that maximizes autonomy and free choice and minimizes the frustrations imposed by physical or mental disability.

Guardianship

Guardianship is the most intrusive of the so-called protective services. It is the ultimate exercise of *parens patriae* powers. Guardianship follows a finding of incompetency and effectively replaces the personhood of the incompetent with that of the guardian. The ward (i.e., the incompetent) is bereft of virtually all rights. He or she cannot vote, drive, marry, contract, sue or be sued, or manage his or her affairs in any way. He or she is not entitled to manage any allowance, cannot give or withhold informed consent for medical treatment, and may not be able to resist "voluntary" admission to a mental hospital, nursing home, or other institution where such arrangements have been made by the guardian.

In some jurisdictions, provision has been made for the office of public guardian. The public guardian is a public official who is named as the guardian for persons found to be incompetent who do not have sufficient estates to pay for the services of a private guardian. Public guardians tend to have bureaucratized offices with assignments of wards to staff on a caseload basis. Caseloads are typically in excess of forty or fifty wards per staff member, a level that makes it impossible for the fiduciary duty of the guardian to be carried out. Wards thus tend to be neglected. No satisfactory system of oversight for public guardians has yet been designed and, for the most part, offices of public guardians rely on institutionalization and more restrictive measures of intervention rather than less.

THE ROLE OF SOCIAL WORKERS AND LAWYERS IN PROTECTIVE SERVICES

Protective-services cases begin with the identification of a problem by family members, friends, neighbors, police, landlords, physicians, emergency-room personnel, or social-service personnel from within or outside the agency.

Too often, the life situation presented is one that has persisted for a long time and where, at the point of reporting, perhaps the life and certainly the well-being of the prospective protective-services client is severely threatened.

The nature of the problem that protective-services clients present typically calls into question the safety of an at-risk individual unless some intervention in his or her life is undertaken. The intervention may be of a medical nature, of a housing nature, of an institutional nature, or some other control over the autonomous conduct of the individual, since it is the autonomous conduct (or the absence of help in the case of someone who is physically or mentally impaired) that has created the risk. This places into conflict the values of safety and freedom.

It is the resolution of that conflict that requires substantial judgment. In an excellent guide series, "Improving Protective Services for Older Americans," published recently by the Center for Research and Advanced Study of the University of Southern Maine, Mary Collins offered a heirarchy of "solutions":

Freedom is more important than safety; safety at home with informal support is preferable to safety with formal interventions; safety with formal kinds of help is preferable to involuntary care; involuntary care in the least restrictive setting with specified time limits and restrictions are preferable to full guardianship or institutional placement. Thus, workers should strive to assist people with their safety and care needs without disrupting their lifestyle or removing their freedom of choice.

If you cannot provide safety in appropriate care at home, you should seek the least restrictive alternative. The formulation suggests the disruption of lifestyle is *more* important than *level* of care.

Marginal help near the home may be far better than sophisticated care far away. Likewise, freedom of choice is more important than safety, except possibly when involuntarily ordered medical treatment has a high probability of restoring the person to health and safety.

The worst possible outcome is one in which the person is made safe but suffers total loss of freedom and maximum lifestyle disruption. This is the case when a public guardian places a person in a distant nursing home or institution.

Within this generalized framework, the social worker is frequently the key "manager" who is expected to do something about the "problem." The process is essentially a four-stage one: The first stage is problem identification. Problem identification breaks down into two parts: First, is this a *prima facie* protective-services case? And second, what is the precise nature of the problem?

The second stage is the stage of solution identification, which is further broken down into the following questions:

What legal relationship appears to be most appropriate in terms of the strengths, capacities, incapacities, and disabilities of the client?

What social, medical, legal, or other services represent specific remedies to meet the precise problems identified in the first stage?

What outcomes are anticipated if the social, medical, legal, and other services are made available for the client, and what time frames can be postulated for the achievement of those goals?

The identification of solutions is further informed by an understanding of the client's desires and preferences, the conflict between safety and freedom, and judgment as to what represents the best interests of the client.

The third stage involves program delivery. Protective-services cases frequently require the aggregation of a variety of services coming from different agencies, organizations, and formal and informal resources, each with a different funding stream and frequently with different eligibility requirements. In this respect, protective-services delivery is little different from the delivery of services for elderly long-term-care patients who, more often than not, present clusters of problems served by different categorical agencies with differing eligibility and funding characteristics.

The final stage is that of assessment to determine whether problems were correctly identified, solutions correctly identified and applied, and hoped-for goals achieved. The assessment process is also utilized to determine the extent to which change has occurred in the life situation, introducing new or modified problems that require adjustment in solutions identified and programs enlisted.

In terms of casework services and case-management services, protective services for the elderly are distinguished by the issue of legal relationships and the resolution of the freedom/safety conflict. The case-management or service-provision model is essentially a common one.

Because assessment of the problem is at the heart of this process, some aids and examples are provided here.

Assessment in protective-services situations is frequently difficult. The prospective client may be uncommunicative, fearful, debilitated, and in need of emergency services. The protective-services worker must develop for himself/ herself criteria that make very clear imminent danger to the safety of the individual or to others. If the individual is completely debilitated, demented, lying in filth, etc., emergency intervention procedures are apparently justified. The situation becomes difficult when, despite apparent dementia and filth, the individual has some ability to get along and wants no part of any intervention. Different jurisdictions make different provisions for emergency detention of mentally deranged individuals. These detentions should be known and sparingly used, but where the emergency is palpable and the danger imminent, workers should not and need not shrink from some form of emergency detention, followed up swiftly with a determination of what less-restrictive alternatives might be available. For those situations that are not urgent, it is important to focus on behavior; the person's wants and preferences; the strengths available through the individual, his family, neighborhood, friends, and other possible supports; and the potential resources that might be available to ameliorate the situation.

Figures 21-1 and 21-2 are two assessment forms, one developed by the Connecticut Department of Social Services and the other by the New York City Human Resources Administration (Project Focus). The Project Focus form is preliminary and has not yet been thoroughly tested and validated. Nonetheless, it is offered here as the result of careful study.[15]

Obviously, the assessment of the potential protective-services client may involve other disciplines, including medicine, psychology, and possibly law.

Where the conclusion is that the problem is not a *prima facie* protective-services case, that is, where no effort will be made to affect legal relationships, the case should no longer be dealt with as a protective-services case. This is not to say that counseling; supportive efforts; the furnishing of homemaker service, chore service, medical service, and housing assistance; or a host of other services should not go forward. It is only to say that protective-services units should not be cluttered up with situations that are service cases for older individuals.

Dealing with the protective-services client calls into conflict the roles that social workers may have identified with. Social workers at one and the same time may find themselves serving as a client's advocate, "protecting his rights," and respecting his or her wishes and preferences. On the other hand, the worker may also be making judgments about what is "in the best interest of the client" and may actively pursue legal interventions that may severely limit the client's range of choices and freedoms. The activity may well represent directions to which the client is opposed. The social worker, for better or for worse, is *not* the client's agent. The social worker may seek involuntary, coercive procedures through judicial intervention that the client may perceive as adverse to his or her interests.

Sometimes, in order to gain access or to obtain consent, social workers may utilize what has been called "authoritative casework" or "professional authority." Caseworkers may "bargain" or use moral persuasion where possible. There are, of course, ethical and legal limits. Workers may seek to persuade but must avoid coerciveness. Workers may seek to assist in management but must avoid decision making. Covert manipulation is to be avoided, and professional authority can never be used to violate civil rights or to act against demonstrated or known wishes. Full disclosure of the worker's activities in behalf of a client should always be made, and the client should provide, at the very least, tacit permission.

There are few formulas for proceeding in many of these difficult cases.[16]

SPECIAL ISSUES

Special issues that should be dealt with include clients who are abused, violent, or whose condition requires emergency intervention. Each of these situations is intimately entwined with legal considerations. How and when to intervene as well as who can intervene are frequently spelled out in statutes dealing with emergency detention, emergency commitment, and temporary detention. Each of these situations has a common thread in the need for emergency action. To be prepared for such eventualities, workers should determine what the law is in their respective jurisdictions, who has the authority to intervene, the nature of the information that must be filed and where it must be filed for emergency intervention, and the most effective ways of securing that intervention. Knowing the law and the procedures, however, is probably not enough. Arrangements should be made in advance through contact with mental-health authorities, Area Agencies on Aging, and the police in order to get to know the personnel involved, what material and information they need, and what is the best way to secure a result.

At the same time, social workers must be cognizant of the extraordinary potential for invasion of clients' civil rights and ought to be prepared to take steps to assure that those civil rights are protected either through location of counsel or some sort of advocate. In some jurisdictions, public defenders are responsible for representing persons confronted with civil commitment, while in other jurisdictions it may fall to community legal services, legal-aid societies, or some element of the private bar. In any event, this area needs coverage as well.

In working with attorneys, keep in mind that they are accustomed to viewing problems of all sorts in a highly structured fashion. In seeking help or advice from an attorney, it is useful to formulate for yourself in advance what you see as the problem or problems and what you believe the remedies are for those particular problems. Lawyers will want to know as precisely as possible what the issues are that the protective-services worker can deal with, what services will right the wrong the client is confronting, who has the resources or authority to deliver what is necessary to right the wrong, and what special attributes of the client may give rise to an entitlement. The lawyer's contribution may take the form of designing a strategy to secure that which is necessary. It must also be clear to the lawyer whom he is representing. The lawyer's advocacy is total. If he is representing the client, he will view the situation through the client's eyes and will look on every effort at restricting the client's freedom of choice in an adversarial way. If he is the social agency's attorney, he will view the situation from the standpoint of the duties and obligations that the agency owes the client, the local, state, or federal agency that provides it money to do certain things, and so on.

The relationship with the courts can be facilitated through a similar understanding of the court's role and range of activity. In protective services, courts play several roles. In the first instance they may be asked to decide upon the competency of an individual or the need for intervention on an emergency or conservatorship basis. While court proceedings are highly ritualistic and heavily surrounded with procedural requirements, they are nonetheless well equipped to decide questions on brief notice, provided they have adequate and sufficient information concisely presented, supported wherever possible by objective evidence. Judges and their clerks are more readily available than is commonly assumed. Protective-services workers above all should not be cowed by the mystique that surrounds the judicial process or the judicial persona. Where emergencies arise, a protective-services worker need not shrink from calling the judge's chambers and asking to speak to the judge's clerk. Good preparation in identifying the problem you wish to solve through judicial intervention, the remedy you are seeking from the court, and the justification for emergency will help immeasurably. Where no emergency exists, courts will appreciate clearly presented petitions outlining all the facts and subsequent support in a hearing by well-presented evidence. Court intervention is an extreme measure. Courts are increasingly disinclined to exercise their power in these situations unless the evidence is compelling. Given the array of legal devices that fall short of court intervention, recourse to the courts should be limited.

Finally, under the rubric of special issues, are those occasional cases that arise among clients who are ill and who refuse to give informed consent for life-saving measures. Where a client is competent and is aware of the consequences of his or her refusal to give informed consent, virtually all jurisdictions will honor that refusal and permit the patient to expire. The social worker's role in situations where the client is apparently aware of the consequences and is sufficiently well-oriented so that he or she can process the information being given to him or her is to support the client in his decision and protect him or her from what may be coercive, if beneficent, behavior on the part of physicians or other providers and to help him or her defend against an incompetency petition.

The more difficult cases are those where the client's orientation and awareness may be less apparent but where nonetheless the expressed wish to forgo treatment is consistent with values held when abilities were less diminished. Here the worker will have to be more sensitive and focus on the discovery and protection of values of individuals of declining or diminished capacity. This may require the search for a "prior explicit statement" by the patient before capacities were diminished or the explication of what Nancy Neveloff Dubler has termed the "sedimented life values of patients," those values being the ones that emerge through the fog of memory loss and even dementia and that are consistent with earlier behaviors, wishes, and preferences.[17]

A number of cases begin to explore the issue of competence and the right to die; knowledge of these cases will undoubtedly be useful to the protective-services worker who confronts such a situation.[18] The courts are stepping gingerly around this issue, which is truly a vexing one. Some are "pull the plug" cases like the Quinlan case, while others involve questions of third-party consents (i.e., consents by surrogates to terminate life-support systems; see *In Re Earl Spring*) or decisions to withhold treatment from retarded or severely demented patients (the *Saikewicz* and *Dinnerstein* cases). None, however, is more vexing than the case of Mary Northern, an elderly lady brought into a hospital against her wishes for treatment of a respiratory infection. Following her admission, it was discovered that her feet were frostbitten. Ms. Northern was advised that gangrene had set in and that if her legs were not amputated she would certainly die. Ms. Northern, who was well-oriented to time, place, and person, demurred. She protested that her legs were not that badly infected, that she knew they would get better, that she had no wish to die, and that the issue was not that she preferred dying to having her legs cut off. It was her firm position that there was nothing wrong with her legs. A petition was filed to have her found incompetent. Despite testimony by examining psychiatrists that she was not incompetent, a court found her to be so and appointed the superintendent of the hospital her guardian. There was additional testimony in this case that if her legs were not amputated she would have only a 10-percent chance of survival. There was further psychiatric testimony that if her legs *were* amputated, there was a 50-50 chance that she would retreat into a psychotic fugue from which she might never emerge. Within a space of two weeks, this case was heard by the Tennessee Supreme Court, which affirmed the decision of the lower court to appoint a guardian but which further required that no action be taken to amputate her legs unless two named physicians asserted that she was in imminent danger of death. In this case, the court appeared to waltz around the problem. Mary Northern was never operated on. She survived for some months after the decision and expired before any surgery took place. Some commentators have suggested that this case is a "right to be left alone case." It undoubtedly presents the most difficult kind of problem that social workers, attorneys, and courts can possibly confront.

FINDING SOLUTIONS

Problems that social workers have encountered in the protective-services arena grow largely out of the lack of clarity, the conflicts between safety and freedom, the ethical dilemmas involved in attempting to help but knowing that precious liberties may be eliminated, and an absence of proper and sufficient services to meet the needs of the physically and mentally impaired who may require what we have come to know as protective services. The solutions are both legislative and nonlegislative. Legislative solutions must be significant alteration of statutes defining incompetency and providing for the imposition of guardianships. John Reagan has outlined an agenda in this area.[19] He suggests first and foremost the narrowing of the criteria for determining incompetency so as to assure that the autonomy of alleged incompetents is maximized by determining whether or not an individual has any recognizable premise for his decisions and whether any reasonable purpose can lie behind the individual's decisions and behavior, however foolish they might appear. While this may appear extreme, given the tendency of courts to permit even single instances of irrational behavior to become the basis for findings of incompetency, modification of criteria in the direction suggested here may well be appropriate.

Second, he suggests requiring behavioral evidence of recent conduct exhibiting inability to manage one's affairs or to give direction to others to carry out that management and threatening vital personal interests. The causes of disability should be eliminated from any evidence since they are irrelevant to determining whether a person has the competence to act on his own behalf or whether his legal capacity should be transferred elsewhere.

Third, Reagan suggests that total guardianship be abolished and that all guardianships be tailor-made to the specific disabilities and impairments of the alleged incompetent. This would mean that all guardianships would be limited and specific and that powers not transferred to a guardian would reside with the ward.

Fourth, Reagan recommends the abolition of public guardianships precisely because they are nonresponsive and, more often than not, harmful to the individual.

And fifth, he recommends that procedural safeguards be assured particularly through the mandatory provision of counsel in all guardianship proceedings.

Provision for protective services and emergency intervention has been vexing state legislators throughout the country. Numerous provisions surface each year. One bill put before the Pennsylvania senate in 1983 is the result of several years' study by the state senate and others. It makes provision for emergency involuntary intervention, imposes obligation to report on findings, severely limits the interventions that courts can authorize, and provides for assuring due-process rights.

Although Reagan's recommendation to eliminate total guardianships would appear to cover the situations provided for by California's conservatorship statute, the steps taken by California appear to provide for some surrogate service without a finding of incompetence and to explicitly assure a number of civil rights to the conservatee. This section of California's probate code deserves attention by other jurisdictions.

While the majority of the states have enacted durable-power-of-attorney statutes, it is recommended that this provision become universal, particularly in the light of America's mobile elderly population and their migration to Sunbelt states.

Finally, protective services would be enhanced by the universal adoption by state legislatures of natural-death acts; only about a dozen states now have them. These acts provide for the filing of an instrument expressing the wish of the "testator" that, in the event of severe illness from which remission is not possible and where no therapeutic purpose can be served, no heroic measures to preserve, maintain, or extend life be taken. Such statutes also provide immunity for physicians and caregivers who fail to take such heroic measures.

Nonlegislative solutions necessarily include the revision of service systems so that services can be requisitioned by protective-services workers much as physicians requisition services in a hospital. This is not unlike the concept operationalized in the Channeling Project on Long Term Care and currently being demonstrated in sites around the country. Protective-services agencies frequently are unable to secure appropriate housing, counseling, homemaker services, chore services, money-management services, friend/advocates (agents), and similar accommodations for their clients. They are left in an impossible situation, attempting to protect the rights of their clients, avoiding excessive intervention, institutionalization, guardianships, or the like, and are utterly without the social-service resources necessary to give effect to the treatment of choice determined in an adequate assessment. Subsumed under that general heading of revised service systems, it is clear that mental-health systems that have traditionally been unresponsive to the needs of deranged, demented, and distressed elderly clients must revise their orientation, services, and relationships with other social agencies serving the elderly.

Finally, some provision must be made either through voluntary organizations or through public social services to develop a cadre of agents who can serve as friend/advocates for those elderly who require assistance to give effect to their wishes, decisions, and preferences.

NOTES

1. *De Praerogative Regis*, 17 Edward 2 c.9 (1324), established in statute law the duty of the sovereign as *parens patriae* to carry responsibility for protection and care of the person and property of mentally disabled people.
2. See, for example, *Bryden's Estate* 211 PA. 633, 636, 61 A. 250, 251 (1905), cited with approval in *Urquhart's Estate* 431 PA. 134, 245 A. 2d 141, 142 (1968) and *In Re Estate of Porter* 345 A. 2d 171, 173 (1975): "A man may do what he pleases with his personal estate during his life. He may beggar himself and his family if he chooses to commit such an act of folly."
3. Adulthood has various benchmarks depending upon context. It may be achieved at age 14 in some jurisdictions for determining contributory negligence, 16 for criminal responsiblity, 18 for voting, 21 for purchase of alcoholic beverages, or no chronological age at all for consent to abortion in the case of a pregnant female.
4. 575 S.W. 2d 8946 (Tenn. 1978).
5. This list of cases draws heavily (although not entirely) from L. Bennett, "Protective Services for the Aged," in Pennsylvania Conference on Protective Services for Older People, 1964, *Proceedings* (Harrisburg: Pennsylvania Citizens Council, Commission on Aging, 1965).
6. L. Shelford, *A Practical Treatise of the Law Concerning Lunatics, Idiots and Persons of Unsound Mind* (London: S. Sweet, 1833).
7. 8 Law Reporter 122 (Mass. 1845).
8. For a fuller discussion of guardianship and *parens patriae*, see P. M. Horstman, "Protective Services for the Elderly: The Limits of Parens Patriae," 40 *Missouri Law Review* 215 (1975).
9. 95 S.Ct. 2486 (1975).
10. See Seminar on Protective Services for Older People, Arden House, 1963, *Proceedings* (New York: National Council on the Aging, 1964); National Council on the Aging, *Guardianship and Protective Services for Older People* (New York: NCOA Press, 1963).
11. G. J. Alexander and T. H. D. Lewin, *The Aged and the Need for Surrogate Management* (Syracuse: Syracuse University, 1972).
12. 364 U.S. 479, 488 (1960).
13. For a fuller discussion of the least-restrictive-alternative doctrine, see D. L. Chambers, "Alternatives to Civil Commitment of the Mentally Ill: Practical Guides and Constitutional Imperatives," 70 *Michigan Law Review* 1108 (1972). Chambers's discussion of the application in a variety of contexts is important because it imparts historical legitimacy to the concept. From the standpoint of legal argument this may be significant in some courts.
14. 364 F 2nd, 657D.C. Circ. (1966).
15. For fuller explication of the Project Focus material, see S. Daiches, *Risk Assessment: A Guide for Adult Protective Services Workers* (New York: New York City Human Resources Administration, 1983) and S. Daiches, *Protective Services Risk Assessment: A New Approach to Screening Adult Clients* (New York: New York City Human Resources Administration, 1983).
16. An excellent review of protective-services-worker roles and relationships with courts can be found in *Guide on Improving Protective Services for Older Americans: Social Worker Role* (Portland: University of Southern Maine, 1982).
17. Outline by Nancy Neveloff Dubler distributed at a seminar entitled Legal and Ethical Aspects of Health Care for the Elderly sponsored by the American Society of Law and Medicine, Washington, 1983.
18. Important right-to-die cases include: *In Re Quinlan* 70 N.Y. 10, 335 A. 2d 647 (1976): *In Re Earl Spring* 405 N.E. 2d 115 (1980); *Superintendent of Belchertown State School v. Saikewicz* 373 MASS. 728, 370 N.E. 2d 417 (1977); *In Re Dinnerstein* 380 N.E. 2d 134 (Mass. App. 1978): *In Re Eichner* (Brother Fox) Ct. of App. 52 N.Y. 2d 363, 420 N.E. 2d 64, 438 N.Y.C., 2d 266 (1981); *Northern v. State* 575 S.W. 2d 8946 (Tenn. 1978).
19. J. Reagan, "Adult Protective Services: An Appraisal and a Prospectus," in National Law and Social Work Seminar, Improving Protective Services for Older Americans, *Proceedings and Prospectus* (Portland, Me., 1982).

STATE OF CONNECTICUT DEPARTMENT OF SOCIAL SERVICES

Protective Services for the Elderly

CLIENT EVALUATION AND FUNCTIONING

Client's Name _____ Age _____ Sex _____

Client's Address _____ Race _____

PHYSICAL ENVIRONMENT

Neighborhood: _____

Shelter: Sound ____ Deteriorating ____ Dilapidated ____

Water ____ Electricity ____ Heat ____ Toilet ____

Food ____ Stove ____

Housekeeping: _____

Hazards _____

Other Observations _____

SOCIAL ENVIRONMENT

Isolated ____ Known & visited by neighbors _____

Relatives _____

Household Composition: _____

PERSONAL APPEARANCE

Dress: ____ Facial Expressions: _____

Gait: ____ Gestures _____

Posture ____ Speech _____

PHYSICAL HEALTH

Client-defined problems _____

(Indicate duration of problems.)

Malnourishment ____ Open sores _____

Lumps ____ Sudden weight loss _____

Persistent cough ____ Severe chest pain _____

Severe headaches ____ Shortness of breath _____

Vomiting ____ Change in bowel habits _____

Blood in urine ____ Vision impairment _____

Vaginal bleeding ____ Hearing impairment _____

Dizziness ____ Other _____

Most recent visit to a doctor _____

Next medical appointment _____

Recent medical problems _____

Medications _____

Comments _____

MENTAL HEALTH

Client-defined problems _____

(Indicate duration of problems.)

Loss of appetite ____ Delusions _____

Insomnia ____ Thought distortion _____

Loss of interest ____ Confusion _____

Hypochondria ____ Impaired judgment _____

Suspiciousness ____ Memory lapses/loss _____

Hallucinations ____ Orientation _____

Feelings of ____ Other _____

Worthlessness _____

Hazardous behaviors _____

Alcohol or other drug use _____

Recent losses of family or close friends _____

Past mental health problems _____

Capacity to consent _____

Other comments _____

CLIENT MOBILITY

Bedridden _____

Partially bedridden _____

Wheelchair _____

Housebound _____

Able to get to yard _____

Neighborhood _____

Public _____

transportation _____

Drives car _____

Other _____

Comments _____

PHYSICAL COMPETENCE

Feeds self _____

Bathes self _____

Dresses self _____

Uses toilet _____

Gets out of bed _____

Climbs stairs _____

Goes outdoors _____

Cooks _____

Shops _____

Light housework _____

Heavy housework _____

ECONOMIC SITUATION

Income ____ Resources _____

Expenses _____

Affairs managed by _____

Comments _____

Other helping persons or agencies involved (specify involvement): _____

Client's perception of problems: _____

Worker's perception of problems (specify nature of protective problem). _____

Recommended action: _____

Obstacles: Does client consent? _____

Is client's ability to consent questioned? _____

Other _____

EMERGENCY: _____

_____ Worker's Name

_____ Date Completed

I, _____, authorize the Department of Social Services to provide the services they may deem necessary to insure my safety. I agree to reimburse the Department if it is later determined that I am to pay for the services provided.

_____ _____ _____
Witness's Name Applicant's Name Date

Figure 21-1. Assessment form developed by the Connecticut Department of Social Services.

507

Client's name _____   Case number [_____]
Date _____

PROTECTIVE SERVICES RISK ASSESSMENT

SECTION I—ENDANGERING CONDITIONS
Instructions: Check all conditions known to be present, then rate the client on each dimension using the scales located along the right hand margin. If the client's life is not endangered on a given factor, circle "O - no life threat." If the set of conditions is immediately life threatening, circle "3 - immediate life threat." Note less hazardous conditions by circling "1" or "2."

RISK FACTORS

1. Neglect

   specify whether by:
   [ ] self
   [ ] other(s)
   [ ] both

   conditions include:
   [ ] dirt, fleas, lice on person
   [ ] skin rashes
   [ ] bedsores
   [ ] ulcerated sores
   [ ] malnourished or dehydrated
   [ ] doesn't get/take medications
   [ ] inadequate clothing
   [ ] fecal/urine smell
   [ ] untreated medical conditions
   [ ] other (specify)_____

   ```
   O.......1.......2.......3
   no life       immediate
   threat        life threat
   ```

2. Abuse

   [ ] words or gestures that put client in
        fear of harm
   [ ] multiple or severe bruises or burns
   [ ] restrained, tied, swaddled, locked in
   [ ] broken bones or wounds
   [ ] rope marks
   [ ] injuries in odd places
   [ ] injuries at several stages of healing
   [ ] other (specify) _____

   ```
   O.......1.......2.......3
   no life       immediate
   threat        life threat
   ```

3. Self endangering behaviors

   [ ] suicidal acts
   [ ] wandering
   [ ] frequenting dangerous place (specify)

   [ ] life threatening behaviors (specify)
        _____

   [ ] refuses medical treatment
   [ ] other (specify) _____

   ```
   O.......1.......2.......3
   no life       immediate
   threat        life threat
   ```

Figure 21-2. Assessment form developed by the New York City Human Resources Administration (Project Focus).

-2-

4. Environmental hazards

[ ] homeless
[ ] no toilet facilities
[ ] no food storage facilities
[ ] no heat
[ ] animal-infested living quarters
[ ] other utilities lacking
[ ] other poor housing condition (specify)

[ ] threatening weather condition (specify)

[ ] other (specify) _____

```
0.......1........2.......3
no life         immediate
threat          life threat
```

5. Intellectual impairments

[ ] faulty reasoning
[ ] can't follow instructions
[ ] incoherent speech
[ ] inappropriate or no response
[ ] disoriented to time and place
[ ] confusion
[ ] memory failure
[ ] loses things constantly
[ ] other (specify) _____

```
0.......1........2.......3
no life         immediate
threat          life threat
```

6. Exploitation

[ ] extortion
[ ] parasitic relationship
[ ] unexplained disappearance of funds or valuables
[ ] servitude
[ ] other (specify) _____

```
0.......1........2.......3
no life         immediate
threat          life threat
```

MANAGEMENT OF DAILY ACTIVITIES

1. Activities of daily living (Check if client does not do)

[ ] transferring from/to bed or chair
[ ] bathing
[ ] grooming
[ ] dressing
[ ] eating
[ ] toileting
[ ] other (specify) _____

```
0. .....1........2.......3
no life         immediate
threat          life threat
```

2. <u>Instrumental activities</u> (Check if client <u>does not</u> do)

[ ] shop for food
[ ] shop for other things
[ ] drive car
[ ] use public transportation
[ ] do housework
[ ] do laundry
[ ] prepare meals
[ ] take medications properly
[ ] other (specify) _____

```
┌─────────────────────────────┐
│ 0.......1.......2.......3    │
│ no life          immediate  │
│ threat           life threat│
└─────────────────────────────┘
```

3. <u>Capacity to manage finances</u> (check if <u>characteristic</u> of client)

[ ] hoarding
[ ] squandering
[ ] failure to pay bills
[ ] many credit purchases
[ ] uncashed checks
[ ] large amounts of cash
[ ] inaccurate/no knowledge of finances
[ ] giving money away
[ ] other (specify) _____

```
┌─────────────────────────────┐
│ 0.......1.......2.......3    │
│ no life          immediate  │
│ threat           life threat│
└─────────────────────────────┘
```

****

ACTION NEEDED

a) If all of the scales in Section I are rated "0 - no life threat", Sections II and III need not be completed. Skip to Section IV— "Action Taken," on page 6.

b) If any scales in section I are rated "1" or "2", but none are "3 - immediate life threat", agency policy and the assessor's judgement will determine whether further assessment is required.

c) Sections II, III and IV should be completed for all clients with any ratings of "3 - immediate life threat" in Section I and for other clients for whom further assessment is required.

****

-4-

SECTION II—AGGRAVATING AND MITIGATING SOCIAL FACTORS
Instructions: Check all conditions known to be present.

1. At the present time, does the client depend for essentials on an unreliable caregiver?

   [] no (skip to question 2)
   [] yes, specify why unreliable below:

         [] sometimes neglects responsibilities
         [] sometimes is incapacitated because of alcohol or drugs
         [] is physically or mentally unable to provide needed care
         [] other_____
         _____
         _____

2. Is any person who lives in the client's household, or has ready access to the client, responsible for any risk factor in Section I— items 1, 2, or 6 (neglect, abuse, or exploitation)?

   [] yes
   [] no

3. Is the client living in unusually isolated circumstances?

   [] yes
   [] no

4. Has a recent change in the client's social environment contributed to the client's endangerment?

   [] no (skip to question 5)
   [] yes, specify changes below:

         [] loss of caregiver
         [] loss of other major social support
         [] move to new environment
         [] other_____
         _____
         _____

-5-   Client's name_____

	Will Provide		
5. How much help will the following social supports provide?	All help necessary	Partial help	Not a potential source of help
a) persons living in the client's household	[] 1	[] 2	[] 3
b) other persons— neighbors, friends, and relatives	[] 1	[] 2	[] 3
c) other agencies, churches, temples, and organizations	[] 1	[] 2	[] 3

If no potential sources of help, skip to Question 6. If help available:
Identify the social support(s)_____

State how the social support(s) will help_____

State the limitations of the social support(s)_____

6. Generally, how willing is the client to accept help?

   [] totally willing
   [] somewhat willing
   [] refuses all help

SECTION III—ASSESSMENT OF CLIENT'S NEED FOR PROTECTIVE INTERVENTION

1. Does the client understand the risk(s) he or she is facing?

   [] yes
   [] partially
   [] no

2. Taking into consideration the client's endangering conditions, social resources, and understanding of the risks he or she faces, assess whether the client needs protective intervention. Use the following criteria:

   a) If the client has social supports that are available, able, and willing to provide all necessary help and he or she will accept this help, the client does not need additional protective intervention (although other forms of help may be required).

   b) If the overall level of endangerment is immediately life threatening, and the client does not have social supports to provide sufficient help or he or she is unwilling to accept such help, the client requires protective intervention.

   c) If you are unable to make either of the above decisions, further assessment is required.

   Does the client require protective intervention?

   [] yes
   [] no

SECTION IV—ACTION TAKEN
Instructions: Complete this section for all clients.

[ ] case not opened
[ ] case referred for service elsewhere
    case referred to:_____

[ ] case opened for protective services
[ ] case opened for other services but not for protective services

If case has been opened, complete the following:

1. Case assigned to:
   worker_____
   unit_____

2. Has an offer of service been made to the client?

   [ ] yes (answer question 3)
   [ ] no (skip questions 3 and 4)

3. Does the client accept the offer?

   [ ] yes (skip question 4)
   [ ] no (answer question 4)

4. Is the client likely to become voluntary with further casework?

   [ ] yes
   [ ] no

5. Types of assistance likely to be provided include:

   [ ] food   [ ] money   [ ] money management
   [ ] shopping   [ ] transportation [ ] housekeeping
   [ ] personal care [ ] shelter   [ ] medical aid
   [ ] psychiatric aid [ ] other (specify_____)

22

Ombudsman Services

Howard Litwin, D.S.W.

Hebrew University, Jerusalem, Israel

Ombudsman programs for the institutionalized elderly are a relatively new phenomenon in the aging network. Mandated by federal law, they have been instituted at both state and local levels, and they encompass a range of roles, tasks, and functions. Nursing-home ombudsmen, as the principal actors in this service system are known, may be salaried professionals or citizen volunteers who act as patient advocates. Social workers sometimes head ombudsman programs. More often, social workers are the staff members of long-term-care facilities with whom the ombudsman makes daily contact. Occasionally, the social worker may become the nursing-home ombudsman's chief adversary.

This chapter describes what nursing-home ombudsmen can realistically be expected to do on behalf of their clients, what ombudsmen do not do, and how social workers interface with this service system.

NEED

With the achievement of greater longevity for significant numbers of older people has come the concomitant problem of how best to care for those aged persons whose health declines and for whom independent living is no longer a feasible option. While efforts have been made to provide alternative home care supports such as home health care, day hospitals, emergency hot lines, and other types of "eldercare," the preferred societal response to those who need long-term care has been institutionalization. Recent government figures indicate that more than 1.3 million individuals reside in 18,200 nursing homes across the country (Health Care Financing Administration, 1981). About 5 percent of persons aged 65 and over live in long-term-care facilities. One in five persons can expect to spend some time in nursing homes before they die (LaPorte and Rubin, 1979, p. 19).

Three types of problems confront the long-term-care population: the physical and mental problems of aging, the consequences of institutionalization, and the vulnerability of this population to abuse. These are the problems that the nursing-home-ombudsman program is called upon to address.

While it is certainly incorrect to equate the aging process with a progressive deterioration of physical and mental capacity, it is nevertheless true that increasing age presents increasing risk of disability. Strokes, cardiac failure, and arterial disease are frequent accompaniments of advancing years (Kannel and Gordon, 1980). Other ailments whose incidence increases with aging include hypertension (Wilkie, 1980), incontinence (Goldman, 1977), and senile dementia (Gruenberg, 1980). The older population is also overrepresented among victims of accidental deaths (Hogue, 1980). To minimize the progression of such impairments and decrease the risk of further disability are primary needs among the institutionalized aged.

Certain consequences of institutionalization exacerbate the already weakened state of the nursing-home resident. Entry to a long-stay facility generally means loss of privacy, stability, and personal possessions. Most of all, it means limitation of one's independence and power to make decisions (Bennett, 1980). As a result:

Severe depression in the form of withdrawal, loss of appetite and lethargy is a very real and significant problem in some nursing home admissions. Some residents completely give up. Sometimes a resident will die within a very short time after admission (Burger and D'Erasmo, 1976, p. 69).

The confines and constraints of institutionalization led Tulloch (1975) to note that *A Home Is Not a Home*.

Nevertheless, nursing-home residents may continue to express choices and make decisions in certain areas. Bennett (1980) notes among these the choice of food, clothing, and friends; religious expression; and control of financial affairs. The preservation of these areas of discretion must be recognized as another important need of the elderly who reside in nursing homes.

Finally, increased utilization of long-term-care facilities for infirm and frail elderly has been accompanied by the rise of abuse of the institutionalized aged. Mendelson (1975) was among the first to call attention to cases of patients "lying abandoned in . . . urine-soaked bed[s], starved, abused at will by aides" (p. 38). She blamed such abuse on the dominance of profit-seeking interests at various levels of the nursing-home industry. Vladeck (1980) has more recently renewed public sensitivity to the tragedy of "slow deaths from indifference, callousness or inadequate nursing services" (p. 153), identifying such phenomena as necessary concomitants of current policy aimed at minimizing costs. Kayser-Jones (1981, pp. 39-55) categorized the most commonly reported incidents of nursing-home abuse as: (1) *infantilization,* when residents are treated like irresponsible, dependent minors; (2) *depersonalization,* when residents are treated mechanically, all alike, and consequently are ignored; (3) *dehumanization,* when residents do not receive compassionate and understanding treatment—a common example being insensitivity to their needs for privacy, as when men and women are bathed together or placed in situations where they must urinate and defecate in the presence of others; (4) *victimization,* including thefts of residents' possessions, punitive restraints, verbal intimidation, and excessive sedation.

As a sample of resident complaints received by the Florida nursing-home-ombudsman program reveals (Henry, 1981), the problems of aging, institutionalization, and abuse may combine to make one's last years difficult at best, intolerable at worst:

A patient had been at a nursing home for three years as a private pay patient and then had to rely on Medicaid. Shortly thereafter the patient was transferred to a hospital because of possible pneumonia. After two days' observation, the hospital could not confirm the home's diagnosis. The patient's relative called to complain that, on release from the hospital on the third day, the nursing home indicated that the patient could not return due to a lack of available beds.

A woman complained that her mother was restrained in a wheelchair by a bed sheet and not released for several hours, with the result that she sat in a puddle of urine. The complainant added that the nursing home did not have a physician's order requesting such restraint.

An elderly resident wandered away from a nursing home on Thanksgiving Day. She was found dead from exposure four days later in a wooded area about one mile from the facility. Police related that they had previously received numerous reports of residents wandering from this facility.

While recognizing that nursing homes have been "characterized by the media as deficient, misdirected and in need of change" (Bennett, 1980, p. 11), nursing-home administrators deny responsibility for the situation. They see themselves as prisoners of unrealistic regulations and constricting mechanisms of Medicaid reimbursement. Regardless of the position with which one chooses to identify, it may be generally concluded that the provision of adequate nursing-home care is frequently overridden by other considerations in the management of the long-term-care delivery system.

LOCAL OMBUDSMAN PROGRAMS

State and local nursing-home-ombudsman programs have different functions and methods of operation. Their repertoires complement one another and together may be viewed as a comprehensive approach to the resolution of nursing-home residents' complaints.

Staff and Operation

The local ombudsman program is usually staffed by a single professional (often a social worker), some support staff, and a cadre of trained volunteers. The volunteers represent diverse interests, backgrounds, and motivations. In Connecticut, for example, volunteers range in age from 21 to over 80. In New York, the volunteer pool includes people with high-school diplomas and others with doctoral degrees. Volunteers are recruited on the basis of their sense of altruism but are maintained in the program through peer support and by supervision from the local program head. Their training consists of lectures, discussions, and facility visits. In a few states—Georgia, for example—volunteers are required to pass written examinations.

In many states, the laws regulating nursing homes include ombudsman-access provisions authorizing volunteers to enter any facility. Lacking such authorization, an ombudsman program must negotiate collaborative arrangements with each facility administrator. Regardless of the mode of entry, local programs are geared toward cooperative resolution of residents' complaints at the facility level. The focus of their intervention is on improving the quality of life of the institutionalized elderly.

Clients—that is, nursing-home residents, their friends and families—may come into contact with a local ombudsman program in a number of ways. Programs advertise through the media, posters, and brochures. Centralized state "hot lines" may channel complaints to local programs. Community advisory-board members and their organizations may serve as conduits of client concern. Most often, however, contact is made through friendly visiting.

Ombudsman volunteers visit long-term-care facilities once or twice a week. During their rounds they attempt to establish a degree of visibility and a measure of trust. By building relationships with the aged residents, they remove initial barriers to communication and open the path for the elicitation of grievances.

Monk and Kaye (1981a) found, however, that despite efforts to establish program visibility, including the wearing of green badges by the volunteers, only a quarter of the residents were aware of the nursing-home ombudsman (pp. 232-236).

Eliciting Complaints

The task of the local nursing-home ombudsman is to receive complaints from or on behalf of aggrieved facility residents, to assess the nature of the complaints and verify their legitimacy, and then to act to effect their resolution. The first step in this process, the receipt of grievances, may be far more difficult than at first appears. The State Nursing Home Ombudsman Committee of Florida warns: "You may find you have created a process for which no complaints immediately surface" (Carter, 1978, p. vi).

There are many reasons for this. Nursing-home patients and their families may be reluctant to complain to a stranger. They may believe that institutionalization has placed them outside the community mainstream and perhaps outside the realm of due process as well. In fact, indignities suffered in the long-term-care facility may only confirm their sense of despair and so may not be resisted. Further, lack of familiarity with long-stay institutions may convince residents that what they are experiencing is the best that can be offered. Finally, and most significantly, residents may not complain out of fear of reprisals from the facility staff. Nevertheless, as the Florida committee maintains, "This lack of reported complaints should not be viewed as proof that there are no problems within the nursing homes in your community" (Carter, 1978, p. vi).

To elicit complaints, ombudsmen must reach out to residents by means of publicity and education, win their trust, and provide them with sufficient confidentiality to minimize their fears of reprisal.

Assessment and Verification of Complaints

Once a complaint becomes known to the ombudsman, the next step is to assess its nature and extent in order to devise appropriate interventive measures. Four types of complaints may be identified: (1) complaints that stem from the personal difficulties of aged residents in adjusting to their new regimen; (2) complaints of lack of fit between residents' individual predilections and the general regulations of the facility; (3) complaints regarding deficient facility procedures; and (4) complaints reflecting inappropriate state policy impacting on the long-term-care delivery system. The following cases illustrative of these four types are adapted from *OmbudsNews*, the newsletter of the New York City Nursing Home Patient Ombudsman Program, and from *Collation*, a publication of the National Citizens' Coalition for Nursing Home Reform in Washington, D.C.:

1. *Personal Difficulty:* A 76-year-old amputee complained to the local ombudsman about a painful prosthesis that did not fit well. The ombudsman subsequently met with the physical therapist in the nursing home and learned that the prothesis had already been changed three times. The patient had become so discouraged that she refused any further therapy. The ombudsman understood that emotional and physical adjustment to the prosthesis was very difficult for her.

Following the meeting, the therapist agreed to consult with a team of mental-health and medical professionals to draw up an appropriate rehabilitation plan for the patient. The ombudsman was enlisted to gain the patient's confidence. On his second visit, the ombudsman explained to the patient that therapy would help her adjust to the prosthesis. With his support, she agreed to return to therapy.

2. *Lack of Fit:* A new resident was not allowed to use his own wheelchair, a wooden chair with a cane back. The nursing home prohibited its use because it lacked the arms and footrest required to protect residents from injury. The resident felt restricted in the new wheelchair issued him by the facility. He became resigned to lying in bed, unable to ambulate, rather than use the facility chair. He told the nursing-home ombudsman that he would sign affidavits releasing the home from responsibility should an accident occur. It mattered that much to him.

The ombudsman approached the medical director with the resident's proposal. Although the doctor was reluctant, the ombudsman stressed the resident's strong desire to use his own wheelchair and his right to participate in decisions about his care. When the ombudsman clarified that, unless there were demonstrated medical contraindications, both she and the resident would continue to pursue the matter, the medical director relented. The resident was allowed the use of the wheelchair he preferred.

3. *Deficient Facility Procedures:* At one facility the ombudsman encountered a problem that affected many patients—those who required specially molded therapeutic shoes. According to established procedures, a contractor visited the facility periodically to make molds of residents' feet. If needs arose between these infrequent visits, it became necessary to transport residents to the contractor's office, some distance away. The journey was time-consuming, expensive, and disruptive for several residents.

The ombudsman brought the complaints of the residents to the attention of the administrator. As a result, a new procedure was instituted. A facility staff member was trained to make molds, which were then sent to the contractor. Shoes were thus produced in a less disruptive and more efficient manner for the residents who needed them.

4. *Inappropriate State Policy:* In testimony before a congressional committee, the ombudsman of a state program described a complaint concerning seven residents who had died in four weeks due to alleged negligence in a new 64-bed intermediate-care facility. A joint investigation was conducted with the state's Department of Human Services. It was determined that the facility had opened without a licensed administrator and had attempted to fill all beds immediately despite a serious lack of trained nurses' aides.

When the Human Services Department did not rule negligence as the cause of the residents' deaths, the ombudsman successfully pressured officials to develop a policy governing the opening of new facilities. The new policy limits the number of admissions per day and per week and requires that only certified, trained personnel be employed when a facility opens its doors. The board that licenses administrators also reviewed and revised its procedures.

The final step in the assessment process is the verification of grievances. In a study of a local ombudsman program in a large northeastern metropolis, Monk and Kaye (1981a) found that roughly a quarter of twenty-five ombudsman volunteers operating in twenty-two nursing homes estimated that over three-fourths of patients' complaints were accurate. Another 41 percent placed the extent of accurate complaints at more than half.

Monk and Kaye also found a critical role for the social worker in the complaint-verification process. Ombudsman volunteers were asked how often they utilized the following verification procedures: personal observation; questioning the administrator; questioning nurses and social workers; questioning aides and orderlies; contacting regulatory agencies; contacting legal services; questioning other residents or their relatives; talking with ombudsman-program staff; using written ombudsman resources; accepting the complaint at face value. Of all these verification procedures, the ombudsman volunteers turned to nurses and social workers second most frequently. They utilized personal observation most often, and turned to outside regulatory or legal organizations least often.

Resolving Complaints

Once a complaint is received and verified, the ombudsman begins the resolution process. The complaint may be brought directly to the attention of the facility administrator or of the home's professional staff. Very often the ombudsman will establish a relationship with the social worker at the facility, who then proceeds to deal with the substance of the complaint. Monk and Kaye found that social-service directors in long-term-care facilities were approached more often by ombudsmen than were other facility personnel. Similarly, social-service directors indicated that, of facility staff, they had the most frequent involvement in patient-related discussions with ombudsman volunteers. The social worker emerges, therefore, as a key figure, if not in the complaint-elicitation stage, certainly in the complaint-resolution process that follows at the facility level.

At the same time, social workers may well perceive the ombudsman volunteer with some degree of apprehension. First, the social worker may be considered a kind of patient advocate in his/her own right. The intrusion of an outside agent into the closed nursing-home environment disturbs the social worker's daily routine, and furthermore raises doubt as to his/her efficacy or role legitimacy. Second, it must be remembered that ombudsman volunteers are goodwilled but nonprofessional change agents. Friction between volunteers and the social worker, as has historically occurred in social services between paraprofessionals and line staff, is therefore to be expected in the nursing home as well. It is thus not surprising that Monk and Kaye found that social workers rated ombudsman volunteers the least effective among the groups of facility staff surveyed. Social workers may well find themselves unwitting adversaries of the nursing-home ombudsman program.

Although ombudsman volunteers seek to resolve residents' complaints in a collaborative and cooperative manner within the facility, they sometimes confront situations that resist consensual solution. The training guide of the California Nursing Home Ombudsman Program therefore attempts to prepare the ombudsman for confrontational possibilities. As part of a training exercise, the manual (California Department of Aging, 1981) presents the following response by an administrator to an ombudsman's petition on behalf of a patient:

"I've done all I can for Mrs. Carey. Yet she continues to disturb and to upset the other patients with all her complaints. I've got 75 other patients to think about, and I can't have her occupying all the aide's time, especially when we're so understaffed. I also cannot have her falling down and injuring herself again. If she won't wait until the aide can come to help her, the only alternative is to restrain her. I have enough problems with staff turnover and I can't force the aides to like Mrs. Carey. Maybe the best thing would be to transfer her to another home" (p. viii).

In this hypothetical situation, the ombudsman would make the problem known to the local program supervisor, usually by a written report or standardized complaint form. With the help of the supervisor, the ombudsman would determine whether state regulations and health codes prescribed minimal patient/aide ratios and, if so, whether the facility is knowingly ignoring them. Pressure could then be brought to bear on the facility by representatives of the health department or such other external agents as the attorney general's staff or the governor's office to correct the situation. The issue of involuntary transfer that is also raised in this example, on the other hand, is one for which there are often few protective regulations.

The same California training guide outlines the investigative procedure in the following stages (p. viii):

1. *Statement of the problem.* What is the problem? Why is it occurring? How did it happen? Who is involved?
2. *Categorizing the complaint.* What type of complaint is it?
3. *Identifying the relevant agencies.* Which agencies have a legal stake in the problem?
4. *Steps already taken.*
5. *Fact gathering.* Through direct observation of the setting and research, such as review of the law, patient's records, interviews, etc.
6. *Reconstruction of events.*
7. *Analysis of the situation.*
8. *Consideration of possible solutions.*
9. *Identifying the obstacles.*
10. *Selecting an approach.* Keeping alternate strategies in mind.
11. *Acting.* Proceeding with the selected plan but remaining flexible with the alternatives.
12. *Follow up and evaluation.* Is the problem solved or ameliorated? Is more information needed?

One helpful tool in the hands of nursing-home ombudsmen is the body of rules and regulations attached to Medicaid reimbursement. The vast majority of long-term-care facilities receive Medicaid payments on behalf of their residents. The regulations provide guidelines by means of which ombudsmen can monitor the care of the institutionalized elderly. Although recent proposals for "regulatory relief" in the nursing-home industry threaten the continuation of these protective regulations, they currently remain in force.

Local programs can achieve impressive results through collaboration. An ombudsman program in rural north Florida is a case in point. The area committee (Florida has eleven district committees and one statewide committee) was comprised, as prescribed by state statute, of experts in gerontology and long-term-care delivery as well as patient representatives. The local nursing-home operators saw the committee as a resource and consulted with it on facility problems. Administrators did not hestitate to request the aid of the district ombudsmen.

Local programs must also be prepared, however, to engage in confrontation, if necessary, to defend residents' rights. Such adversarial activity is most fruitfully effected when backed up by a statutorily empowered state ombudsman.

STATE OMBUDSMAN PROGRAMS

When a problem arises that is not covered by existing regulations, the locus of ombudsman activity switches from the local to the state program. While local programs deal best with case advocacy, or interventive efforts on behalf of aggrieved individuals who reside in nursing homes, the state program is invoked in matters of issue advocacy. This form of advocacy comes into play when more than one resident or facility are affected by the same problem.

Established and funded by state legislatures, state ombudsman programs are generally located within departments of aging in state governments. A few states sponsor their ombudsman programs through human-services departments or through the governor's office. Only one state, Michigan, contracts its state program to a voluntary advocacy organization.

State ombudsman programs centralize and monitor the documentation of all resident complaints to determine whether the complaints reflect patterns or idiosyncratic circumstances. State programs also monitor the degree to which problem or issue areas recur. On the basis of these statistical data, a state ombudsman can identify gaps in the implementation of nursing-home regulations, suggest the strengthening of existing protective legislation, propose areas of required concern, and provide support for litigation against offenders.

Complaints are recorded in a variety of fashions for transmission to state programs. A few states, like Ohio, are beginning to implement computerized management information systems to track complaint patterns. Others still depend on periodic reports from local programs. State complaint-codification schemes vary, but most include the following resident-centered issues: resident rights; resident abuse, nursing-home regulations and their enforcement; Medicaid discrimination; upgrading of nursing-home staffs; relocation trauma; boarding-home standards (adult homes, RCFs); consumer education relating to long-term-care facilities; mental health needs of long-term-care-facility residents; resident funds abuse; resident participation in facility governance. Most also include such facility-centered issues as: food and nutrition; administration; environmental safety; facility sanitation; interpersonal relations (residents); personal care (e.g., help with washing and dressing); health care; personal allowances; protection of personal property.

A few state ombudsman programs, like the one in New Jersey, maintain staffs of analysts and investigators to keep abreast of developments in the long-term-care delivery system. Most states, however, rely on collaboration among government departments and agencies to fulfill their mandates. Cooperation must sometimes be forged with the very departments that may be targets of complaints—for example, a state health-facilities licensing office whose investigations are essential to the ombudsman in the complaint-verification process but whose laxity may itself constitute a source of problems. Which issues do state ombudsmen deal with, therefore, and how do they perceive them?

A comparative study of state nursing-home ombudsman programs (Monk, Kaye, and Litwin, 1982) found that ombudsmen dealt most frequently with issues of residents' rights, consumer education, and nursing-home regulations and their enforcement. Issues presenting the most difficulties for state ombudsmen, on the other hand, included the upgrading of nursing-home staffs, boarding-home standards, and discrimination against Medicaid-supported patients. On the facility level, state ombudsmen reported that complaints of poor food, deficient health care, and failure to protect residents' personal property were dealt with most frequently. Protection of property proved to be the most difficult problem to resolve, followed by facility administration and health care.

EFFECTIVENESS OF OMBUDSMAN PROGRAMS

State ombudsmen view state programs as most effective in the provision of information to legislators and program planners. Such information can be used to bring about changes in the long-term-care delivery system. State ombudsmen view local programs as most effective in alerting facility staffs to patient's needs. State ombudsmen's ratings thus reflect the different focuses of state and local programs and underscore the complementarity between them.

As Monk, Kaye, and Litwin discovered, however, the long-term-care network maintains a more guarded estimation of the program's success. State commissioners of health and welfare, state offices on aging, and citizens' organizations concerned with the elderly rate the ombudsman program as only moderately effective. Long-term-care provider associations view the ombudsman as hardly effective at all. All consider the program successful in the protection of individual patients' rights and the fostering of greater accountability among facility staffs. The program is considered to be much less effective when addressing partisan policy advocacy.

Effectiveness ratings, of course, should be viewed with some caution. The realm of long-term care is hardly a neutral one. Each of the varying components of the delivery system has a different stake in how the system works. Views of the ombudsman program are likely to vary depending upon the rater's particular interests. It is understandable, therefore, that those least appreciative of the program's efforts, the long-term-care-provider associations, are also those who are most confronted by ombudsmen, whether local volunteers or state officials. Evidence thus suggests that "perceptions of ombudsman program function and performance may be heavily influenced by one's own affiliation and normative stance in the long term care system" (Monk, Kaye, and Litwin, 1982, p. 158).

How do the consumers of ombudsman services, the nursing-home residents, view the program's effectiveness? Monk and Kaye (1981b) found that, among residents who presented grievances to a volunteer ombudsman, almost half believed that their problems had been solved, while 39 percent were sure that they had not been. There was general agreement, on the other hand, that ombudsmen were more successful in the expressive domain—that is, in their display of sensitivity and respect—than in the instrumental domain of actual problem resolution.

Differences emerged when the study controlled for various characteristics of the nursing-home population. Men were more willing to seek help than were women, and those with higher education even more so. Residents of proprietary homes were less likely to complain than were residents of not-for-profit institutions. This last point is particularly relevant, since the proprietary residents rated the quality of their care to be worse than did the residents of the voluntary facilities and since 77 percent of all homes are run for profit (Bennett, 1980, p. 25).

Despite group differences, it was generally not the ombudsman to whom aggrieved patients turned when a problem arose, if they dared to turn to anyone at all. The ombudsman program has a significant way to go, therefore, in developing sufficient visibility and competence to fulfill its mandate as a mediator and resolver of residents' complaints.

The black residents in long-term-care facilities identified in the Monk-Kaye study (1984) were significantly younger, more likely to be female, had received less education, and were receiving more skilled nursing care than the white respondents.

Both black and white users of ombudsman services perceived volunteers to have been more effective in displaying affective or compassionate qualities than in performing practical competencies. Both groups agreed also that ombudsmen made a positive difference. Black residents, in particular, were more emphatically convinced that ombudsmen were needed to contend with patient grievances and used their services more often. Monk and Kaye assume that a greater activist orientation toward the ombudsman program among black residents may be due to a specific ethnic effect, namely, the salience of advocacy and a greater civil-rights consciousness in the black community that is spilling over into long-term-care institutions and canceling handicaps in educational attainment.

LINKS TO THE AGING NETWORK

Nursing-home ombudsman programs are intended to constitute an integral link in the aging-services network. As such, they should be part and parcel of the system of Area Agencies on Aging, established to provide a community-based focus to the planning and delivery of services for older people (Fall Creek and Gilbert, 1981). Experience shows, however, that many ombudsman programs view the AAAs as obstacles to the successful implementation of their work. Conversely, AAAs do not seem to recognize ombudsman services as part of their interventive repertoire.

State nursing-home ombudsmen cite several reasons for the strained relations between the AAAs and ombudsman programs. Foremost among them is the AAAs' role as contractors for the delivery of concrete or direct services such as meals, transportation, counseling, and homecare. Local ombudsmen services depart from this service pattern in at least three ways: (1) ombudsmen offer mediational rather than direct services; (2) ombudsman programs are attached administratively to AAAs, requiring supervisory as well as financial assistance; and (3) they focus on institutional services, which have not tended to be the main interest of the Older Americans Act under which the AAA service network is mandated. In addition, some AAAs would prefer to see the funds required for ombudsman programs (1 percent of Title III-B funds for social services or $20,000, whichever is larger) utilized instead for the purchase of concrete community services. Thus while nursing-home-ombudsman programs should be seen as one link in the chain of aging services, they have not yet fully attained such status in many communities.

THEORY

The major theoretical issue underlying the ombudsman program is whether it would operate better in a collaborative mode, as an impartial mediator, or in an adversarial advocacy stance, championing the nursing-home residents' cause. This issue is hardly unique to the long-term-care setting. The collaborative-versus-contest strategy choice is a major philosophical and methodological dilemma affecting the development and delivery of social services.

The debate over the relative efficacy of the collaborative- or the contest-strategy orientation has its roots in sociological theory. The collaborative orientation may be traced to the consensual approach of structural sociology, which maintains that all societies have the same functional prerequisites (Parsons, 1951). Societal structure is seen to be basically sound and self-corrective. When dysfunction appears, enhanced consensus-building reestablishes a functional balance or equilibrium. As Etzioni (1968, pp. 7, 8) notes:

> The structural functional approach tends to perceive the main source of social problems in technical failures of the social system; that is, in ad hoc aberrations in the social equilibrium which are expected to occur occasionally in any system of inter-related but heterogeneous parts. . . . The correctives are seen to lie in strengthening or repairing existing socialization and social control processes and in resocializing or rehabilitating deviants.

The source of dysfunction is not in the societal structure itself but in the pathology of individuals. As such, structural functionalists believe that social problems are best corrected through adjustment rather than transformation of society (Etzioni, 1968, p. 9). Focus on the consensus-building, adjustment, and self-correcting tendencies of society provides the basis for what is essentially a collaborative social orientation, the same approach that underlies the classical ombudsman concept and is carried out through impartial mediation.

The conflict school of sociology, on the other hand, espouses a wholly different explanation of the nature of society as well as a distinctive prescription for the amelioration of societal dysfunction. The root of the difference lies in the conflict sociologists' perception that the source of most social problems is in the existence of, as Horton (1968, p. 41) puts it, "illegitimate social control and exploitation." For conflict theorists, society as a concept has no inherent existence except as a tool for those in power. Furthermore, social problems constitute problems primarily because those in power do not really want to solve them (Skolnick and Currie, 1982). Empowered classes, in this view, tend to benefit from the continued existence of many social ills.

Since, as this perspective holds, social problems are really disguised political issues, personal troubles are distinguishable from the public issues of contradictory institutional arrangements (Mills, 1956). Notions of collective consciousness give way to notions of class consciousness and class strife. The logical approach to societal correction that stems from this approach, therefore, is through fundamental social change. The approach of the conflict theorist implies an adversarial base to intergroup relations and provides a theoretical framework for the development of confrontational advocacy strategies and contest orientations.

The heart of the debate is the question of the acceptance of the status quo as reflected in social structure and social values or its total rejection. When problems arise, those of the former persuasion seek adjustment and amelioration within the existing social parameters. Those of the latter school, on the other hand, cite the same problems as proof of the need for basic social change and reform. The two sides of this theoretical dichotomy constitute the end points of a collaborative/contest continuum.

Nursing homes may be viewed as microsocieties. When dysfunctions periodically occur, solutions could follow either of two opposing routes. Structuralists would recommend an impartial ombudsman to help uncover the ad hoc aberrations and restore the state of equilibrium. Conflict theorists, on the other hand, would view the same dysfunction as proof of exploitative behavior by nursing-home operators, for which redress could be effected only through an adversarial campaign. The two approaches are as difficult to reconcile as they are independently to affirm. How then does the ombudsman program coordinate such diverse theoretical underpinnings?

As noted earlier, the ombudsman program operates both a locally based, quality-of-life-oriented approach and a state-level, patients' rights approach. The former is based mostly in a collaborative mode, reflecting a structuralist perspective. The latter does not hesitate to engage in advocacy as would befit a contest perspective on society. The program thus attempts a two-pronged approach that can maximize a range of theoretical perspectives. The degree to which it succeeds on both fronts, however, is as dependent on the development of public policy in this area as it is on its theoretical bases.

POLICY

The ombudsman, who originated in Scandinavia during the nineteenth century, was first conceived as an independent, impartial officer of the legislature who responded to citizens' complaints of public maladministration. His function was to investigate and recommend appropriate avenues of redress. The power of the position, however, was informal, rooted in the prestige of the officeholder and effected by means of persuasion. The ombudsman was not empowered to reverse or revise administrative action (Gellhorn, 1966; Rowat, 1968).

The nursing-home-ombudsman program in the United States has evolved over the last decade from at least three separate mandates. President Nixon initially proposed a plan to upgrade the state of long-term care in 1971. Point 6

directed the Department of Health, Education and Welfare to assist the states in establishing investigative units which will respond in a responsible and constructive way to complaints made by or on behalf of individual nursing home patients (Mendelson, 1975, p. 235).

In 1972 the Health Services and Mental Health Administration of HEW awarded demonstration contracts for four states and the National Council of Senior Citizens for the development and implementation of state nursing-home-ombudsman programs. The Administration on Aging (AoA) assumed responsiblity for the ombudsman initiatives in 1973 and granted two additional states the funds to establish demonstration projects.

Several unpublished state reports indicate that the early ombudsmen saw their roles as advocates for the aged and as harbingers of systemic reforms. They hoped to spur new legislation and new facility regulations. However, as Regan (1977, p. 703) notes, "the partisan position recommended for the office in these reports [was] inconsistent with the neutrality traditionally associated with an ombudsman."

The seven demonstration projects were followed by funding, administrative, and programmatic changes. The Older Americans Act Amendments of 1975 directed AoA to set up yearly grants for the appointment of state ombudsman-development specialists. The intent was to spur "the development of voluntary community action groups as the new ingredient in the process of settling complaints of nursing home patients" (Regan, 1977, p. 704). The focus thus shifted to an ombudsman program-building process, in contrast to the earlier demonstration projects' advocacy recommendations. Policymakers were apprehensive about excessive costs, not to mention the political unpopularity of a patient-advocacy focus. Newly approved state ombudsman programs subsequently operated as model projects subject to the discretionary funding of the Commissioner on Aging.

The 1978 amendments to the Older Americans Act and the rules and regulations that derived from them clarified several ambiguities concerning the status and function of the ombudsman. They required states to operate ombudsman services for residents in all long-term-care facilities, including skilled-nursing facilities, intermediate-care facilities, nursing homes, and similar adult-care facilities. Programs may be carried out directly by the state or they may by contracted to public or private nonprofit organizations, as long as the contractee does not also provide long-term care or certify its operation. The new regulations also stipulated that each state use 1 percent of its Title III-B allotment or $20,000, whichever is larger, each year to operate a long-term-care ombudsman program.

Current legislation mandates that each state: (1) investigate and resolve complaints made by or on behalf of long-term-care residents; (2) monitor laws, regulations, and policies with respect to long-term-care facilities; (3) provide information to public agencies on problems of long-term-care residents; (4) promote citizen involvement in the ombudsman program; and (5) carry out other activities deemed appropriate by the Commissioner on Aging. Other relevant concerns are less explicitly treated in the regulations, such as access to facilities, access to residents and patient records, confidentiality, disclosure of records and files, and the establishment of a statewide uniform reporting system to collect and analyze information on complaints and conditions in long-stay institutions.

Ombudsman programs are also affected by the extent of state legislation regulating nursing-home matters in general and ombudsman provisions in particular. Many states have mandated ombudsmen access to long-stay facilities and to patients' records but others have not. Some state statutes impacting on the ombudsman program concern quality of care and patients' rights. To the degree that statutes exist, ombudsmen are equipped with the authority to engage in advocacy. In their absence, ombudsmen must rely on consensual persuasion. The extent of statutory empowerment thus directly affects the particular approach a given state program will assume.

The different focuses and the still somewhat diffuse statutory mandates behind the long-term-care ombudsman program have allowed room for diversity in its implementation at state and local levels. An increase in the program's effectiveness in the future may be tied to a strengthening of its statutory mandate and a clarification of its scope and responsibility.

REFERENCES

Bennett, C. (1980). *Nursing home life: What it is and what it could be.* New York: Tiresias Press.

Burger, S. G., and D'Erasmo, M. (1976). *Living in a nursing home: A guide for residents, their families and friends.* New York: Seabury Press.

California Department of Aging. (1981). *A core training program for California's long term care ombudsmen.* Sacramento: California Department of Aging.

Carter, P. (1978). *Nursing home ombudsman committee resource manual.* Jacksonville: State of Florida.

Etzioni, A. (1968). *The active society: A theory of societal and political processes.* New York: Free Press.

FallCreek, S., and Gilbert, N. (1981). Aging network in transition: Problems and prospects. *Social Work,* **26**(3), 210-216.

Gellhorn, W. (1966). *Ombudsmen and others: Citizens' protectors in nine countries.* Cambridge: Harvard University Press.

Goldman, R. (1977). Aging of the excretory system: Kidney and bladder. In C. E. Finch and L. Hayflick (Eds.), *Handbook of the biology of aging.* New York: Van Nostrand Reinhold.

Gruenberg, E. M. (1980). Epidemiology of senile dementia. In *Second conference on the epidemiology of aging.* Bethesda, Md.: National Institutes of Health.

Health Care Financing Administration. (1981). *Long term care: Background and future directions.* Washington, D.C.: U.S. Department of Health and Human Services.

Henry, R. A. (1981). *Annual report of the long term care ombudsman committee.* Jacksonville: State of Florida.

Hogue, C. C. (1980). Epidemiology of injury in older age. In *Second conference on the epidemiology of aging.* Bethesda, Md.: National Institutes of Health.

Horton, J. (1968). Order and conflict theories of social problems. In F. Lindenfeld (Ed.), *Radical perspectives on social problems: Readings in critical sociology.* New York: Macmillan.

Kannel, W. B., and Gordon, T. (1980). Cardiovascular risk factors in the aged: The Framingham study. In *Second conference on the epidemiology of aging.* Bethesda, Md.: National Institutes of Health.

Kayser-Jones, J. S. (1981). *Old, alone, and neglected: Care of the aged in Scotland and the United States.* Berkeley: University of California Press.

LaPorte, V., and Rubin, J. (Eds.). (1979). *Reform and regulation of long term care.* New York: Praeger Publishers.

Mendelson, M. A. (1975). *Tender loving greed: How the incredibly lucrative nursing home "industry" is exploiting America's old people and defrauding us all.* New York: Vintage Books.

Mills, C. W. (1956). *The power elite.* New York: Oxford University Press.

Monk, A., and Kaye, L. W. (1981a). *Ombudsmen services for the aged in long term care facilities.* New York: Brookdale Institute on Aging and Adult Human Development.

Monk, A., and Kaye, L. W. (1981b). *The utilization of patient advocacy services in long term care facilities for the aged: Ethnic perspectives.* Paper presented at the 11th Annual Conference of the National Caucus and Center on Black Aged, Washington, D.C., May 28.

Monk, A., and Kaye, L. W. (1984). Patient advocacy services in long term care facilities: Ethnic perspectives. *Journal of Long Term Care Administration,* 5-10.

Monk, A., Kaye, L. W., and Litwin, H. (1982). *A national comparative analysis of long term care ombudsman programs for the aged.* New York: Brookdale Institute on Aging and Adult Human Development.

Parsons, T. (1951). *The social system.* Glencoe, Ill.: Free Press.

Regan, J. J. (1977). When nursing home patients complain: The ombudsman or the patient advocate? *Georgetown Law Review,* **65**.

Rowat, D. C. (Ed.). (1968). *The ombudsman: Citizen's defender* (2nd ed.). London: George Allen and Unwin.

Skolnick, J. H., and Currie, E. (Eds.). (1982). *Crisis in American institutions* (5th ed.). Boston: Little, Brown.

Tulloch, G. J. (1975). *A home is not a home: Life within a nursing home.* New York: Seabury Press.

Vladeck, B. C. (1980). *Unloving care: The nursing home tragedy.* New York: Basic Books.

Wilkie, F. L. (1980). Blood pressure and cognitive functioning. In *Second conference on the epidemiology of aging.* Bethesda, Md.: National Institutes of Health.

23

Services for the Dying

Richard A. Kalish, Ph.D.

University of New Mexico

First came Feifel's (1959) seminal book on the meaning of death. Exactly a decade later Kübler-Ross (1969) described the dying process and subsequently contributed her charisma to the improved treatment of dying persons. By the time another decade had elapsed, the market had been saturated by self-help books and proof-of-life-after-death books. Along with these books, there appeared books on the history of death (Ariés, 1981; Choron, 1963), on death and philosophy (Choron, 1964; Koestenbaum, 1971), on death and theology (Reimer, 1974; Thielicke, 1970), on death and the law (Shaffer, 1970), on funerals (Pine, 1975), on bereavement (Caine, 1974; Parkes, 1972), on dying patients (Brim et al., 1970; Garfield, 1978), and on uncounted other concerns.

During the past few years, several single-authored college textbooks have appeared (Kalish, 1984; Kastenbaum, 1981); descriptions of how to establish institutions for the dying have been published (Koff, 1980); two journals are in regular publication (*Death Studies, Omega*); and a national membership organization has been founded (Forum on Death Education and Counseling). These events seem to have announced the emergence of the topic from its previous taboo status to general acceptance, even to health-related and government bureaucracies.

Thus in twenty-five years the issues of death and dying have shifted in emphasis from innovation and exploration to institutionalization and bureaucratization. The period from the mid-1950s to the mid-1970s laid the groundwork by challenging the taboos and pointing out potential paths for possible services; from the mid-1970s to the present, the emphasis has been on planning, developing, and funding improved services. In 1967, Cicely Saunders began St. Christopher's, the first facility in the modern hospice movement; within fifteen years, with an unknown number of hospices in varying stages of development, the major issue in the United States has become the potential of third-party payments. Again: from innovation and exploration to institutionalization and bureaucratization.

But, in spite of the pejorative implications of terms such as institutionalization and bureaucratization, it is these procedures that have signaled the success of the first quarter century of the death-awareness movement. The frustration and upset reflected in the early work of Feifel, Kastenbaum, and numerous others have provided the basis and the impetus for vast improvements in the delivery of services to the dying, to their survivors, and to individuals whose work roles bring them into substantial contact with death and the dying process.

WHO ARE THE "ELDERLY DYING"

The definition of "older person" can be controversial, but for our present purposes we can select an arbitrary operational definition: an older person is anyone age 65 or over. Whether the individual is ill or healthy, self-accepting of the age status or rejecting of it, viewed by others as old or not, are irrelevant for present purposes.

The definition of "dying" is much more complex. An elderly woman has a major heart attack, recovers, and returns to her former activity level albeit on medication; three years later she has a second major coronary from which she dies within hours. When did her dying trajectory begin?

An older man has a severe automobile accident, is narrowly saved from death by surgery at the hospital, loses the use of both legs, and commits suicide three weeks later by a lethal ingestion of pills; his death occurs forty-five minutes after he swallows the pills. When did his dying trajectory begin?

An elderly man has a stroke, is rushed to the hospital, and is declared clinically dead. However, he is resuscitated, eventually recovers, returns home with only modest loss of function, and dies two years later of cancer. Or an older woman is dying of cancer, an illness from which she was declared incurable six weeks earlier; she undertakes a regimen of natural food, exercise, and meditation, and the symptoms go into remission. Two years later she dies of a stroke. When did the dying trajectory of these two people begin? Is it appropriate to consider someone as dying when they don't die?

If a friend of yours was diagnosed as pregnant but the diagnosis was later found to have been in error, would you tell others that your friend had been pregnant but no longer was? If a friend of yours was diagnosed as terminally ill but the prognosis was incorrect, would you later tell others that your friend was dying?

Usually when we think of a dying person we visualize someone in a hospital or institution who is ill and who will die in a reasonably defined future from the illness or from a complex of medical problems of which the illness is one. The image, of course, is inaccurate. Paula was diagnosed as having terminal cancer; she had decided against continuing cobalt treatment and was leading a fairly normal life with relatively little pain, although diminished energy, until one morning, after having enjoyed a dinner party with close friends, she was found to have died in her sleep.

Pattison (1977) defines a dying person as someone who has entered the living-dying interval. Subjectively, this interval begins when the dying person learns of it; objectively, it begins when someone such as the physician of the dying person might have known it, had that person had the information that was potentially available. For the purposes of the potential service provider, the issue often reduces itself to the awareness of the person who will die or to a family member of that person. However, for certain kinds of health or legal services, the awareness of the dying person may be less important than the perceptions of the service provider. And there are occasions when the dying person has no awareness at all of impending death: he or she is comatose, disoriented, or suffering cognitive impairment; he or she has been successfully protected from knowledge of his or her prognosis.

Not only is the theoretical definition of "older dying person" of necessity vague, but the operational definition of the population to which services are to be provided is also vague. It then becomes necessary to contemplate those characteristics of older dying persons that make them appropriate targets for the kinds of services being considered. However, in spite of these warnings, there will be times in the pages ahead when this author will be implicitly defining as "older dying persons" those individuals whose dying trajectory is somewhat predictable, who are aware of their prognoses, and whose symptoms are now evident either to them or to others.

THE NEEDS OF THE ELDERLY DYING

The needs of the older dying person are, in a broader context, identical to the needs of the not-yet-dying person (this expression is used in an attempt to reduce the psychological distance between persons defined as "dying" and persons not so defined). To use one familiar theoretical model, the older dying person—like everyone else—will try to satisfy physiological needs, safety and security needs, love and belonging needs, esteem and self-esteem needs, and self-actualization needs (Maslow, 1954). Or, to apply another framework, this individual has needs that can be viewed as psychological, social, spiritual, health-related, financial, and legal.

However, although the more broadly defined needs of the older dying person are the same as the needs of anyone else, the circumstances faced by this individual lead to two kinds of differences that require attention: first, the relative importance of these needs may differ considerably from those of other people; and second, the ways in which the needs can best be satisfied may also differ considerably.

Consider the circumstances faced by a dying 80-year-old man who has been a gourmet cook all his adult life. He has always required food for survival, just as anyone else does, but his own unique circumstances had led to a strong want — perhaps "need" is an appropriate term — for fresh, creatively prepared food served in a pleasant atmosphere. Now, as he is dying, he receives his nutrition by tube, and the atmosphere in which it is served would reduce anyone's appetite to zero. Well-prepared food is no longer a priority for him, but, since he depends on its ingestion to survive, it is just as much a need of his as it is of any reader of this book.

Now, for the sake of discussion, let's assume he has a temporary remission of symptoms. He leaves the hospital, returns home, and entices a member of his gourmet club to visit him and cook for him. His needs are being satisfied now as they had been satisfied for years, and his love of good food returns. This doesn't alter the significance of responding to his hunger need, but it does mean that the priority of food and the way the hunger need is satisfied are once again altered.

We could offer other examples, ranging from the need for oxygen to the need for power or for self-actualization. The point is that, as we consider needs, it is not that a person is dying or that a person is elderly that in some universal fashion affects his/her needs. Rather, it is the circumstances that accompany the dying process or the status as "elderly" that determines how the need — which may be universal — is satisfied in its unique fashion.

Lesson number one, then, is that service providers cannot define a population as "older dying persons" and then respond to them in a unitary fashion. Because they are older, they may have more dietary restrictions than younger dying persons would have; because they are dying, they may view the role of food in their lives as less important than an older nondying person would. These two probability statements may suggest some programmatic emphases for these people that would improve delivery systems, but they are only probability statements and they cannot replace an understanding of the unique personal, social, and situational characteristics that are found in the persons to be served.

The Uniqueness of the Older Dying Person

The older person who is dying must face everything that older persons face and everything that dying persons face, with the very real possibility that advanced age and the dying process are interacting, each worsening the other. As a dying person, this individual must cope with present losses, with imminent future losses, with the possibility of social isolation, with reduced functional capacities, with questions regarding the meaning of life and the purpose of limited futurity. As an older person, this individual has already had to cope with many of these same issues, although at differing levels of intensity and with differing resources available.

The research and speculative literature suggests that older people find death to be less anxiety-arousing, although more salient, and that overall they handle the imminence of their own dying better than do the nonelderly (see Kalish, 1984, for review). Thus it appears that older dying persons have already experienced more loss and stress than younger dying persons; at the same time, evidence suggests that their general level of upset and anxiety concerning death and dying is less than that of younger persons, perhaps because of these experiences of loss.

What is it, then, about being both elderly and dying that has unique effects upon the individual? Some thoughts come to mind. We know, for example, that older people are more likely to be dying from chronic diseases, especially cardiovascular conditions and cancer, and relatively less likely to die from accidents and suicide. We know, too, that chronic illnesses have a different dying trajectory than acute conditions, that they require different kinds of medication, and that their victims require a different kind of personal and health-care plan.

We also know that older people are likely to have different family supports than younger people. Older men are likely to receive most of their support from their wives; older women, much more likely to be widows, will receive most of their support from their adult children (Cartwright, Hockey, and Anderson, 1973). The nonelderly will likely receive most of their support from spouses or others of their own age, although occasionally from older parents or younger adult children.

And we know that older people perceive their own futurity in a different light than the nonelderly. They recognize that if they don't die soon "of this" they are likely to die a little later "of that." The nonelderly may see death as cheating them of a well-deserved opportunity for considerably more life; the elderly tend to see imminent death as something that had been anticipated, more or less, all along (Kalish, 1984). These statements differentiating the elderly and the nonelderly are, of course, more valid for the old old than the young old, and they speak to tendencies and not universals in any event.

These three circumstances—cause of death, family supports, and perceived futurity—have been outlined only as examples of circumstances that are much more likely to affect the need systems of older dying persons than of younger dying persons or of older nondying persons. They are typical of the kinds of circumstances that must be taken into consideration in planning programs.

The research evidence, then, suggests that a larger proportion of older persons than of younger persons have come to terms with their death and will be more concerned with the dying process in terms of pain, discomfort, and isolation from others. The research also produces the realization that we cannot make the same assumptions about family supports of older dying persons that we would tend to make about nonelderly dying persons; for example, the wife of an elderly dying man is much less likely to be working full-time than the wife of a younger man, but she is also less likely to have the physical strength to help him bathe and the physical endurance to serve all of his needs.

While there is no substitute for a healthy combination of experience and sensitivity, being familiar with the research findings can be useful in alerting health and social-work professionals to look for age-related circumstances in the lives of the dying elderly. What should always be avoided in applying research findings is to permit them to establish a self-fulfilling prophecy.

Demographic research on suicide has some interesting practical implications also. Most people are aware that suicide rates go up among the elderly; most people are also aware that suicides are frequently attributed to a combination of feelings of hopelessness and helplessness, which are obviously related to depression; and most people know that depression is high among the elderly. What is less well known is that the suicide rates of white males continue to rise during the later years, while rates for older black men and for older white and black women increase very slightly or not at all or even diminish. And white males living alone have the highest suicide rates of all. Thus the research data help us to focus our attention on the group primarily at risk, but they do not indicate which particular individual is likely to make a serious suicide attempt.

Views from the Hierarchy of Needs

The familiarity and general acceptance of Maslow's hierarchy of needs makes it a useful model with which the needs of the dying elderly can be discussed. Meeting and satisfying the five sets of needs described by Maslow is particularly difficult for dying older persons. For example, the most basic needs of all, those necessary for survival, can be satisfied by almost all of us without having to turn to service programs or the care and support of others. This isn't always true for elderly dying individuals during the later stages of the dying process. As a function of the particular set of health conditions that have produced the terminal diagnosis, breathing may be difficult, pain is often great, temperature regulation is frequently difficult to maintain, and the individual—especially in the final days of life—may suffer from thirst if the condition is not alleviated regularly.

When people are asked to anticipate their own death, they indicate that fear of pain becomes especially strong, and this fear is just as strong for older persons as it is for younger or middle-aged people (Kalish and Reynolds, 1981).

Safety and security needs obviously come under attack during the dying process, no less so for the elderly than for other age groups. It is well-known that health professionals struggle harder to maintain the life of a nonelderly person than they do for an elderly person (Kastenbaum, 1981), and this knowledge is often recognized by the dying older person, undoubtedly to his or her consternation. The dying process generates feelings of vulnerability and uncertainty. Unless support persons — either family, friends, or health-care professionals — are in attendance, the fear of abandonment may become overwhelming. The lyrics of a song written particularly for dying persons expresses this well: "Teach me to die, hold on to my hand" (Teach Me to Die, by Deanne Edwards). And Avery Weisman (1977), whose clinical writings on dying persons have yet to be improved upon, proposes that dying people need *safe conduct*: cautious and prudent behavior and guidance through peril and the unknown. If physicians or other health professionals are unable to accomplish this task, they should turn it over to others who are both willing and competent to do so.

Safety and security needs in the older dying person are also unmet when anxiety is aroused concerning legal and financial issues. Caring for survivors, appropriate distribution of property, and paying health-care costs are all issues that may lead to a sense of vulnerability and insecurity, especially since the person whose survivors or property or costs are at stake will not be present to verify that the "right" thing has been done.

Older dying persons also have the same needs for love and esteem as anyone else. Because they are sometimes isolated from family and community supports, the difficulties of having their love needs met are frequently greater than those faced by persons still living in the community or by younger dying people whose family members may be more responsive. And esteem needs are also more difficult to meet at this point in life: triumphs and successes are now often many years in the past, and the kind of act that produces either esteem or self-esteem is much more difficult to accomplish.

The need for self-actualization of the older dying person leads to some challenging thoughts. First, the idea that personal growth can be enhanced by the dying process is certainly not a new one. Historically, there was an era when people believed they were judged in the hereafter not so much by how they lived as by how they died (Ariés, 1981). Nearly two decades ago, Zinker and Fink (1966) described the process of growth in a dying person.

Personal growth at this point in life could come through a variety of sources: improving one's handling of difficult interpersonal relationships, including re-establishing contact with someone with whom great tension had arisen years earlier; coping courageously with the pain, discomfort, and anxiety brought about by the terminal condition; responding to new spiritual awareness; accomplishing tasks that the health condition led others to believe were impossible.

This is just one approach to ordering the needs of the dying older person. Other systems can be applied just as readily.

The Need for Death with Dignity

Articles, talks, workshops, and classes on death and the dying process seem unanimous that the dying person needs a dignified death. Is dying with dignity the acceptance of death that designates the final stage in Kübler-Ross's (1969) work? Or is it "not go[ing] gently into the good night," as expressed so ardently by Dylan Thomas?

Weisman (1972) has described the importance of enabling a person to die an *appropriate* death, which means enabling that person to live the remainder of his or her life as nearly as possible as the individual wishes. The focus shifts from how to die to how to live, which picks up the point that so many people seem to be missing today: the issue is not so much how to die as how to live until death. We have observed some people who are so consumed with helping others die with dignity that the entire focus of their interactions is around the dying process, not the enrichment of the remaining living process.

Weisman (1972) was also among the first to point out that the social worth of older persons was lower than that of the nonelderly, and that therefore the dying elderly were less likely to receive the care and attention that the dying nonelderly received. Also, the elderly were more likely to receive pessimistic prognoses for their conditions. Since staff members appear less likely to provide services for persons whom they consider of lower social worth and for persons whose future life expectancy is least, these two attitudes can produce a self-fulfilling prophecy through reduced care and attention for terminally ill elderly persons.

To counter this tendency, it is necessary to provide optimum health care and optimum human care for dying elderly persons (even for those who apparently are not aware of the care), which will improve the likelihood that everyone can die an appropriate death.

Another issue that has emerged recently is what Kastenbaum (1982) has defined as the "image of terminal self-actualization" that requires "the terminal phase of life to be . . . exalted, fulfilling—something special, well beyond the ordinary dimensions of daily experience" (p. 164). This is sometimes extended to include altered-states-of-consciousness (ASC) experiences similar to those induced by mood-enchancing or psychotropic drugs. These states include feelings of total well-being or enhanced pleasure, of being physically outside one's body, of having been transported elsewhere in a mystical fashion, of having died or been about to die and then being "pulled back" from death to life. While Shneidman (1971) urged that death and the dying process be "deromanticized" and Garfield (1979) found that only slightly over 20 percent of a population of dying cancer patients had had an altered-state experience, others have encouraged the use of interventions to make the dying process a conscious one or, as one advocate stated, to "live your dying" (Keleman, 1974).

On the one hand, the encouragement of adding richness to the months, weeks, days, and hours prior to death by providing opportunites for self-actualization and for ASC experiences can only be applauded. It is likely that these experiences would be more common if the dying process were made less painful and less isolated, conditions that could be achieved by removing the restrictions on the use of certain drugs and by providing greater opportunities for personal relationships with family members, friends, and health caregivers.

However, to assume that self-actualizing or ASC experiences are needs of the dying places a burden on both the dying person and everyone in his or her milieu that may only add to the already existing pressures while accomplishing relatively little. And, as Kastenbaum (1982) emphasizes, it may be a recycling of the denial of death. "Dying will be all right as long as we are healthy, vibrant and creative. Death will be all right, too, as long as it is not death" (p.165). This coincides with the views of theologian Paul Ramsey (1975), who discusses the "indignity of the 'dignity of death'" when the cruel and destructive aspects of dying are ignored in favor of peace, naturalness, and potential for transcendence.

Another View of Needs

One pair of investigators spoke with caregivers of the dying—health professionals, clergy, and others—to learn what they perceived as the qualities that enable people to die an appropriate death (Augustine and Kalish, 1975). Three interrelated factors emerged from this study: (1) open communication concerning dying between patients and intimates; (2) physical and psychic closeness in these relationships; and (3) specific religious beliefs, with particular emphasis on transcendent meaning. To the extent that one of these was lacking, the others were also somewhat diminished.

There is little difficulty applying these qualities to the circumstances faced by the elderly. Open communication is more likely to have to take place with people of a younger generation than with age peers. In addition, both people in general (Kalish and Reynolds, 1981) and health professionals in particular (Kastenbaum, 1982) place less value on the lives of older persons than on those of the nonelderly, which suggests that less time and energy will be dispensed in developing open communication.

The closer these relationships are and the more opportunity for personal interaction that exists, the greater will be the capacity of the dying older person to draw strength from the relationships. Often, however, the older person has already lost through death and other processes those very persons who might have provided the kind of closeness now required. It is also interesting to speculate on the extent to which the surge in the divorce rate will affect intimate relationships that the elderly of the future will have available.

The consideration of religious beliefs and transcendent meaning is more complex. This does not refer to an uncritical acceptance of the community's mores but to the "capacity . . . to experience awe, wonder, and even terror through a kind of cosmic, nonego-centered awareness of the mysterious depths of life and reality" (Augustine and Kalish, 1975, p. 10). To communicate these experiences and their significance to others requires both a set of shared symbols and, often, shared experiences. Older people may find communication, or communion, more readily available with others of their generation, since membership in the same age cohort improves the likelihood of shared experiences.

In this context, the concerns of communication, intimacy, and meaning pervade all three of the desired qualities.

The issue for the practitioner is not only to be aware of these possibilities for growth but to be aware of how his or her attitudes and behavior can improve or stifle opportunities for growth. Elderly dying persons are highly vulnerable to those few remaining individuals who are still important to their well-being, among whom are health and social-service professionals. When the latter communicate lack of interest, assumptions of incompetence, impatience, or limited caring, the patient may internalize this communication as a lack of his or her own worth rather than the ineptitude of the professional. Conversely, those professionals who communicate that competence is necessary for their approval are also reducing the potential freedom of the dying person, who may fear failure. To encourage growth in these last weeks, or even hours, of life, the professional must accept the individual with all his or her present limitations, provide encouragement for growth-producing activities without making them an issue, and offer assurance that the individual will not be abandoned. Add to these factors the previously discussed concerns of open communication, close relationships, and meaning, and the scene is set for the improvement of personal growth.

Developing Open Awareness

Since most professionals who work with the dying appear to prefer an open-awareness, open-communication context to the alternatives, the obvious question arises for the practitioner: How can I achieve that situation in my day-to-day interactions with dying persons?

The response inevitably must be prefaced with two comments: first, each individual and each setting must be viewed on its own merits; and second, when in doubt, the professional should be cautious and trust his or her intuition. Not that these two suggestions are always correct or even always helpful, but they appear to be more successful than their alternatives.

Nonetheless, some generalizations can be made. For example, when the dying person has limited cognitive awareness, it is difficult or even impossible to know whether your words will be understood. There seem to be three modal possibilities: you will be understood; you will be misunderstood; you will have no impact at all. If the situation is either the first or the third of these possibilities, your course is clearer than if it is the second. What you need to consider is whether you risk more by (a) communicating nothing of the prognosis, (b) communicating a falsely optimistic prognosis, or (c) communicating an accurate prognosis.

In instances in which you believe you will receive no response to your statement or in which you won't be able to interpret the response accurately, you might consider saying something like this: "Mr. J., I think you know that you have been very sick recently. It seems possible that your sickness is going to get worse and you may not recover from it. In fact, it is even possible that you will die from this sickness. However, I want you to know that everyone at this hospital/hospice/agency will continue to look after you. We will take care of you and visit you and do everything we can to see that you are comfortable and without pain. I know your family and friends will be doing the same. (Note: Use the latter sentence only if it is likely to be true.) You will not be abandoned or forgotten."

This is the message that needs to be communicated to all dying persons. It is a combination of straight talk and caring. Sometimes, of course, the dying person responds with anger when he or she hears this message. It is not the task of the health or social-work professional to force a person to accept his or her own death. As Avery Weisman commented a number of years ago, our obligation is to give the individual enough information so that he or she can ask relevant and intelligent questions *if* he or she wishes to ask them. This avoids the Scylla of saying nothing or pretending everything is all right and the Charybdis of the you-*will*-accept-your-death attitude that one occasionally finds today.

Some elderly dying persons have come to terms with their own death and do not need more information; they are likely to need reassurance that they will not suffer or be abandoned. These are both legitimate fears, but they relate to the dying process, not to the meaning of death, and this difference must be recognized. Others will deny their impending death, and that is their right, but experience suggests that even the initial burst of anger or depression at being told of a terminal prognosis can be the first step to a willingness to cope effectively with the concerns.

MODELS OF SERVICES FOR OLDER DYING PERSONS

If there's a need, there must be a service to meet it; if there's a service, there must be a professional to staff it; if there's a professional, there must be a funding program to support it. These axioms of service and service providers are not always supported by either necessity or reality. And even necessity and reality may be perceived differently as philosophies, fads, and funds appear and subsequently disappear.

There are, to my knowledge, no service programs or service-program models developed specifically for older dying persons, and perhaps there should be none. Those that exist include either the nonelderly dying or the nondying elderly, and it is unusual when more than a minority of the persons served are both elderly and dying.

This in no way implies that the elderly dying are not served in any meaningful fashion. During the past dozen years, the number of persons, both professional and nonprofessional, who are sensitive to the needs of the elderly dying has increased greatly. Throughout the country there are now social workers, chaplains, physicians and nurses, volunteers, psychologists and psychiatrists, librarians and many others who are capable of responding at a personal level to a dying individual. Above and beyond individual interventions, many hospitals and other agencies have developed programs for dying persons. At the same time, the topics of death and bereavement are frequently on the agenda of senior centers and long-term-care facilities.

Given the lack of models specifically for the elderly dying, I will outline three models that are not directed at any age group but that are frequently of value in serving the elderly population: a self-help, community-based organization; a volunteer-staffed, community-based organization; and a hospice.

Make Today Count

Make Today Count is a national organization with chapters all over the country. Begun by Orville Kelly shortly after he was diagnosed as having terminal cancer, the organization has grown rapidly as local chapters are begun either by cancer patients or their families or, less frequently, by clergy or health or social-work professionals. A national office is maintained at 218 South Sixth Street, Burlington, Iowa 52601.

The purpose of the organization is to provide those suffering from cancer and their family members with the social and emotional support that derives from meetings with others who face similar circumstances. During the regular chapter meetings, participants exchange experiences, offer encouragement, respond to difficulties with the specific issues of the mutilating effects of surgery or the side effects of radiation therapy, and try to make each day matter (Kelly, 1978). Referrals are often self-generated, but also come through health professionals, social workers, clergy, friends, and family members.

All ages are served through Make Today Count, although the elderly constitute a smaller proportion of the participants than might be anticipated based on the number of older persons who suffer from life-threatening cancer conditions. However, no membership statistics exist regarding age, and no published attempt has been made to evaluate the outcome of this organization's program. The assumption is implicitly made that if enough people wish to participate in the organization's program to keep the local chapters active, this provides a kind of de facto positive evaluation of their value.

Centers for Attitudinal Healing

Like chapters of Make Today Count, Centers for Attitudinal Healing are located in many communities around the country. Each center establishes its own model while retaining loose and informal ties with the initial center, located in Tiburon, California.

The Sante Fe, New Mexico, Center is typical. It was begun by a Santa Fe businesswoman who worked with the local hospital and interested lay persons in the area. Clergy, health professionals, social workers, and others were eventually contacted as sources of support and referral. All time is donated.

The present program consists of one evening gathering each week, attended by persons who are known to be suffering from life-threatening conditions, their family members, and a small number of volunteers who are referred to as facilitators. Following a meal, donated in part by a different local restaurant each week, the group gathers in what they call "a love circle," which permits each participant to say a little about himself/herself. This particular center has a spiritual orientation, without denominational focus and including Eastern as well as Western theology and philosophy.

The major portion of the evening is devoted to small-group discussions, with about ten persons—at least one of whom is a facilitator—in each group. Facilitators receive careful screening and meet twice a month for informal and unstructured training-discussion sessions. The issues that are aired in the discussions range from concerns that the participants have about their own death or the dying process of a family member to what happened at work that day. The facilitators do not attempt to adhere to any topic, nor do they interpret or probe or function as psychotherapists. They are what they are called: facilitators.

The Santa Fe Center for Attitudinal Healing attempts to reach people without regard to family status, age, or ethnicity. Because it operates in northern New Mexico and wishes to expand its activities into the rural areas of that part of the state, it has tried to be especially responsive to Hispanic and Native American cultural expectations, since these groups are especially numerous in northern New Mexico. While a significant proportion of the persons served by this center are elderly, no special effort is made to reach such individuals and no special programming has been developed for them.

Both the Make Today Count chapters and the Centers for Attitudinal Healing are grass-roots operations, each one being initiated by one or several interested persons in a community and maintained in the same manner. Professionals, other than as volunteers or participants, are not included; costs are minimal; resources are normally thin; work tends to fall disproportionately on one or a few unpaid persons who may, after a period of time, burn out, at which point the future of the chapter/center may become tenuous. However, if paid professionals were to take over an operation, the financial costs to the participants could become prohibitive and the likelihood of volunteers working at the same level alongside the paid professional would possibly diminish.

Hospices

In contrast to the two models described above, the hospice cannot function without substantial investment in well-paid professional workers. While often begun by community volunteers and continuing to depend on volunteers for some tasks, the hospice requires professionals as directors, health-care staff, and volunteer directors, as well as other personnel.

The basic hospice model is well-known. In effect, it is a service for persons who have been diagnosed as terminally ill and whose physicians believe that the more traditional hospital stay and medical treatment are no longer relevant. The hospice program focuses on the personal well-being of the dying individual, aiming to improve opportunities for living at home as long as possible, to keep pain and discomfort to a minimum without diminishing conscious awareness, to ensure as much time as possible with loved ones, and to enhance the patient's assurance that he/she will not be abandoned by either professionals or family members.

This is accomplished through a judicious use of trained volunteers, modest use of professionals, involvement of family members in the caregiving process, and health education for both the patient and the family members. Hospice care appears to be both cost-effective and care-effective, and so it is approved both by those whose major concern with health care is cost containment and by those whose major concern is patient satisfaction. (For additional information, Koff, 1980, and Davidson, 1978, are useful and practical sources; for a description of several hospice programs and an analysis of the most significant issues, Wass, 1978, is most helpful.)

However, within the basic parameters for hospices in general there are numerous variations: outpatient versus outpatient plus inpatient; working through available resources, such as the Visiting Nurse Association, versus developing its own staff; integrated with one inpatient facility versus involved with numerous inpatient facilities; under the control of a hospital or long-term-care facility versus free-standing; serving a limited geographic area versus serving a fairly large geographical area; being almost exclusively an operation for cancer patients versus being open to anyone who finds the service appropriate; and so forth.

The proportion of older persons served by hospices, both through inpatient and outpatient programs, is substantial, although considerably lower than would occur if these institutions served a random cross-section of all dying persons. The one available study of mental-health training in hospices understandably did not request information concerning older persons. However, it was found that the "special problems of grown children of the terminally ill parents" received less attention in the training offered than all but four of the thirty-two categories of training needs and was viewed as calling for additional training by more hospices than any of the other categories (Garfield, Larson, and Schuldberg, 1982).

The reasons that the elderly are relatively underserved by hospices are several: first, hospice programs are for the most part not set up to provide lengthy inpatient services, which is what the dying trajectory of the elderly often requires; second, hospices are normally not set up to handle persons who are cognitively impaired; third, hospices often prefer to work with persons who can be attended to at home, through the hospice volunteer program, which normally means that at least one available caregiver must be in the home, a requirement often not met by elderly dying persons. It is also possible that the elderly retain a more traditional view of what constitutes appropriate health care and are less likely to seek newly developed models.

FUTURE TRENDS

With the continued graying of America and with anticipated increases in life expectancy, there is every likelihood that the proportion of dying persons who are elderly will increase during the years ahead. This increase will slow down during the period in which the relatively small number of Great Depression babies reach their later years, then will speed up rapidly when the Baby Boom babies enter their 70s and 80s. Cures for heart disease, stroke, and cancer would only delay the timing by a decade or more.

Given the history of humanity, it would appear unlikely that services would be increased commensurately with the needs. And, in fact, as I have stated elsewhere in this chapter, it does not appear that the elderly dying require their own unique service model. The issue that arises is that of providing appropriate medical, psychological, social, and spiritual services for dying persons in response to the family status, cognitive competence, and nature of the illness of the individual, not in response to age. Certainly this has already occurred to some extent, as evidenced in the development of the three service models previously described and of their many counterparts.

What seems to be required now is an analysis of why older persons do not participate in these programs more than they do. If it is because the programs are unresponsive to the elderly, one set of interventions is suggested; if it is because older persons are unresponsive to the programs, another set of interventions may be contemplated.

There is little doubt that, during the past fifteen years, the consciousness of the public concerning the needs of both the elderly and the dying has been raised substantially. This trend is likely to continue before it reaches a plateau. By the end of the decade, hospices will probably be as well recognized as nursing homes are today, and counseling programs directed at dying persons will be viewed as no more unusual than those directed at troubled married couples. And the same trend will probably be found among health-care professionals, social workers, and others. Although perhaps such consciousness will never be as great at it "should" be, it will still be considerably greater than it now is.

It then seems obvious that our capacity to improve services for the elderly in general and for the dying in general may accomplish all that is necessary to improve services for the elderly dying.

REFERENCES

Ariés, P. (1981). *The hour of our death.* New York: Knopf.

Augustine, M. M., and Kalish, R. A. (1975). Religion, transcendence, and appropriate death. *Journal of Transpersonal Psychology.* **7**, 1-13.

Brim, O. G., Freeman, H. E., Levine, S., and Scotch, N. A. (Eds.). (1970). *The dying patient.* New York: Russell Sage.

Caine, L. (1974). *Widow.* New York: Morrow.

Cartwright, A., Hockey, L., and Anderson, J. L. (1973). *Life before death.* London: Routledge and Kegan Paul.

Choron, J. (1963). *Death and western thought.* New York: Collier.

Choron, J. (1964). *Modern man and mortality.* New York: Macmillan.

Davidson, G. W. (1978). *Hospice, development and administration.* Washington: Hemisphere.

Feifel, H. (Ed.). (1959). *The meaning of death.* New York: McGraw-Hill.

Garfield, C. A. (Ed.). (1978). *Psychosocial care of the dying patient.* New York: McGraw-Hill.

Garfield, C. A. (1979). The dying patient's concern with "life after death." In R. J. Kastenbaum (Ed.), *Between life and death.* New York: Springer.

Garfield, C. A., Larson, D. G., and Schuldberg, D. (1982). Mental health training and the hospice community. *Death Education,* **6**, 189-204.

Kalish, R.A. (1984). *Death, grief, and caring relationships.* Monterey, Calif.: Brooks/Cole. 2nd ed.

Kalish, R. A., and Reynolds, D. K. (1981). *Death and ethnicity: A psychocultural study.* Farmingdale, N.Y.: Baywood. 2nd ed.

Kastenbaum, R. J. (1981). *Death, society, and human experiences* (2nd ed.). St. Louis: Mosby.

Kastenbaum, R. J. (1982). New fantasies in the American death system. *Death Education,* **6**, 155-166.

Keleman, S. (1974). *Living your dying.* New York: Random House.

Kelly, O. E. (1978). Living with a life-threatening illness. In C. A. Garfield (Ed.), *Psychosocial care of the dying patient.* New York: McGraw-Hill.

Koestenbaum, P. (1971). *The vitality of death.* Westport, Conn.: Greenwood Press.

Koff, T. H. (1980). *Hospice: A caring community.* Cambridge, Mass.: Winthrop.

Kübler-Ross, E. (1969). *On death and dying.* New York: Macmillan.

Maslow, A. H. (1954). *Motivation and personality.* New York: Harper & Row.

Parkes, C. M. (1972). *Bereavement.* New York: International Universities Press.

Pattison, E. M. (1977). The dying experience-retrospective analysis. In E. M. Pattison (Ed.), *The experience of dying.* Englewood Cliffs, N.J.: Prentice-Hall.

Pine, V. R. (1975). *Caretaker of the dead: The American funeral director.* New York: Irvington.

Ramsey, P. (1975). The indignity of "death with dignity." In P. Steinfels and R. M. Veatch (Eds.). *Death inside out.* New York: Harper & Row.

Reimer, J. (Ed.). (1974). *Jewish reflections on death.* New York: Schocken.

Shaffer, T. L. (1970). *Death, property, and lawyers.* New York: Dunellen.

Shneidman, E. S. (1971). On the deromanticization of death. *American Journal of Psychotherapy,* **25**, 4-17.

Thielicke, H. (1970). *Death and life.* Philadelphia: Fortress Press.

Wass, H. (Ed.). (1978). The hospice: Special issue. *Death Education,* **2**, 1-230.

Weisman, A. D. (1972). *On dying and denying.* New York: Behavioral Publications.

Weisman, A. D. (1977). The psychiatrist and the inexorable. In H. Feifel (Ed.), *New meanings of death.* New York: McGraw-Hill.

Zinker, J. C., and Fink, S. L. (1966). The possibility of psychological growth in a dying person. *Journal of General Psychology,* **74**, 185-199.

PART VII

POLICY, PLANNING, AND OPERATION OF SERVICES

24

Models of Services for the Elderly

Sheldon S. Tobin, Ph.D.

State University of New York at Albany

Ron Toseland, Ph.D.

State University of New York at Albany

The many preceding chapters in this volume have provided the reader with not only an introduction to generic concepts regarding gerontological services for the elderly but also with a wealth of information on specific treatment interventions and programs. Here the task is to pause and reflect on ways to synthesize some of the preceding content, and, more specifically, to discuss models of social services for the elderly. Principles for the development of a comprehensive model will be offered, but only after discussing general approaches to the classification of services and the complexity of matching services to needs, which is surely one reason for model building. The use of brief case vignettes will help to anchor our discussion of how to translate discrete services into rational models. Then, after a presentation of some principles for comprehensive models, some specific kinds of models will be reviewed that are, in varying degrees, comprehensive.

CLASSIFYING SERVICES

The organization of this volume reflects one way that services for the elderly can be classified. In Part IV, community-based services were considered; in Part V, home-based services; and then in Part VI, long-term-care and institutional-based services. Because topics covered within each of these three sections suggest a progression from services for the least impaired to the most severely impaired elderly, there was an implicit association of community-based services with the least impaired, of home-based services with those with greater impairments, and of long-term-care and institutional-based services with the severely impaired. With only slight modification of this trichotomy, however, each focus of service delivery can become appropriate for all levels of impairment.

For three general levels of impairment, as shown in Table 24-1, services can be identified within each of the three kinds of geographical distinctions. A previous effort to show how services can be organized in various ways for individuals with the same general levels of impairment led to a trichotomy of home-based services, congregate-organized services, and congregate-residence services (Tobin, 1975; Tobin and Lieberman, 1976; Tobin, Davidson, and Sack, 1976). The differences between the earlier trichotomy and the present one makes it apparent that there is no absolute way to classify the geography of services. Yet it is sensible to consider how elderly with the same general level of impairment can benefit from the use of differing organizing principles to make rational the current array of uncoordinated services. For the severely impaired, for example, care outside of institutions can be organized primarily around services delivered into the home or around medically oriented, as well as psychiatrically oriented, community or congregate day-care treatment programs. The boundaries between classes of services, as well as between service components within each class, are obviously quite permeable. Additionally, sets of services can be clustered, as when services are delivered by a multipurpose senior center or through a case-management system or when elderly live in a retirement village. Still, the trichotomy is useful.

A geography of services provides one way for planners and practitioners to understand the terrain of service delivery. Currently, a variety of services exists in all communities that needs to be coordinated if individual elderly are to benefit from their presence. Beyond a way of identifying available, but not necessarily accessible, services, a geography of service reaffirms the importance of having diverse services for individuals with similar levels of impairments. Two elderly persons with similar levels of impairment may need very different kinds of services because of, for example, the presence or absence of family able and willing to provide assistance in caregiving. For the elderly person with such family members, home-based services may suffice, but for another elderly person who does not have these supports, an enriched congregate environment may be necessary. In turn, the family that is overburdened from caregiving may need respite care (a vacation or holiday from caregiving), which can be organized by providing a bed in a congregate facility for the elderly person. A twenty-four-hour homemaker, in turn, may provide sufficient assurance to the anxious family when a case-management system offers around-the-clock backup to the homemaker.

Table 24-1. A Classification of Services for Older Persons (Focus of Service Delivery)

Degree of impairment	Community-based	Home-based	Congregate residential and institutional-based
Minimal	Adult Education Senior Centers Voluntary Organizations Congregate Dining Programs Individual and Family Information and Referral, Advice, and Counseling	Home Repair Services Home Equity Conversion Share-A-Home Transportation Telephone Reassurance	Retirement Communities Senior Housing Congregate Residential Housing with Meals
Moderate	Multipurpose Senior Centers Community Mental Health Centers Outpatient Health Services Case Management Systems (Social/ Health Maintenance Organizations, etc.)	Foster Family Care Homemaker Meals-on-Wheels Case Management for Family Caregivers and Elderly Impaired Members	Group Homes Sheltered Residential Facilities Board and Care (Domiciliary Care) Facilities Respite Care
Severe	Medical Day Care Psychiatric Day Care Alzeheimer Family Groups	Home Health Care Protective Services Hospital Care at Home	Acute Hospitals Mental Hospitals Intermediate (Health Related) Nursing Facilities Skilled Nursing Facilities Hospice Care in a Facility

DISCRETE AND INTEGRATING SERVICES

Discrete services for older persons have existed since antiquity (Beattie, 1976). In modern industrial society, particularly since the inception of social security, there has been an enormous increase in programs and services for both the young old and the old old. These programs and services, however, have not arisen as part of a carefully thought-out plan for meeting the needs of older persons (Kahn, 1976). Rather, these programs and services have been developed, in large part, in a Band-Aid, patchwork fashion, as needs were identified and political pressures were sufficient to bring about the development of specific programs and services. The Older Americans Act of 1965 reflects how political pressures result in statements of intent but not with organizing principles for service delivery (Estes, 1979). Some subgroups among the elderly were targeted as particularly needy and discrete services identified for development, but integrating mechanisms were not identified. Funding nutrition programs and multipurpose senior centers can be interpreted as only a modest attempt to develop ways of organizing or integrating services. Indeed, several of the services discussed earlier in this volume, and some that appear in Table 24-1, are programs that do attempt to integrate services such as one-step intake services, multiservice centers, and case management. Yet the Older Americans Act when amended in 1973 (P.L. 93-29) did not mandate any forms of service integration but rather focused upon a clearer specification of programs that needed to be coordinated for specific subgroups among the elderly. At the same time, however, the Allied Service Bill of 1974 (92nd Cong., 2nd Sess.; S. 3643, H. R. 15856), did go beyond the listing of services to encompass the need for integration of services. To integrate services, Frank Carlucci, who was then Under Secretary of the Department of Health, Education, and Welfare, emphasized in 1974 the need for common intake and case management: "a comprehensive assessment of a person's multiple need for services at a single entry point, then [taking] responsibility for seeing to it that appropriate services are provided."

It is now almost one decade later and little has been done to attain the lofty goal of integrating services. Case management exists more in word than deed, and whereas coordination has replaced service integration as the *lingua franca,* it also is more of a cliché that refers to a desired outcome rather than to the reality of the achievement of service integration through adequate funding. All but a few direct practitioners must still function in a fragmented nonsystem of services. Yet service integration for those who can benefit from alternatives to institutional care has been shown to be effective (Applebaum, Seidl, and Austin, 1980; Eggert, Bowlyou, and Nichols, 1980; Hodgson and Quinn, 1980). In these times of austerity, however, the favorable experiences of the three cited programs—the Wisconsin Community Care Organization, Access in Monroe County, New York, and Triage in Connecticut—have not led to a national program but rather to the newest set of demonstration projects, the channeling grants of the Health Care Finance Administration.

The purpose of the National Long Term Care Channeling Demonstration Program is to identify the most efficient and effective methods for utilizing community-based long-term resources for clients 65 and over who have unmet service needs and fragile informal supports. Ten states are participating in this initiative, which has been designed to assess the costs associated with various kinds of delivery systems as well as the impact of comprehensive assessment and case management on client well-being. A standard design has been developed for all ten sites that includes randomizing clients into either a treatment (experimental) group or a control group. A standardized instrument is used for screening, and clients who are assessed to be appropriate for the program are randomly assigned to either the control or treatment group. Those in the control group are referred to the current system and followed by the researcher. Those in the treatment group are given a comprehensive assessment by the channeling staff, who make an in-person assessment, again using a standard instrument. A care plan is developed and case managers then arrange for the delivery of services according to the care plan. A reassessment is conducted every six months unless the client situation changes, necessitating a reassessment within a shorter period of time. Because the program will be operational through March 1985, results cannot be expected until sometime thereafter.

Until coherent and rational service systems are developed, when knowledgeable persons describe services for the elderly, the narrative is more likely to be a catalogue of services rather than a description of a coherent system of services (Beattie, 1976; Gelfand and Olsen, 1980; Gold, 1974; Holmes and Holmes, 1979; Lowy, 1979). Cataloguing and detailing the usefulness of services, as well as how they can function for individual elderly, however, is useful because it familiarizes practitioners and planners with the diversity of services currently available to older people, suggests gaps in services, and raises issues about organizing services.

Development of models for the integration of services has occurred most often in relation to services that prevent unnecessary institutional care — services that are alternatives to institutional care. Witness the Morris (1971) proposal for a local personal care organization that would be developed and funded through nonprofit corporations that would purchase care for all beneficiaries within a substate area. The intent of his proposal was to create for each beneficiary a package of social and health services that would be tailor-made to meet his/her particular needs. The optimism of the early 1970s is reflected in the translation of the Morris model into legislation proposed by Kennedy and Mills (in H. R. 13870, 93rd Cong., 2nd Sess., 1974). (See also U.S. Congress, 1971a, 1971b.) Among other attempts to consider ways of organizing services are those included in a conference report on the topic edited by Pfeiffer (1973), and also Bell (1973), who, like Morris, advocated that services should be coordinated by one public agency in each geographical area. He identified five services that need to be coordinated: health maintenance, home help, mobile meals, transportation, and counseling. Some, but insufficient, attention has been given to how services need to be modified for minority elderly (Adams, 1980) and differences in urban and rural areas (Birren, 1976; Nelson 1980; Rose, 1976).

MATCHING SERVICES WITH NEEDS

Basic to all models of service delivery is the assumption that an array of services are available for the direct-service worker to provide to individual clients as needed. The geography of services presented initially in this chapter reflects this assumption. Comprehensive taxonomies for organizing services for the elderly, however, as noted earlier, are relatively rare. A quite ambitious and laudatory attempt was undertaken by Golant and McCaslin (1979), who built on Lawton's (1972) formulations for assessing the functional status of individual elderly. They based their taxonomy on Lawton's dimensions of competence and independence to generate levels of functioning. In their schemata, competence is measured on seven levels of increasingly complex tasks: (1) life maintenance, (2) functional health, (3) perception and cognition, (4) physical self-maintenance, (5) instrumental self-maintenance, (6) effectance, and (7) social-role performance. Independence, in turn, similar to one dimension of our typology, is measured on three levels: (1) services for those whose impairments necessitate institutional care or its equivalents, (2) services that provide alternatives for preventing premature institutionalization, and (3) services for the comparatively well elderly. Using these two dimensions, Golant and McCaslin categorized a variety of services that are available to meet the needs of older persons. Because Golant and McCallin have been so ambitious, and thus so comprehensive, their classification system is rather complex. Indeed, our simpler system becomes rather complex when focusing on individual cases.

The following case vignettes illustrate the diversity of services that can be developed to meet the needs of the heterogeneous population of the elderly. They also illustrate ways that service integration can occur, including through individual inititative in the marketplace, within a retirement community, by medically oriented sheltered housing, and by case management. Additionally, gaps in service are evident, particularly in the last illustration, that of Mrs. Jansen, who remained in a costly hospital bed for five weeks while awaiting nursing-home placement.

The first two vignettes illustrate the different ways that services are organized for those whose degree of impairment is minimal. In the first case, Mrs. Larandi relies on a number of community and home-based services to keep her functioning at an optimal level while living in her own home. In the second case, Mr. and Mrs. Texter rely on several community-based and home-based services while residing in a retirement community.

Mrs. Larandi is a 69-year-old widow who lives in her own home in an ethnic community in a large city. Except for her chronic arthritis, which affects her knees and makes walking somewhat painful, Mrs. Larandi is in good health. She does, however, utilize several community services in addition to the outpatient services she receives at the local hospital for her arthritis. To utilize her leisure time productively, she is involved with RSVP. Through this program, she works for a local hospital's patient-services department four hours a day, three days a week. Two other days during the week she has her lunch at the senior citizens center, where she remains to play bingo with her friends during the afternoon. She also uses the home-repair service that is available through the senior center and is considering becoming involved in the home-equity-conversion program. This program allows her to use the equity she has accumulated in her home to pay her taxes and her heating bill so she can continue to live in her own home.

Mr. Texter is 73 and Mrs. Texter 72. When Mr. Texter retired twelve years ago, they moved to Leisure World, a retirement community in a Southwestern state. Although they miss having more contact with their children and grandchildren, who continue to live in the community from which they migrated, both Mr. and Mrs. Texter are very pleased that they moved away from the frigid weather of North Central States. Not only have they made many new friends, but they enjoy the self-contained nature of Leisure World, which has a wide variety of services to meet their needs. For example, when Mr. Texter had difficulty with retirement benefits he was receiving, he received help in straightening out the problem from a worker at the residents service office (information and referral), which is centrally located in the community center at Leisure World.

For Mr. Texter's hearing problem and for Mrs. Texter's glaucoma, they rely on private physicians who have offices in the community. They are both involved with a variety of leisure-time activities through the men's club and the women's club, which are housed in the fitness center at Leisure World. Because they have no transportation, they rely on the senior van service, which takes them on shopping trips to two medium-sized cities some distance from Leisure World.

The next two case examples illustrate the different ways that services may be arranged for those who are moderately impaired. With the help of a variety of support services, both Mrs. Bishop and Mr. Fendel are able to function at optimal levels and avoid being institutionalized.

Mrs. Bishop is a 77-year-old widow who lives in a one-bedroom apartment in a rent-controlled building in a large urban area. Almost seven years ago, Mrs. Bishop was hospitalized for a short time for agitation and sleeplessness. Her condition, diagnosed as a severe depression, was stabilized with Lithium. Since that time, she is seen monthly by a worker at an after-care community mental health clinic, where her Lithium blood level is monitored and her prescription is renewed. Because of her chronic arthritis and hearing difficulties, she found it increasingly difficult to keep her clinic appointments. Her Department of Social Services (DSS) adult-services worker arranged for a light to be attached to her bell so she could be aware when someone was at her door even if she did not hear the doorbell ring. The DSS worker also arranged for escort services to take her to and from her clinic appointments. Since she qualifies for Meals-on-Wheels, and had difficulty preparing meals for herself, this service was begun two years ago. Through Title XX of the Social Security Act, she was also eligible for homemaker services. The homemaker helps her with her household chores three hours a day, three days a week. On days the homemaker does not come, two neighbors in her apartment building look in on her. She gave both these neighbors keys to her apartment, just in case "something should happen and I can't answer the door."

Mr. Fendel, who was a migrant farm worker, fell on icy pavement last year just before his seventy-sixth birthday. He received treatment for his broken hip at the community hospital. Because he had no family in the area to care for him, Mr. Fendel could not return to his apartment. However, since he was able to get around with the help of a walker, his medical social worker at the hospital decided that Mr. Fendel might be a good candidate for a supportive living program sponsored by the Visiting Nurse Association (VNA). This program provides sheltered housing, in which Mr. Fendel could have his own room while sharing kitchen facilities with three other persons. Although he had a little difficulty getting adjusted, Mr. Fendel has done quite well in the new setting. The building, which was recently rehabilitated, was designed with the needs of the physically handicapped in mind. A homemaker and the Meals-on-Wheels service, which he obtained with the help of his medical social worker and a VNA nurse, who acted cooperatively in planning for Mr. Fendel's discharge from the hospital, are perfect for Mr. Fendel's needs. In case of an emergency such as falling down, the VNA has a nurse's aid stationed in the building twenty-four hours a day. In addition, there is a registered nurse available during the day. Other services, such as physical and occupational therapy, are available from the central office of the VNA if they are needed in the future.

The last two case examples illustrate the ways services may be organized for the severely impaired older person. In the first case, the availability of a caregiver makes it possible for Mrs. Hunter to remain at home. In the second case, despite a variety of community-based and home-based services, it was not possible for Mrs. Jansen to remain at home.

After some "periods of forgetfulness" and a serious incident in which the gas range was left on, Mr. Hunter decided to seek help for his wife. He was referred by his family physician to a geriatric unit in a state hospital fifteen minutes by car from his home. After a home visit, psychological testing, and a medical evaluation, the geriatric screening team decided that Mrs. Hunter, age 63, was suffering from Alzheimer's Disease. Because of her proximity to the hospital, it was decided that she should attend the day treatment program, which operates six hours each week. This program, designed especially for those with Organic Brain Syndrome, was especially useful because it gave Mr. Hunter some relief from the burdens of caring for his wife. It also provided supportive counseling, including involvement in a group for family members of patients with Alzheimer's Disease, for Mr. Hunter, who was psychologically devastated by the rapid deterioration of his wife's condition. After several months, further diagnostic testing was ordered by the geriatric team's physician and a CAT Scan revealed two small lesions, one in the frontal lobe and one at the base of Mrs. Hunter's brain. The latter was inoperable. The diagnosis was changed, and after some deliberation it was decided to change Mrs. Hunter's plan of care and involve her with a home-based hospice program. A worker from the geriatric team, acting as case coordinator, stayed involved with Mr. and Mrs. Hunter. In addition to coordinating a variety of services, including medical care, SSI, and legal counseling to prepare a will, the worker helped Mr. Hunter to cope with his wife's illness.

Eight months after Mr. Hunter had contacted his family physician, Mrs. Hunter died at home. The worker from the geriatric unit had several contacts with Mr. Hunter following his wife's death. These were designed to ensure that he was successfully coping with the loss of his wife. Through these contacts he was helped to become involved in a men's club at a local senior citizens center.

Mrs. Jansen is an 81-year-old, black female who resided with her brother in subsidized senior housing in a poor, high-crime, urban area. For eight years, Mrs. Jansen has suffered from Alzheimer's Disease. At first, only her short-term memory was impaired, but in recent years the disease has progressed and she is no longer oriented to person, place, or time. In the last six months she has also become incontinent. She received homemaker services as well as Meals-on-Wheels. These services would have been insufficient, however, to maintain Mrs. Jansen at home due to the severity of her confusion, if it were not for the devoted attention of her husband, who provided twenty-four-hour care for Mrs. Jansen.

Unfortunately, while the homemaker was attending to Mrs. Jansen, Mr. Jansen went out shopping for groceries and was mugged by two teenagers, who robbed him and knocked him to the ground. Because of the injuries he sustained, he had to be hospitalized, creating an emergency situation for Mrs. Jansen, who could not be left unsupervised in her apartment. An adult-protective-service worker at the county social service office became involved immediately after the problem was reported by the homemaker. Placement in a nursing home was the only alternative, but because a nursing home bed was not immediately available the protective-service worker advised the Jansens' physician to hospitalize her, which he did. Although Mrs. Jansen was needlessly occupying a costly hospital bed, nursing homes were reluctant to accept her because of her mental impairment and intermittent incontinence and, also, because she was a Medicaid patient. Mr. Jansen was recovering nicely and wished to care for his wife at home, but the Jansens' physician advised against it because of Mr. Jansen's immobility and the burden of caregiving and told Mr. Jansen that "it was time for her to go to a home." After three weeks in the hospital she was accepted into a voluntary sectarian home.

The case examples illustrate that many different kinds of service arrangements are necessary to meet the diverse needs of older persons. In addition to the general rule of developing a flexible and diverse service-delivery system to meet the unique and disparate needs of different older persons, a variety of questions should be resolved when considering models for organizing services for older persons.

FROM CLASSIFICATION TO MODELS

To translate classifications of services for the heterogeneous elderly to models first necessitates a statement of purposes. The case vignettes suggest that goals vary by functional status. For the relatively unimpaired, services should enhance well-being and prevent deteriorations; for the moderately impaired, they should facilitate activities of daily living, enhance the caregiving of informal supports, prevent further deterioration, and, whenever possible, restore lost functioning; and for the severely impaired, in addition to the goals for the impaired, services should limit unnecessary and premature institutional care and, when necessary, offer appropriate institutional care. To be effective, a service system must be accessible to the target population, receptive to the idiosyncratic needs of clients, and able to provide options and multiple services for each client, both simultaneously and in appropriate sequence, as needed. Thus goals, in turn, can be achieved only by a system of services that is coordinated so that diverse parts function in concert to assure that service-delivery goals are attained and planned so that resources may be allocated and distributed rationally, giving major attention to client needs.

This set of goals can be applied to all human services, not only social services. Social services, according to Kahn (1973), pertain to "programs that protect or restore family life, help individuals cope with external and internal problems, enhance development and facilitate access through information, guidance, advocacy, and concrete help of several kinds" (p. 19). Focusing on social services *per se*, however, does not resolve issues of who should be provided with social services, what social services should be provided, and how social services should be delivered. Stated another way, a social-service model for the elderly could focus on people of all ages, including the elderly, or specifically on the elderly, and if on the elderly, on all the elderly or on elderly identified as more in need; could encompass all possible social health services or be concentrated in specific services to meet the most unmet of needs; and could be fully coordinated and planned or partially so, through, for example, informal arrangements. (For a fuller discussion of these issues, see Tobin, Davidson, and Sack, 1976.)

PRINCIPLES FOR A COMPREHENSIVE MODEL

Any comprehensive model must answer three questions: For whom? What? And how? These three questions will be discussed in order.

For Whom?

The elderly could be served as part of the larger society. Indeed, Neugarten (1983) has argued for an age-irrelevant society in which chronological age becomes extraneous. With adjustments of Social Security by the cost of living index, the percentage of elderly below the poverty level now approximates the percentage for other age groups (about 15 percent). Moreover, because the elderly receive a diversity of in-kind benefits, the elderly may now be considered to be relatively advantaged. For example, whereas the amount of chronic impairment among the elderly is similar to the amount among other age groups, the elderly receive Medicare. The graying of the federal budget (Hudson, 1978) reflects the increased expenditures for the elderly. Thus, in years past, providing services to all the elderly, through age-based entitlement, was sensible because attributed need could be demonstrated by population statistics. This particularistic approach, however, is no longer valid, and increasingly advocated are universalistic approaches using demonstrated need — that is, need-based programs (Etzioni, 1976). Illustrations of the argument for basing programs on need rather than age occur in our vignettes. Mrs. Hunter, for example, was only 63 when diagnosed as afflicted with Alzheimer's Disease, whereas Mrs. Jansen was 81.

Kutza and Zweibel (1983) have contrasted the arguments for each approach. An age-based (or attributed-need) allocative policy is attractive because of political expediency, administrative efficiency, simplicity of measurement, and lack of stigmatization. A need-based policy, on the other hand, more efficiently targets the most needy. In turn, Ozawa (1976) has shown that SSI, a need-based program, does not stigmatize elderly recipients as does welfare programs for the chronically poor. Because of the political viability of programs for the elderly, Austin and Loeb (1983) argue that age is relevant and, for this reason, Kutza and Zweibel (1983) advocate programs that combine age and need, such as mandating group eligibility of the elderly for those receiving SSI or Medicaid. This kind of combination is certainly better than recent programs, such as those of the Administration on Aging, that have disproportionately benefited the more affluent (U.S. General Accounting Office, 1977b; Estes, 1979; Estes and Newcomer, 1978; Kutza, 1981; Nelson, 1983). Apparently funding through Title XX of the Social Security Act has not heretofore proved an effective remedy to maldistribution for the most needy among the elderly (Gilbert, 1977; Gilbert and Specht, 1979; Schram, 1983; Schram and Hurley, 1977).

A concrete example of how the age-based program has not reached those with the greatest need is the nutrition, or congregate dining, program for the elderly (Title III-C of the Older Americans Act, formerly Title VII). This program was funded to redress nutritional and social-interaction deficiencies. Although great numbers of the elderly have participated in this program, the evidence suggests that those who have participated have been the healthier and the more socially active. Tobin and Thompson (1981) have referred to one aspect of this phenomenon as the "countability paradox" because, in their study of programs in one community, those nutrition sites with greater numbers (and thus judged more successful by the local office on aging) had fewer impaired participants than programs with fewer participants (that were judged as less successful by the group that allocated funds for dining sites). Where accounting is based on numbers rather than need, it is easy, and perversely sensible, to exclude those with impairments because they make the well elderly feel uncomfortable, create additional management problems, and necessitate consideration of programs beyond recreational activities.

Determining eligibility by need rather than by age, however, does not resolve two other kinds of questions. Should personal assets also be used, such as a means test, in determining eligibility? And, independent of eligibility considerations, do the special needs of the elderly dictate special kinds of service systems?

Regarding the first of these two questions, there are at least two reasons why means tests may not be appropriate in determining eligibility for the chronically impaired. First, means tests generally stigmatize individuals. Second, few families have the resources necessary to provide homecare for their impaired elderly members. Currently, for example, there may be as many as double the percentage of families providing care at home for their elderly members as there are elderly with comparable functional statuses in nursing homes. The percentage of elderly in nursing homes is approaching 6 percent, but 8 percent of all the elderly are homebound (about 3 percent are bedridden) and certainly more than 4 percent are not homebound but need surveillance to remain in the community. The value of family caring, in turn, is much greater than the cost of agency services. In this "shared function" (Litwak, 1978) by family and agency, for example, the average monthly cost or value by both family (including friends) and agencies for those greatly impaired is $407, but the value of family and friends caregiving is $287 and agency cost is only $120; for the extremely impaired, the total cost is $845, with the value of family and friends caregiving placed at $673 and agency costs for their services at $172 (U.S. General Accounting Office, 1977a). The task, therefore, is to facilitate family and friends caregiving to the greatly and extremely impaired elderly so that all costs are not covered through agency and public expenditures. Because very few can afford this kind of monthly outlay of dollars, the solution in Great Britain has been to provide a modest Constant Attendance Allowance to families, regardless of income or assets (Moroney, 1976). Thus advocated is eligibility determined not by age or income through a means test but through assessment of need. The distinction between means and needs assessment, as well as the problems in needs assessment, has been cogently discussed by Austin and Loeb (1983).

Regarding the second question, whether the needs of the elderly dictate special services for them, it can be argued that the elderly are too often screened out of services, that family caregiving to the elderly may necessitate special kinds of programs and knowledge, and that the impairments and kinds of services needed for the elderly also demand speical expertise that can be gained only in age-specific programs. Cook (1983) has detailed the following steps in deciding whether the organization and delivery of services should be age based: the "specialness" of the problem, the importance of the special problem, the likelihood of successful targeting, the probability of ameliorating the problem, and the probability of minimizing unintended side affects. These steps, or criteria, in decision making do suggest the usefulness of an age-specific strategy in the organization and delivery of services, particularly for the more chronically impaired elderly. Because dependency from impairments rises precipitiously beyond age 75, priority should be given to the old old—that is, the most vulnerable—using a criterion of attributed need or a combination of age as a reflection of attributed need and demonstrated need.

A service system designed specifically for the most vulnerable and impaired elderly, as noted earlier, must also attend to issues of prevention. Unless consideration is given to the needs of the less impaired, predominantly young old, all resources will be allocated for the severely impaired elderly with no attention to prevention. There are three kinds of prevention: primary prevention refers to reducing the incidence of a disease; secondary prevention to reducing the effects of acute illness through early detection and vigorous intervention; and tertiary prevention to limiting the effects of chronic illness by stabilizing and enhancing functioning and, also, to reducing the likelihood of acute flare-ups. If resources are not specifically allocated for prevention, services will be concentrated for more desperate situations. Moroney (1976) found that, in Great Britain, personal-care services were almost exclusively used for those elderly without viable family supports. From the social workers' perspective, families with elderly could continue to manage for a time even if severely overburdened by caregiving. Whereas prevention of deterioration in family caregiving was an explicit goal, it could not be achieved if resources allowed only for attention to crisis and emergency situations.

For the severely impaired, however, institutional care can absorb all resources, leaving little for community-based services. Alternatively, prevention of institutionalization can lead to a focus on community alternatives without allocations for those who need institutional care. Other modern societies, as now we are, have confronted the reality that shifting resources from insitutional to community-based services can eventuate in the prevention of institutionalization but leave only benign neglect and custodial care for those who can no longer remain in the community. Given the reality of limited resources, this may be a deplorable necessity, but to have it occur without a rational debate on long-term care policies is to relinquish our responsibility to make the most critical of decisions.

What?

Services that can be provided in a comprehensive social-service system are too numerous to mention. Listed in Table 24-1 were only some of the services that can be provided to the elderly. The vignettes incorporated, among others, the following services: volunteer activities, senior centers, home repair, home equity conversion, information and referral, retirement communities, case management, homemaker and home-health services, sheltered housing, day treatment, hospice care, hospital care, and nursing-home placement. Must, however, a comprehensive system provide all possible services? It may not be feasible to do so. A classic example is that of homemaker. No society can provide all the homemaker services that every citizen desires. Even a comprehensive system would, therefore, have to confront the issue of rationing services. In addition, it is certainly necessary to echelon services so that more intense and more expensive services with less usage are developed for larger population bases than more everyday services. The corollary is in medical services, where primary-care physicians must be available in every community, secondary medical services, such as general hospitals, distributed among larger groups of people, and specialized tertiary-care facilities developed for even larger population bases. Rationing and echeloning of services, therefore, must be incorporated into any comprehensive system. This consideration of rationing and echeloning of services is particularly relevant to the case of Mrs. Jansen, who lingered in a costly bed in an acute general hospital while awaiting placement in a skilled-nursing home.

Most clear is that income maintenance must be provided to meet basic daily survival needs; and where there is heightened vulnerability and impairment, medical and social-service needs must then additionally be met. Any attempt to meet social-service needs must go beyond a proliferation of discrete services and include one or more strategies for assuring the availability of an appropriate mix of discrete services and those services that provide for their integration. A distinction between discrete services and integrating services has been noted earlier in this chaper and is reflected also among the diverse earlier chapters in this handbook. How to accomplish integration is our next question.

How?

The "how" in this context of models of social services for the elderly refers to service integration at the delivery level and to coordination and planning, as well as allocation, at the organizational level. Some solutions to service integration, as just noted, have been covered in this volume and were also reflected in the vignettes. The Texters, who were minimally impaired, lived in a retirement village in which the senior center functioned as a one-step multipurpose center but without decentralized common intake and case management. Mrs. Bishop, who was moderately impaired, had a Department of Social Service worker who functioned for her as case manager. Mrs. Fendel, also with moderate impairment, benefited from the service integration provided within medically oriented sheltered housing that Sherwood et al. (1981) found to limit nursing-home usage. Mrs. Hunter's case manager was a worker on the geropsychiatric team.

An alternative to a coherent professional system is, of course, to use the marketplace. Even if cash were provided for the purchase of service, when the purpose is to enhance the shared function of formal supports and the family for the impaired elderly member, would it best be given to the primary family caregiver or to the older person? Frankfather, Smith, and Caro (1981) argue that too much attention to the caregiving family diminishes the autonomy of the older person. They also apply this argument to professional case managers who they perceive as intrusive and likely to impose their own bias, which can result in supportiing family members at the expense of the elderly person—as was apparently the case in the Blenkner, Bloom, and Nielsen (1971) social experiment but not in Goldberg's (1970) study. If a case-management system is advocated for the integration of services for individuals and their families, then professional judgment obviously must include a sensitivity to the wishes of clients, and professional judgment of need must be tempered by a principle of minimal intervention (Kahn and Tobin, 1981).

Can, however, any kind of case-management system be comprehensive? No primary-care system can control the specialized services provided in a tertiary-care agency or facility. Thus the interaction between primary-care and tertiary-care providers can never be simple. Kane and Kane (1980), in their excellent study of long-term care in diverse modern societies, quickly discovered the many dynamic tensions among providers at different levels of service and among providers at the same service level. In Great Britain, for example, a major mechanism for assuring coordination among community-based care, hospitals, and long-term-care facilities was the lodging of authority to place the elderly person in a long-term facility in the hands of the community-based social worker. Only when the community-based worker judges that community care no longer assures independent living is institutional care provided.

Ownership of all services by an integrating provision mechanism, such as by a case-management system, is indeed not feasible. For coordination at the organizational level there must be formal agreement among service providers, particularly between providers who integrate services and discrete-service providers. To be sure, decentralized local-care services can increase accessibility for clients, capitalize on informal supports, respond to clients and family needs, and increase local autonomy, but at the same time must assure the delivery of more centralized services—the more costly secondary and tertiary services. Only, however, through centralized planning and allocation of resources can there be the capacity to assess the total needs of large segments of the population; a balancing of priorities among conflicting organizational demands; a setting of uniform standards and common objectives, increasing efficiencies; increasing coordination; and an assuring of formal commitments among agencies.

Coordination among agencies can take many forms, including hierarchical, egalitarian, and reciprocal relationships. It can also extend from informal agreements to collaborating through formal agreements to confederations to federations. Such complexities often suggest how simple it is to favor market place coordination. Yet through formal as well as informal agreements that include mechanisms for reimbursement for services, a great amount of coordination can be developed (Davidson, 1976; Tobin, Davidson, and Sack, 1976).

DESIGN OPTIONS FOR MODELS

The optimum model for service provision emerges from the previous discussion of some basic principles. Still, as noted in the discussion, optimum solutions to the questions for whom, what, and how do not permit an ideal model. There are none; there are, at best, trade-offs. Recent volumes edited by Meltzer, Farrow, and Richman (1981) and Callahan and Wallack (1981) contain a diversity of solutions to the financing of long-term care reflecting the kinds of trade-offs necessary in the real world. Our task, however, is to ignore reality for a moment and to advocate a more idealized model, but one that can accommodate rules of eligibility based on need and personal resources.

Tobin, Davidson, and Sack (1976) contrasted a preferred option for the design of services with two effective alternative designs. As shown in Table 24-2, reproduced from that monograph, the preferred model focuses on the most vulnerable among the elderly. Services for these elderly would not be restricted to the elderly with the lowest incomes because elderly above the poverty level need costly services even with moderate degrees of impairments if independent community living is to be assured. A full set of services would be provided through service integration, decentralized coordination would be extensive, and planning and allocation would be centralized.

The two effective alternatives vary on the five dimensions, but both contain mechanisms necessary for service integration. In turn, from the discrete options within each of the three general models, further models can be proliferated that combine solutions for the five dimensions. Given the realities of human services, for example, partial coordination may be preferred because of the need for dynamic tensions among providers with different missions and different expertise. This is most apparent, as noted earlier, in relationships among community-care

Table 24-2. Options for Configurations: The Preferred and Two Other

Central Questions	Preferred Design Options	Effective Alternatives	
I. Service delivery components			
Who	Elderly-Vulnerable Services as a right of all elderly, with priority given to the vulnerable	Universal-Vulnerable Services as a right to all in need, with the vulnerable elderly given priority	Low-Income Elderly Services provided only to low-income elderly
What	Full Service Comprehensive social service strategy providing social services, including income maintenance	Centralized I & R Broad social service strategy relying on disparate providers to meet service and income needs	Limited Service A limited range of services available at the neighborhood level with decentralized I & R
How	Social Integration A system which features decentralized intake, multipurpose centers, and professional integrators	Confederation A loose association of agencies which together provide a relatively full range of services through centralized intake without professional integrators	Neighborhood Nonprofessional A system which features decentralized intake and multipurpose centers through nonprofessional integrators
II. Organizational components			
Coordination	Full Coordination A system with formal inter- and intra-level agreements, with shared staff, intake, and information	Partial Coordination A system with formal intra-level agreements and informal inter-level agreements, with shared intake and information, but with separate staff	Informal Coordination A network with informal intra- and inter-level agreements, with agency-specific intake and staff and shared information
Planning and allocation	Centralized A system with centralized point planning, common objectives, and pooled resources	Cooperative A system with separate planning and decentralized decision making, with a combination of agency-specific and stated objectives, with some pooling of resources	Autonomous Community A system with decentralized planning at the neighborhood level, with agency-specific objectives and little pooling of resources

providers, hospitals, and long-term-care facilities. A "fully" coordinated system could too easily lead to domination by hospitals.

The design options detailed in Table 24-2 do not provide a fine-grained set of models. Returning to Table 24-1, it is possible, however, to build models from a variety of integrating services. Among community-based services, the multiple service center is a natural setting for service integration; among home-based services, diverse housing options and case management also offer rare opportunities for service integration; and all the kinds of institution-based services can likewise provide these opportunities. To single out only two kinds of special facilities, enriched group living for a dozen or so elderly has been found to be an excellent alternative to institutional care in other countries, and Sherwood et al. (1981) have similarly shown that medically enriched housing is effective for those with chronic impairments regardless of age.

A FINAL COMMENT

Models for the provision of services for the elderly are probably as varied as the elderly themselves. It is possible, however, to develop logical classification systems for the varied and uncoordinated services that currently are available for the elderly, as was discussed in the initial section of this chapter. Case vignettes were useful for illustrating how services with differing geographical organizing principles can meet the needs of elderly individuals with similar levels of impairment and also a variety of ways services can be integrated. Principles can, and were, identified that must guide the development of service-integration models. These principles must answer three kinds of questions. For whom among the elderly are services to be provided? What services must be provided to meet the needs of these elderly? And how can these services be integrated in their delivery and, at the organizational level, how can they be coordinated and planned? A modest attempt was made to develop an optimum model, as well as two alternative models that contained many design options. Albeit the accumulated knowledge permits the construction of optimum and also sensible alternative models, trade-offs would be necessary even in an ideal world. In a less-than-ideal world, obviously characteristic of the current state of affairs, alternatives that at least provide for some beneficial integraton are to be preferred over simplistic solutions that maintain the current fragmented nonsystem of services for the elderly.

REFERENCES

Adams, J. P., Jr. (1980). Service arrangements preferred by minority elderly: A cross-cultural survey. *Journal of Gerontological Social Work,* **3**(2), 39-57.

Applebaum, R., Seidl, F. W., and Austin, C. D., (1980). The Wisconsin community care organization: Preliminary findings from the Milwaukee experiment. *Gerontologist,* **20**(3), 350-355.

Austin, C. D., and Loeb, M. B., (1983). Why age is relevant in social policy and practice. In B. L. Neugarten (Ed.), *Age or need: public policies for older people.* Beverly Hills, Calif.: Sage Publications.

Beattie, W. M., Jr. (1976). Aging and the social services. In R. Binstock and E. Shanas (Eds.), *Handbook of aging and the social sciences.* New York: Van Nostrand Reinhold.

Bell, W. G. (1973). Community care for the elderly: An alternative to institutionalization. *Gerontologist,* **13**(3), 349-354.

Birren, J. E. (1976). The aged in cities. In B. D. Bell (Ed.), *Contemporary social gerontology.* Springfield, Ill.: Charles C. Thomas.

Blenkner, M., Bloom, M., and Neilsen, M. (1971). A research and demonstration project of protective services. *Social Casework,* **52**(10), 483-499.

Callahan, S. S., and Wallack, S. S. (Eds.). (1981). *Reforming the long-term care system.* Lexington, Mass.: Lexington Books.

Cook, F. L. (1983). Assessing age as an eligibility criterion. In B. L. Neugarten (Ed.), *Age or need: public policies for older people.* Beverly Hills, Calif.: Sage Publications.

Davidson, S. M. (1976). Planning and coordination of social services in multiorganizational context. *Social Service Review,* **50**(3), 117-137.

Eggert, G. M., Bowlyow, J. E., and Nichols, C. W., (1980). Gaining control of the long term care system: First returns from the ACCESS experiment. *Gerontologist,* **20**(3), 356-363.

Estes, C. (1979). *The aging experience: A critical examination of social policies and services for the aged.* San Francisco, Calif.: Jossey-Bass.

Estes, C., and Newcomer, R. (1973). *State units on aging: discretionary policy and action in eight states.* San Francisco, Calif.: University of California.

Etzioni, A. (1976, November/December). Old people and public policy. *Social Policy,* pp. 21-29.

Frankfather, D. L., Smith, M. J., and Caro, F. G. (1981). *Family care of the elderly: public initiatives and private obligations.* Lexington, Mass.: Lexington Books.

Gelfand, D. E., and Olsen, J. K. (1980). *The aging network.* New York: Springer.

Gilbert, N. (1977). The transformation of social services. *Social Service Review,* **51**(12), 624-641.

Gilbert, N., and Specht, H. (1979). Title XX planning by area agencies on aging: Efforts, outcomes and policy implications. *Gerontologist,* **19**(6), 264-274.

Golant, S. M., and McCaslin, R. (1979). A functional classification of services for older people. *Journal of Gerontological Social Work,* **1**(3), 187-209.

Gold, B. D. (1974). The role of the federal government in the provision of social services to older persons. *Annals of the American Academy of Political and Social Sciences,* **415**, 55-69.

Goldberg, E. M. (1970). *Helping the aged: A field experiment in social work.* London: George Allen & Unwin.

Hodgson, J. H., Jr., and Quinn, J. L. (1980). The impact of the Triage health care delivery system upon client morale, independent living and the cost of care. *Gerontologist,* **20**(3), 364-371.

Holmes, M., and Holmes, D. (1979) *Handbook of human services for older persons.* New York: Human Sciences Press.

Hudson, R. (1978). The graying of the federal budget and its consequences for old age policy, *Gerontologist,* **18**(10), 428-440.

Kahn, A. J. (1973). *Social policy and social services.* New York: Random House.

Kahn, A. J. (1976). Service delivery at the neighborhood level: Experience, theory, and fads. *Social Service Review,* **50**(1), 23-56.

Kahn, R. L., and Tobin, S. S. (1981). Community treatment for aged persons with altered brain function. In *Clinical Aspects of Alzheimer's Disease and Senile Dementia.* New York: Raven Press.

Kane, R. L., and Kane, R. A. (1980). Alternatives to institutional care of the elderly: Beyond the dichotomy. *Gerontologist,* **20**(3), 249-259.

Kutza, E. A. (1981). *The benefits of old age: Social welfare policy for the elderly.* Chicago: University of Chicago Press.

Kutza, E. A., and Zweibel, N. R. (1983). Age as a criterion for focusing public programs. In B. L.

Neugarten (Ed.), *Age or need: Public policies for older people*. Beverly Hills, Calif.: Sage Publications.

Lawton, M. P. (1972). Assessing the competence of older persons. In D. P. Kent, R. Kartenbaum, and S. Sherwood (Eds.), *Research planning and action for the elderly*. New York: Behavioral Publications.

Litwak, E. (1977). Theoretical base for practice. In R. Dobrof and E. Litwak, *Maintenance of family ties of long-term care patients*. U.S. Department of Health, Education and Welfare.

Lowy, L. (1979). *Social work with the aging: The challenge and promise of the later years*. New York: Harper and Row.

Meltzer, J., Farrow, F., and Richman, H. A. (Eds.). (1981). *Policy options in long-term care*. Chicago: University of Chicago Press.

Moroney, R. M. (1976). *The family and the state: considerations for social policy*. London: Longman Group.

Morris, R. (1971). *Alternatives to nursing home care: A proposal*. Washington, D.C.: Government Printing Office.

Nelson, G. (1980). Social services to the urban and rural aged: The experience of area agencies on aging. *Gerontologist*, **20**(2), 200-207.

Nelson, D. W. (1983). Alternative images of old age as the basis for policy. In B. L. Neugarten (Ed.), *Age or need: Public policies for older people*. Beverly Hills, Calif.: Sage Publications.

Neugarten, B. L. (1983). *Age or need: Public policies for older people*. Beverly Hills, Calif.: Sage Publications.

Ozawa, M. N. (1976). Impact of SSI on the aged and disabled poor. *Social Work Research and Abstracts*, **14**, 3-10.

Pfeiffer, E. (Ed.). (1973). *Alternatives to institutional care for older Americans: Practice and planning*. Durham, N.C.: Center for the Study of Aging and Human Development, Duke University.

Rose, A. M. (1976). Perspectives on the rural aged. In B. D. Bell (Ed.), *Contemporary Social Gerontology*. Springfield, Ill.: Charles C. Thomas.

Schram, S. F. (1983). Social services for older people. In B. L. Neugarten (Ed.), *Age or need: Public policies for older people*. Beverly Hills, Calif.: Sage Publications.

Schram, S. F., and Hurley, R. (1977). Title XX and the elderly. *Social Work*, **22**(3), 95-102.

Sherwood, S., Greer, D. S., Morris, J. N., and Mor, V. (1981). *An alternative to institutionalization: The Highlands Heights experiment*. Cambridge, Mass.: Ballinger Publishing.

Tobin, S. S. (1975). Social and health services for the future aged, Part II. *Gerontologist*, **15**(1), 32-37.

Tobin, S. S., Davidson, S. M., and Sack, A. (1976). *Effective Social Services for Older Americans*. Ann Arbor: Institute of Gerontology, University of Michigan-Wayne State University.

Tobin, S. S., and Lieberman, M. A. (1976). *A last home for the aged: Critical implications of institutionalization*. San Francisco, Calif.: Jossey-Bass.

Tobin, S. S., and Thompson, D. (1981). The countability paradox. In *Controversial Issues in Gerontology*. New York: Springer.

U.S. Congress. Senate. Special Committee on Aging. (1971a). *Alternatives to nursing home care: A proposal*. Washington: Government Printing Office.

U.S. Congress. Senate. Special Committee on Aging. (1971b). *Making services for the elderly work: Some lessons from the British experience*. Washington: Government Printing Office.

U.S. General Accounting Office. (1977a). *Home health: The need for a national policy to better provide for the elderly*. Washington: General Accounting Office.

U.S. General Accounting Office. (1977b). *Local area agencies help the aging but problems need correcting*. Washington: General Accounting Office.

25

Funding and Monitoring Social Services for the Elderly

Gary M. Nelson, D.S.W.

University of North Carolina, Chapel Hill

In 1981, $173.3 billion in direct federal expenditures were made for programs benefiting the elderly and another $38.4 billion in federal tax expenditures. The elderly use these resources to secure goods and services that are essential to maintaining adequate standards of well-being. In a time of diminishing resources, increasing pressure is being put on finding out what the services secured by the elderly and provided by the helping professions accomplish and how they can be made more efficient and effective. In this chapter, the issues of funding and monitoring social services for the elderly are examined. The examination is not restricted to categorical social-service programs. Such categorical programs as the Title XX Social Services Block Grant Program and the Older Americans Act are usually targeted to the poor or near-poor elderly. Rather, the focus is on how social services for the elderly in general are funded and secured and how they are to be monitored. Service monitoring as presented here concerns client-outcome monitoring—the detection of sought changes in client behaviors, social conditions, or feelings, thoughts, and attitudes.

Publicly funded social services are but one among many forms that social benefits for the elderly may assume. The traditional policy dilemma in social welfare has been whether benefits should be offered to the beneficiary in cash or in kind. The major types of cash benefits targeted to the elderly include Social Security, Supplemental Security Income (SSI), tax-assisted private pensions, and tax subsidies. In-kind benefits take the form of goods such as housing and food stamps and services such as homecare, counseling, training, health care, and day care. Not all benefits fall neatly into these various packages. Rein and Rainwater (1981) refer to health-care entitlement programs such as Medicare and Medicaid as restricted-cash-benefit programs. Health-care entitlement programs are rapidly becoming a major funding source for homecare social services to the elderly.

Both policy strategies, the provision of cash and in-kind benefits, have a common objective of ensuring that the elderly have access to the services that they need. Cash and restricted in-kind health-care benefits allow for more consumer choice in the selection of the service and the service provider, and they place more responsibility for monitoring services on the consumer and the individual practitioner. Publicly provided social services have generally involved a restriction of client choice as to what interventions would be most suitable to meet his or her needs, and they are often characterized by a monopoly in the provision of the designated service. Publicly provided social services are defined as involving the performance of certain functions in the client's behalf and as being nontransferable in relation to their immediate market value to recipients (Gilbert and Specht, 1974). Professionals, both clinicians and planners, most often select those services that they see as appropriate for the elderly. The primary responsibility for monitoring such public social services has been placed with the agency funding the particular service or set of services.

In reviewing the various issues and developments in the area of funding and monitoring of social services to the elderly, this chapter is organized around several key areas. First, a conceptual framework for identifying and understanding the place of social services in aging policy is developed. In this conceptual framework, alternative strategies for funding the service needs of the elderly and for monitoring those services are identified. The implications of different approaches to funding social services for client-outcome monitoring requirements are reviewed. Second, monitoring issues are examined from the perspectives of the funding agency, the professional involved in providing the service, and the consumer who receives it. In conclusion, recommendations are made concerning future social-service funding and monitoring strategies for services for the elderly.

SOCIAL SERVICES IN THE CONTEXT OF AGING POLICY

When we speak of social services for the elderly, it is not readily apparent what types of programs and policies fall under that heading. Lee and Estes (1979) identify eighty federal programs that provide benefits to the elderly. The federal government uses seven categories for grouping the various benefit programs: employment and volunteer services; health care; housing; income maintenance; social-service programs; training and research programs; and transportation

(U.S. Congress, 1980). The major social-service programs that fell under the service grouping included Title XX and Older American Act senior centers and social-service and nutrition programs. Title XX is now referred to as the Social Service Block Grant Program. Other social-service programs worth noting and included in this group were the Legal Services Corporation and Senior Opportunities and Services (SOS). The SOS program has under the Reagan administration been collapsed into the Community Services Block Grant Program.

This identification and categorization of social services to the elderly is too limiting. The social-service programs most notable for their absence in this categorization are community mental-health programs and social services funded under such health-care programs as Medicare and Medicaid and by the Veterans Administration. As the major health-care entitlement programs are opened up to fund community-based services in long-term care, there is a very real prospect that they will shortly become the primary sources of social-service funding in the country. Additionally, one should not restrict the discussion of social services to direct public categorical health and social-service programs. While conventional analysis of social-welfare measures dichotomizes the provision of social services into two sectors, private and public, we need to look more closely at the private sector and the public use of that sector to provide social services to the elderly. For instance, the funding of an income-tax deduction to families for the care of their dependent elderly members may be seen as an indirect social-service strategy. Under this strategy, an income-tax deduction is given to a specified family member(s) in exchange for services rendered to keep the elderly person in the community. Families are then able to use these additional resources to privately secure services for an elderly family member. Other individuals are able to privately secure social services because publicly provided or assisted cash benefits such as Social Security, state and federal retirement benefits, "private pensions," and tax subsidies provide them with the financial wherewithal to do so. Other elderly individuals have private insurance benefits that enable them to secure necessary health and, increasingly, social-service benefits.

How does the social-welfare dollar break down in terms of resources allotted to cash, restricted-cash, and in-kind benefits? Direct federal outlays for the elderly in the fiscal year 1981 amounted to $173.3 billion or 23.7 percent of the federal budget. Some 71 percent of these expenditures were for unrestricted cash benefits, 25 percent were for restricted-cash health-care entitlements under Medicaid and Medicare, and the remaining 4 percent was divided primarily between the in-kind benefits of housing, food stamps, and categorical social-service programs. Direct social-service benefits, principally the Older Americans Act and the Title XX Social Service Block Grant programs, accounted for roughly 1 percent of the federal elderly social-welfare dollar. Federally legislated tax subsidies or, as they are perhaps more familiarly known, tax expenditures amounted to an additional $38.4 billion in 1981 (Olson, 1982; White House Conference on Aging, 1981).

In the overall scheme of federal public policy for the elderly, directly funded social-service programs have played a very limited role. The primary role of government has been to secure adequate incomes for the elderly through various income-transfer programs and secondarily to ensure a minimum of health-care coverage through restricted health-care entitlement programs. Essentially what this points up is that, in public policy for the elderly, the primary service strategy has been to provide the majority of elderly individuals with adequate incomes so they can purchase their own services and respond to their needs as they see fit. Given adequate incomes, elderly individuals prioritize their own service needs and employ their own service providers to meet those needs. Under this policy approach, the major responsibility for monitoring the quality and effectiveness of social services lies with the consumer and private practitioners. Additionally, this income-based strategy has freed family members of the elderly individual from a major responsibility for financial assistance and has enabled them to respond more fully to the personal-care service needs of that individual.

PRESSURES FOR ACCOUNTABILITY

The public funding of social-welfare programs is undergoing severe criticism. In-kind programs in particular are bearing the brunt of this criticism and cost cutting. The criticisms are directed at the objectives of traditional programs and at their alleged inefficiency and lack of state and local accountability. There is a growing current of thought in public-policy discussions that favors state and local over federal funding and administration of social programs and private, consumer-controlled and incentive-based provision of care. Government provision of categorical social-service programs is seen by many as the social-service system of last resort. Nowhere is this point better made than in the chapter on "Social Benefits and Services for the Elderly" in the *Final Report* of the 1981 White House Conference on Aging. The government's role as outlined in this document is viewed as limited and only appropriate when private efforts are either unavailable or insufficient for the task. Quoting from the *Final Report*, "It is sufficient for our purposes to recognize that all agree that government solutions are appropriate when there is evidence that people can't handle a problem themselves, though they may disagree on what and how much evidence is needed to know when this threshold has been reached" (White House Conference on Aging, 1981, p. 97). However, even then the authors of the *Final Report* argue that, on grounds of efficiency, government services are but a pale substitute for private efforts. "Although large industries and organizations often can provide economies of operations because of their size, this is usually not true of government programs with their legions of administrators, planners, evaluators, and auditors. When it comes to providing for the unique needs of a frail elderly person or the transportation needs of an elderly couple, a dedicated family or caring neighbor, if available, is more flexible, sensitive, and efficient than even the best-designed government program" (p. 97).

This growing preference for nongovernmental or at least less bureaucratic interventions is no doubt an outgrowth of the real and perceived waste and inefficiency of categorical programs for the elderly. While individually these programs often have praiseworthy goals and produce benefits for many elderly individuals, seen as a whole they are often characterized by duplication in services, failure to sufficiently target resources to those in need, and wasteful and functionally overlapping bureaucracies. In her indictment of the "aging enterprise," Estes holds that agencies associated with the enterprise ". . . are far more interested in struggling over existing resources than in considering the results of their programs or services" (Estes et al., 1979, p. 3). These developments reflect a strong animus against bureaucratic aspects of the welfare state but not against state provision of services. "The contradiction between wanting more government services and less government may be only apparent. More precisely, we suggest that the modern welfare state is here to stay, indeed that it ought to expand the benefits it provides—but that alternative mechanisms are possible to provide welfare-state services" (Berger and Neuhaus, 1977, p. 1).

PROGRAM FUNDING AND IMPLICATIONS
FOR SERVICE MONITORING

The criticisms of traditional service approaches to the problems of the elderly are to be taken seriously. Those points of criticism that are valid need to be identified and to the degree possible used to modify present social-service intervention strategies. The alternative mechanisms we use to fund social programs for the elderly have direct implications for the way in which the services obtained by the elderly are to be monitored. Accordingly, we should review the different funding options available to policymakers in delivering social benefits and services to the elderly and their implications for different monitoring models and requirements. There are perhaps three basic strategies employed by government to ensure that the elderly receive the services they need. The first strategy involves providing the elderly person with an income sufficient to enable the individual to privately purchase the services that he or she needs. This is not a nonservice approach to the problems of the elderly as some people argue. Rather, the difference between this approach and a categorical service program is that the locus of control for the service selection, payment, and monitoring lies more with the individual and less with the agency or program. The second strategy involves the use of restricted cash funding, most notably in health care, to purchase health and personal-care services. The third strategy involves the funding of social services through categorical service programs such as the Older Americans Act, Mental Health, or the Title XX

Social Services Block Grant Program. The objective of ensuring that the elderly receive necessary services is and can be reached by using any one or a combination of these strategies.

Each one of these social-service strategies has very different funding and monitoring requirements and characteristics. An income-based approach to services requires simply that a check or checks be sent to the individual and that the individual choose how he or she will spend that income to meet his or her own needs. Service monitoring in this situation is primarily the responsibility of the individual and the helping professional. Free-market advocates hold that the individual will, in the process of choosing services, stimulate competition on the part of providers that will improve the overall quality of services and ensure provider accountability. However, individual practitioners also have a responsibility for setting professional standards and monitoring their own practices. Additional monitoring in this model may be assisted by government use of the regulatory process whereby government requires that institutions and service providers meet certain basic health and safety standards.

An income-based strategy encourages self-responsibility, self-help, and the continued and expanded provisions of informal support services to the elderly. In addition to retirement benefits, tax subsidies in the areas of family care of dependents, housing, and general income maintenance free additional resources for the elderly individual that can be used for privately securing needed services. Adequate income also frees family members from financial assistance and enables them to devote more time to the personal-care needs of elderly family members. Family members have been found to provide approximately 80 percent of all personal-care services to the elderly (U.S. National Center for Health Statistics, 1972). Tax expenditures or subsidies are simply revenues foregone to the treasury, either state or federal, through the use of various tax exclusions, credits, and deductions. Responsibility for monitoring the targeting of tax subsidies lies with Congress. Monitoring of the use of retirement income and subsidies for social services lies primarily with the elderly consumers and their families. Helping professionals have a responsibility to monitor their own practices.

The second strategy for delivering services to the elderly involves the use of restricted cash grants. Restricted-cash-grant programs such as Medicaid and Medicare make available certain prescribed services on the basis of whether or not the individual meets certain eligibility criteria — income in the case of Medicaid and age in the case of Medicare. Funding under such arrangements is usually made directly to the provider, who is reimbursed for providing identified reimbursable services to entitled individuals. In the case of Medicare, the elderly individual may be required by the doctor to pay him or her in full and request reimbursement from Medicare. The consumer under this funding arrangement has control — albeit limited — over the type of service and the provider who will deliver it. The identification of client needs and the prescription of services to meet those needs is a function of public-policy decisions about what is reimbursable, of professional judgments about what the client needs, and of limited client choice in relation to service options and providers. Co-payments as well as concern for the quality and effectiveness of the services place a responsibility on the consumer to monitor his or her use of services. Individual fee-based services place additional responsibilities on practitioners to closely monitor their practices.

The third social-service strategy and the one that most people think of first when considering service strategies involves the funding of categorical service grants for the elderly. In this service strategy, planners, politicians, and clinicians decide what in the lives of elderly individuals constitutes a need and what services should be developed to address those needs. In some cases these decisions may be informed by needs assessments or various types of client participation in the planning and decision-making process. The clients' choices of services are largely limited to what services providers make available and whether or not individuals meet provider-defined functional- or financial-eligibility criteria. The only choice available to clients in such situations may be whether to accept or not accept the proffered service.

Each of these strategies is marked by varying levels of consumer involvement in the identification of individual needs and choice in the selection of services to meet those needs. The continuum ranges from a maximum of consumer choice in the use of cash to purchase needed services to a minimum of consumer choice in the use of publicly provided in-kind services. The key argument for a cash approach to meet service needs of the elderly is that it provides for a maximization of individual welfare by allowing the individual optimum choice in spending resources as he or she pleases. A rational person, it is argued, will achieve a higher level of satisfaction if given $100 to spend rather than $100 worth of goods and services, the nature of which has been determined by others. The key point or assumption here is that the consumer is rational and informed and able to make decisions in his or her own best interest and ultimately in the best interest of those who are financing the benefit.

The argument for in-kind benefits rests on the control it provides over individual consumption patterns. While limiting consumer sovereignty and freedom of choice, in-kind benefits as social services may offer a degree of protection to the wary or uninformed consumer. It is assumed that the uninformed consumer lacking in basic knowledge about what choices are available to him will not be able to act in his or her own best interest. In between directly funded social services and cash grants are restricted cash grants. Restricted cash grants such as Medicaid and Medicare allow the individual some choice in the selection of health-care services. While the consumer has some choice as to which provider to seek services from and whether or not to accept provider-prescribed services, it is the provider who, upon assessing the client, decides what the client needs and requests and receives reimbursement directly from the government for providing reimbursable services.

CURRENT PRACTICE IN MONITORING

There is mounting pressure to make social services more accountable. Even without this pressure, policy analysts, agency directors, and social-service practitioners need feedback on the results of their efforts. The present monitoring practices for social-service programs for the elderly focus primarily on such information as the number of clients served, the characteristics of clients, the number of meals served, and the number of transportation rides given (Estes and Noble, 1979). McCartney (1979), in examining evaluation efforts pertaining to programs of the Administration on Aging, found that almost no assessment had been made of Area Agency on Aging efforts in evaluation, quality control, and the monitoring of standards. A central problem of service programs for the elderly and of human-service programs in general lies in the finding that agencies often lack outcome-oriented objectives either for system development or client change (U.S. Department of Health and Human Services, 1980). A review of information-system applications and case studies of good practice in these systems reveals an almost total focus on such programmatic activities as agency use of multiple-funding sources, detailing of client characteristics, counting and costing out-of-service units, and identification of service types and service providers. With the exception of information systems like that of the On Lok Health Services Program of San Francisco, the typical program on aging information system possesses no real capacity to monitor program impacts as they pertain to individual clients or to detect broader impacts on the social condition of the elderly (National Association of State Units on Aging, 1982). A review of the self-audit guide developed for the National Association of State Units on Aging also reveals that little or no attention is devoted to providing guidelines for conducting a program audit on the agency's capacity to conduct client-outcome monitoring (National Association of State Units on Aging, 1979).

The general absence of client-outcome monitoring systems from the field of aging cannot be explained by any one set of circumstances. Certainly, one issue concerns the dissemination of the program technology needed to conduct client-outcome monitoring. Yet perhaps key to the development of client-outcome-monitoring capabilities is the need for federal, state, and local administrators to change their accountability stance and to call for outcome monitoring. Additionally, human-service professionals in the field of aging need to change their accountability stance and develop the necessary skills to conduct outcome monitoring in their own practices. Social work and other helping professions have been remiss in developing and applying the necessary research methodology for evaluating and monitoring their own practices. Elderly consumers have a right to expect and demand efficient, quality services. The elderly can and should play a central role in monitoring the outcomes of services that are developed to enhance their well-being.

CLIENT-OUTCOME MONITORING

The primary purpose of client-outcome monitoring is to improve service delivery, to help make services more effective, and to modify or eliminate activities that are ineffective (Millar and Millar, 1981). The concern in client-outcome monitoring is with the client who has gone to an agency or to an individual practitioner for social services. The client-outcome monitoring process does not concern itself with elderly clients in the community who may need the service but do not enter the service system. Client-outcome monitoring procedures do not include general community needs-assessment activities. The term *client outcome* refers to the condition of the elderly client subsequent to service provision and the extent and direction of change experienced by the client. The term *monitoring* refers to the regular collection and analysis of outcome information. The collection and analysis of outcome information is done on a standardized basis with outcome reports being developed annually or perhaps semi-annually, quarterly, or monthly. Special, one-time-only studies of programs would more appropriately fall in the province of program evaluation.

Client-outcome monitoring is generally seen as an agency management tool. However, this conceptualization is too restrictive. Again, the majority of elderly individuals obtain social services outside of traditional public social-service agencies. Client-outcome monitoring can also be a practitioner-centered and consumer-centered methodology for improving the efficiency, effectiveness, and quality of gerontological services. Agency-centered client-outcome monitoring can be developed to generate comprehensive, relatively low-cost information about the effects of agency services on client populations on an ongoing basis. In this fashion, agencies can increase their accountability to government and elderly consumers alike. Practitioner-centered client-outcome monitoring addresses the need of those in the helping professions to be responsible for evaluating their own individual private or public practices with the elderly and to provide evidence of the effectiveness of their work. Consumer-centered client-outcome monitoring entails establishing a meaningful role for elderly consumers in assessing the efficiency, effectiveness, and quality of services delivered to the elderly. In this manner, elderly consumers play a central role in holding agencies and the helping professions accountable for their services.

What is the utility of client-outcome monitoring? Client-outcome monitoring can be used to provide important information about the effects of gerontological services to human-service managers, practitioners, and consumers. Outcome data increase the overall utility of management-information systems, make in-depth program evaluation easier, and are an integral part of an effective case-management system. Examples of additional needs that client outcome monitoring addresses include the following (adapted from Millar and Millar, 1981, pp. 4-6):

1. *Helping to identify improvements in procedures, programs, policies, and*

practice. Analysis of outcome information can point to either program or practitioner changes that may improve service outcomes or reduce service costs without significantly changing outcomes. For instance, outcomes among individual practitioners or programs using different interventions with the same type of clients can be compared. Such comparisons may enable program managers and practitioners to detect which services and service mixes yield the greatest improvements.

2. *Motivating employees and service practitioners to improve performance.* Agency employees and in particular direct-service practitioners who work with the elderly are the keys to the effective and efficient delivery of gerontological services. Perhaps pivotal to gaining practitioner acceptance of the concept of outcome monitoring is the building in of the expectation that practitioners should be involved in evaluating their own practices and that successful practice will be rewarded. Superimposing a management-derived and management-controlled client-monitoring system without the involvement of the practitioner in that process may prove to be counterproductive for improving employee performance. Outcome data can be used to improve employee performance by: (a) identifying staff development needs and modifying interventions, (b) setting performance targets for individual program units and individual practitioners, and (c) structuring monetary and nonmonetary incentives for both individual practitioners and groups of employees.

3. *Holding contractors and practitioners accountable for results.* There is a need to hold individual practitioners and agency service providers accountable for outcome performance. To date, the interest in performance monitoring in gerontology has focused on holding service providers accountable only for such process outcomes as the number and unit cost of delivered services. Client-outcome data should be used in the selection of service providers through a competitive bidding process during the period of contract renegotiation.

4. *Enhancing quality assurance activities.* Often quality assurance focuses on the maintenance and presence of staffing, procedural, and physical-facility standards as indicators of service quality. These standards, however, in and of themselves do not assure quality services. Client-outcome measures like client satisfaction with services can act as additional quality assurance checks.

5. *Aiding budget preparation and justification.* Budget proposals that can demonstrate discernible client outcomes are likely to have a strong competitive advantage over those that cannot. Such performance data can also play a central role in any internal agency resource-reallocation process.

6. *Providing feedback on the effects of agency program, procedure, or policy changes.* Ongoing client-outcome monitoring can enable program managers and practitioners to detect possible effects of changes in program policies or procedures. For instance, a homecare service program that shifts its client outreach efforts from a primary focus on hospital-based intake and referrals to a broader communitywide referral network is likely to experience changes in the incoming client mix and subsequently change in client outcomes.

7. *Assisting in answering nonroutine management questions.* Responding to information requests from federal, state, and local officials, the legislature, and the press is easier for program managers and practitioners if they have access to client-outcome data for their specific programs. Rather than vague references to broadly stated goals and objectives, answers can be specific and concrete and place the program in the best possible light.

AGENCY-CENTERED CLIENT-OUTCOME MONITORING

There are gaps between public expectations for better social services and the government's or even the private sector's ability to provide them. Unless we begin to keep score, to measure our client outcomes, it is difficult or impossible to know whether we are winning or losing in our efforts. Agency client-centered outcome monitoring can provide us with the tools necessary to help us develop effective social services. The Urban Institute, a nonprofit policy research and educational organization, has developed a guide for state and local client-outcome monitoring systems (Millar and Millar, 1981). The guide also has direct application to private profit and nonprofit service agencies. In the guide, entitled *Developing Client Outcome Monitoring Systems,* major steps for developing client outcome monitoring procedures are identified (Millar and Millar, 1981, p. 9). They are:

Step 1. Obtaining and conveying top-management commitment
Step 2. Establishing a client-outcome monitoring working group
Step 3. Choosing which programs to monitor
Step 4. Determining specific information uses and specific analyses and reports that are needed
Step 5. Selecting the outcome indicators and the data collection approaches
Step 6. Designing the data collection process
Step 7. Implementing the data-collection process
Step 8. Maintaining the client-outcome monitoring procedures

This framework for guiding an agency in the development of client-outcome monitoring procedures involves often complex design and implementation decisions within each step. Four processes critical to client-outcome monitoring that overlap and intertwine with a number of the Urban Institute procedural steps are: (1) the statement of client-outcome objectives and the setting of performance indicators; (2) the place and importance of assessment in the selection of outcome objectives and performance indicators; (3) the role of case management in assuring that the prerequisites of client-outcome monitoring are in place and in tracking client progress; and (4) the development of an action plan for utilizing client-outcome information.

Goals and Client-Outcome Objectives

There are differences between organizational goals and client-outcome objectives. Goals are a general statement of desired organization outcomes. They are often not time-limited and frequently embrace broadly stated social ends. Improving self-sufficiency among the elderly would be an example of a program goal. Program goals do not identify specifically what is to be achieved nor how we are to distinguish a successful program from an unsuccessful one. Client-outcome objectives, in contrast, are "quantifiable, time limited statements of planned results" (Altman, 1979). Client-outcome statements should have five components. They should specify who will do what, to what extent, under what conditions, and in what time frame (Bloom and Fischer, 1982; Altman, 1979).

Who?

Client-outcome objectives need to be stated in terms of outcomes for clients and not in terms of what the practitioners will do. An objective that states that a home-health aide will provide assistance twice weekly to improve elderly client self-sufficiency is not a client-outcome objective. The concern is with what the elderly individual will do and not the process activities that the provider is engaged in.

Will Do What?

A measurable program indicator needs to be identified that will detect the presence of change in client performance either in overt behavior or in a cognitive change such as improvement in life satisfaction. Returning to the example of improved self-sufficiency, elderly self-sufficiency could be specified to mean an increase in functioning in activities of daily living (ADL). An ADL instrument measures client functioning in bathing, toileting, transfer, continence, eating or feeding, and walking. The instrument can be scored to categorize various levels of functional independence or dependence.

To What Extent?

Here the purpose is to establish a client-outcome performance target—called a criterion level—that would be acceptable. A criterion level pertains to how well a planned activity or behavior has to be performed to be considered successful. A central problem here concerns the availability of standards, norms, or targets for client-outcome measures. Such client norms and standards are in most cases still undeveloped. However, even without them, an agency can still compare its own performance from one period in time to another. If, for instance, 40 percent of the elderly clients are functionally self-sufficient in four of six ADL areas, a client-outcome indicator or performance target may be to increase that to 50 percent.

Under What Conditions?

A particular client outcome may be desired only under certain conditions or in specified situations. It is helpful when thinking about the conditions for the behavior to occur to consider the following: (1) where it should occur; (2) when it should occur; and (3) with whom? Performance targets of improvements in ADL no doubt vary from situation to situation and from one population to another. If you are talking about performance targets for elderly individuals who are homebound, your targets are going to be quite different from targets for an elderly nursing-home population.

In What Time Frame?

Here you will want to set a reasonable time frame for achieving your performance target. The time frame is a function of the nature of the problem being dealt with, the urgency associated with it, and the intervention used to treat that problem.

Assessment

Program managers need to be able to clearly identify the theories and assumptions behind the design of programs and program objectives. Unless there is a thorough understanding of the client, the system, and the nature of the problem, there is little basis for selecting a particular intervention or setting a client-outcome objective. Systematic assessment with a preference for instrumental assessment is essential to define client concerns and problems, to specify desired changes, and to identify social-service interventions to effect these changes. Instrumental assessments that yield quantifiable client measures through client records, observation, client self-reports, or standardized measures are also necessary for establishing client-outcome performance targets and tracking progress toward those targets. Again, in order to establish a measure for improved elderly self-sufficiency as conceptualized by successful completion of ADL, a standardized ADL measurement instrument would be used. Kane and Kane (1981) provide a valuable service to professionals concerned with serving the elderly by reviewing the state of the art in elderly-assessment methodology. Their text, *Assessing the Elderly,* serves as an important resource for both program managers and clinicians concerned with client-outcome monitoring in the field of aging.

Case Management

Case management for both the clinician and the program manager can be viewed as the pivotal service methodology for overseeing and maintaining client-outcome monitoring procedures. Elderly individuals often experience multiple problems. In order to ensure that elderly clients receive appropriate services to match specific needs, it is often essential for a case manager to oversee and track the client's progress through the service system. The term *case manager* refers to a social-service clinician who manages his/her own caseload or to an individual with the title of case manager who monitors a large number of clients as they work their way through the social-service system.

Steinberg and Carter (1983) identify five client-level phases in the case-management process. They are: (1) client entry into the service network, (2) client assessment, (3) client goal setting and service planning, (4) client-care-plan implementation, and (5) review and evaluation of client status. The role of the case manager, either clinical case manager or program case manager, is crucial in that such a person is perhaps the only one in a position to ensure that the necessary prerequisites of client-outcome monitoring are in place. The client-outcome monitoring prerequisites from the case manager's perspective include (1) the performance of client assessments that provide baseline outcome information and the basis for program and individual client objectives; (2) the assurance that client program objectives are outcome-oriented; (3) the assurance that similar people are matched with similar program interventions; and (4) availability of a methodology for tracking and monitoring client progress in relation to program performance targets. The case manager is the person who is in the key position for detecting problems and calling them to the attention of the program manager. The case manager reviews client progress against client or program performance objectives and if necessary calls for reviews of client care plans or calls for client termination.

Use of Outcome Information

All performance-monitoring systems are marked by a data component, an analytic component, and an action component (Altman, 1979). The data component provides the framework for measuring and collecting the monitored performance information. The analytic component provides the framework for

Table 25-1. Summary of Changes in Client Condition Across Functional Assessment Fields
(Percentages)

		Social Resources	Economic Resources	Mental Health	Physical Health	Activities of Daily Living	Change Across all Problem Fields
Elderly services	Improved	30	10	25	18	20	21
	Unchanged	52	74	66	61	62	64
	Worsening	18	16	9	21	18	15
		100	100	100	100	100	100

Note: Hypothetical data for elderly clients using OARS Multidimensional Functional Assessment Questionnaire. Duke Center on Aging, Duke University, Durham, North Carolina, 1975.

determining what analyses and reports are needed and preparing such reports for dissemination to relevant decision-makers. To understand the potential use of client-outcome data, you are referred to the earlier listing of basic uses for such data. If the client-outcome performance targets are not reached, the information may be used to pinpoint needed improvements in procedures, programs, or policies. If the problem is seen as in part a function of staff motivation, program managers may seek ways for motivating employees to improve performance. If the client-outcome report comes at the end of a contract period, the agency may want to entertain competitive bids for contracts to provide the service in the future.

When agencies lack norms or standards for developing client-outcome measures, a fairly common situation, an appropriate starting point for an agency or practitioner would be to establish its own norms or standards. An example would have a local department of social services, using the OARS Multidimensional Functional Assessment measure, derive functional outcome measures for a sample of its elderly service clients and develop its own functional outcome norm (Table 25-1). A department of social services would develop its own normative outcomes by performing several quarterly measures or by drawing upon similar data from other departments of social services. By analyzing the data in the various functional areas and looking at the average or normal rates of improvement, performance targets could be set for the various functional areas. Here an important use of outcome data can be for establishing future performance targets for the agency.

PRACTITIONER-CENTERED CLIENT-OUTCOME MONITORING

I appeal to you. . . . Measure, evaluate, estimate, appraise your results, in some form, in any terms that rest on something beyond faith, assertion, and "illustrative case."

State your objectives and how far you have reached them. . . . Let time enough elapse so that there may be some reasonable hope of permanence in the results which you state (Cabot, 1931).

Human-service practitioners recognize at least intellectually the importance of these ideas. The above quote was taken from a social-work conference over fifty years ago. The importance of accountability in services to the elderly is too important to be left only to program managers. The responsibility for client-outcome monitoring when left to program managers has not been assumed on any significant scale. If there is to be accountability for social services for the elderly, it will come only through the joint efforts of program managers, practitioners, and consumers.

Practitioner-centered client-outcome monitoring employs the methodology of single-system designs to evaluate social-service interventions. Single-system designs involve the repeated collection and monitoring of information on a single system over time. The "systems" referred to in the context of practitioner-centered monitoring include individual, family, and group systems. Each is treated as a single unit for the purposes of client-outcome monitoring. The "design" reference concerns a systematic plan for collecting and monitoring client-outcome data. Practitioner-centered client-outcome monitoring is particularly well suited to both private independent clinical practice and to private profit or nonprofit agency-based practice. Independent private clinicians and private-profit and nonprofit agency providers do not feel the same pressures as public agencies for accountability. The basis for their accountability efforts is more likely to stem from concern for profitability, maintenance of a service market, and a desire to demonstrate quality professional practice standards. The practitioner-centered client outcome monitoring methodology has significant utility for professionals who seek to improve the efficiency, effectiveness, and quality of their services to the elderly.

Bloom and Fischer (1982, p. 3) have identified the basic characteristics of single-system designs and underscored their applicability for practitioner-centered client-outcome monitoring. Those characteristics are partially revised in the following to represent the major steps for implementing single-system client-outcome monitoring designs.

Step 1. Specifying problems through assessment
Step 2. Specifying measurable client-outcome goals
Step 3. Obtaining a clear definition of the intervention
Step 4. Baselining: Establishing client outcomes prior to intervention
Step 5. Designing data collection
Step 6. Implementing repeated-outcome measures
Step 7. Analysis of data

Many of the characteristics or requirements for conducting practitioner-centered monitoring are similar to agency-centered monitoring requirements. Client assessment, preferably instrumental assessment, is essential for objectively specifying client problems, developing a preintervention client baseline, and setting client-outcome performance targets or objectives. Case-management methods are essential for assuring that repeated outcome measures are administered, that client progress is monitored, and that client interventions are revised or terminated as indicated by client progress toward targeted outcomes. The major differences between practitioner-centered as opposed to agency-centered monitoring are that the primary responsibility for conducting client-outcome monitoring and assuring effective, quality services lies more with the practitioner in relation to his/her clients than with the agency program manager.

The heart of single-system outcome monitoring involves measurement of problem states and repeated measures over time to see if changes occur before, during, and following the practitioner's intervention. Again, a wide array of measurement tools have been developed to measure an individual client's functional dimensions, feelings, family interaction patterns, and community involvement and participation. A key feature of single-system designs is the baseline. Baseline data are taken in the assessment process to help identify change targets as a basis for comparison with data collected following the social-service intervention. Data analysis for single-system designs relies more on visual presentations of data and less on statistical methods of data analysis. Collected data is placed on charts and graphs and visually inspected for changes in data patterns (trends, slope, and level of data) (Bloom and Fischer, 1982). The helping professional who uses the client-outcome monitoring techniques embraced in single-system designs is committed to conducting practice as an empirically based problem-solving experiment and to learning and looking for new and more effective approaches to social-service interventions.

Practitioner-centered outcome monitoring can be illustrated with a hypothetical case involving a client presenting a problem of severely impaired mental functioning. An assessment of the elderly individual reveals that the client is experiencing a severe depression and refuses to eat. The client also exhibits serious confusion. The outcome objective for the client identifies an intervention plan combining home-delivered meals, a friendly visitor, and regular counseling sessions. The client-outcome criterion calls for a reduction within four weeks of the level of mental impairment from severe to moderate as measured by a short, portable mental-status questionnaire. Figure 25-1 maps client preintervention baseline status using a short, portable mental-status questionnaire and post intervention changes. Client-centered outcome monitoring using single-system designs can effectively capture client outcomes.

CONSUMER-CENTERED CLIENT-OUTCOME MONITORING

The only party directly and ultimately concerned with effective, quality gerontological social services is the elderly individual. Consumer monitoring of social services assumes two basic forms: consumer participation in agency-based decision-making and consumer education. Consumer participation in

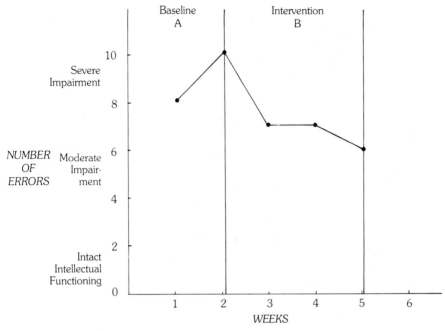

Figure 25-1. Hypothetical data on elderly mental status using the short portable mental status questionnaire from the multipurpose senior services project comparison group assessment instrument multipurpose senior services project, Sacramento, California, 1980.

client-outcome monitoring focuses primarily on public, agency-based social-service-provision models. The decisions or choices as to what services are to be provided, to what elderly, by which service providers, and whether or not to monitor for client outcome are often made by an elite of experts. The objective for this consumer-based monitoring strategy is to make such social-service programs responsive to participant-defined needs and demands for accountability. The consumer-education strategy for client-outcome monitoring focuses on the elderly individuals themselves. The objective of this strategy is for the elderly to make informed choices when selecting needed social services. The strategy, while certainly applicable to all elderly, has special relevance for the majority of elderly who privately purchase social and health services from private nonprofit or profit-based providers.

Consumer Participation

Consumer participation in policy formation is an accepted but not always practiced principle of a democratic society. Since the 1960s consumer participation has been encouraged in public social-welfare programs beginning with the War on Poverty. The Older Americans Act and the Title XX Social Services Block Grant programs have historically called for consumer participation through a variety of avenues such as advisory boards and public hearings. However, Van Til and Van Til (1970), in their study of changes in citizen participation in the 1960s, noted a shift from client activism to a more traditional citizen-participation model where nonelite consumers joined with elite professionals in a minimal advisory capacity. Additionally, service programs under the thrust of the New Federalism have become increasingly decentralized and consumer-participation efforts more fragmented and diluted. Estes argues that consumer participation has been characterized by advice without influence. Elderly consumers run the risk of being co-opted by the agencies they advise. In analyzing the role of Older Americans Act state and area agencies on aging advisory boards, Estes (Estes et al., 1979, p. 215) observed that they were likely to serve the following functions: (1) legitimation of the organization's or planner's efforts; (2) sharing in the public symbols of authority and public responsibility without the transfer of substantive power; (3) advocating expansion of the organization's or planner's programs by petitioning for resources at state or local levels; and (4) shielding the organization's or planner's decisions from opposition and criticism.

How does one increase elderly consumers' effectiveness in monitoring social-service programs? First, elderly consumers, like aging-network program managers and planners, need to change their stand on social-service monitoring from a primary concern with the activities of programs to one that addresses the outcomes, the actual improvements in the welfare of the elderly. Yet, in order for elderly consumers to be able to provide advice with influence, they need to be directly involved in the decision-making process, including the defining of the problems and needs of their constituency, the implementation of service interventions, and ultimately the monitoring of social services for client outcomes. The major dilemma in the delivery of public social services to the elderly concerns the issue of who controls these crucial service decisions. Because social-service choices for the elderly are limited under categorical service models, a shift to a consumer focus on client outcomes may ensure service accountability in a way that has been extremely difficult to achieve under traditional consumer-participation approaches.

Consumer Education

Consumer education as a client-outcome monitoring strategy is most beneficial to individuals who have choices in purchasing needed social services in old age. The middle- and upper-middle-income elderly who are provided significant public cash benefits under Social Security, publicly assisted "private pensions," various tax subsidies, and restricted cash benefits under Medicare are able to exercise a considerable degree of choice in the selection of social services. The objective of a consumer-oriented service-monitoring strategy is to ensure effective and quality services through informed choice. Informed consumer choice involves three components: (1) knowledge of the aging process; (2) knowledge of the range of self-help and social-service interventions available to meet age-associated needs; and (3) knowledge about what choices are available in the selection of service providers.

An example of a successful organization that both advocates effective, quality programs for the elderly and monitors those programs is the 13.5-million-member National Retired Teachers Association and the American Association of Retired Persons (NRTA-AARP). State AARP chapters and retired teachers associations work at local, state, and national levels to enhance the quality of life for the elderly. A major thrust of NRTA-AARP is to educate the elderly about the aging process and about policies that affect them and to actively engage them in self-help and political organizing. An example of these consumer-education efforts can be found in the Fall 1982 issue of the AARP *Chapter News.* That single issue had articles on (1) recognition, prevention, and treatment of hypothermia and hyperthermia; (2) a successful campaign to reduce utility rates in Missouri; and (3) references to a number of energy-related background papers of interest to the elderly and guides to energy-assistance offices in the various states.

Another example of an education-based approach to enabling people to effectively use services can be found in the Duke ADRDA Family Support Network (ADRDA stands for Alzheimer's Disease and Related Disorders Association). The ADRDA Family Support Network operates out of the Center on Aging at the Duke University Medical Center in Durham, North Carolina. The Duke ADRDA Family Support Network is a self-help intervention designed to assist family caregivers of Alzheimer's victims in effectively caring for afflicted family members. The orientation is to provide families with an understanding of the disease and information on where and how help can be obtained. The first Alzheimer's Family Support group in North Carolina was initiated in March 1980. The organization has since expanded to include over twenty-eight support groups representing over 3,000 North Carolina family caregivers. The groups, while facilitated by professionals, are organized and run by lay individuals. The groups have open monthly meetings that provide forums for family, friends, and health professionals to share information, discuss mutual problems, and present caregivng tips and coping techniques. The participants receive written and mailed information about medical care, financial/legal planning, nursing care, and such community facilities and programs as day care, nursing homes, and respite care (Gwyther, 1983). The program also has a telephone hot line to provide individuals with information and assistance.

FUTURE DIRECTIONS

Our concern that the elderly receive effective, quality social services extends to all elderly, not just those in select public programs. The responsibilities for monitoring gerontological social services must extend to the programs that develop social services, the practitioners who implement services, and the elderly who utilize them. A client-outcome monitoring strategy that relies on only one approach is not likely to succeed.

Outside the area of long-term care, the pressure for monitoring client outcomes in the social services has been insufficient. Fiscal pressures on Older Americans Act and Title XX Social Service Block Grant Programs have resulted in perhaps a more refined monitoring of program activities and client-population characteristics but little if any measurable progress in client-outcome monitoring. Without client-outcome feedback it is impossible to know what staffing standards should be used for social-service programs or what additional training that staff needs. It also makes little sense to establish quality-of-care standards for the social services without knowing what the client outcomes are for those services. Finally, in the absence of client-outcome information it is impossible to make informed judgments about how to reallocate resources in periods of fiscal retrenchment.

There are, however, some bright spots in social-service client monitoring. They are to be found in the area of long-term care. Increasingly, states are requiring that comprehensive assessments and case management be used to help ensure that elderly individuals receive the appropriate level of care. In 1981, some twenty-nine states were conducting some preadmission screening of nursing-home applicants. The typical composition of a state screening team includes a social worker, a nurse, and, in a number of states, a physician (Knowlton, Clauser and Fatula, 1982). Such nationally recognized long-term care programs as the National Long Term Care Channeling Demonstration Program, the New York Nursing Homes Without Walls programs, and projects Access and Triage have met with a measure of success in monitoring client outcomes, particularly in the areas of client placement and cost containment (Eggert, Bowlyow and Nichols, 1980; Hodgson and Quinn, 1980; New York State Council on Home Care Services, 1982). While many of these demonstration projects have focused on client outcomes other than placement and cost containment, the standards and practices that regulate quality assurance and accountability are generally inconsistent and inadequate in the field of long-term care (Trager, 1980). Kane and Kane (1980) have speculated that we run the risk of replicating many of the problems experienced by the mental-health profession if, in implementing deinstitutionalization and diversion from institutions, we do not concern ourselves with what happens to the individuals who are put back into or kept in the community. There is no reason to believe that the problems of inappropriate care, inadequately paid and trained staff, and patient abuse that have characterized the history of nursing homes won't also characterize community care of the elderly. Unless client-outcome measures are applied to the areas of care quality and client satisfaction with services, client dissatisfaction and inappropriate client care will be hard to detect other than through an occasional newspaper exposé.

In the last decade commentators on aging policy have spoken of the increasing movement of social services to the community (Maddox, 1980). It should be noted, however, that the majority of social services for the elderly have always been in the community if one refers to services secured privately by the elderly themselves or provided to the elderly by caring families and communities. What has moved into the community is a growing public and professional assumption of familial and community responsibility for the care of the elderly and, to a certain extent, the elderly's own responsibility for self-care. In many instances it would appear that there is an attempt to shift the elderly from high-technology health care to high-technology social care in the community. This in part reflects a ". . . high regard for professional expertise and limited confidence in the competence and responsibilities of families to deal with impaired [family] members" (Maddox, 1980, p. 505).

A number of recent efforts have been made to moderate the movement to professionalize community-based services for the elderly. Such efforts are likely to become more prevalent in the future. Perhaps the most notable and controversial proposal in this area is the suggested use of vouchers under Medicare. Additional moves to shift the locus of control for the selection of social and health services to the elderly consumer include the use of tax subsidies and home-equity conversions to provide additional resources to the elderly individual for his own self-care. These and other initiatives would allow the consumer more choice in the selection of services and service providers. Many argue that by increasing consumer choice in the selection of services the potential abuses and excesses that may accompany professional agency-based service strategies will be minimized. Such efforts are perhaps more in keeping with some of the major tenets of American culture, which emphasizes maximizing both individual freedom and individual responsibility. These less bureaucratic and yet no-less-public initiatives to ensure that the elderly obtain needed social services call for increased accountability on the part of professionals for their practice and increased knowledge on the part of consumers as to their service options.

REFERENCES

Altman, S. (1979). Performance monitoring systems for public managers. *Public Administration Review,* **39**(1), 31-35.

Berger, P. L., and Neuhaus, R. J. (1977). *To empower people: The role of mediating structures in public policy.* Washington: American Enterprise Institute.

Bloom, M., and Fischer, J. (1982). *Evaluating practice: Guidelines for the accountable professional.* Englewood Cliffs, N.J.: Prentice-Hall.

Cabot, R. C. (1931). Treatment in social casework and the need for criteria and tests of its success or failure. In National Council of Social Work, *Proceedings of the national conference of social work, 1931.* New York: The Council.

Eggert, G. M., Bowlyow, J. E., and Nichols, C. W. (1980). Gaining control of the long term care system: First returns from the ACCESS experiment. *Gerontologist,* **20**(3), 356-363.

Estes, C. L., et al. (1979). *The aging enterprise: A critical examination of social policies and services for the aged.* San Francisco: Jossey-Bass.

Estes, C. L., and Noble, M. (1979). Accountability, bureaucracy, and the Older Americans Act. In C. L. Estes, et al., *The aging enterprise: A critical examination of social policies and services for the aged.* San Francisco: Jossey-Bass.

Gilbert, N., and Specht, H. (1974). *Dimensions of social welfare policy.* Englewood Cliffs, N.J.: Prentice-Hall.

Gwyther, L. (1983). Alzheimer's disease. *North Carolina Medical Journal,* **44**(7), 435-436.

Hodgson, J. H. Jr., and Quinn, J. L. (1980). The impact of the Triage health care delivery system upon client morale, independent living and the cost of care. *Gerontologist,* **20**(3), 364-371.

Kane, R. L., and Kane, R. A. (1980). Alternatives to institutional care of the elderly: Beyond the dichotomy. *Gerontologist,* **20**(3), 249-259.

Kane, R. A., and Kane, R. L. (1981). *Assessing the elderly: A practical guide to measurement.* Lexington, Mass.: Lexington Books.

Knowlton, J., Clauser, S., and Fatula, J. (1982). Nursing home pre-admission screening: A review of state programs. *Health Care Financing Review,* **3**(3), 75-87.

Lee, P. R., and Estes, C. L. (1979). Eighty federal programs for the elderly. In C. L. Estes et al., *The aging enterprise: A critical examination of social policies and services for the aged.* San Francisco: Jossey-Bass.

McCartney, D. (1979, November). *Synthesis of evaluative procedures pertaining to programs of the Administration on Aging.* Paper prepared for the Federal Council on Aging.

Maddox, G. L. (1980). The continuum of care: Movement toward the community. In E. W. Busse and D. G. Blazer (Eds.), *Handbook of geriatric psychiatry.* New York: Van Nostrand Reinhold.

Millar, R., and Millar, A. (Eds.). (1981). *Developing client outcome monitoring systems.* Washington: Urban Institute.

National Association of State Units on Aging. (1979). *Aging unit information system self-audit guide.* Washington: NASUA.

National Association of State Units on Aging. (1982). *Information systems applications in programs on aging: Case studies in good practice.* Washington: NASUA.

New York State Council on Home Care Services. (1982). *Annual report to the governor and legislature, April 1981-April 1982.* New York: The Council.

Olson, L. K. (1982). *The political economy of aging: The state, private power, and social welfare.* New York: Columbia University Press.

Rein, M., and Rainwater, L. (1981). *From welfare state to welfare society* (working paper no. 69). Cambridge: Joint Center for Urban Studies of MIT and Harvard University.

Steinberg, R. M., and Carter, G. W. (1983). *Case management and the elderly.* Lexington, Mass.: Lexington Books.

Trager, B. (1980). Home health care and national health policy. *Home Health Care Services Quarterly,* **1**(2), 1-103.

U.S. Congress. House of Representatives. Select Committee on Aging. (1980). *Future directions for aging policy: A human service model.* Washington: Government Printing Office.

U.S. Department of Health and Human Services. Office of Planning and Evaluation. (1980). *Exploratory evaluation of Administration on Aging programs.* Washington: Department of Health and Human Services.

U.S. National Center for Health Statistics. (1972). Home care for persons 55 and over, United States, July 1966-June 1968. In *Vital and Health Statistics*, series no. 10, no. 73. Washington: Government Printing Office.

Van Til, J., and Van Til, S. B. (1970). Citizen participation in social policy: The end of the cycle? *Social Problems*, **17**(3), 313-323.

White House Conference on Aging. (1981). *Final report: The 1981 White House Conference on Aging*, vol. 1. Washington: The Conference.

26

Information Needs, Information Resources, and Program Management

Martin McCarthy, Jr., Ph.D.

New Jersey Department of Higher Education

Most of what human-service workers do involves the collection, assessment, communication, or use of specialized information. The focus may be an individual client, an extended family unit, a service program, or a relationship with another agency. The common thread is always access to and then the filtering and processing of relevant information. Information is needed at the client, program, agency and service-network levels and information resources are as important as staff and funding resources for program management.

A structured assessment process is the first step in identifying information needs and matching those needs with available and desired information resources. Planning is required for the design and implementation of information systems. Evaluation and positive and corrective feedback are the final steps in the routinization and day-to-day use of the information resources available to a program or agency. This ASSESSMENT⟶PLANNING⟶IMPLEMENTATION ⟶EVALUATION cycle is the same whether it is applied to the information needs of a program or to the service needs of an individual client. The stages of the process may proceed in a structured or in an informal way, but the sequence of stages is familiar to service workers and program managers in geriatrics, gerontology, and long-term care.

This chapter presents some simple methods for identifying typical information needs for programs and agencies providing gerontological services. In addition, two broad categories of information resources are considered. Useful *information sources* for program-management purposes are presented, along with a discussion of computer-based *information systems.* Since office automation and microcomputer systems are evolving at a rapid rate, the emphasis is on prescriptive advice rather than on detailed description of particular systems. The discussion also focuses on the process of technological innovation within and among organizations. The chapter concludes with some highly condensed case studies of computer-based information systems in gerontological-services agencies and a listing of on-line information utilities.

COMMUNICATION WITHIN THE AGING-SERVICES NETWORK

Two factors are driving forward the development of an extensive network of services for elderly people. The first and more important factor is simply the increasing numbers of older people. The second factor is a political ideology that places a measure of responsibility for the health and welfare of citizens on government. The responsibility is being met, in part, by public funding of remedial and supportive services, and in a limited way by the provision of direct services by governmental and quasi-governmental agencies.

Gerontology is a young field. Its early growth was encouraged by the federal legislation embodied in Lyndon Johnson's Great Society program. The Older Americans Act was passed by Congress in 1965 and has been amended several times during the intervening years. In addition to funding provisions the legislation established a set of administrative structures and responsibilities. At the federal level, the Administration on Aging (AoA) and the National Institute on Aging (NIA) were created. The AoA is concerned with gerontological services, while the NIA has a research mission. At the state-government level State Units on Aging were mandated, with responsibility for distributing federal and state funds and administering and monitoring programs.

Smaller-scale units for the provision and administration of services to the elderly have been set up in forty-four of the fifty states. These Area Agencies on Aging (AAA) range in size from a few employees to over a hundred. Often they are part of county governments. The responsibilities of the AAAs include the planning, coordination, and evaluation of service programs within their geographic areas. Some State Units on Aging and many of the smaller Area Agencies on Aging provide direct services to elderly persons. More typically, the AAAs fund programs through contract or grant mechanisms. At the community-program level, the great majority of services are currently provided by private nonprofit or governmental entities, although the emergence of quasi-public agencies is an interesting recent trend. The range of community-service activities includes information and referral, transportation, recreation, home-delivered meals, housekeeping, and visiting. Home health care and case management are usually available only on a limited basis. As long-term community care continues to become an increasingly important issue, supportive services can be expected to grow.

A number of organizations have collateral relationship with the aging-services system. A network of Long Term Care Gerontology Centers was set up by the Administration on Aging in 1980. The centers, affiliated with universities, are located in eleven regions around the country. The planning and development of cost-efficient and replicable service models is an important activity of these resource centers. In addition, their responsibilities include identification of policy issues, the development of options and priorities in long-term care, and the provision of training resources, curriculum materials, research and evaluation services, and consultation on information systems. Clients include the State Units on Aging, Area Agencies on Aging, and regional and local entities.

The National Association of State Units on Aging (NASUA) is a training and technical assistance resource center for the state agencies. The National Association of Area Agencies on Aging (N4A) performs a similiar role for Area Agencies on Aging. Both also function as advocates regarding legislative, regulatory, and policy issues in aging. In addition, these organizations have sponsored projects and published studies regarding information systems at the service-program level. A National Data Base on Aging, containing information about all program activities and services supported by the State Units and Area Agencies across the country, has been developed by the two agencies. A national sample of one-third of the Area Agencies on Aging will be surveyed annually to update the information base.

Figure 26-1 illustrates the relationships of these key elements of the aging services network.

One of the defining characteristics of a network is communication, with regular, patterned exchanges of information and other resources among the constituent parts. There are, of course, multiple formal and informal linkages among agencies at the federal, state, area, and community levels. The relationships among these levels in the network is hierarchical, with an emphasis on reporting, funding, and policy issues. It is important that information flow and policy development be a mutual, two-directional process rather than merely "top-down." Information available to entities low in the hierarchy can help them affect policy development at higher levels in the network.

At the Area Agency and community-program levels, the emphasis on service provision often leads to flatter hierarchies with horizontal linkages among entities. Coordination and consensus building, within local government and across agencies and providers, are important issues here. Case-finding, client referral, and data-sharing are common specific needs at the community program and Area Agency levels of the network. Information exchange among regional agencies is required to create and maintain new linkages and to establish new programs.

The organizations involved in the aging-services network have become more

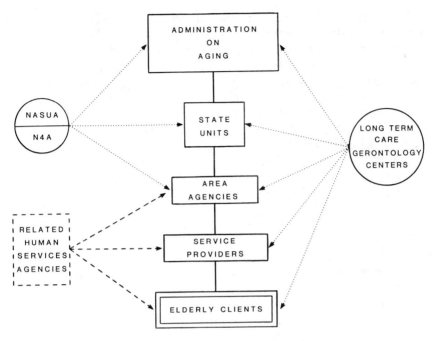

Figure 26-1. The aging services network.

interdependent, and coordination and planning mechanisms have evolved considerably over the past two decades. For instance, priority-based planning and the targeting of services for population subgroups, such as minority elderly, the frail and homebound, low-income groups and others, are common practices now. These kinds of initiatives require information about local demographic trends and service-utilization patterns for planning at the local level. Feedback and periodic reassessment are required at all levels of the network to determine and to revise service priorities. The circulation of reporting and planning information among levels provides the basis for these policy decisions.

It is important for organizations to identify patterns and trends and to respond to them. But organizational resources can be dissipated in finding and accessing needed data and then sorting and filtering out what is really useful. Broskowski (1976) cites three "laws of information" that describe the exact opposite of how an effective program information system would function. These are:

1. The information you have is not what you want.
2. The information you want is not what you need.
3. The information you need is not what you can get.

Concurrent with the growing importance of information in the aging-services network has been the increasing power of computer and telecommunications technology to process and transfer information. Information flow in and among levels of the network is heavy now. As the computerization of program management and reporting systems proceeds the multiple levels will become even more interconnected. Data communication linkages among programs and with other service-resource systems will also become more common and increasingly important in day-to-day functioning.

The assessment of agency and systemwide information needs, along with the planned development of information and communication resources, can at least partly assure that the right kind of data are collected, stored and retrieved, and processed, utilized, and communicated in a timely fashion.

ASSESSMENT

To help assure a positive outcome, the assessment and planning stages of the transition to a new system are best accomplished by an information-resources planning group. Stages of the assessment process are as follows:

Form information resources planning committee
Identify information needs of program
Identify information sources and data elements
Review current office systems and procedures
Match information needs with available resources
Identify unmet information needs
Prepare assessment report

It is important to involve potential users of the system from the start. The committee should include representatives of program administrators, service workers, and supporting staff. Their multiple perspectives and concerns will provide a more complete view of the issues. The task of the committee is to identify needs and resources and to develop systems-design alternatives. The committee director is to coordinate the information-systems planning study, implement the recommended systems, and act as a facilitator for users at a later time. An internal or external consultant familiar with small-computer systems can be an invaluable asset to the group. Various subgroups of the committee can have differing responsibilities, as determined by interest, aspirations, and experience. Two reports should be prepared—an assessment report and a planning report. These reports can be used to develop and justify detailed recommendations for the acquisition of information systems.

Information technology can have strong and deep impacts on program activities. Accordingly, existing administrative structures must be clearly under-stood and altered, if necessary, to make them rational and systematic. If management automates an organization with underlying administrative problems, the result will be a more complicated set of automated problems, with added costs of time and expense required for undoing and redoing later on.

Identifying Information Needs

The assessment process can proceed either forward, with a focus on what data is available to the organization, or backward, with a focus on what outputs are required and how information is used to produce management reports, policy decisions, planning documents, and so on. There are seven essential categories of information required for program management:

1. Client data
2. Staffing data
3. Program data
4. Fiscal data
5. Reporting data
6. Evaluation data
7. Planning data

The first four categories are fundamental, since they are also the primary sources for reporting, evaluation, and planning data. Detailed discussion of the kinds of information subsumed under these category headings will be provided later in the section on information sources.

To consider only the input side of the management-information picture is a common mistake. Not all available data are useful, and not all useful data are collected. The specification of existing and desired *information inputs* should *follow* the assessment of *information needs*. The process is relatively straightforward. Samples of internal and external reports, important memoranda and letters, planning proposals, grant proposals, and contracts forms should be reviewed. These documents should represent functional areas of program responsibility. Then statements of the problems and benefits associated with the principal documents, as well as listings of useful but not presently available information, should be collected from management, supervisory, and service staffs. Regularities in content and format of these information outputs should be noted. The review of documents and written statements will provide a summary perspective on the information needs of an organization.

The next stage of the assessment of information needs is also simple. Brief interviews should be conducted with samples of staff from all levels within the program or agency. Knowledge gained from the earlier review of documents can be used to structure the interviews. The process of information flow within the program should be mapped—from the initial stages of client contact, to the recording of information on office forms, to the aggregation of data across service workers, to the generation and use of reports. Typical sequences of events and the number of steps and kinds of information-handling activities should be identified. More detail regarding problems and gaps in available information should be probed for. In this way those procedures and reports that are useful and that fit in most easily with ongoing program activities can be identified.

During the survey and interview phases of assessment, data on information outputs should be collected in a format that will simplify the later development of an assessment report. Smaller programs may require mostly qualitative, descriptive information for assessment purposes, while larger agencies will have to collect quantitative data as well.

Identifying Information Sources

A similar set of activities is involved in the delineation of information inputs. The definition of an "important" office form will vary from agency to agency, but typical examples would be client registration and intake forms, assessments of service needs, log sheets for recording client contacts and staff activity, billing schedules, accounting records, and program-service summaries. Statements regarding problems, benefits, and information deficits should be collected as before, with special attention to data-collection procedures. Depending on the number of forms involved, the staff interviews can be obtained at the same time as the other materials or on a later occasion. The findings from the review of forms and staff interviews can be incorporated into an information-sources section of the assessment report.

Many but not all important information sources for program management exist on paper forms. Most agencies collect client, program-resources, fiscal, and reporting data this way. However, much useful evaluation and planning information comes to administrative staff through informal sources such as conversations, press reports, television programs, and the like. Table 26-1 presents some specific data elements relating to client characteristics and service area demographics. Additional details about information sources and representative data-collection methods for the seven categories of program-management information follow.

1. *Client data* include demographic information about clients, financial data for determining program eligibility, descriptions of functional limitations, relevant clinical data, and descriptions of service needs. This information is usually collected from the client during intake or may be provided by referral sources. Forms designed for these purposes are widely available and can be adapted for a particular program.

Table 26-1. Client Characteristics and Service Area Data Elements

Client characteristics

Name
Address—residence location
Telephone number

Date of birth—age
Sex
Marital status—household composition
Ethnicity
Religion
Language spoken

Referral source
Service needs
Service received
Functional limitations
Transportation arrangements
Income category—above or below eligibility levels
Health insurance
Relatives or other contact persons

Service area demographics

Persons by age, sex and race
Population age 60+ and age 75+
Persons age 60+ living alone
Unrelated individuals age 60+
Persons age 65+ with transportation disability
Households age 60+ by number of persons

Elderly below or near poverty level
Elderly living in substandard housing

Changes in decennial and five year census figures
Estimated elderly population at risk—future need for services
Estimated elderly population in need—present service needs
Elderly population served
Service utilization trends

Inventory of service resources and locations

2. *Staff data* provide descriptions of the characteristics of program workers. Job functions, classification titles, relevant skills, education, licensing, and training experience would be included here. These data are generally available from personnel records.
3. *Program data* include information about the type of facility, numbers of staff and clients, process data on program and service-worker caseloads, allocations of staff time across project areas, utilization rates for service categories, and so on. The transaction data are usually recorded by staff

in daily-activity logs and then aggregated across functional units within the agency.

4. *Fiscal data* are essentially about funding sources and amounts of program income and expenses. Grant and contract budgets, reimbursement schedules, units-of-service costs, program and materials costs, in-kind payments, and staff salaries are included under this heading. Accounting and budget records are used to develop this information.

5. *Reporting data* are usually derived from the preceding three information categories. Individual client and staff data are collated from tally sheets, service-program logs, and similar sources. Administrative workers then aggregate the data according to service-type, program, and worker categories.

6. *Evaluation data,* whether formative or summative, derive from measurement of the effects of services on clients' status. Information from the categories just listed will be combined with these outcome measures to determine program effectiveness and efficiency. Sources for information about service efficacy are clients themselves and their kin, as well as program staff and related service providers.

7. *Planning data* include information from the previous categories, as well as information about changes in the external environment of the program. The internal administrative activities of the agency and external reporting requirements provide data related to the first aspect of planning. Hard data about shifting environmental conditions and changing service-area demography can be developed from sources like the federal census of population and housing, regional and county planning agencies, health-systems agencies, and service utilization reports from other provider agencies. Perceptual information about changing service needs and trends, available financial and staffing resources, and potential impacts of new governmental regulations is often obtained from discussion with other providers and from public hearings. Sources here include program staff, administrative staff from related agencies, advisory councils of service consumers, and religious, community, and political leaders, as well as the media. Descriptive and evaluative information about new service programs is available from journals and from bibliographic data bases.

Reviewing Office Procedures

The assessment of information needs and data sources results in a description of the kinds of information required for program management. The next question that arises is how to best access and process this information. The answer starts with a third aspect of the assessment process, a review of office procedures. While some procedures are performed by clerical workers, others by service workers and administrative staff, certain information-handling activities are common to all offices. These fundamental activities are data collection, typing, filing, and budget preparation, as well as internal and external communication. Table 26-2 shows how these activities are performed in offices using manual procedures and in offices using computer systems.

It is important to find out *how* these fundamental processes take place, *who* does them, *where*, and *when*. Clusters of related activities — such as typing, filing, and document reproduction and distribution — should be reviewed to see which procedures can be integrated with others. Secretarial and supporting staff can be involved in preliminary design of information systems by having them describe their office responsibilities. In particular, areas where a strain or unsatisfied need exists should be identified. The same survey/interview approach used in earlier assessments can be employed here.

Table 26-2. Information-Handling Activities

Activity	Manual Procedures	Computer Systems
Data collection	Paper forms	Interactive programs
	Data sheets	Data entry software
		Numeric keypads
		Bar code readers
		Scanning devices
Typing	Typewriters	Word-processing software
	Copying machines	Mailing list programs
Filing	Folders	Computer files
	File indexes	Data base management software
	File cabinets	
Budget preparation	Accounting sheets	Accounting programs
	Calculators	Spread-sheet programs
	Charts	Graphics display programs
Office communication	Telephone calls	Electronic mail
	Notes	Office calendar/
	Memoranda	Meeting schedule programs
	Meetings	
External communication	Telephone calls	Computer mail
	Letters	Computer conferencing systems
	Reports	Data base searching
	Meetings	

Matching Information Needs with Available Information Resources

The categories of information needed and desired can be matched up with the data elements collected in a cross-tabular format. The presence or absence of information can be seen by examining the individual cells of the table. This is one way to identify gaps or limitations in program management information, and this section of the assessment report can be of particular value for revising data collection and office procedures. Information-collection deficiencies should be evaluated in terms of "lost" opportunity costs and what the potential usefulness would be if the information were available. These information deficits should be ranked in order of importance, and then mechanisms to address and satisfy these unmet needs incorporated during the planning of program information systems.

Preparing the Assessment Report

The three-stage assessment process may be more or less detailed depending on characteristics of the program or agency. The report ought to present a fairly complete sense of the information needs of the program, sources of required management data, current information-handling capability, and procedures within the agency. This codification of the survey and interview material will provide a foundation from which useful and efficient information systems can be developed. Since systems planning will be based on the report, it is important that the design phase proceed from a complete and reliable base of descriptive data.

PLANNING

Most gerontological-services agencies now use manual office systems with typewriters, calculators, copying machines, and filing cabinets in managing day-to-day program activities. Some innovators may use computerized systems for word processing and data processing, but many more do not. The intent of this chapter is to facilitate the transition from manual procedures to micro-computer-based information-handling systems for these agencies. The key to success is an orderly, gradual progression, integrating new technology into existing program structures. The development process can be modular and incremental, proceeding one step at a time, but the changeover ought to proceed within the context of some organization-wide plan. This structured approach allows for both flexibility and coherence.

The information-resources planning group has responsibility for developing a systems design and comparing alternative approaches to realizing that design. The following list details the stages and activities involved in systems planning.

Define desired applications
Review product literature and arrange demonstrations
Review systems in place in other agencies
Develop system specifications
Compare alternative system configurations
Prepare planning report and develop consensus
Prepare recommendations and make purchase decision

The most pressing or the most easily satisfied needs can be addressed first, either as individual projects or as parts of a larger multistage plan. In any case, it is important that hoped-for benefits be realizable and fairly immediate. The basis of the modular approach is system compatibility. Various hardware, software, and data components can be acquired and developed separately if necessary. However, the ability to access and fit the components together over time is required. Careful attention to communications and software compatibility across equipment vendors and software manufacturers is necessary to assure this.

A simpler alternative is to purchase from a single manufacturer a system that can be expanded or upgraded within the same product line. If reliable, internally compatible equipment is selected, this choice will often save time, effort, and cost. But a clear, written statement of needs and desired capabilities is still a prerequisite to information-systems design and the selection of a vendor.

All information systems, however beautiful or overwhelming in their complexity, include five basic elements. Some of the interrelated parts have been mentioned previously.

1. *Hardware,* or the equipment itself includes the work stations, floppy-disk drives, hard-disk, memory, and processing units.
2. *Software* includes both computer programs and the operating system, an intermediary program that controls input and output functions and establishes communication between an applications program and the hardware.
3. *Data* may be in text, numeric, or image form. Information must either be collected and entered into the system for storage or retrieved from an external source.
4. *Personnel* or users of the system need to be trained in how to use the equipment and the computer programs. They also need to be able to learn independently and extend their usage of the system.
5. *Procedures* structure the relationship between users and the system itself. In effect, these procedures are the "software" that control the enterprise. Accordingly, they should be rational, flexible, and clear.

Defining Applications

Certain generic information-handling capabilities are of value to any geron-tological-service program. These applications were originally referred to in Table 26-2 and are described in detail below. Any office system considered for purchase should have all of the capabilities listed.

Word Processing

Word processing can be done on most microcomputer systems. A dedicated word processor is a special kind of microcomputer with a labeled keyboard and software designed to manipulate text. Commercial word-processing systems have generally been easier to use and more flexible than microcomputers for these purposes. Second- and third-generation word-processing software for microcomputers is now coming on-line, however. These new programs take advantage of user-definable function keys so that office staff do not need to type in complex combinations of escape and control characters to manipulate text. Any word processing system considered should be able to insert, delete, and replace individual characters and words, move blocks of text within and between document files, and format text quickly and easily. Recently developed software will allow the display screen to be split into "windows," each of which can be used to create or edit text. The transfer of text and data between windows is possible. Many software vendors have spelling-check routines, with extensive vocabularies, that can identify possible typing errors and reduce the proofreading time for documents. Word-processing output can often be transferred to computerized typesetting equipment via communications linkages for the production of printed reports as well.

Most commercial word processors now have computing capabilities available as an option, and can run many of the same kinds of programs previously available only on microcomputers. In effect, the two kinds of systems are beginning to converge. Useful capabilities have become more a function of the software and less a function of the hardware or equipment itself. Since word processing is likely to be a high-volume and fundamental support-staff capability, software that is integrated with or at least easily compatible with other required program applications should be sought.

Data-Base Management

Data-base management is essentially the electronic filing and retrieval of text and data. Instead of being stored in folders in filing cabinets, letters, memo-randa, reports, and budget proposals are saved in files on disk or tape. Documents can be located using indexes based on file names. Depending on software capabilities, key words and phrases can also be searched for within the entire set of files. Related sets of documents can be retrieved in either way.

List-processing and records-processing programs are variants of data-base-management programs. To give a functional example, a subset of clients from a program's mailing list could be identified from information contained in the client-data-base file, such as service category and length of time since last clinic visit. This group of service recipients could then be sent an individually addressed form letter asking them to call and schedule a follow-up appointment. Monthly billing schedules can sometimes be incorporated into these kinds of list-processing and data-base programs.

Many data-base programs also offer forms-creation and data-entry routines to assist in the process of data collection.

Accounting and Spread-Sheet Programs

Accounting and spread-sheet programs are used to prepare budget documents and financial plans. The table format or template is laid out by the user and computational formulas specifying relationships between fiscal variables are defined. The program will then calculate marginal totals after numeric data have been entered into the rows and columns of the table. Information needs to be entered only once and can be edited or revised later. For example, new data can be added each year to update a service-program budget, or accounting formulas can be changed or trends projected over time to answer "what if . . ." kinds of questions. These programs can be an important part of the solution to the complex problems resulting from multiple funding sources. Information in spread-sheet displays should be accessible and transferrable to graphics programs and word-processing files.

Graphics Display Programs

Graphics display programs can often be combined with data-base management and spread-sheet programs to translate numeric data into pie charts, bar graphs, or trend lines. Graphics displays are particularly valuable as illustrations and as summary statements in program reports and planning documents. They are easy to understand but have been expensive and time-consuming to produce by hand.

"Integrated software" is now available, which makes it relatively easy to pass data from numeric tables to charts and then embed both the tables and the resulting figures in text documents. Related programs also assist in project planning, activity scheduling and resource coordination activities. This kind of software can represent a worthwhile investment resulting in greater ease of use of programs and improved communicability for documents. The defining characteristic of these integrated sets of program applications is a common "user interface." Instead of learning different commands for the word-processing, data base, spread-sheet graphics and other functions, the user only needs to know one consistent and related set of instructions for all applications.

Communication Functions

Communication can take place between microcomputers and word processors within an office network or between a program office and an external computer system. "Electronic mail" has advantages over the telephone. It can be asynchronous in that the person to whom the message is addressed does not have to be in the office to receive it. The receiver can check a computer mailbox when convenient and read or respond to the message directly. Electronic mail also allows for immediate and simultaneous distribution of messages or documents to multiple persons in a network. Some office-mail systems have meeting-scheduling programs that can record and coordinate individual calendars with respect to available time periods and meeting locations.

External communications can also enable quick transfer of reports, data, or documents between agencies. Devices called modems can automatically dial a telephone number or answer an incoming call from another computer system. Service program descriptions and evaluations stored in remote data bases such as the Mental Health Abstracts at NIMH and the Social Science Citation Index, for example, can also be accessed over dial-up lines.

Many office automation companies and computer manufacturers are experimenting with speech recognition and speech production systems. These applications are the early beginnings of computer systems that can understand and respond to spoken instructions. While somewhat expensive and limited now, they will become more flexible and less costly. It is interesting to speculate about the possible uses of voice controlled systems in the context of gerontological services, as small computer systems become increasingly common in homes and offices.

Summary

To sum up, word-processing and electronic-filing programs are basic applications that will save time and effort and increase the productivity of support staff. They are extremely cost-effective in that the quality of typed work will improve, work volume will increase, and turnaround time will decrease, particularly for documents requiring multiple revisions. The spread-sheet and graphics software are more useful for management and professional staff. They are what are called "decision-support" tools. Alternate courses of action can be developed and compared to each other with regard to costs, for instance, and the consequences of decisions or trends can be projected over time. Telecommunications capability makes possible the exchange of both incoming and outgoing information. Large data files can also be stored and processed on mainframe computers at remote sites, or subsets of larger files can be down-loaded for processing on a microcomputer.

As the network of aging services continues to evolve, computerized communication and data linkages among service providers and between these programs and state and area agencies on aging will become commonplace. These linkages can be expected to lead to rapid and simplified reporting procedures as well as to access to information resources external to individual agencies.

A wealth of packaged software is available for both microcomputer and work-processing systems. Computer programs designed specifically for the management of human services agencies will probably be available within the next few years. In the meantime, the best approach is to use packaged programs and adapt these to the specific needs of the service provider. It is most reasonable to buy integrated software with computer programs that are mutually compatible and allow for the quick and easy exchange of data between applications. Typing of commands or cursor selection of functions listed on functional menus is generally required now. However, newer systems display iconic images representing filing cabinets, printers, and so on at the screen margin of the terminal. The images signify various activities and a device called a "mouse" moves the screen pointer to the function to be performed. This approach is easy for non-typists to learn and also provides fast execution of functions. Technology is now available that process data and text by touching function areas on a display screen or by writing on an electronic tablet.

A discussion of specific applications in the context of service program information-handling needs should be the first section of the planning report. When combined with the assessments and the procedures study, this will provide the front end of the agency's information-systems plan.

Planning Information Systems

Certain basic mechanisms are involved in all information-handling technology. Information can enter into a computer system by way of a keyboard, a bar code reader, an optical scanner, or a communications linkage. *Storage* means that information entered is permanently saved. Word processing is simply typing, with the text stored on a machine readable medium, such as a floppy disk, rather than on paper. The stored document can then be edited and printed; retyping after corrections have been made is not required. *Retrieval* is the capability to locate and access information in text or numeric files. It is often useful to retrieve material from one or more text files that are then edited, merged together, and saved or printed as a new document. *Processing* is the manipulation of stored information by means of computer programs. The software, whether for word processing, accounting, or telecommunications, is itself retrieved and loaded into computer memory from a storage medium such as disk or tape. The myriad of computer systems and applications programs all function in terms of these three mechanisms. A glossary of technical terms relating mostly to microcomputer systems is given in the Appendix.

Computer systems exist in small, medium, and large sizes. These categories correspond to microcomputers, minicomputers and, mainframes. Differences between the three classes of systems exist in memory size, processing speed, numbers of operations performed per unit of time, and storage capacity. There is some overlap between the system types. The microcomputers of the 1980s often have greater capabilities than the minicomputers of the 1970s and the mainframes of the 1960s.

An important trend in information-processing is the development of what are called "distributed resource" or "distributed intelligence" systems. These systems are essentially networks of compatible microcomputers; usually they are linked to a minicomputer or have communication with large mainframe systems. Each work station on the network can load software, data, or text from an external source for local processing. The resulting work product can then be printed, forwarded to another station for editing, or directed to centralized storage on a larger system. Maximum flexibility is assured by combining local processing on the microcomputer and storage on a centralized fixed disk with access to other systems, both small and large, through communications.

A "local area network" (LAN) is similar to the distributed resources concept. The difference is that microcomputers and word processors from different vendors are linked together on the same network. Access to and transfer of text and data files across different systems is possible. The LAN will provide compatibility across different manufacturers' equipment, but various hardware and software elements are necessary to link the microcomputers into the network.

The initial step in systems planning is to gain an awareness of technological opportunities. A confusing richness of computer equipment and software exists now, and the cascade of available products has only begun. Commercial sources, advertising material, and descriptions of systems and software in magazines and journals can be used to get a sense of what is available. But detailed evaluations of products are also important. The planning committee should discuss the needs of the agency with vendors and have them demonstrate the capabilities of their products. It is often a good idea to bring specific tasks to the vendor and have program-management applications demonstrated on the system under consideration. For instance, secretaries could try a word-processing and filing software package, or an administrator could review an accounting and budgeting spread-sheet program. The results of the evaluations should be recorded in a straightforward and consistent format that will allow later comparisons across different products lines.

It is also useful to talk with computer users in other service agencies about the computer systems and program packages they have acquired. This kind of interaction will provide information about actual performance, real-world benefits and limitations, product reliability, and the extent of available training and support. In addition to helping to develop a sense of what works well, these conversations and equipment demonstrations by users will provide new ideas about the kinds of information systems best suited to the needs of the organization.

The next part of systems design is the development of system specifications. This involves listing out the types of applications, numbers of users, approximate work volume, data-storage requirements, frequency of updating files, preferred locations for terminals, work stations and printers, estimated system growth potential, and similar issues. A mix of hardware and software components that will meet these requirements can be developed in consultation with two or three vendors. To start, the kinds of applications software needed should be identified and then what operating system the programs will run under determined. The final step is to select a hardware manufacturer whose computer systems have the desired capacity and who will support the software and operating system selected. In particular, the printer should be compatible with the software chosen.

The following dimensions must be considered in comparing computer-system configurations across vendors.

Cost
Capabilities
Performance
Ease of use
Support
Reliability
Maintenance
Expandability
Compatibility

Cost should be the first consideration, since it determines the limits of feasibility. Purchases can often be justified to program administrators in terms of cost savings in staff time, reductions in various categories of expenditures, or longer-term cost-avoidance. *Capabilities* are the software-based functions that the new system can perform. *Performance* refers to considerations such as system-response time, processing time, and memory and storage capacity. *Ease of use* is important in terms of staff access to and effective operation of the system. Support involves both training and post-sales consultation. *Reliability* is particularly important for electromechanical devices such as printers and disk-drive units. *Maintenance* and prompt response to service requests are important. The reputation of a vendor in the support and maintenance area should be carefully investigated with users. A maintenance contract is definitely needed for centralized, multiuser systems. *Expandability* and *compatibility* are fundamental considerations in later system development. Attention should be paid to estimated future-growth requirements during the systems-design phase. Product lines should be selected that will allow for the addition of memory, storage capacity, work stations, printers, and new functionality at a later time. Upward compatability or the transfer of data and programs across systems is particularly important. It is not a good idea to buy into a closed-ended, noncommunicating, stand-alone system, even if the price is low.

When comparisons of various systems have been incorporated into the planning report, the information-resources committee can discuss and consider alternative approaches. If the needs of the organization have been identified and equipment evaluations properly addressed, consensus should come easily within the committee. The final phase of the systems-planning effort will be the development of a set of recommendations that will form the basis for the purchase decision.

IMPLEMENTATION

A series of related activities take place during the system implementation phase. These activities are:

Train staff
Design forms
Install equipment
Adapt software
Prepare documentation
Parallel run of old and new systems
Test and debug new system
Change over to new system

Some activities, such as preliminary staff training and the design of data-collection forms, can begin even before the new equipment is delivered. Staff should be prepared for the differences in office routine that will follow the introduction of the new system. Affected personnel should have a chance to review the system design and proposed applications.

Two possible avenues can be considered for getting information into the system. The first is to simply modify existing paper forms for use with the computerized system and to develop new forms as required. Program staff, in collaboration with a computer-systems consultant, can contribute substantially to this process. Modular, integrated sets of forms should be prepared, and the forms indexed with a client identification number so that repetitive information does not have to be obtained from clients and recopied by staff with each service contact. Early editions can be tested with clients and revised as needed. This "test and revise" cycle may have to take place a few times with the new system before a final easy-to-use form has been prepared.

The second approach to forms design is appropriate for data-entry programs that will reside on the computer system. Commercial software packages can be purchased and adapted, or a computer programmer can prepare the prompting and data-capture routines that will make direct entry of data possible. In either case the interactive prompts should be simple and logical. The person at the keyboard ought to be able to select activities from menus and respond quickly to information-entry requests. Error-checking subroutines that will flag out-of-range or inappropriate data values are good insurance against typing mistakes. A client data base of linked demographic, service contact, and cost data can be constructed and updated in this way.

Depending on the size of the system and contractual agreements, the manufacturer, retailer, or program staff will install and test the equipment. An electrical contractor may be needed to install coaxial, twisted-pair, or fiber-optic cable if a network of communicating work stations has been decided upon. If commercial software has been purchased, agency staff with relevant experience or aptitude can begin to adapt the programs for the specific needs of the service workers and administrative staff. The other alternative in software customization is to hire a programmer. Many software-development consultants are commercially available. However, college and graduate students familiar with microcomputer systems will often work on a part-time basis, and this approach can be quite cost-effective. Whether the software adaptation or the software development route is chosen, two kinds of documentation should be prepared. The first level of documentation consists of descriptions of program logic and listings of the actual programming statements. The second level of documentation includes a functional discussion of what the software does and detailed instruction in how to use it. This user-oriented documentation will help to prepare staff for the "hands-on" phase of training.

Extended training for all affected staff on the features available and the actual use of the system can begin after the purchase decision has been made. The usual approach in the case of smaller systems is for vendors to provide system guides, software manuals, training diskettes, and other standard educational materials. Hardware and software manufacturers sometimes offer a toll-free telephone number for user consultation and problem-solving. Training classes for particular applications such as spread-sheet packages and word processing can also be purchased at additional cost. These classes can be held either on-site or in a vendor's training center. With larger networks, more staff training will be required. Since the level of investment is higher on these more complex systems, the manufacturer will often provide extensive training without charge to staff from the purchasing organization.

When the system and software are in place and staff have been trained in the new procedures, the actual implementation process can begin. Unless the primary uses of the new system are for word-processing or other fairly straightforward activities, it is a good idea to continue the older manual procedures in parallel with the new automated system. During this testing and debugging phase, the manual systems already in use can provide backup assurance and thus minimize the impact of any problems or failures with the new equipment. If newly installed hardware components are going to fail, it is most often early on, during the warrantee period; software problems are also likely to be identified during the first three months of system operation.

The testing phase of implementation will be a time when staff are accommodating themselves to the computer-based system. Learning costs may be relatively high and reduced efficiency can be expected. Program management and the information resources committee can anticipate these difficulties and provide a supportive rather than a critical environment to staff users during this transitional period. As the incidence of system and people problems is reduced, the older manual procedures can be gradually discontinued and reliance placed on the new information system. Increased productivity and efficiency can be anticipated.

EVALUATION

Information-processing systems evolve through cycles of vision and revision as usage increases, new technology becomes available, and additional capabilities are desired. During the later stages of implementation, structured evaluations can be initiated that will allow use feedback and measure the degree to which the system satisfies design criteria. Some of the activities involved in system evaluation are:

Obtain use feedback
Correct problems
Reinforce progress
Document system changes
Plan for later development

One primary measure of system acceptance is to see how many hours per day the equipment is actually used. If there are design, implementation, or training problems, usage may be low. Or staff may discover additional uses for the system and have to compete for access. Detailed evaluations of the utility of software applications should be carried out during the evaluation phase.

Paper forms are the simplest reporting method, and will also provide written records of problems and suggested improvements. Another possibility is to create a small number of on-line files for positive and negative comments. Difficulties with the system can then be identified on a continuing basis, and positive aspects of user experience can be sought and obtained. This approach is easily implemented in multiterminal networks and will allow the information-resources committee to review user evaluations and reply to questions quickly. New ideas about how to use the system that have tested out successfully can be broadcast back to staff to help increase efficiency and productivity. Positive user experiences can be reinforced and progress rewarded by encouragement and public acknowledgement.

Both major and minor changes in system procedures should be incorporated into the written documentation. Training manuals will need to be revised accordingly. Since a predominantly nonliterate, unrecorded culture of system lore can be expected to build up over time, the information-resources committee should survey and interview staff periodically. These kinds of assessments can be quite useful in the later modification and development of the system. Interaction between staff users and a constructive, responsive information-resources planning committee will also promote a sense of ownership. As new technology becomes available and as demand for additional services grows, the system can be upgraded and expanded in line with user and management suggestions. It is reasonable to expect a useful product life cycle of five to eight years or longer with a planned program of system monitoring and development.

ORGANIZATIONAL INNOVATION

The days of manual data-collection and information-handling systems are passing. Agency-wide plans will need to be developed, budgets will have to be modified, service program and clerical staff will require retraining, and subtle and powerful changes in the social environment of the office will occur. When systems are properly planned, the disruptions in routine will be outweighed by increases in productivity and quality of work life by a ratio of one to three or better.

Two important considerations are involved in moving new initiatives forward. The first is simply maintaining an awareness of the opportunities presented by new information technology. Microcomputer systems and their associated software are the areas where the most significant growth can be anticipated and the largest and most immediate gains realized. Developments here should be monitored on a regular basis by the information-resources committee. The incremental costs for adding work stations and new applications programs to a well-designed network are low.

The second critical consideration is marketing a proposed innovation to decision-makers and staff in both the program and agency environment. A certain amount of selling will be required, whether the technology is a completely new venture or an adaptation or conversion of an existing system. Various characteristics of the product, the program, the staff, and the internal and external agency environment have to be taken into account in marketing an innovation. Table 26-3 lists some factors affecting the acceptance of a new product. These variables can be used in the development of marketing strategies directed at management and other personnel.

A few words about "technophobia" and "organizational resistance" are in order. People have a tendency to resist changes they do not understand and participate in. A new information system may be seen as a threat to job security, or as leading to loss of status or to the downgrading of older skills. Most human-services agencies and workers can benefit substantially from information technology. If staff are properly prepared and trained, the introduction of new systems and procedures will not alienate them. The information-resources committee should identify possible fears and potential people problems early on, as well as later during training, implementation, and system evaluation. It is quite useful to have staff express their negative feelings and doubts. Changes in goals, plans, and procedures should be made in response to valid objections. The support of administrative staff at higher levels of the agency is a necessary,

Table 26-3. Factors Promoting Acceptance of Innovations

Characteristics of the Product

　　Relative advantage over other products or approaches
　　Improved performance, immediate and tangible gains
　　Conformity with existing organizational goals, values, and procedures
　　High demonstrability and ease of transfer
　　High understandability and ease of use
　　High reversibility, relatively low cost and low risk

Characteristics of the Innovator

　　Highly cosmopolite, with orientation and contact outside organizational social system
　　Highly professional, willing to consider, discuss new ideas
　　Personal sense of security, willing to face threat of change and its consequences
　　Above average economic, social, educational status
　　Successful, earlier innovations have attracted attention and increased upward mobility

Characteristics of the Organization

　　Available funding resources and staff time
　　Social climate supports change and some risk-taking, rewards new ideas
　　Administrative and collegial support for the innovation
　　Consultative, participatory style of decision-making
　　Good formal and informal communication patterns
　　Interactive relationship with external environments

but not a sufficient, condition for the acceptance of an innovation. All levels of the organization have to be included in the process of consensus-building.

In general, to accomplish change within an organization the driving forces have to be increased and the restraining forces decreased. As Bowers and Bowers (1977) note *communication* and *participation* are the two most important mechanisms to achieve this. While clear statements of needs, system capabilities, and goals are the responsibility of the information-resources planning committee, important detailed information can be developed from staff, preferably in an interactive way so that mutual exchange of views is possible. Staff people should be actively involved in fact-finding, problem identification, solution generation, and planning.

In addition to the intra-agency factors involved in the acceptance of an innovation, there can be beneficial influences from outside organizations. The office-automation revolution is in its early phases. We need to be able to learn from the positive and negative experiences of other agencies. As noted earlier, discussion with staff from other agencies and hands-on demonstrations of the exact office application wanted can be very valuable. There can also be substantial benefits involved in *not* being the first user of a new product or system. Evaluations provided by people from other agencies can provide validity and legitimacy to recommendations for and against various systems and software products.

DESCRIPTIONS OF GERONTOLOGICAL INFORMATION SYSTEMS

This section presents selected case studies of information systems used in services agencies in the aging network around the United States. Since computer-based systems are relatively new resources for program management, only bits and pieces of an idealized information system can be identified within the case studies. Although appropriate technology exist now, no one agency has implemented a complete range of management systems on a computer. Information resources can be expected to evolve quickly within organizations as these technologies develop further and their benefits in terms of labor and cost-savings become accepted.

AGENCY:	Broome County Office for the Aging Governmental Plaza Binghamton, N.Y. 13902 607/772-2411
APPLICATIONS:	An integrated client-demographic, service-transaction and unit-cost data base, with 8,000 records on an IBM mainframe. Word processing and meal program nutrient analysis on an IBM Personal Computer system.
HARDWARE:	An IBM 4341 computer system with disk and tape storage owned by the

county government supports the client data base. Access to the mainframe is by direct connect terminals.

An IBM PC with dual floppy-disk drives and a dot-matrix printer is located in the Nutrition Program offices.

SOFTWARE: ADABASE, a natural-language query system produced by Software A.G. is used on the mainframe, along with FAMIS, countywide financial accounting management information system.

The IBM PC has WORDSTAR word-processing software and DBASE II file management and data-retrieval programs.

AGENCY: Center for Geriatrics, Gerontology and Long Term Care
Columbia University Medical Center
100 Haven Avenue
New York, N.Y. 10032
212/781-0600 or 0601

APPLICATIONS: A FORTRAN program for scoring the Comprehensive Assessment and Referral Evaluation (CARE) developed by Dr. Barry Guland is available on the Columbia IBM 4341 system. The CARE is a multifocus survey instrument standardized on probability samples of community-based elderly in both the United States and Great Britain. The program is designed to score twenty-two problem area scales covering mental, physical, and social problems, and service needs of elderly persons. It is easily adaptable for microcomputer usage.

Consultation on management-information systems in gerontology, program administration and evaluation, computerized case management, and forms design is also provided by center staff.

HARDWARE: Two DEC-20 minicomputer systems are accessed through terminals connected to the Columbia University Computer Center. Two IBM 4341 mainframes are also used, one at the New York State Psychiatric Institute and another at the Columbia downtown campus.

A DEC-MATE II word processor with a CPM-based 8-bit processor, dual disk drives and a high-speed matrix printer are located at the center. A DEC WPS-78 word processor with two disk drives and a letter quality printer is also networked into the Columbia system.

SOFTWARE: Another CARE scoring program using SPSS is available and can be adapted for special needs. DEC word-processing and list-processing software are used in the Center. MULTIPLAN spread-sheet analysis software is run on the DEC-MATE II microprocessor.

AGENCY: Connecticut Community Care
719 Middle Street
Bristol, Conn. 06010
203/589-6226

APPLICATIONS: Computerized case management, a service coordination, assessment and monitoring program is provided for elderly persons living in Connecticut. The focus is on the development of long-term planning to maintain the client in the most suitable community or institutional environment.

The Comprehensive Community Care Information System is a management-information system for processing clinical and administrative information on the 3900 clients receiving case-management services in multiple locations across the state. Provider transactions and accounting services are also included within CCCIS.

HARDWARE: A Hewlett-Packard 3000 Series minicomputer with three 120 megabyte disk drives, a 600-line-per-minute printer, one 8100-byte-per-inch tape drive, and multiple data-entry terminals.

SOFTWARE: Advanced data-entry and data-base-management software form Hewlett-Packard. FORTRAN and COBOL programs developed by data-processing staff and independent consultants.

AGENCY: Essex County Division on Aging
19 High Street
Orange, N.J. 07050
201/678-9700

APPLICATIONS: A model client-tracking, unit-cost services-reporting system for Area Agencies on Aging. Includes forms-processing and file-updating procedures as well as a menu-driven report generator. The forms-processing software assigns name and number codes to services, maintains contract and budgeting information, registers new program participants, and records service units and expenditures. Demographic analyses, service reports, client assessments, and case-management plans can be produced from the data base.

HARDWARE: An ALTOS AC8 8000 series microcomputer that will support multiple concurrent users, with two 500-kilobyte floppy disks and a 40-megabyte hard disk, a CENTRONICS 180-character-per-second dot-matrix printer and two ADDS Regent display terminals.

SOFTWARE: An OASIS operating system from Phase One Systems, control and sort programs and multiuser COBOL. Much of the software is adapted from earlier projects supported by Administration on Aging grants to TSDI, a New York City-based consulting firm.

AGENCY: Long Term Care Gerontology Center
University of Kansas College of Health Sciences
39th and Rainbow Boulevard
Kansas City, Kans. 66103
913/588-1203

APPLICATIONS: The Long Term Care Information System is a comprehensive, cross-referenced listing of the programmatic activities and staff resources of the long-term-care centers across the United States. Network activities are updated on a quarterly basis. Dial-up access to the center activities and product files may become available at a later time.

Statewide Nursing Home Admission Assessments and Follow Up Assessments are stored in an additional data base and used to evaluate institutional placement decisions.

Client registration, service reporting, and care-planning software has also been developed for Area Agencies on Aging.

HARDWARE: A COMPUPRO Level C multiuser microcomputer system with both 8- and 16 bit programming capability. Two 1.2-megabyte floppy disks, a 20-megabyte hard disk, a HAYES Smartmodem, and four VISUAL 200 terminals are also included in the system.

SOFTWARE: Packaged software includes WORDSTAR for text processing, SUPERCALC for financial analysis, and DBASE II for data-base management and forms generation.

AGENCY: Ohio Commission on Aging
50 West Broad Street
Columbus, Ohio 43215
614/466-7649

APPLICATIONS: Centralized accounting and grants-management services, unit-cost data, and report generation are available for the twelve Area Agencies on Aging in the state. The individualized fiscal data base for each Area Agency also includes demographic and population data from the 1980 federal census.

Modeling and forecasting software to assist the state and Area Agencies with resource allocation decisions is under development.

HARDWARE: A DEC-20 minicomputer from the Ohio Department of Administrative Services is used on a time-sharing basis by the Commission on Aging and the AAA's. Grants of $3,000 to $5,000 are available to the Area Agencies to assist them in the purchase of Digital Equipment Company VT100 compatible microcomputers (such as the DEC Rainbow) terminals and printers.

SOFTWARE: An Interactive Business Management systems financial-accounting package was purchased by a consortium of five state agencies. The Commission on Aging then modified the software so that multiple funding accounts could be debited and credited, one for each area agency.

AGENCY: Orange County Office for the Aging
60 Erie Street
Goshen, N.Y. 10924
914/294-8801

APPLICATIONS: Client tracking and demographic files and fiscal-management programs are resident on a Honeywell minicomputer. Data regarding the agency's funding applications cycle, state-mandated four-year plan, mailing and volunteer lists, and text and budget documents are stored and processed on an Apple microcomputer.

HARDWARE: The county-government-owned Honeywell System 6 minicomputer is linked into an IBM mainframe. Communication with this system is over a leased telephone line using a terminal.

The Apple II Plus microcomputer at the Office for the Aging includes two floppy-disk drives and an Epson dot-matrix printer.

SOFTWARE: APPLEWRITER word processing, VISICALC spread-sheet programs, and VISI-SCHEDULE project-management software are used on the Apple. The DBMASTER data-base package is also used for list and records processing and file management.

AGENCY: City of Phoenix Aging Services Division
320 West Washington
Phoenix, Ariz. 85003
602/262-4789

APPLICATIONS: A bar code reader system is used to track 8000 elderly clients in the city's nutrition programs. Visually coded identification cards are issued to all program participants. The ID codes are scanned upon arrival at the nutrition center. At the end of the day the bar-code reader is attached to a modem and a remote APPLE microcomputer automatically calls the nutrition site and extracts the client data from the reader's memory. Demographic and service reports are then generated on an APPLE system.

HARDWARE: An APPLE II microcomputer with a CORVUS 10-megabyte hard disk, a

	HAYES Chronograph, and a RACAL-VADIC auto-dial modem. TELXON 787 bar-code readers with 16K of memory and TELXON DCM-387 direct-connect modems are used at the twenty nutrition sites.
SOFTWARE:	The DBASE Base II data-base-management package is used to aggregate meal-count data across the nutrition-program sites and produce the reporting information on the Apple system.

AGENCY:

Region One Area Agency on Aging
1366 East Thomas Road
Phoenix, Ariz. 85014
602/264-2255

APPLICATIONS: Monthly financial reports are generated from data supplied by nineteen sub-contractors. Year-to-date expenditures for each provider are compared with program budget allocations.

Individual-client-level data files for SSI-related State Supplemental Payment program costs may also be developed.

HARDWARE: Two IBM Personal Computers with dual floppy-disk drives share access to a CORVUS 10-megabyte hard disk.

SOFTWARE: VISICALC financial analysis programs are used to prepare the budget reports. BPI Accounting System software is also in use by the agency.

AGENCY:

Southeastern Queens Consortium on Aging Services
c/o The Jamaica Service Program for Older Adults
8931 161st Street
Queens, N.Y. 11432
212/657-6500

APPLICATIONS: Computerized case-management services link nine community-based agencies. Service tracking for elderly clients and agency fiscal management including accounting and general-ledger applications are provided.

HARDWARE: A DATA GENERAL CS-40 minicomputer with 192K of memory and 20 megabytes of hard-disk storage, one 315-kilobyte floppy disk, terminals, and printers.

SOFTWARE: The case-management and fiscal-management programs were written in COBOL. The software was custom designed by TSDI and is similar to that developed for the Essex County Area Agency on Aging.

ORGANIZATIONAL VALUES AND GOALS

An implicit assumption underlies the advice presented in this chapter. Simply put, it is that the incorporation of computerized information systems into gerontological-services programs can directly influence the quality of life of elderly clients, as well as the quality of work life of program staff. By reducing staff time spent in information-finding and administrative tasks, these resources can increase the quantity of direct services available to the elderly and job satisfaction among service workers. An investment in the development of information resources at the agency and program level is an efficient way to improve the quality of gerontological services. A purely economic value system is not adequate and not appropriate for human-services planning decisions. Instead of being limited by "bottom line" considerations, information systems can be used to develop and explore funding and alternate service-delivery approaches within an agency. Both information resources and economic systems are human creations and are best used to improve the living situations of clients and workers.

The use of information systems as tools to survey and measure the impacts of these same technologies is also highly recommended. The important considerations involved are asking the right questions and investing the required times and effort to ensure valid and reliable responses. This process of meta-evaluation will enable management to see how organizational goals are being impacted by the new technology. Measures of client and staff satisfaction with the process as well as the outcome of service procedures can be valuable program-guidance mechanisms.

APPENDIX 26-1: INFORMATION SYSTEMS CONCEPTS AND VOCABULARY

Baud rate is a measure of the speed at which data is transferred between computer systems. Common data-transfer rates over telephone lines are 300, 1,200, 2,400, and 9,600 bits per second. These data rates correspond to 30, 120, 240, and 960 characters per second. Rates of 1 million bits per second and higher can be achieved with direct connections between systems using coaxial cable and fiber-optic technology.

Bits and bytes are units of information. A bit represents a 1 or a 0 (a digital "yes" or "no") and a byte is a collection of 8 or 16 bits. Text or numeric characters are represented as individual *bytes*, and storage capacity is typically expressed in thousand-byte (kilobyte) units. Since there are approximately 2,000 characters on a typical 8½-×-11-inch typed page, a floppy disk that holds 320 kilobytes of data will store about 160 pages of typewritten text.

A *chip* is an integrated circuit made up of many thousands of transistors. With Very Large Scale Integration (VLSI) the room-sized assemblies of vacuum tubes characteristic of the first generation of computers have been reduced in size to silicon wafers smaller that a fingernail. Costs for these components have undergone the same kind of shrinkage, from millions of dollars to less than ten dollars, while power and processing speed have increased exponentially.

The most common 8-bit chip, the Zilog Z80, is often found in earlier generations of microcomputers. The Intel 8088 is a 16-bit processor with an 8-bit data path, and is used in the IBM Personal Computer and the DEC Rainbow.The Intel 8086 is a second-generation 16-bit chip with a 16-bit data path for faster input-output and a clock speed of 8 mega-hertz for faster processing. It is used in the WANG professional microcomputer, among others. A math coprocessor like the Intel 8087 will provide rapid processing of numeric data. Since the coprocessor is segregated off from the central processor, it can perform these operations in parallel with and virtually independent of the CPU. The Motorola 68000 series chip has a 32-bit processor and a 16-bit data path. It is used in the Apple MacIntosh and in multitasking, multiuser microcomputer systems. Overall, a larger bit size means that larger "chunks" of information can be processed, leading to greater efficiency and speed.

A *data base* is an integrated collection of computer files. The files in turn are made up of individual records or sets of data fields. By using simple logic statements such as "and," "or," "not," "greater than," "less than," individual data elements can be retreived from multiple files and joined together to produce reports. For instance, demographic data on individual clients in one file could be joined with service-usage data from a second file to generate a report describing the age and income characteristics of high-service-usage elderly clients.

A *disk* can be either a flexible-floppy disk or a fixed-hard disk. Although 8-inch floppy disks are fairly common, they are being replaced by 5¼-inch or smaller diskettes with equivalent storage capacities. Double-sided, double-density technology makes it possible to store a megabyte of information or more on a single diskette.

Winchester technology hard disks can store 20 million or more bytes of data. Access time is the amount of time required to read and write information on the disk. In addition to increased storage, access time is substantially reduced with hard disks.

Memory is typically available in 64K segments, and 128K is the minimum amount needed for running most useful programs. 256-kilobyte memory chips are now being produced, and these memory sizes are required with the newer generations of integrated software. Microcomputer programs typically access both data and processing instructions from disks and shuttle this information back and forth between program memory and storage media.

RAM is *random access memory*. This memory area can have either data or program instructions written into it and can be erased and reloaded as needed. ROM is *read only memory*. Also called firmware, ROM is permanent memory storage. System start-up program instructions in ROM are always available and do not need to be loaded each time the computer system is powered on.

A *modem* is a modulator-demodulator. This device translates keyboard input or stored data into electrical signals or auditory tones. An acoustic coupler is a modem that connects to a telephone handset. Both modems and couplers are used to transfer data between computer systems at rates between 300 and 9600 baud. Half-duplex operation means that data is being sent over the telephone line in only one direction at a time; full-duplex transmission allows for the simultaneous sending and receiving of data between systems.

An *operating system* is the control software that orders the movement of information between the keyboard, disk storage areas, the central processing unit, RAM and ROM, the display unit, and peripheral devices such as printers and modems. Common operating systems include CPM 80 for 8-bit machines, CPM 80-86 for running both 8- and 16-bit programs on the same microcomputer system, and Concurrent CPM for multitasking or performing multiple operations simultaneously. PC-DOS was developed by Micro-Soft for the IBM Personal Computer; MS-DOS is a very similar form of PC-DOS that operates on many other 16-bit systems. UNIX is a multiuser operating system developed by Bell labs that may become increasingly important as microcomputers become more powerful and multiuser networks become more common.

Certain operating systems will function only with certain hardware, and the choice of an operating system thus determines what software programs are available. Many of the newer 16-bit machines will support multiple operating systems, however.

A *port* is a channel that connects the computer to the outside world. Data is sent and received through these connectors either serially (one bit at a time) or in parallel (several bits at a time). Telephone communication is usually done serially and printing is very often accomplished through parallel ports.

Printers are evolving at a fast rate. Dot-matrix printers are inexpensive and fast with print speeds of up to 240 characters per second. These printers will also produce graphic displays. Multiple-character sets, italic type styles, and multicolor printing are available with these machines. High-density dot-matrix printers can strike over characters a second or third time to produce correspondence-quality output. The cleanest and highest quality impact printing is provided by daisy wheel printers. These letter-quality printers are usually slower (30 to 60 characters per second) and more expensive. Ink jet printers are very quiet with speeds ranging from 30 to 150 characters per second. High quality color graphics can also be produced. Laser printers are based on electronic print technology and are extremely fast. In addition, they can provide multiple type faces and sizes and graphics output for electronic publishing applications. Laser printers can be cost efficient in multiuser networks.

APPENDIX 26-2: INFORMATION UTILITIES

BRS/After Dark
1200 Route 7
Latham, N. Y. 12110
800/833-4707

This bibliographic data-base supplier provides dial-up access to social-science and medical-data files, as well as electronic mail services. The After Dark facility is available to microcomputer users between 6 p.m. and midnight and on weekends. Access charges are considerably lower than the business-day rates for regular subscribers.

Compuserve
Consumer Information Service
5000 Arlington Center Boulevard
P.O. Box 20212
Columbus, Ohio 43220
800/848-8199

Multiple consumer, business, entertainment, and news data bases are available. Electronic mail, programming languages, and user group conferences are also accessible with a subscription.

Computer Users in Social Services
Network and Newsletter
Dick Schoech, Coordinator
P.O. Box 19129
University of Texas at Arlington
Arlington, Tex. 76019

The CUSS network publishes a quarterly newsletter for the exchange of information and experiences with social-service uses of computer systems. A regional skills bank and software reviews are included along with articles and reports on information systems. Network dues are $5 for students and $10+ for others. A newsletter subscription is included with membership.

Electronic Information Exchange System
New Jersey Institute of Technology
323 High Street
Newark, N.J. 07102
201/596-2929

EIES is an electronic mail and computer conferencing system accessible over dial-up telephone lines. University-level courses in technology and management are also available. Subscriptions are available on a limited basis to eligible organizations and individuals.

Dialog Information Retrieval Service
3460 Hillview Avenue
Palo Alto, Calif. 94304
800/227-1927 or 800/982-5838

Another large collection of business, govenrment, medical, public service, and social-science data bases. Subscription rates are higher for the regular business-day services than for the Lockheed Knowledge Index, a subset of consumer-oriented files available evenings and on weekends.

GTE Telenet
8229 Boone Boulevard
Vienna, Va. 22180
703/442-1000

Data communications, electronic-mail services, and access to computer data bases are available through TELENET and TELEMAIL. Business, off-peak, and night rates are available to direct subscribers and intermediary service organizations such as AMA/NET, the American Medical Association's medical information network.

MCI Mail
2000 M Street N.W.
Washington, D. C. 20036
202/293-4255

A commercial electronic mail service providing on-line delivery of messages to subscribers with dial-up access. Four-hour and overnight delivery of printed material can be provided to non-subscribers. The annual subscription fee is $18, and charges for the electronic mail and hard copy mail service are reasonable.

NewsNet
945 Haverford Road
Bryn Mawr, Pa. 19010
800/345-1301

Full text retrieval of 100 newsletters on various subjects, in addition to electronic mail communication with newsletter publishers. Hourly rates.

NEXUS and LEXIS
Mead Data Central
P. O. Box 933
Dayton, Ohio 45401
800/227-4908

The NEXUS data base provides access to more than 100 full-text publications including the *New York Times* and other newspapers, magazines, and wire services. LEXIS includes complete listings of court decisions and regulatory proceedings. Subscribers to these services are usually business, media, and legal firms, as well as government agencies.

Source Telecomputing Corporation
1616 Anderson Road
McLeon, Va. 22102
800/336-3366

Consumer-information, electronic-mail, and computer-conferencing services. Rates are somewhat higher than Compuserve.

ACKNOWLEDGEMENTS

I would like to thank Erma Ferraro, Amanda Billups, Sharon Schley, and Karen Fernicola of the Department of Higher Education for their help with the preparation of the manuscript, tables, and charts. Suzy Seibert, David Wilder, Vicki Ashton, Ann Cortese, Lew Dars, and Charles Watts reviewed drafts of the chapter and made substantive contributions as well.

REFERENCES AND BIBLIOGRAPHY

Adler, D. A., and Edwards, C. N. (1981). Issues encountered in an attempt to implement a second-generation management information system. *Public Health Reports,* **96**(4), 369-375.

Association of Long Term Care Gerontology Centers. (1983). *Long term care gerontology centers.* Tampa, Fla.: University of South Florida Medical Center.

Bowers, G., and Bowers, M. (1977). Cultivating client information systems, *Human Services Monographs,* Series 5. Rockville, Md.: Department of Health and Human Services.

Broskowski, A. (1976). Management information systems for planning and evaluation in human services. In N. C. Schulberg and F. Baker, *Program evaluation in the health field,* vol. 2. New York: Human Sciences Press.

Chapman, R. (1976). *The design of management information systems for mental health organizations: A primer.* Washington, D.C.: United States Government Printing Office.

Connecticut Community Care, Inc. (1982). *Annual Report.* Bristol, Conn.: CCC Inc.

Evans, C. (1979). *The micro millennium.* New York: Viking Press.

Feigenbaum, E. A., and McCorduck, P. (1983). *The fifth generation.* Reading, Mass.: Addison-Wesley.

Heise, D. R. (Ed.). (1981). Microcomputers and Social Research. *Sociological Methods and Research,* **9**(4), 395-535.

Hiltz, S. R., and Turoff, M. (1978). *The network nation.* Reading, Mass.: Addison-Wesley.

Human Interaction Research Institute. (1976). *Putting knowledge to use: A distillation of the literature regarding knowledge and change.* Washington, D.C.: Institute of Mental Health.

Kanter, R. M. (1983). *The change masters.* New York: Simon & Schuster.

Landau, R., Bair, H. J., and Siegman, J. H. (1982). *Emerging office systems.* New York: Ablex.

Mullins, C. J., and West, W. T. (1982). *The office automation primer.* Englewood Cliffs, N.J.: Prentice-Hall.

National Association of Area Agencies on Aging and the National Association of State Units on Aging. (1982). *A profile of state and area agencies on aging.* Washington, D.C.: N4A and NASUA.

National Association of State Units on Aging. (1982). *An information specialist's guide to the older Americans act network on aging.* Washington, D.C.: NASUA.

National Association of State Units on Aging. (1982). *Introduction to information systems for the network on aging.* Washington, D.C.: NASUA.

National Association of State Units on Aging. (1981). *Information systems planning, development and operation: A guide to good practice for management of state and area agencies on aging.* Washington, D.C.: NASUA.

National Association of State Units on Aging. (1982). *Information systems applications in programs on aging—case studies of good practice.* Washington, D.C.: NASUA.

National Association of State Units on Aging and TSDI, Inc. (1981). *Uniform descriptions of services for the aging.* Washington, D.C.: NASUA.

National Committee on Vital and Health Statistics. (1980). *Long term health care—minimum data set.* Hyattsville, Md.: National Center for Health Statistics.

National Science Foundation. (1983). *The process of technological innovation: Reviewing the literature.* Washington, D.C.: United States Government Printing Office.

Ouichi, W. G. (1981). *Theory Z.* Reading, Mass.: Addison-Wesley.

Rosen, A., and Fielden, R. (1982). *Word Processing.* Englewood Cliffs, N.J.: Prentice-Hall.

Scott, H. D., Cook, S. A., Laufer, D., and Thornberry, H. (1976). Some successes and failures with long term data systems: The Rhode Island experience. *Medical Care,* **14**(5), Supplement.

Simon, H. A. (1981). *The sciences of the artificial.* Cambridge, Mass.: MIT Press.

Smith, H. T. (1983). *The office revolution.* Willow Grove, Pa.: Administrative Management Society Foundation.

Taylor, J. B. (1981). *Using microcomputers in social agencies.* Beverly Hills, Calif.: Sage Publications.

RECOMMENDED PERIODICALS

Microworld
Electronic Office
Auerbach Publishers
6520 North Park Drive
Pennsauken, N.J. 08109

Microworld is a guide to available hardware and software for microcomputers. Detailed product descriptions are included and are updated yearly.

The *Electronic Office* series includes discussion of management and planning issues, in addition to reviews of new office technology. It is also published and updated yearly.

DATAPRO Reports on Mini-Computers
DATAPRO Reports on Office Systems
DATAPRO Automated Office Solutions

Datapro Research Corporation
1805 Underwood Boulevard
Delran, N.J. 08075

In addition to product descriptions and discussions of management issues, the DATAPRO Reports include user evaluations of systems and hardware. The user surveys are quite detailed and are conducted yearly. A monthly newsletter on new product announcements is also provided.

A multitude of microcomputer magazines can be purchased at newsstands, in computer stores, and by subscription: The best include *Byte, Interface Age, Personal Computing, Personal Software,* and *Popular Computing. Infoworld,* published in Menlo Park, California, is highly recommended.

Index

About the Editor

ABRAHAM MONK is Brookdale Professor of Gerontology at the Columbia University School of Social Work in New York City and director of the Brookdale Institute on Aging and Adult Human Development at Columbia University. He is also associate director of the Long Term Care Gerontology Center of Columbia University's faculty of medicine.